The Nervous System

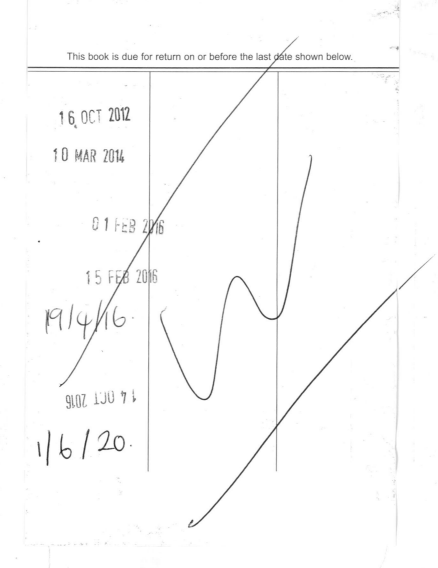

Commissioning Editor: Timothy Horne
Development Editor: Lulu Stader
Project Manager: Janaki Srinivasan Kumar
Designer/Design Direction: Charles Gray

SYSTEMS OF THE BODY

The Nervous System

BASIC SCIENCE AND CLINICAL CONDITIONS

SECOND EDITION

Adina Michael-Titus

Centre for Neuroscience and Trauma
Blizard Institute of Cell and Molecular Science
Barts and the London School of Medicine and Dentistry
Queen Mary University of London
London, UK

Peter Shortland

Centre for Neuroscience and Trauma
Blizard Institute of Cell and Molecular Science
Barts and the London School of Medicine and Dentistry
Queen Mary University of London
London, UK

Patricia Revest

Centre for Medical Education, Institute for Health Sciences
Education,
Barts and the London School of Medicine and Dentistry,
Queen Mary University of London
London, UK

Illustrations by Robert Britton

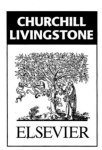

CHURCHILL
LIVINGSTONE

ELSEVIER

EDINBURGH LONDON NEW YORK OXFORD PHILADELPHIA ST LOUIS SYDNEY TORONTO 2010

CHURCHILL LIVINGSTONE
ELSEVIER

First Edition Elsevier Limited, 2007.
Second Edition © 2010, Elsevier Limited. All rights reserved.

ISBN 9780702033735
Reprinted 2011 (twice)

British Library Cataloguing in Publication Data
A catalogue record for this book is available from the British Library

Library of Congress Cataloging in Publication Data
A catalog record for this book is available from the Library of Congress

Notice
Knowledge and best practice in this field are constantly changing. As new research and experience broaden our knowledge, changes in practice, treatment and drug therapy may become necessary or appropriate. Readers are advised to check the most current information provided (i) on procedures featured or (ii) by the manufacturer of each product to be administered, to verify the recommended dose or formula, the method and duration of administration, and contraindications. It is the responsibility of the practitioner, relying on their own experience and knowledge of the patient, to make diagnoses, to determine dosages and the best treatment for each individual patient, and to take all appropriate safety precautions. To the fullest extent of the law, neither the Publisher nor the Editors/ Authors [delete as appropriate] assumes any liability for any injury and/or damage to persons or property arising out of or related to any use of the material contained in this book.

                                                              The Publisher

ELSEVIER   your source for books,
            journals and multimedia
            in the health sciences
www.elsevierhealth.com

Printed in China

The diseases of the nervous system represent one of the most important challenges in modern medicine. Medical schools worldwide have adopted various strategies in the teaching of neuroscience. One of the more recent approaches combines anatomy, physiology and pharmacology, in order to achieve an integrated view of the various pathologies. The problem-based learning method in medicine is based on this concept of integration.

This book is part of the Systems of the Body series, which has been designed to provide a teaching tool for medical curricula that use problem-based learning. The aim of our book is to cover the basic science required to understand the structure and function of the nervous system, and its major pathologies, at a level appropriate to medical students in the first years of training. The volume comprises two parts. The early chapters offer an introduction to the general organization of the nervous system, and the cellular and molecular mechanisms that govern its function. A separate chapter is devoted to the clinical examination of the nervous system. The later chapters, which form the main body of the book, are built around clinical cases. The chapters start with clinical scenarios, which prompt an exploration of specific issues, thus allowing us to introduce and discuss the knowledge that is required for the diagnosis and treatment of the conditions presented. To reflect the rapid pace of research in neuroscience, the information in the second edition has been updated throughout the text, and figures modified as appropriate.

Our experience of teaching medical students guided us throughout the writing of this text, and we tried to present complex concepts in an accessible and clear manner. Our wish was not only to present the facts, but also to increase the students' awareness of the many unresolved issues in neuroscience. It is our hope, therefore, that this book will not only assist students in the learning process, but also stimulate their interest and enthusiasm for the fascinating field of neuroscience.

We would like to express our thanks to the various people who have supported us throughout the writing of this book.

Michael Parkinson encouraged us to write this volume, and Lynn Watt provided guidance in the initial phases of the project. Very special thanks go to Dr Lulu Stader, who helped us, cajoled us and kept us on track, so that the work could be completed. Her expertise, understanding and support, and her sense of humour, were invaluable.

Many thanks are due to our colleagues, Dr Gregory Michael, Dr Julian Millar and Dr Sadashiv Karanth, who provided some material and made comments on parts of the manuscript, and to Dr Joshi George, who reviewed the Clinical Examination chapter.

ADDICTION   301

ORGANIZATION OF THE NERVOUS SYSTEM

1

Chapter objectives

After studying this chapter you should be able to:

1. Describe the basic organization of the peripheral and central nervous systems.

2. Name and identify the major nervous system structures and describe their primary functions.

3. Describe the organization and functions of the autonomic nervous system.

Introduction

The nervous system, which consists of the brain, spinal cord and peripheral nerves, is a highly specialized and complex structure. It is an information-processing system that regulates all the physiological functions of the organism. In addition, the nervous system performs unique functions that operate independently of other systems in the body. These underlie consciousness, memory, rationality, language, and the ability to project our mental images forwards or backwards in time. Representations of the external world are transmitted, transformed and manipulated by the nervous system to subsequently affect behaviour. Thus, the nervous system has four important functions:

1. sensory (gathering of information from the external environment)

2. integrator (of information from all sources for assessment)

3. effector (to produce a motor response)

4. internal regulator (homeostasis for optimum performance).

The net results of all these functions are as follows: first, the creation of a sensory perception of the external world; second, behaviour; and finally, the creation of knowledge that can be used to guide future behaviour in response to changes in the surrounding environment.

In order to appreciate how the nervous system produces behaviour, it is necessary to understand how it is organized functionally and anatomically. The experience of examining a brain is very much like the experience of buying a car. Before buying a car, you inspect it and then take it for a test drive to make sure that it operates normally and runs smoothly without faults. Then you open up the bonnet to look at the engine. Unless you happen to be a trained mechanic or have an interest in car engines, you might be able to name a few parts, e.g. the radiator, the battery and the fan belt, but not the rest of the mass of wires, spark plugs and assorted boxes. Moreover, knowledge of the name does not always indicate what the function is, or how all the different parts combine to burn petrol to make the car run. It is the same with the nervous system; you may be able to name some of the parts, such as the cortex, cerebellum and brainstem, and have a rough idea of what some of the different parts do, but have little idea of how they accomplish a task such as reading this sentence. And when the car breaks down, we call the automobile rescue services. When the nervous system breaks down or misfires, we call in the neurologists, neurosurgeons or psychiatrists.

Although the anatomy of the nervous system appears complex and daunting, its organization is governed by a set of relatively simple developmental, organizational and functional rules that bring order to it. The functional rules are summarized in Table 1.1.

The aim of this chapter is to provide a functional overview of the neuroanatomy of the brain, spinal cord and

Table 1.1 Principles underlying the functioning of the nervous system

Behaviour is produced by processing of information in a sequence of 'in → integrate → out'
Separate sensory and motor divisions exist throughout the nervous system
The nervous system has multiple levels of function
The nervous system is organized both in parallel and in series
Most neural pathways relaying information decussate from one side of the central nervous system to the other
The nervous system regulates activity through excitation and inhibition
There is both symmetry and asymmetry in brain anatomy and function
Some of the functions of the brain are located in specific regions of the brain, while others are distributed

nerves. To do this, it is necessary to consider the basic parts of the nervous system, to identify what they do, and how they are related. Finally, we can see how the different parts interact, using the principles outlined in Table 1.1, to produce behaviour.

The nervous system comprises two parts: the peripheral nervous system (PNS) and the central nervous system (CNS). These two systems are anatomically separate but are functionally interconnected and integrated (Fig. 1.1). The PNS consists of nerve fibres that transmit specific sensory and motor information to the CNS, which comprises the spinal cord, brainstem and brain. The CNS is housed within the bony structures of the vertebral canal and skull, for protection. Additional mechanical buffering protection of the CNS is afforded by the surrounding meninges and ventricular system.

Overview of brain anatomy

The CNS comprises six anatomical regions: the cerebral cortex, the diencephalon (thalamus and hypothalamus), the midbrain, the pons and cerebellum, the medulla, and the spinal cord (Fig. 1.2). The best way to understand the anatomy is to look at the external and internal topography, to identify anatomical structures and their relationships, and then to define the functions of the identified structures.

Meninges

If we open the skull and look inside, the first thing seen is the membranes that cover the brain, called meninges. These membranes surround and protect the CNS. There are three layers: the dura mater, arachnoid and pia mater. The dura mater forms folds that separate different brain regions from each other and demarcate anatomical

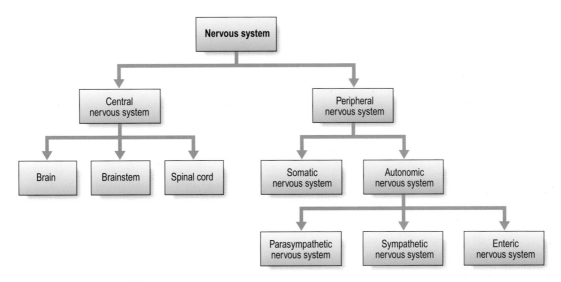

Fig. 1.1 Overview of the anatomical organization of the nervous system.

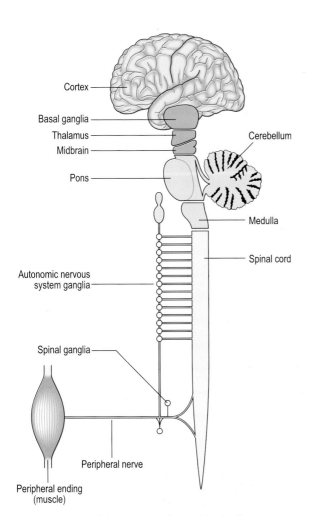

Fig. 1.2 Major parts of the nervous system. Light shading: structures of the supratentorial level. Dark shading: structures of the posterior fossa level. No shading: structures of the spinal level.

boundaries within the skull cavity. These layers are described in more detail in Chapter 12.

Cortical lobes

When the meninges are removed, one can observe the gross anatomy of the CNS. Anatomically, the cortex is described according to lobes that are named in relation to skull bones. Thus, there are four lobes visible from the outside of the brain: the occipital, temporal, parietal and frontal lobes. In addition, there is one other lobe that cannot be seen from the outside of the brain: the limbic lobe. It comprises the medial portions of the frontal, parietal and temporal lobes, forming a rim around the corpus callosum (a fibre tract that connects the two cortical hemispheres). Another cortical area, the insula, lies buried in the medial wall of the lateral fissure, overlain by parts of the frontal, parietal and temporal lobes; it is functionally associated with the limbic lobe. The lobes are divided into regions that are associated with specific functions (see Table 1.2).

Surface features: sulci and gyri

The surface of the cortex is highly convoluted and is subdivided into fissures (deep grooves), gyri (elevated folds; singular = gyrus) and sulci (singular = sulcus; shallow grooves between folds). The folds massively increase the surface area of the cortex. The longitudinal fissure separates the two cortical hemispheres, and the lateral fissure (of Sylvius) separates the temporal lobe from the parietal and frontal lobes. The central sulcus and the parieto-occipital sulcus define the boundaries of the frontal and parietal, and parietal and occipital, lobes respectively. On the lateral surface of the hemispheres, the boundaries between parietal, occipital and temporal lobes are established by continuing the line of the parieto-occipital sulcus downwards, to the inferior surface of the hemisphere, and the line of the lateral fissure backwards to meet this line (Fig. 1.3B).

The pattern of sulci and gyri is extremely variable, and defining even the major sulci and gyri is not easy. In general, the surface of each lobe can be divided into three gyri by two sulci. The sulci provide landmarks for identifying lobes and functional areas of the brain. The main lobes, gyri and sulci are shown in Figure 1.3. The central sulcus marks the position of two important functional areas: primary somatosensory cortex and primary motor cortex. The latter lies anterior to this sulcus in the precentral gyrus; the former lies posterior in the postcentral gyrus.

On the medial surface (see Figs 1.3C and 1.5), the cingulate sulcus follows approximately the curvature of the corpus callosum, extending through both the frontal and parietal lobes. Below this sulcus is the cingulate gyrus (functionally associated with the limbic lobe). This sulcus terminates by passing upwards to form a sulcus that continues onto the lateral surface of the hemisphere as the postcentral sulcus (Fig 1.3B). The central sulcus is usually the sulcus immediately anterior to this sulcus (on the lateral surface). The gyrus in between these two sulci is the postcentral gyrus, which contains the primary somatosensory cortex. Anterior to the point where the cingulate sulcus crosses (to the lateral surface of the brain) is the paracentral lobule, which contains the lower limb primary motor and somatosensory cortical function regions. The gyri (lingular and cuneus) either side of the calcarine sulcus in the posterior part of the brain are associated with vision.

On the inferior surface (Fig. 1.3A) of the temporal lobe, the most medial gyrus is the parahippocampal gyrus, which expands at its anterior end to form the bulbous, hook-like uncus. These are evolutionarily old parts of the cerebral cortex and are concerned, in part, with the olfactory (smell) system and with memory. In the orbitofrontal cortex (the part that sits above the orbit in the skull) is located the olfactory gyrus. These structures form part of the limbic system, which is involved in emotional processing and perception.

Also visible from the underneath of the brain are the cerebellum and brainstem, which together form the hindbrain. The cerebellum is the broccoli-like structure that lies above the fourth ventricle at the back of the head and below the occipital cortex. It is the largest part of the hindbrain. The function of the cerebellum is coordination of movements. This includes muscle tone, movement range, smoothness and equilibrium. The cerebellum is considered in more detail in Chapter 9.

Brainstem

The brainstem is located within the posterior fossa of the skull and consists of three parts: midbrain, pons and medulla. These relay information to and from the periphery to higher centres such as the cortex and cerebellum. The brainstem also receives direct input from the cranial nerves. The functions of these nerves and the internal anatomy of the brainstem are described in Chapter 6.

Medulla

On the ventral surface of the medulla are the pyramids (see Fig. 6.1) that contain descending motor fibres from the cerebral cortex that form the corticospinal tract (CST), also called the pyramidal tracts of the spinal cord. The pyramidal decussation is where most of the CST fibres cross to the other side to become the lateral CST. The decussation marks the location of the spinomedullary junction, i.e. the end of the spinal cord and the beginning of the brainstem. Lateral to the rostral part

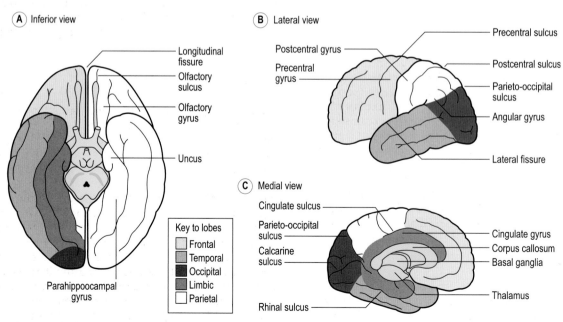

Fig. 1.3 Main gyri, sulci, fissures and lobes of the brain.

of the pyramids are two oval swellings that identify the inferior olivary nuclei (ION), which are functionally associated with the cerebellum. They provide a surface landmark for the emergence of cranial nerves IX–XII; nerve XII emerges between the ION and the pyramids, whereas nerves IX–XI emerge laterally to the ION.

On the dorsal surface of the brainstem, the medulla consists of two parts, the open and closed medulla, due to the emergence of the central canal from the spinal cord opening into the fourth ventricle. The point at which this occurs is called the obex. The closed part of the medulla shows a pair of gracile and cuneate tubercles that mark the position of the gracile and cuneate nuclei (see Fig. 6.1), which transmit sensory information to higher brain centres.

Pons

The ventral pons has a transversely ridged appearance, with a shallow groove running along the midline called the basilar sulcus, which contains the basilar artery. The ridged appearance is due to fibres entering the cerebellum from the nerve cells in the pons, which, in turn, are the recipients of a major input from the cerebral cortex (see Fig 6.1). The trigeminal nerve is the only nerve to emerge from this ridged region, while cranial nerves VII and VIII exit at the cerebellopontomedullary angle. The position of cranial nerves VI–VIII identifies the pontomedullary junction on the ventral surface.

The pons is sharply demarcated both rostrally and caudally from the other parts of the brainstem. The open medulla and pons together form the floor of the fourth ventricle, which is diamond-shaped. The closure of the rostral part of the fourth ventricle to form the cerebral aqueduct and the cerebral peduncles demarcates the transition from pons to midbrain.

Midbrain

The midbrain (see Fig. 6.1) is short, and very little of it can be seen in the undissected brain. Ventrally, the cerebral peduncles are located lateral to two small circumscribed mounds, the mamillary bodies (part of the hypothalamus). The peduncles are large bundles of fibres descending from the motor cortex to the brainstem and spinal cord, and comprise chiefly the pyramidal and corticopontine fibre systems. The dorsal surface of the midbrain is called the tectum and has two paired swellings, the inferior and superior colliculi, which are involved in auditory and visual reflexes. These are buried beneath the overlying cerebral hemispheres. Two cranial nerves exit the midbrain, cranial nerve III at the midbrain–pons junction and cranial nerve IV on the dorsal surface.

Spinal cord

The spinal cord connects the brain to the PNS. It is the part of the CNS located outside the skull, below the foramen magnum but within the vertebral column. The spinal level of the nervous system extends from the skull to the sacrum. The spinal cord receives input from the periphery, relays it to the brain and sends response signals back to the periphery. The spinal cord is not segmented; rather, the distribution of the peripheral nerve spinal roots gives it a functional segregation. The details of spinal cord function are described in Chapter 4. The spinal cord consists of grey matter and white matter, like the brain (except that in the spinal cord the white matter is on the outside). The grey matter contains cells and is surrounded by white matter that contains mainly bundles of axons ascending and descending in the spinal cord.

Internal anatomy of the brain

The easiest way to see the various anatomical structures deep inside the brain is to cut it open. However, what is seen depends on the plane of section; the same structures look different in different planes (see Box 1.1).

Sagittal sections

If the brain is split in two at the midline, cutting along the sagittal fissure, the cerebrum is divided into its two hemispheres, as shown in Figure 1.5. In this plane, below the corpus callosum we can see most of the deep (subcortical) structures of the brain, the thalamus, the hypothalamus and the ventricular system. Moving laterally in this plane, adjacent sections would also reveal the appearance of the basal ganglia nuclei that are located on top of the thalamus and form part of the lateral walls of the ventricular system. The basal ganglia are more easily viewed in frontal and horizontal sections (see Figs 1.7 and 1.10). In the upper part of Figure 1.5, they are obscured by a thin membranous sheet, the septum pellucidum (which is torn in this specimen). Most of these structures can be seen in the MRI image shown in the lower part of Figure 1.5.

Coronal sections

Frontal (coronal) sections are the easiest plane to visualize, because their orientation is such that viewing them is just like looking at another person face-on. When sectioning from front to back, the very first section seen in a coronal series would be just the tips of the frontal lobes, which are located right behind the forehead. In Figure 1.6 we have moved backwards a little, to the first section containing internal structures. In these sections, the white matter (axons) appears white and the grey matter (cell bodies) appears grey. The first thing to notice is the corpus callosum. This major pathway connects the two hemispheres and serves as a useful landmark, because it appears in all coronal sections in which deep structures are present.

Below the corpus callosum are the front ends of the two lateral ventricles, separated by the septum pellucidum. The masses of grey matter that form the lateral walls of the

Brain topography

Anatomical descriptions of images and tissue sections are based on four anatomical planes, sagittal, horizontal, transverse and median (Fig. 1.4). The horizontal (axial) plane is a plane across the brain that would be horizontal if the patient were standing up. The median plane is one that slices the brain vertically along the midline into two symmetrical halves; sagittal sections are vertical planes through the brain parallel to the median plane. The coronal (frontal) plane is one slicing the brain vertically across (e.g. from ear to ear).

In addition, structures towards the front of the brain are termed anterior (or rostral) and those towards the back are posterior (or caudal). Those towards the top of the brain are termed superior and those towards the bottom are termed inferior. Structures located laterally are further away from the midline, and those located medially are nearer the midline.

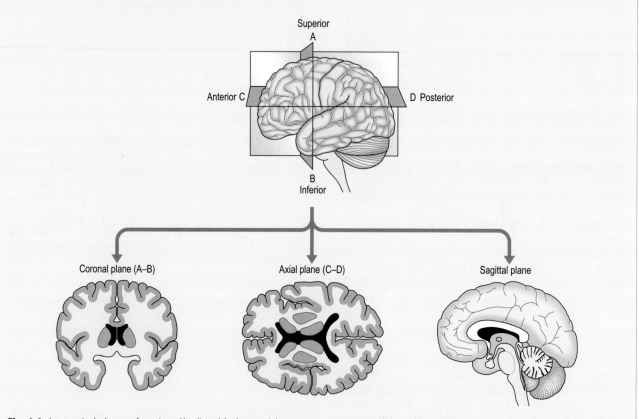

Fig. 1.4 Anatomical planes of section. Shading: black, ventricles; grey, grey matter; yellow, white matter.

lateral ventricles are the caudate nuclei (part of the basal ganglia). The rule for identifying them is simple: if the lateral ventricles are visible, so is the caudate. This applies throughout the curved extent of the lateral ventricles, as the caudate follows them the whole way.

The caudate appears to be joined by threads of grey matter to another nucleus, the putamen. These two nuclei are almost always divided by a band of axons called the internal capsule, which is a major pathway for connections between the thalamus and the cortex. In the rostral brain, these two nuclei are continuous at the base, so that in reality the caudate and the putamen are a single nucleus, divided in half by the internal capsule; hence

they are commonly called the striatum. Early anatomists did not realize this, so they were named separately, and the small ventral bridge below the internal capsule which connects them was named the nucleus accumbens. The nucleus accumbens and the septal nuclei are associated with conscious 'reward' and motivation and are part of the limbic system. These structures are involved in the mediation of the effects of addictive drugs such as cocaine, heroin and amphetamines.

In the next most caudal section, shown in Figure 1.7A, the nucleus accumbens has disappeared and the caudate and putamen are no longer connected. The caudate nucleus is decreased in size, and medial to the putamen

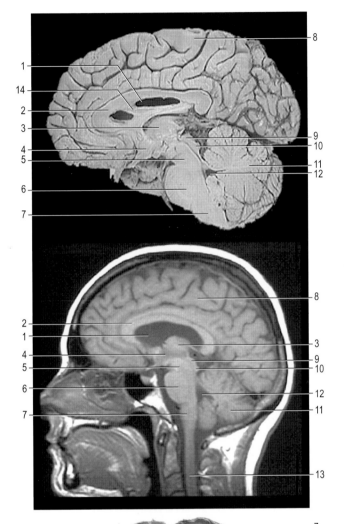

1. Lateral ventricle.
2. Corpus callosum.
3. Thalamus.
4. Hypothalamus.
5. Midbrain.
6. Pons.
7. Medulla.
8. Paracentral lobule.
9. Superior colliculus.
10. Inferior colliculus.
11. Cerebellum.
12. Fourth ventricle.
13. Spinal cord.
14. Septum pellucidum.

Fig. 1.5 Midsagittal section of the brain shown in a gross specimen (top) and at the equivalent level on a magnetic resonance imaging scan (bottom).

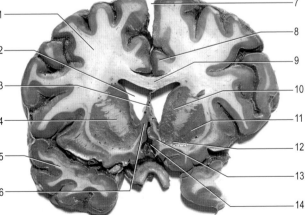

1. Frontal lobe.
2. Lateral ventricle.
3. Septum pellucidum.
4. Anterior limb of internal capsule.
5. Temporal lobe.
6. Septal nuclei.
7. Longitudinal fissure.
8. Cingulate gyrus.
9. Corpus callosum.
10. Caudate nucleus.
11. Putamen.
12. Nucleus accumbens.
13. Hypothalamus.
14. Third ventricle.

Fig. 1.6 Coronal section of the brain.

there is the emergence of a new set of basal ganglia nuclei, the globus pallidus external (GPe) and internal (GPi). We can clearly see the diagonal openings that connect the lateral ventricles with the midline third ventricle. The septum here is very small, and suspended from it like two pieces of fruit are tracts called the fornices (fornix for one tract). The third ventricle is below the fornices. The fornix connects

the mamillary body to the hippocampus (in the temporal lobe). Its inferior part can be seen adjacent to the third ventricle above the hypothalamus. Below the hypothalamus at the base of the brain is the optic tract. Below and between the putamen and GPe and just above the temporal lobe is a white matter tract called the anterior commissure, which connects the temporal lobes of each hemisphere. In the

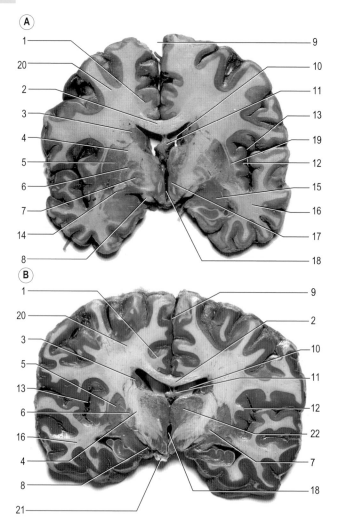

1. Cingulate gyrus.
2. Corpus callosum.
3. Caudate nucleus.
4. Internal capsule.
5. Putamen.
6. Globus pallidus external.
7. Globus pallidus internal.
8. Optic tract.
9. Longitudinal fissure.
10. Lateral ventricle.
11. Fornix.
12. Insula cortex.
13. Lateral fissure.
14. Anterior commissure.
15. Amygdala.
16. Temporal lobe.
17. Hypothalamus.
18. Third ventricle.
19. Claustrum.
20. Frontal lobe.
21. Mamillary bodies.
22. Thalamus.

Fig. 1.7 Coronal section of the brain.

medial part of the temporal lobe is a circumscribed region of grey matter, the amygdala. The amygdala is a specialized form of cortex, and is part of the limbic system. It deals with the emotional significance of experiences. The insula cortex is also visible at this level. The insula appears to play a role in language and in the integration and perception of sensory stimuli such as pain and is part of the limbic system. Between the insula and putamen is a nucleus called the claustrum. The function of the claustrum is unclear but it has connections with the hippocampus, amygdala, caudate nucleus, premotor, prefrontal, auditory and visual cortices, suggesting a role in integration of multiple modalities to contribute to perception. The claustrum is separated from the insula by the extreme capsule and from the putamen by the external capsule.

Moving further caudally, (Fig. 1.7B), another major nucleus appears: the thalamus. The thalamus is a heterogeneous group of nuclei that are the gatekeepers for any information passing to and from the cerebral cortex. The thalami are located on either side of the slit-like third ventricle. This provides another anatomical rule: if the third ventricle is visible, so is the thalamus. The thalamus is located medial to the internal capsule (posterior limb),

while the putamen and globus pallidus remain lateral to it; this relationship is always preserved and is more easily seen in horizontal sections. The ventral surface of the pons has also been cut, showing the transverse cerebello-pontine fibres. The two swellings above it are the mamillary bodies at the base of the midbrain.

In the next section (Fig. 1.8), the globus pallidus and putamen have disappeared. The caudate nuclei are very small and the thalami are larger. A new structure visible here in the medial temporal lobe, shaped like a sea-horse, is the hippocampus. At this level, more of the ventral surface of the brainstem has been sectioned. Medial to the hippocampus on either side are diagonally running white matter tracts that pass through the midbrain, pons and medulla. These are the pyramidal tracts. Also visible in the midbrain region is the substantia nigra, which has been cut obliquely.

Figure 1.9 is the last section of this series and now a lot has changed. The posterior part of the left lateral ventricle is visible as a long diagonal slit comprising the posterior and inferior horns (and associated choroid plexus). The lateral ventricle, like many other structures in the brain, curves back and loops under itself like a big C. The hippocampus, which is involved in memory formation, is clearly

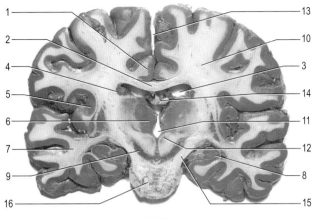

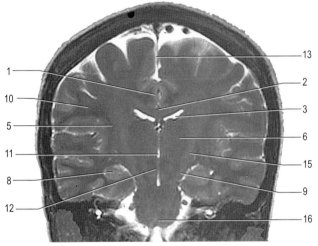

1. Cingulate cortex.
2. Corpus callosum.
3. Lateral ventricle.
4. Caudate nucleus.
5. Insula cortex.
6. Thalamus.
7. Temporal lobe.
8. Hippocampus.

9. Substantia nigra.
10. Frontal lobe.
11. Third ventricle.
12. Red nucleus of midbrain.
13. Longitudinal fissure.
14. Fornix.
15. Pyramidal tract.
16. Pons.

Fig. 1.8 Coronal section of the brain shown in a gross specimen (top) and at the equivalent level on a magnetic resonance imaging scan (bottom).

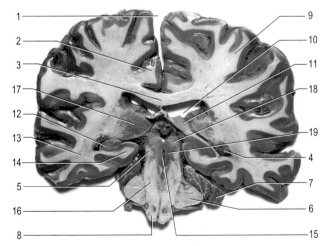

1. Longitudinal fissure.
2. Cingulate cortex.
3. Splenium of corpus callosum.
4. Choroid plexus in inferior horn of lateral ventricle.
5. Midbrain.
6. Middle cerebral peduncle.
7. Cerebellum.
8. Medulla.
9. Parietal cortex.

10. Posterior horn of lateral ventricle.
11. Fornix.
12. Hippocampus.
13. Temporal lobe.
14. Parahippocampal gyrus.
15. Cerebral aqueduct.
16. Pons.
17. Thalamus.
18. Superior colliculus.
19. Peri-aqueductal grey region.

Fig. 1.9 Coronal section of the brain.

visible on the medial side of the lower part of the lateral ventricle, and is connected to the fornix, which runs inside the ventricles. This section is at the junction of brainstem and cerebrum, which is called the midbrain. The midbrain can be identified by the cerebral aqueduct, which connects the third and fourth ventricles. Below the midbrain is the pons, with the two middle cerebellar peduncles (tracts of white matter) connecting the pons to the cerebellum.

Horizontal sections

MRI and CT scans are often viewed in the horizontal plane. All the major subcortical nuclear structures are related to the positions of the ventricular system and internal capsule.

Figure 1.10 shows a brain cut at two different levels, the right superior to the left. Both are cut at the level

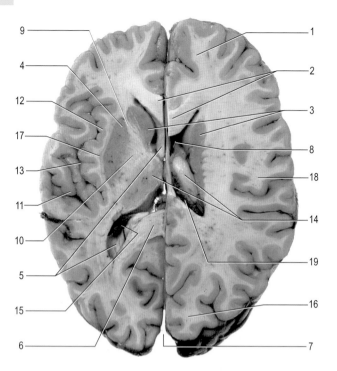

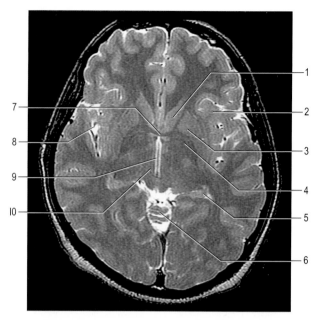

1. Frontal lobe.
2. Genu of corpus callosum.
3. Caudate nucleus.
4. Putamen.
5. Fornix.
6. Splenium of corpus callosum.
7. Longitudinal fissure.
8. Anterior horn of lateral ventricle.
9. Anterior limb of internal capsule.
10. Posterior limb of internal capsule.
11. Temporal lobe.
12. Insular cortex.
13. Lateral fissure.
14. Thalamus.
15. Posterior horn of lateral ventricle.
16. Occipital lobe.
17. Claustrum.
18. Parietal lobe.
19. Choroid plexus.

Fig. 1.10 Horizontal section of the brain at the level of the lateral ventricles.

1. Caudate nucleus.
2. Insula.
3. Putamen.
4. Internal capsule.
5. Hippocampus.
6. Vermis of cerebellum.
7. Anterior commissure.
8. Lateral fissure.
9. Third ventricle.
10. Hypothalamus.

Fig. 1.11 Horizontal section of the brain at the level of the third ventricle shown in a gross specimen (top) and the equivalent level on a magnetic resonance image scan (bottom).

of the lateral ventricles. The caudate nuclei protrude into the anterior part of the lateral ventricles to form its lateral wall, and on the left, the putamen is separated from the caudate by the anterior limb of the internal capsule. The white matter tract immediately anterior and posterior to the ventricles is the corpus callosum, which crosses in and out of the plane of the page. Remember that in the sagittal plane it curves like a C from front to back; in this horizontal section, it was cut through twice, at the front end (genu) and back end (splenium). At this level, on the left, the true shape of the internal capsule is revealed in horizontal section. It is V-shaped. It has an anterior limb and a posterior limb. We can also see the third ventricle and the thalamic nuclei on either side. The channel between the lateral ventricles and the third ventricle is visible, the foramen of Monro. Also visible in the left ventricle are the cut parts of the fornices.

In Figure 1.11, which is inferior to Figure 1.10, the lateral ventricles are now absent but the third ventricle is visible. The two globus pallidus nuclei (GPe and GPi) are

medial to the putamen, which is medial to the insula cortex, and caudal to the caudate nucleus on each side. The anterior commissure is a horizontal band of white matter joining the hemispheres (see Fig. 1.7A), and just below that are the two white dots that mark the position of the columns of the fornix. The hypothalamus makes up the walls of the third ventricle, and the hippocampus is also visible in the inferior horn of the ventricle.

Ventricular system

The ventricles are irregularly shaped cavities within the brain that contain cerebrospinal fluid (CSF). The main functions of the CSF are to provide buffering support during rapid head movements and to provide buoyancy to CNS structures, so that they are, in effect, weightless.

The ventricular system of the brain consists of two lateral ventricles, and the midline third and fourth ventricles, connected by the cerebral aqueduct (Fig. 1.12). The lateral ventricles are the largest cavities and are located deep within the brain. They are symmetrical structures. Each communicates with the third ventricle through the interventricular foramen (of Munro) and the latter is connected to the fourth ventricle via the cerebral aqueduct.

CSF drains from the fourth ventricle through a median and two lateral apertures in its floor (giving it a

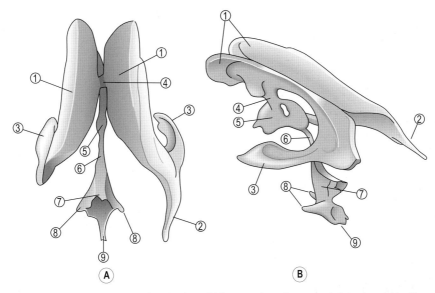

Fig. 1.12 Anatomy of the ventricular system from the (A) superior and (B) posterolateral aspects. 1, lateral ventricle; 2, posterior horn; 3, inferior horn; 4, interventricular foramen (of Munro); 5, third ventricle; 6, cerebral aqueduct; 7, fourth ventricle; 8, lateral aperture (of Luschka); 9, median aperture (of Magendie).

space. These apertures are the only means by which the CSF can enter the subarachnoid space. The cerebellum forms the roof of the fourth ventricle and is called the superior medullary velum.

All the ventricles contain variable amounts of choroid plexus, which is the main source for the production of CSF (see Chapter 12). If the flow of CSF becomes blocked (especially in the cerebral aqueduct), there is a rise in intracranial pressure. If this happens in infants, they may develop severe brain damage and hydrocephalus.

Forebrain

This is the largest part of the brain (80% by volume) and comprises the cerebral cortex, the limbic system and the basal ganglia. The forebrain is concerned with perception, cognition, motivation, memory, emotion and control of higher motor functions.

The architecture of the cortex differs between the cerebral cortex and limbic cortex. The limbic cortex is evolutionarily older and comprises only three or four cell layers of grey matter, whereas the rest of the cortex, called neocortex, is evolutionarily more recent and comprises six layers. The cortex is made up mostly of pyramidal cells and granule cells; simplistically, granule cells (in layer 4) receive sensory input and pyramidal cells (layer 6) provide output. The other layers connect to other areas of the cortex on the same side of the brain via association fibres and to the contralateral side via commissural fibres.

The cortex can also be divided into areas that have a single function, such as touch, vision, hearing, taste and smell or the production of movement. These are called primary areas (see Table 1.2). Their function is to receive and start the initial processing of information. The rest of the

Table 1.2 Functions of brain lobes

Lobe	Important functional areas	Function
Frontal	Primary motor cortex	Control of movement
	Broca's area	Speech
	Motor association cortex	Intelligence, intuition, movement planning, rationalisation and motivation
Parietal	Primary somatosensory cortex	Somatosensation
	Parietal Association cortex	Spatial awareness of surroundings
	Taste cortex	Taste sensation
Temporal	Primary auditory cortex	Hearing
	Wernicke's area	Language comprehension
	Temporal association cortex	Object and face recognition
Occipital	Primary visual cortex	Vision
	Visual association cortex	Visual spatial awareness, colour perception
Limbic	Medial temporal lobe (uncus)	Emotions (fear, anxiety), memory
	Medial prefrontal cortex	Personality, working memory, emotional behaviour
	Cingulate cortex	Cognition, emotional affect
	Orbitofrontal	Smell, emotional behaviour

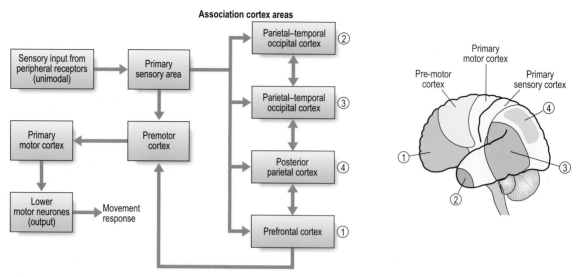

Fig. 1.13 Intercortical connections of primary, higher-order and association cortices used in processing a sensory stimulus to produce a behavioural response. Inset shows the location of the various association areas.

cortex, which carry out diverse types of sensory integration required for purposeful movements. They make the link between sensations and (re)action by making connections with motor areas. These include the posterior parietal cortex, which integrates sensory and visual stimuli; it is associated with the cognition of the body itself and the awareness of objects surrounding it, and is critical for attention to external events. The parietal–occipital–temporal association region coordinates somatosensation with visual and auditory cues to produce perceptual recognition, or movements in response to visual or auditory stimuli. The prefrontal association cortex occupies most of the rostral part of the lateral frontal lobe and is important in the planning of voluntary movements. The limbic association area is associated with the medial and inferior surfaces of the brain and is devoted mostly to memory, motivation and emotion. All the association areas feed into the higher-order motor areas, which then project to the primary motor cortex, which ultimately exerts control over the motor neurones (Fig. 1.13).

It is important to recognize the locations of the major functional areas of the cortex, particularly the primary somatosensory, visual, auditory and motor cortices. Selective damage to these regions leads to discrete neurological deficits (Figs 1.14 and 1.15).

Hemisphere specialization

The anatomy of the brain appears symmetrical, in that most regions of the sensory and motor cortices are the same on both sides of the brain, and damage to one region leads to a contralateral deficit. However, some of these regions, particularly in the frontal, temporal and parietal lobes, differ in size. For example, primary auditory cortex is larger in the right temporal lobe than in the left; conversely, Wernicke's area (auditory association cortex)

is larger on the left than on the right. Similarly, the left parietal lobe is larger than the right but the right posterior parietal region is bigger than the corresponding area on the left. Also, the left facial somatosensory cortex area is larger than the right. Broca's area on the left is also different from that on the right. This is because there are regions in the frontal and parietal lobes that have dramatically different functions in the left and right brain. These are associated with 'higher functions', such as language, analytical and intuitive thinking, and spatial orientation, artistic and musical ability (Fig. 1.16). Much of what is known about hemispheric asymmetry comes from patients with brain lesions or who have had surgery to control diseases such as epilepsy or cancer.

The hemisphere that contains the centres for language production and comprehension is called the dominant hemisphere; in most people, this is the left hemisphere. Damage to the left hemisphere gives rise to difficulties in speech comprehension or production that do not occur if the lesion is in the right hemisphere. Lateralization of language function can be determined using the Wada test. If a patient has the speech centres in the left hemisphere, then anaesthetic injected into the left carotid artery will block speech perception and production.

Another asymmetry occurs in writing. Most people are right- or left-handed. Very few people are ambidextrous. Handedness and cerebral dominance are thought to be linked. Ninety per cent of the population are right-handed and have left cerebral dominance, and the few individuals who have their speech control in the right hemisphere tend to be left-handed. However, 97% of the population, including three-quarters of left-handers, have their language centres in the left hemisphere.

In addition to speech production, the left hemisphere is important in language articulation and comprehension, mathematical calculations and cognitive functions such as analytical and rational thinking. For example, damage

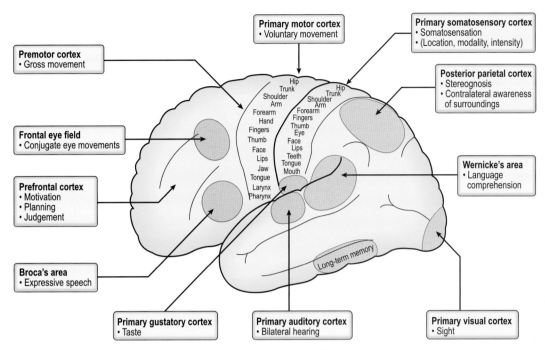

Fig. 1.14 Functional anatomy of specific cortical areas on the lateral surface of the brain.

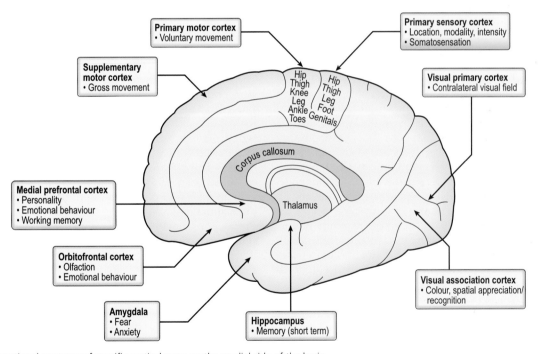

Fig. 1.15 Functional anatomy of specific cortical areas on the medial side of the brain.

to the left parietal lobe causes difficulties in copying movements (ideomotor apraxia), naming objects, reading (alexia), solving mathematics problems (dyscalculia) and language, whereas the same lesion in the right hemisphere causes difficulty in copying drawings (agraphia), assembling puzzles (constructional apraxia) and spatial navigation, such as finding the way to the shops or work, because the landmarks used as a guide are no longer familiar. In some patients, damage to the right posterior parietal cortex results in a contralateral neglect syndrome. The patient fails to recognize the left side of the body as theirs. They may fail to wash or dress the left side of the body, and if presented with a stimulus such as pain, they may report it hurting, but not them.

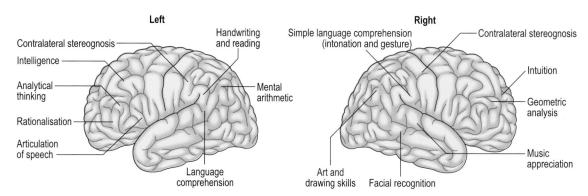

Fig. 1.16 Hemispheric specialization of function.

Studies of lesions in the right brain have shown that it is essential for the processing of non-verbal sound patterns such as music; for example, patients with right-sided strokes can speak but often cannot sing properly. Lesions in the right hemisphere in regions corresponding to Wernicke's area produce deficits in music perception, appreciation of tone and the emotional nuances of speech. Poetry, for example, may seem meaningless after a right area lesion.

Although these studies tell us that there are differences between the two sides of the brain, it is not clear what this means. Brain areas are more similar than they are different. However, if the hemispheres process information differently, this implies that they 'think' differently. There are various speculative theories as to why the brain evolved like this. One is that the left hemisphere is important in the control of fine movements, and this is important in the control of production of speech, which involves fine control of the muscles of the larynx, tongue and oral cavity. The left hemisphere is also involved in the production of actions; damage leads to an inability to copy movements. Finally, another link between language and movement occurs in the representation of language areas. Verbs are 'doing' words that describe actions or states, whereas nouns are names of things. Verbs appear to be processed only in the left hemisphere, while nouns are processed in both hemispheres. Thus, the left hemisphere not only has a role in the production of actions but has a role in the production of mental representations of actions in the form of words.

If the left hemisphere is involved in fine motor control, what about the right hemisphere? One idea is that the right hemisphere is specialized for spatial movement relative to the surroundings, so that at a higher level it can produce mental images of such movements. Damage to this lobe would impair such abilities. This is indeed the case.

One last controversial idea about asymmetry is that the left hemisphere is critical for language interpretation, and this is what sets humans apart from other animals. Evidence for this comes from 'split-brain' studies (Box 1.2), in which the corpus callosum was surgically sectioned in an attempt to reduce the severity of fits in patients with severe epilepsy. This meant that the two hemispheres could no longer communicate with each other. Such patients were shown two pictures of related objects, to both hemispheres. Then several more pictures were shown and patients were asked to select a picture that had an inferred relationship with the first two objects. For example, if the first two pictures were of rain and clouds, the third might be an umbrella. The right brain cannot make the connection, but the left can. The same is true if words, rather than pictures, are used. The ability to infer leads to the ability to believe, and this sets humans apart from other animals. Parrots can be trained to talk but they cannot infer or believe things.

Limbic system

The limbic lobe, situated on the medial side of the brain, surrounds the rim of the ventricles (see Figs 1.3C and 1.15). The cingulate and parahippocampal gyri, together with their associated nuclei, the hippocampus, the amygdala, the septal nucleus, and insula comprise the limbic system. The limbic system is evolutionarily old; it can be found in fish, amphibians, reptiles and mammals. It controls emotional behaviour and the internal factors that motivate animals and people to adapt to a constantly changing external environment.

Emotions have three components: a visceral sensory component caused by endocrine and autonomic stimuli (a 'gut feeling'), a motor component involving the facial muscles to communicate the pleasantness or unpleasantness of the situation to others, and a cognitive–evaluative component to consciously assess the situation. Pathology involving damage to the limbic system can elicit inappropriate behavioural patterns. These patterns include motivational behaviour relating to nutrition and fluid balance, sexual courtship behaviours, and expressions of mood and affect. Memory is an important component of these patterns, and lesions within several limbic areas affect memory.

Input to the limbic system comes from the association cortex areas, the olfactory cortex and the medial temporal lobe regions, and is ultimately passed on to the hypothalamus, which controls the endocrine system and the autonomic nervous system. The connections of the limbic system and the functions of the various nuclei are detailed in Figures 1.17, Figure 1.18 and Table 1.3.

Box
1.2 **'Split-brain' syndrome**

The brain houses two minds, not one, but they only orchestrate into a single personality if the two cerebral hemispheres communicate. Under normal conditions, both halves receive nearly identical information on the world, and life proceeds as though nothing is different about perception. Both hemispheres share the same knowledge base and reactive inclinations. Thus, consciousness is controlled by both hemispheres, and there is crossing over of functions so that one never normally experiences a dissociation of information. However, 'splitting' the brain, by sectioning the corpus callosum, and thereby disconnecting the hemispheres, reveals separate functions. In the early 1960s, researchers showed that when a cat had its optic chiasm and corpus callosum severed, two independent learning centres were established, one in each hemisphere. The same effect was seen in humans. It was concluded that the brain had 'two separate realms of conscious awareness; two sensing, perceiving, thinking and remembering systems'.

Severing the corpus callosum was used by surgeons to treat chronic intractable forms of epilepsy. To the casual observer, the split-brain patients appeared normal and their seizures disappeared. However, psychological testing revealed that if the patient held up an object like a comb in the left hand, they could not say what it was. When it was transferred to the right hand, the patient had no trouble at all in communicating its identity. The same happened with words. If a card with a printed word like 'ring' was visible only in the patient's left visual field, they could not read it, yet vision in the left eye was fine. When the word

was in the right field, the patient immediately recognized it. In order to explain these observations, it was necessary to understand certain basic rules of perception. Right and left worlds of touch and sight project to opposite cerebral hemispheres. Sounds project to both hemispheres simultaneously, so the patient could be cued by the doctor's voice. Many things that people learn and think about are non-verbal: music, art, spatial relationships and geometry. To test the functions of the right hemisphere of split-brain patients, psychologists constructed a screen with a slot under which a patient could reach and touch objects, but not see them. Then he focused a picture of one object in the patient's left field of view (signalling the right hemisphere) and asked them to match the picture to the objects that they could feel behind the screen with the left hand. The patients passed the matching test, with scores similar to those of any normal person. However, when the same task was performed with the right hand, the patient failed to choose correctly because the right hand is controlled by the left hemisphere, which cannot see the object, as it is not in the right visual field.

It is now recognized that cutting only the anterior three-quarters of the corpus callosum and the anterior commissure, and leaving the splenium (posterior part) intact is sufficient to stop seizures completely or render them responsive to drugs. At the same time, psychological tests show results identical to those of normal subjects, suggesting that the cerebral hemispheres totally integrate if just a small fraction of the corpus callosum remains intact.

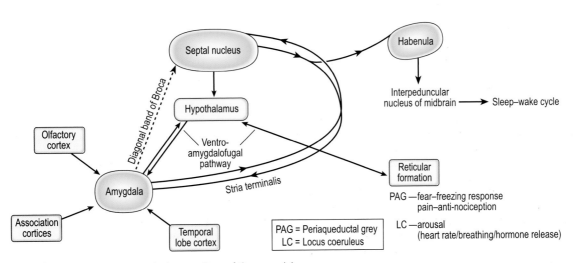

Fig. 1.17 The limbic system: neuroanatomical connections of the amygdala.

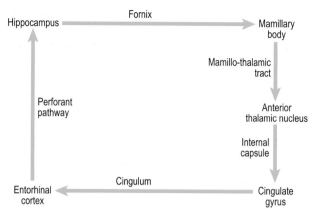

Fig. 1.18 The limbic system: The Papez circuit for emotions. Neuroanatomist James Papez demonstrated that emotions are not a function of any specific brain centre but involve a circuit comprising the hypothalamic mamillary bodies, thalamus, cingulate gyrus and hippocampus. Damage to any of these structures affects emotions and the ability to create memories.

Table 1.3 Functions of limbic system structures

Structure	Function
Hippocampus	Memory acquisition and recall; formation of long-term memory
Amygdala	Emotional content of stimuli; fear, anxiety and danger
Septal nucleus	Pleasure and reward
Cingulate cortex	Affective significance

The hippocampus and amygdala are found in the uncus of the medial temporal lobe. The amygdala is necessary for self-preservation. It is a collection of subnuclei. Clinical studies have shown that when stimulated it gives rise to fear and anxiety or euphoria, depending on which part is stimulated. This is the structure that is responsible for the feelings of fear or dread when you are walking home late at night and hear footsteps behind you. Another important role is in recognizing the emotions indicated by other peoples' facial expressions. The amygdala receives input from the hippocampus, olfactory cortex and temporal lobe association cortex, and aminergic input from septal and brainstem nuclei. Its main outputs are to the septal nucleus and hypothalamus, via the stria terminalis and diagonal band of Broca (septal nucleus only), temporal cortex, and other autonomic and brainstem reticular formation centres, and the nucleus accumbens (via the ventral amygdalofugal pathways). Damage to the amygdala is rare, but experimental studies show that bilateral damage may produce an inability to perceive situations as dangerous, which can have disastrous consequences for people and animals. Such lesions produce the Klüver–Bucy syndrome (Box 1.3).

The hippocampus is involved in the production of long-term memories and the recall of such information. Long-term

In the 1930s, Heinrich Klüver and Paul Bucy found that bilateral temporal lobectomy in monkeys produced a dramatic effect on the animals' responses to fearful situations. The bizarre behavioural abnormalities could be placed into five categories: visual agnosia, oral exploration of all objects, hypermetamorphosis (a compulsion to touch everything, and place each found object into the mouth), altered and increased sexual behaviour and emotional changes, including fearlessness and decreased facial expressions usually associated with emotion. This constellation of symptoms is called the Klüver–Bucy syndrome. Nearly all the symptoms of the Klüver–Bucy syndrome reported in monkeys have also been found in humans with temporal lobe lesions. In addition to visual recognition problems, oral tendencies and hypersexuality, people appear to have 'flattened' emotions.

memory is stored as a modification of connections between neurones, and is analogous to information stored on the hard drive of a computer. The hippocampus allows humans to compare the conditions of a present situation, such as danger, with similar past experiences, in order to decide which is the best option to guarantee survival. The hippocampus is part of the hippocampal formation, which includes the dentate gyrus and subiculum. The dentate gyrus is at the tip of the hippocampus, and the subiculum is at the base and is continuous with the entorhinal cortex of the parahippocampal gyrus. There is a one-way flow of information through the hippocampus. Information arrives via the perforant pathway from the entorhinal cortex to the dentate gyrus, which passes information to a region called CA3 (CA stands for cornu Ammonis or 'ram's horn' because of its shape), and then to the CA1 region and on to the subiculum, which is responsible for the output projection to either the nuclei of the mamillary bodies (part of the hypothalamus) via the fornix or back to the sensory cortex via the entorhinal cortex. Somewhere along these pathways, memories are created. Bilateral damage to the hippocampi impairs the formation of new memories, and nothing can be retained; information is soon forgotten. The hippocampus is also damaged in disease states such as dementia and epilepsy (see Chapters 13 and 14), and is a pathological hallmark of rabies.

The septal nuclei are the anterior thickenings of the septum pellucidum, and are located immediately anterior to the anterior commissure. Stimulation of this area evokes pleasurable sensations, particularly sexual ones. It has been suggested that this is the location of the orgasm centre, and that women have four centres, while men only have one! Inputs are from the amygdala, hippocampus, mesolimbic dopaminergic system and olfactory tract. Outputs are to the hypothalamus (via the medial forebrain bundle), hippocampus and habenula (via the stria terminalis) and reticular formation.

The cingulate cortex evaluates the affective significance of events, i.e. whether they are harmful or beneficial. Anatomical studies have revealed prominent afferent input to the cingulate motor areas from the limbic structures and the prefrontal cortex, which can send information about motivation and the internal state of subjects, as well as cognitive evaluation of the environment. The anterior cingulate cortex is also involved in pain perception, receiving input from the posterior insula cortex. Other important inputs are from the anterior thalamic nucleus, which receives its input from the mamillary bodies forming the Papez circuit, involved in the cortical control of emotion (see Fig. 1.18). The anterior cingulate gyrus communicates between the prefrontal cortex and subcortical areas of the limbic system. Bilateral destruction releases the 'rage centres' of the amygdala and hypothalamus from any prefrontal inhibitory influence.

The limbic system is tightly connected to the prefrontal cortex, and together they funnel emotional input to the hypothalamus. There is frontal lobe asymmetry in regard to emotional processing. Activation in the left prefrontal regions may be part of a mechanism that inhibits 'negative' affect (e.g. sadness and disgust); conversely, the right prefrontal regions may inhibit positive emotions (e.g. happiness). People with increased left prefrontal activity are described as more 'optimistic' and more adept at minimizing negative emotions. Lesions of the left prefrontal neocortex are more likely to be associated with depression than lesions in the homologous location in the right hemisphere. During the Wada test, when the left hemisphere is temporarily anaesthetized, patients report negative changes in mood (e.g. sadness). PET studies have indicated increased left-side orbitofrontal blood flow during self-generated sadness.

Orbitofrontal cortex

The orbitofrontal cortex is anatomically linked with the limbic system and the anterior temporal lobe cortex, and mediates the conscious perception of smell. The orbitofrontal cortex interacts with the limbic system in support of higher-order functions such as association, integration and regulation of central autonomic processes, mood and affect, and those motor patterns that are under limbic control. Orbitofrontal lesions interfere with motivation and arousal. Prefrontal leucotomy patients are typically unmotivated and lethargic. Orbitofrontal lesions reduce the sensation of chronic and intractable pain, and sometimes reduce the expression of anger and frustration when expected rewards are not received. In the past, such findings gave impetus to the use of prefrontal leucotomy as a treatment for intractable emotional problems and psychosis. Orbitofrontal lesions interfere with the prediction of reward. Humans with orbitofrontal lesions are unable to anticipate the future positive or negative consequences

of their actions, although immediately available rewards and punishments do influence their behaviour. A classic case of damage to the prefrontal and orbitofrontal lobes is that of Phineas Gage (see Box 15.7).

Basal ganglia

The basal ganglia are a group of large subcortical nuclei found in the forebrain. They are located above and anterior to the thalamus (see Figs 1.6, 1.10 and 1.11). They comprise the caudate nucleus, putamen and globus pallidus. The caudate nucleus fuses at its anterior end with the putamen to form the corpus striatum, so called because, as these two structures become anatomically separated by the anterior limb of the internal capsule, strands of grey matter can be seen connecting them (see Fig. 1.6). At the bottom of the anterior part of the striatum is the nucleus accumbens. This structure, although anatomically part of the basal ganglia, is considered to be part of the limbic system, and is involved in reward systems that are involved in addiction mechanisms. The body of the caudate runs over the thalamus and then curves to pass into the temporal lobe, where it becomes caudate tail and ends at the amygdala, another nucleus that is functionally part of the limbic system. The subthalamic nucleus and substantia nigra (in the midbrain) are functionally associated with the striatum and the globus pallidum. The basal ganglia are concerned with the initiation and maintenance of actions, and are involved in decision-making about what the body is going to do next. The basal ganglia work via four circuit loops that start and end in the cortex:

- a motor loop, concerned with learned movements and involved in the correct sequencing of actions for the execution of learned motor programmes

- a cognitive loop, concerned with motor intentions and advanced planning for later movements

- a limbic loop, concerned with the emotive aspects of movement

- an oculomotor loop, concerned with voluntary saccadic eye movements.

Damage to basal ganglia structures results in movement disorders (see Chapter 10).

Diencephalon

The diencephalon connects the midbrain to the forebrain. It is located deep within the brain and comprises the epithalamus, thalamus, subthalamus and hypothalamus. The epithalamus forms the roof of the diencephalon and consists of the pineal gland (an endocrine gland involved in circadian rhythms and the onset of puberty) and the habenular nuclei, whose functions are associated with the limbic system, as it connects to the septal nuclei via a tract called the stria terminalis thalami. The subthalamus tract called the stria terminalis thalami. The subthalamus is located dorsolateral to the hypothalamus and has two notable cell groups: the subthalamic nucleus and the zona incerta. The former is part of the basal ganglia circuitry (see Chapter 10), while the latter is a rostral extension of the brainstem reticular formation.

Thalamus

This bullet-shaped structure is the largest nuclear mass in the whole body and, together with the hypothalamus, forms the lateral wall of the third ventricle. The two thalami face each other medially across the third ventricle and touch at the inter-thalamic adhesion. The thalamus is the gateway to the cortex and functions in the coordination and integration of sensory, motor and autonomic information. The thalamus is divided into 12 sub-nuclei that have reciprocal connections with the cortex (except for the inhibitory reticular nucleus) via four thalamic peduncles that are incorporated into the corona radiata, a white matter tract in the brain. The thalamic input to the cerebral cortex is the first step in generating sensory perception. This input is integrated along with other sensory input to the association cortex, and initiates appropriate responses.

The thalamus contains a sheet of fibres called the internal medullary lamina that divides the thalamus into three nuclear groups: the anterior, medial and lateral groups. The anterior and medial groups are associated with the limbic system. The lateral part of the thalamus receives restricted sensory or motor input, and is further subdivided into dorsal and ventral nuclei, based on function and projection.

Additionally, thalamic nuclei can be divided into three functional relay groups: specific, association and diffuse nuclei (Table 1.4). Specific nuclei process either a single sensory modality or input from a motor region, and project to a specific cortical region. Each receives reciprocal input from the region to which it projects. The association nuclei are reciprocally connected to association cortex areas of the brain, and are predominantly involved

Table 1.4 Functional organization of the thalamus

Nucleus	Functional group	Inputs	Outputs
Anterior	Association nucleus	Hippocampus Mamillary body	Cingulate cortex
Medial dorsal	Association nucleus	Amygdala Olfactory cortex Hippocampus	Prefrontal cortex Hippocampus
Lateral dorsal	Association nucleus	Amygdala Olfactory cortex Hippocampus	Cingulate cortex Other limbic regions
Lateral posterior	Association nucleus	Superior colliculus pretectum	Occipital, parietal, temporal association cortex
Pulvinar	Association nucleus	Superior colliculus pretectum	Occipital, parietal, temporal association cortex
Medial geniculate	Specific nucleus	Inferior colliculus	Primary visual cortex
Lateral geniculate	Specific nucleus	Left and right eyes	Primary auditory cortex
Ventral posterior	Specific nucleus		
Ventroposteromedial		Trigeminothalamic tract	Primary somatosensory cortex
Ventroposterolateral		Medial lemniscus	Primary somatosensory cortex
Posterior nucleus		Spinothalamic tract Superior colliculus Inferior colliculus	Primary somatosensory cortex Parietal association cortex Temporal association cortex
Ventral lateral	Specific nucleus	Globus pallidus	Primary motor cortex Supplemental motor cortex
Ventral anterior	Specific nucleus	Globus pallidus	Premotor cortex
Intralaminar	Diffuse nucleus	Spinal cord (spinothalamic tract) Reticular formation Cerebellar nuclei Globus pallidus Superior colliculus (deep layers)	Cerebral cortex Striatum
Reticular thalamic	Diffuse nucleus	Reticular formation Corticothalamic efferents Thalamocortical afferents	Dorsal thalamic nuclei (GABAergic)

in sensory integration and the control of emotional aspects of behaviour, and the memory of stimuli. The diffuse nuclei have widespread projections to all functional divisions of the cortex and other thalamic nuclei. They are involved in arousal, and regulate the level of cortical excitability. The intralaminar nuclei are housed in the internal medullary lamina and are considered to be a rostral extension of the reticular formation. The reticular nucleus is the only nucleus that does not directly project to the thalamus. It receives collateral input from the cortex and thalamus. It is physically separate from the other thalamic nuclei and its role is to modulate the activity of other thalamic nuclei, via activation of GABA-ergic synapses. If the thalamus is the gateway to the cortex, the thalamic reticular nucleus is the gatekeeper. It is active during sleep, to inhibit information passing to the cortex.

Hypothalamus

This is the most ventral part of the diencephalon. It lies anterior and inferior to the thalamus, and extends from the optic chiasm to the caudal border of the mamillary bodies. The pituitary gland is connected to the hypothalamus by the infundibulum and is functionally related, as the posterior pituitary gland is a direct outgrowth of the hypothalamus.

The hypothalamus is composed of numerous nuclei that form the major control centre of the visceral system. It integrates activity from the limbic, autonomic and endocrine systems. It regulates the basic survival systems: sleep–wake cycles, thermoregulation, fluid intake, growth, metabolic energy expenditure and reproduction. The hypothalamus receives input from neural and circulatory systems. The neural input is from autonomic structures such as baroreceptors, which relay information about blood pressure (via the solitary nucleus), and chemoreceptors, which give information about the chemical constituents of the fluid cavities. Also, the level of neural arousal is signalled by pathways arising in the brainstem reticular formation and medial forebrain. The hypothalamus also receives input from the limbic and olfactory systems. Circulatory input arrives in the form of blood-borne information concerning temperature, osmolarity, blood sugar and pH levels, as well as hormonal levels that regulate growth, reproduction and feeding behaviour. The hypothalamus has reciprocal connections with many parts of the brainstem and cortex, especially the basal, frontal and medial cortical areas, and the reticular formation. It is therefore considered to be part of the limbic system. It also has an important role in regulating hormone secretion from the pituitary gland. It is a critical player in regulating body homeostasis and in regulating appropriate behaviour in physical and social environments. Its control of stress, sex, thirst and hunger is mediated by release of hormones from the pituitary gland, which act on specific target organs to induce release of other hormones that act on body tissues and feed back to the hypothalamus and pituitary gland to regulate their activities.

The hypothalamus can be divided in the sagittal plane into anterior (supraoptic), middle (tuberal) and posterior (mamillary) regions. The hypothalamus is also divided into three regions in the coronal plane: lateral and medial (with respect to the position of the fornix) and periventricular, which surrounds the third ventricle (Fig. 1.19). The nuclei of the periventricular zone participate in neuroendocrine control, autonomic responses and biological rhythms, and response to stress (Box 1.4), while the lateral nuclei are concerned with arousal mechanisms and motivational behaviour. The medial zone nuclei are involved in homeostasis and reproduction. The organization of these nuclei is summarized in Table 1.5.

The suprachiasmatic nucleus controls the circadian rhythms (body clock) of the body, via connections with the pineal gland, using a genetic pacemaker that is indirectly modulated by light. This may regulate sleep cycles. The medial preoptic nuclei and lateral hypothalamic area are also involved in sleep behaviour. Damage to these areas results in insomnia and hypersomnia.

Temperature is regulated by the preoptic and posterior nuclei. Cells act like miniature thermostats, and are extremely sensitive to skin temperature changes. The correct body temperature is maintained by feedback circuits using behavioural or reflex mechanisms. For example, if one enters a room that is too cold, the heating is turned up, or extra clothes are put on to warm the body, or body heat is generated by shivering. If one is too hot, heat is lost by reflex measures, such as sweating, or by behavioural means, such as undressing.

The thirst centres reside in the supraoptic nucleus. Cells here are extremely sensitive to fluid volume and osmolarity. If the blood volume drops or the osmolarity is too high, water must be ingested. This is triggered by the release of vasopressin from the pituitary gland. Vasopressin acts on the kidney and leads to retention of water. The kidney signals back to the hypothalamus via the secretion of renin into the bloodstream, which leads to the formation of angiotensin II. This peptide feeds back to the hypothalamus by stimulating the subfornical organ, in the lining of the lateral ventricles. This stimulates the thirst centres and ultimately leads to more water intake.

The hypothalamic control of eating and hunger is less well understood than other functions of the hypothalamus. Based on lesion studies, it was initially thought that there were two discrete centres for hunger and satiety, in the lateral and ventromedial hypothalamic regions. Bilateral lesions of the former cause starvation behaviour, while damage to the latter causes overeating and obesity. This is an oversimplification, as lesions of the lateral hypothalamic region damage the medial forebrain bundle, leading to neglect syndrome; that is, there is no motivation to eat. Lesions of the ventromedial hypothalamus affect connections to the periventricular nucleus, disrupting satiety input signals from the digestive tract, and giving the impression that the body is still hungry.

The hormones oxytocin and vasopressin are made in the paraventricular and supraoptic nuclei of the hypothalamus, and are released at axon terminals that travel in

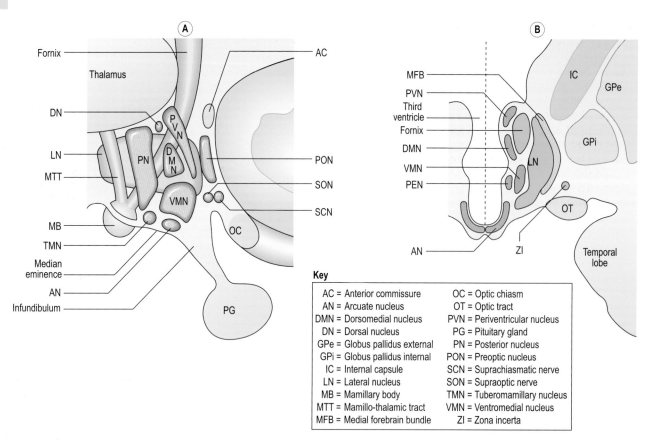

Key

AC = Anterior commissure	OC = Optic chiasm
AN = Arcuate nucleus	OT = Optic tract
DMN = Dorsomedial nucleus	PVN = Periventricular nucleus
DN = Dorsal nucleus	PG = Pituitary gland
GPe = Globus pallidus external	PN = Posterior nucleus
GPi = Globus pallidus internal	PON = Preoptic nucleus
IC = Internal capsule	SCN = Suprachiasmatic nerve
LN = Lateral nucleus	SON = Supraoptic nerve
MB = Mamillary body	TMN = Tuberomamillary nucleus
MTT = Mamillo-thalamic tract	VMN = Ventromedial nucleus
MFB = Medial forebrain bundle	ZI = Zona incerta

Fig. 1.19 Anatomical organization of the hypothalamus. (A) Lateral view. (B) Midline view.

> **Box 1.4 Stress**
>
> Nearly 60% of medical complaints seen by doctors are thought to be stress-related. Stress is defined as any external stimulus, physical or psychological, that threatens homeostasis. Stress both helps and harms the body. The body goes through three stages in response to a sudden stressor. First, there is a degree of shock, and this is followed by a stage of resistance, in which the body fights back. This is via activation of the sympathetic autonomic nervous system and the release of adrenaline, whose effects are felt almost immediately, e.g. increased heart rate, and put the body on a state of alert to deal with the immediate situation. Adrenaline also stimulates the periventricular nucleus in the hypothalamus to induce release from the adrenal cortex of the stress hormone cortisol, whose functions are two-fold. In
>
> the short term, some of its effects are to help cope with the stress response, e.g. mobilizing energy reserves for delivery to muscles, and enhancing feeding to replenish energy sources after mobilization and use. The longer-term effects are to counteract the stress response, by re-establishing the homeostasis by feedback inhibition of the hypothalamus. However, if there is too much cortisol produced for too long, the third stage, exhaustion, ensues, and this has deleterious effects on the body, as its defence systems begin to break down. For example, chronic stressful situations such as a high-pressured job or a messy divorce lead to elevated cortisol and adrenaline levels in the body. This may lead to impaired immune function, chronic hypertension, obesity and atherosclerosis.

---

the median eminence to the posterior lobe of the pituitary. Damage to these structures can result in diabetes inspidus and Cushing's disease. In contrast, the functional connection with the anterior lobe is vascular, and originates in the arcuate, preoptic, periventricular and ventromedial nuclei. These either promote or inhibit the release of various hormones from the anterior pituitary,

such as adrenocorticotrophic hormone (ACTH), thyroid-stimulating hormone, growth hormone, prolactin, follicle-stimulating hormone and luteinizing hormone. Damage to the pituitary gland causes various clinical syndromes. Pituitary dysfunction results in hypothyroidism or hyperthyroidism (thyrotoxicosis), due to failure of thyroid regulation. Infertility is due to failure of gonadotrophic hormones, while growth hormone dys-regulation results in acromegaly or dwarfism.

Peripheral nervous system

The PNS includes all the neuromuscular structures outside the skull and vertebral column. It can be divided into the somatic nervous system, consisting of nerve fibres that transmit information from skeletal muscle, the skin and the visceral organs, and the autonomic nervous system (ANS), which regulates automatic (involuntary) efferent control over visceral organs (see Fig. 1.1).

Somatic nervous system

The major structures of the PNS are the peripheral receptors, the neuromuscular junction, the peripheral nerves (trunks and plexuses) and their associated sensory ganglia.

Peripheral receptors

Receptors can be classified by sensory modality as mechanoreceptors, chemoreceptors or photoreceptors (Table 1.6 and Fig. 1.20). Each receptor is generally specialized to be sensitive to a specific type of stimulus.

The senses of smell, taste, vision and hearing have specialized receptors. Auditory and visual receptors are detailed in Chapters 7 and 8. Olfactory receptor cells have several hair-like cilia that are stimulated by odour molecules in the air. These generate action potentials that are transmitted to the mitral cells of the olfactory bulb, which then relay information to the primary olfactory cortex in the orbito-frontal and medial temporal lobe regions, where conscious appreciation of smell begins. There are connections from this region to the limbic system and hypothalamus that evoke emotional and memory responses to odours.

Taste is detected by the taste buds on the tongue. Each taste bud has around 100 receptors that respond to sweet, sour, salt and bitter stimuli. A substance is tasted when the chemicals in food are dissolved in the saliva and enter the pores of the taste buds to stimulate the hair cells, which then relay signals to the gustatory cortex (in the parietal lobe) and the limbic cortex, for emotional labelling. Taste and smell are intimately linked to give the perception of flavour. Loss of smell leads to a reduction in taste sensation, manifested as a lack of flavour.

Sensory mechanoreceptors in the skin can be encapsulated or unencapsulated. Encapsulated endings 'tune' the axon to respond to a particular kind of stimulus. They are either rapidly adapting (RA), i.e. they stop firing quickly in response to a constant stimulus, or slowly adapting (SA), i.e. they do not stop firing. For example, if a pen is placed in the palm of your hand, the RA receptors fire on contact to let you know that something has landed in your hand. If the pen remains stationary, they will stop firing immediately, but the SA fibres (Merkel's

Table 1.5 Location of hypothalamic nuclei

Sagittal subregion	Coronal subregion		
	Lateral	Medial	Periventricular
Anterior	Supraoptic	Medial preoptic	Suprachiasmatic
	Lateral preoptic		Anterior Periventricular nucleus
Middle	Lateral hypothalamic area	Ventromedial	Arcuate
		Dorsomedial	Paraventricular
Posterior	Lateral hypothalamic area	Mamillary body	Posterior hypothalamic
	Mamillary body		
	Tuberoinfundibular		

Table 1.6 Classification of peripheral receptors

Receptor type	Receptor end organ	Sensory modality
Mechanoreceptors	Hair follicles	Light touch
	Pacinian corpuscles	Vibration
	Ruffini endings	Skin stretch
	Merkel cells	Pressure
	Meissner corpuscles	Velocity
	Muscle spindles	Muscle length, joint position
	Golgi tendon organs	Muscle tension
	Free nerve endings	Pain
	Auditory hair cells	Hearing
	Cupulae, maculae hair cells	Balance and motion
Chemoreceptors	Taste buds	Taste
	Olfactory receptor cells	Smell
	Visceral chemoreceptors	Pain
Photoreceptors	Rods	Vision
	Cones	

and Ruffini's) keep firing to tell the brain that the pen is still there. Accurate manipulation of objects requires cooperation between all receptor types and the motor system. The ability to identify objects placed in the hand (without seeing them) is called stereognosis.

The receptors in skeletal muscle are the muscle spindles and the Golgi tendon organs. The muscle spindle is the major stretch receptor that monitors the length of the muscle, and just like cutaneous afferents, it has RA and SA components. The Golgi tendon organ monitors the

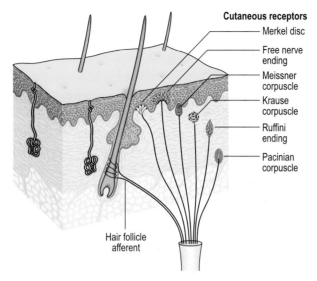

Fig. 1.20 Types of peripheral receptor found in skin.

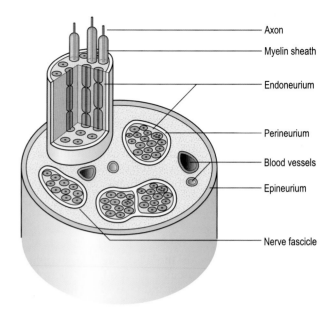

Fig. 1.21 Anatomical structure of a peripheral nerve.

The mnemonic 'C3, 4, 5, keeps you alive' refers to the function of the phrenic nerve. Each phrenic nerve innervates half the diaphragm, and paralysis of both, as can occur in spinal cord injury at high cervical levels, is often fatal. Unilateral damage does not affect the other side because of its separate nerve supply. Unilateral damage can be detected radiographically by observing asymmetry of the diaphragm position. Normally, during inspiration, the diaphragm dome is forced downwards by the muscle fibre contraction (as well as the action of the external intercostal muscles), but on the paralysed side the dome rises as it is compressed by the displaced abdominal viscera, which are being compressed on the active side. During expiration, the dome returns to its original position in response to positive pressure in the lungs.

force exerted by a muscle during contraction. They are found at the muscle–tendon interface. They are described in more detail in Chapter 9.

Pain and temperature sensory afferents do not have any specialized receptor organs; they use 'free nerve endings'. They are polymodal, i.e. they respond to more than one kind of stimulus, e.g. chemical, thermal or mechanical stimuli. Free nerve endings are found in all parts of the body except the interior of the bones and the interior of the brain itself. In the cornea of the eye there are only free nerve endings; therefore, abrasions of the cornea can be extremely painful.

Peripheral nerves

Nerves are conduits for axons connecting the peripheral receptor ultimately to a neurone in the spinal cord. The cell body of the sensory axon is housed in a specialized structure called a ganglion. Nerve fibres can be either myelinated or unmyelinated, and in the latter case the nerve fibre covering is called a neurolemma. Nerve fibres are bound together by connective tissue called endoneurium, and gathered into bundles called fasciculi, which are enclosed in a connective tissue sheath called a perineurium. The whole nerve is encased in a tough coat called the epineurium (Fig. 1.21). This arrangement provides mechanical strength and support for the nerve. The epineurium is continuous with the dura mater, while the arachnoid and pia mater are continuous with the perineurium and endoneurium respectively.

Nerve fibres are classified according to their diameter, and this is proportional to their conduction velocity, the speed at which impulses are transmitted. There are two commonly used systems. The Lloyd–Hunt system is used for afferents only, and divides them into groups I–IV, while the Erlander–Gasser system is used for afferents and efferents, and separates them by size into groups A, B and C. Table 1.7 summarizes the generally accepted view concerning human nerves. There are four main fibre groups/classes:

1. The fastest fibres, both sensory and motor, mediate postural reflexes (e.g. monosynaptic reflexes) and are group I or Aα.

2. Sensory fibres from specialized encapsulated endings responsive to low-threshold stimulation are group II or Aβ.

Table 1.7 Classification of peripheral nerve fibres

Class (group)	Myelin	Diameter (μm)	Conduction velocity (m/s)	Function/type of sensation
Afferents				
Aα (I)	Yes	12–20	> 72	Joint receptors
Aα (I)	Yes	12–20	> 72	Joint receptors
Ia				Muscle spindle
Ib				Golgi tendon organ
Aβ (II)	Yes	6–12	30–72	Low-threshold mechanoreceptors (Pacini corpuscles, Ruffini endings, Merkel cells, Meissner corpuscles, hair follicles)
				Secondary 'flower-spray' endings in muscle
Aδ (III)	Yes,	1–6	5–29	Mechanical pain
	thin			Muscle flexor reflex afferents
				Autonomic afferents
C (IV)	No	< 1	0.5–2	Temperature, muscle and visceral pain
Efferents				
Aα	Yes	12–20	> 72	Motor to skeletal muscle fibres
Aγ		5–8	30–48	Motor to muscle spindle (Ia) fibres
B	Yes, thin	< 3	3–30	Autonomic preganglionic efferents
C	No	< 1	0.5–2	Autonomic postganglionic efferents

3. Sensory fibres from non-specialized endings responsive to higher-threshold stimuli are group III or Aδ.

4. Sensory fibres from unmyelinated fibres are group IV or C.

The muscle spindles are unique among sensory endings in that they have their own motor supply (Aγ fibres).

The somatic nervous system consists of 31 pairs of spinal nerves and 12 pairs of cranial nerves. The spinal nerves innervate all parts of the body and neck. At the level of the cervical and lumbar enlargements, spinal nerve fibres intermingle with each other in the brachial and lumbosacral plexuses to form peripheral nerves that have multiple spinal nerve contributions. The organization shows bilateral symmetry. Spinal nerves are formed by the union of dorsal and ventral roots; thus, most spinal nerves are mixed nerves containing both sensory and motor fibres. However, the first cervical spinal nerve does not have a sensory root, and the fifth sacral and coccygeal spinal nerves do not have ventral roots. Dorsal roots transmit sensory information from skin, muscle, joints and, in some cases, viscera to cells in the grey matter of the spinal cord. The dorsal root contains a swelling called the dorsal root ganglion that houses the cell bodies of all the sensory neurones that send axons into the spinal cord. Ventral roots transmit motor and autonomic information to the periphery (Fig. 1.22).

Spinal nerves divide into dorsal and ventral rami. Each ramus contains both sensory and motor fibres, just like a spinal nerve. The dorsal rami serve sensorimotor functions of the posterior body, while the cervical, lumbar and sacral ventral rami do not project directly to body structures; they merge with adjacent rami to form four major plexuses that have important motor functions (Table 1.8). The thoracic ventral rami project directly to the ribcage and stomach muscles.

The cranial nerves that innervate the face and head originate from different parts of the brainstem. Three cranial nerves are purely sensory, five are motor only and four are mixed. Four contain autonomic (parasympathetic efferent) fibres (see Chapter 6).

Dermatomes

Each spinal nerve innervates a specific skin region called a dermatome (Fig. 1.23), and the muscles innervated by a single ventral root are called a myotome. Most muscles are innervated by axons from two spinal segments (although the intrinsic muscles of the hand are unisegmental). Muscles sharing a common primary action are supplied by the same segment, and opposing muscles by segments in sequence with the former. For example, in elbow movement, spinal cord segments C5 and C6 supply the bicep flexors and C7 and C8 innervate the triceps extensors. There is some functional overlap at the boundaries between adjacent dermatomes and myotomes. This acts as a sort of biological 'damage insurance', for if one spinal nerve is damaged, not all of the sensory information for that skin region will be lost, as some is carried

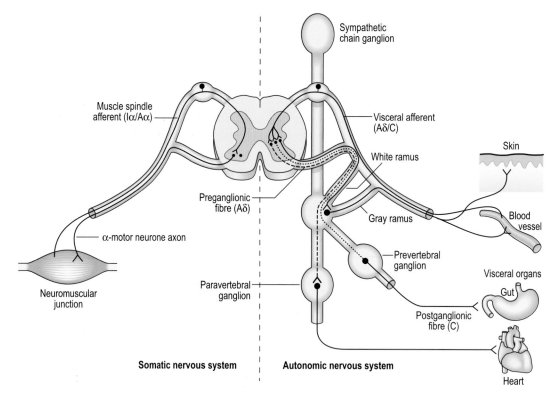

Fig. 1.22 Comparison of reflex circuitry in the somatic and autonomic nervous systems.

Table 1.8 Main functions of nerve plexuses

Plexus	Function	Main peripheral nerves	Clinical deficit
Cervical (C1–C5)	Respiration	Phrenic	Respiratory paralysis (see Box 1.5)
Brachial (C5–T1)	Movement of the hand	Radial	Wrist drop
		Median	Ape hand (unable to grasp objects)
		Ulnar	Claw hand (unable to spread fingers)
Lumbar (L1–L4)	Movement of the leg and foot	Femoral	Unable to extend knee and flex hip
Sacral (L4–S4)		Sciatic	Unable to flex knee and extend hip
		Peroneal	Foot drop

in nerves of the adjacent spinal nerves. Thus, in reality, for a sensory or functional deficit to be seen, more than one spinal root must be damaged. Thus, knowledge of the skin regions corresponding to particular dermatomes plays an important role in the clinical diagnosis of peripheral nerve lesions (Table 1.9). Diseases that damage the nerves or muscles are called neuropathies and myopathies (Box 1.6).

Autonomic nervous system

The autonomic nervous system (ANS) consists of peripheral afferent and efferent neurones that regulate the body's internal environment and control exchanges between the internal and the external environment. Together with the endocrine system, the ANS regulates homeostasis and controls a myriad of body functions and behaviours. As homeostasis is a prerequisite for survival, the ANS is an evolutionarily primitive neural system. Much of its normal function is accomplished involuntarily, without conscious intervention, through a series of reflexes that require input from viscera, smooth muscle, cardiac muscle and secretory glands.

It comprises three spatially segregated divisions:

1. the enteric system, which controls the smooth muscle function of the gut

2. the parasympathetic division, which is involved in rest and recuperation

3. the sympathetic system, which acts as the body's alarm system for stress and danger, as well as preparing the body for increased levels of activity; it is involved in flight, fright and fight reactions.

The basic organizational plan of the ANS is illustrated in Figure 1.24. ANS fibres are found in peripheral and some

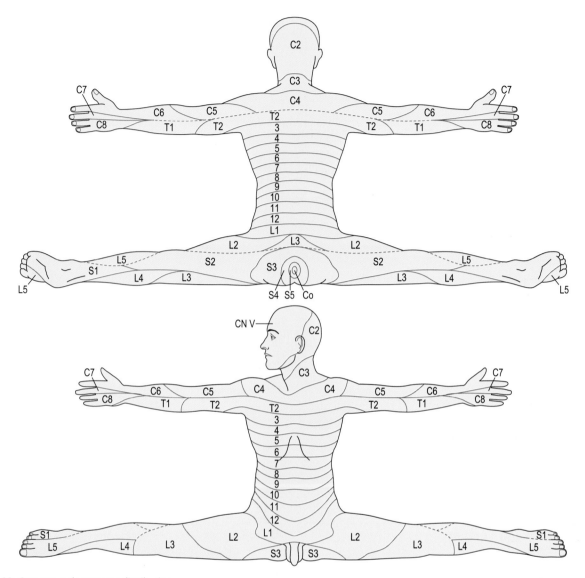

Fig. 1.23 Cutaneous dermatome distribution.

cranial nerves. The afferents arise from visceral organs and blood vessel walls and have cell bodies located in spinal or cranial ganglia (Table 1.10). Their function is to initiate visceral reflexes.

Most visceral sensations do not reach the level of consciousness, and those that do, such as nausea and hunger, are poorly localized and are transmitted via sympathetic afferents. Parasympathetic afferents are more concerned with reflex activity control such as the cough or pupillary light reflexes. The afferents connect to neurones of the spinal cord, brainstem reticular formation and solitary nucleus. This latter nucleus integrates sensory information from internal organs and coordinates motor output via interactions with parasympathetic brainstem nuclei and reticulo-spinal tracts. It also relays information to the hypothalamus, which is the main gatekeeper of ANS preganglionic function. The hypothalamus and reticulospinal

tracts have axons that converge on the common output neurone, the preganglionic neurone.

A key feature of the ANS is that the efferent output consists of two neurones: the preganglionic and postganglionic neurones. The cell bodies of the former are located within the CNS at either the craniosacral or thoracolumbar levels (see Fig. 1.24), while the latter are the true effector (motor) neurones but are located outside the CNS, in peripheral ganglia. Preganglionic fibres leave the CNS in the ventral roots, while postganglionic fibres are only found in peripheral nerves or nerve plexuses. Thus, visceral reflexes are disynaptic and thereby differ from the reflexes in the somatic nervous system, where monosynaptic reflexes occur. Other differences from the somatic nervous system include the speed of motor system action: somatic α-motor neurones rapidly excite skeletal muscle, whereas ANS actions are more slow and widespread

Table 1.9 Functions of some specific dermatomes and myotomes

Root	Skin area	Motor function
C5	Lateral shoulder (over deltoid muscle)	Shoulder abduction (e.g. beer drinking!)
		Body rotation
C6	Lateral forearm, thumb and index finger	C5 and C6 forearm flexion (e.g. biceps)
C7	Middle finger	Finger (C7) and forearm extension (C7–C8)
C8	Ring and little finger	Digit abduction/adduction (C8–T1)
T1–T12	Skin overlying ribs	Breathing (external and internal intercostals)
T6–T12		Production of speech (stomach muscles)
L2	Anterior thigh skin	Hip, thigh and knee extension, thigh adduction
L3	Anterior knee skin	
L4	Medial lower leg skin	
L5	Lateral lower leg skin, toes 1–3	Ankle and toe dorsiflexion
S1	Toes 4 and 5, sole of foot	Ankle plantar flexion

Box 1.6 Neuropathies and myopathies

Peripheral neuropathy is a disease of the nerves and disrupts the flow of information between the central and peripheral nervous systems, producing sensorimotor deficits. A mononeuropathy affects a single nerve, whereas polyneuropathy affects several nerves. There are a variety of causes: direct trauma or entrapment (e.g. carpal tunnel syndrome), infection (e.g. HIV), toxicity (e.g. anti-cancer or anti-HIV drugs), genetic (e.g. Friedrich's ataxia), metabolic (e.g. diabetes), neoplasm or idiopathic (e.g. Guillain–Barré syndrome). The common symptoms are pain and paraesthesia of the affected area, with a temporal profile that is acute, chronic or relapsing.

The cardinal feature of myopathy is motor weakness, although the muscle reflexes may appear normal on examination. Myopathies can be caused by tissue degeneration, toxicity or inflammatory disease. Genetically inherited myopathies, called muscular dystrophies (e.g. Duchenne's dystrophy), involve progressive wasting and weakness of the muscles. Peripheral myopathies are non-painful.

in effect. The ANS balances excitatory and inhibitory effects to achieve coordinated and graded control. A good example of this is the male penile erection. Activation of the parasympathetic system is initially needed to erect the penis through engorgement with blood, while activation of the sympathetic system is needed to maintain the erection and achieve orgasm and ejaculation, and the whole process is coordinated by the CNS. Any male will know the effects of increased anxiety or nervousness on 'performance'—impotence or premature ejaculation!

The effects of the two systems on target organs are largely antagonistic or reciprocal (see Fig. 1.24); they cannot act strongly at the same time, and the CNS inhibits activity in one division while the other is active, so that if levels of activity in the sympathetic system are high, activity in the parasympathetic system will be low. However, some targets—glands—only receive a single innervation. For example, sweat glands have only a sympathetic innervation, while salivary and lacrimal glands only have a parasympathetic innervation. Many other anatomical and functional differences exist between the two divisions (see Table 1.9); for example, sympathetic preganglionic fibres terminate in paravertebral or prevertebral ganglia, but not both, whereas parasympathetic preganglionic motor fibres terminate in terminal ganglia located in or near the effector organ. The paravertebral chain ganglia are also known as the sympathetic trunk ganglia, and comprise 20–25 pairs that run along the vertebral column. The prevertebral ganglia are located along the abdominal aorta, especially around the celiac, superior

and inferior mesenteric arteries, and innervate the gut. Sympathetic system effects are widespread, while parasympathetic effects are more localized.

There are similarities and differences in their pharmacology: both divisions use acetylcholine (ACh) as a neurotransmitter in pre- and postganglionic motor fibres, just like the somatic motor system. ACh acts on nicotinic ACh (ionotropic) receptors of the preganglionic cells to evoke fast excitatory postsynaptic potentials that trigger action potentials, in the same way as occurs at the neuromuscular junction. However, ACh can also act on postganglionic muscarinic ACh (metabotropic) receptors that produce slower excitatory postsynaptic potentials, which do not produce action potentials unless repetitive activation occurs. The sympathetic postganglionic fibres use mostly noradrenaline to activate their targets. Parasympathetic fibres release ACh, which has very localized effects on its targets. Sympathetic fibres release noradrenaline, which activates either α- or β-adrenergic receptors. Noradrenaline has global effects because it is also released from an endocrine gland, the adrenal medulla. The adrenal medulla, essentially a modified sympathetic ganglion, secretes adrenaline (80%) and noradrenaline (20%) into the bloodstream. This accounts for the 'adrenaline rush' experienced when people encounter life-threatening or thrilling situations. The widespread action of bloodborne catecholamines such as noradrenaline and adrenaline, and the high degree of neuronal divergence in the sympathetic system (see Table 1.10), lead to a whole-body action. This, together with the

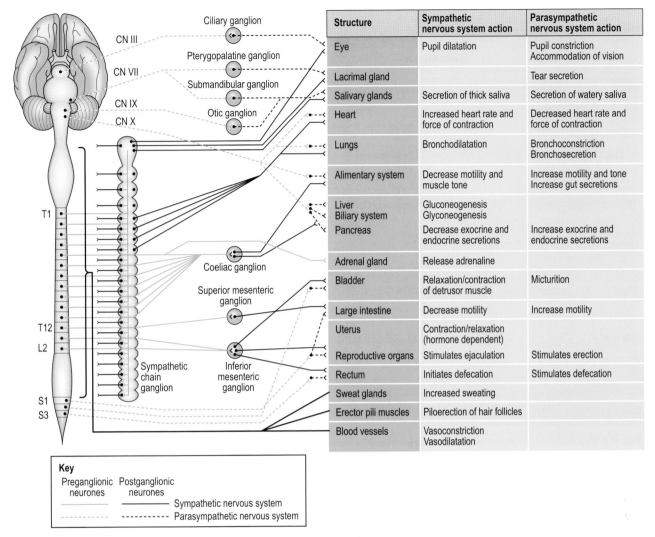

Structure	Sympathetic nervous system action	Parasympathetic nervous system action
Eye	Pupil dilatation	Pupil constriction Accommodation of vision
Lacrimal gland		Tear secretion
Salivary glands	Secretion of thick saliva	Secretion of watery saliva
Heart	Increased heart rate and force of contraction	Decreased heart rate and force of contraction
Lungs	Bronchodilatation	Bronchoconstriction Bronchosecretion
Alimentary system	Decrease motility and muscle tone	Increase motility and tone Increase gut secretions
Liver Biliary system Pancreas	Gluconeogenesis Glyconeogenesis Decrease exocrine and endocrine secretions	Increase exocrine and endocrine secretions
Adrenal gland	Release adrenaline	
Bladder	Relaxation/contraction of detrusor muscle	Micturition
Large intestine	Decrease motility	Increase motility
Uterus	Contraction/relaxation (hormone dependent)	
Reproductive organs	Stimulates ejaculation	Stimulates erection
Rectum	Initiates defecation	Stimulates defecation
Sweat glands	Increased sweating	
Erector pili muscles	Piloerection of hair follicles	
Blood vessels	Vasoconstriction Vasodilatation	

Fig. 1.24 Functional organization of the autonomic nervous system. CN, cranial nerve.

multiple release sites for neurotransmitters associated with the numerous varicosities along their terminal axons, contributes to the diffuse action of the sympathetic division.

The effects of drugs that work on the different receptor systems associated with the sympathetic system are shown in Table 1.11. Generally, a drug that enhances the actions of noradrenaline is called a sympathomimetic drug, while drugs that are agonists at muscarinic ACh receptors have a parasympathomimetic profile. Sympathomimetics are primarily used to treat hypotension and cardiac arrest. They can also be used to dilate bronchioles in asthma attacks or cases of anaphylactic shock. Adrenergic drugs are also used in local anaesthetic injections to constrict blood vessels, increasing the duration of effect of the anaesthetic drug by slowing down the rate of its washout. β-Blocker drugs (sympathetic antagonists) are primarily used to treat hypertension and heart disease. Propranolol, a non-selective β-adrenergic antagonist, is used to slow the heart rate. Parasympathomimetic

drugs are also used to treat urinary incontinence or stimulate bowel function after surgery.

Clinical signs and symptoms of autonomic nervous system dysfunction

Autonomic dysfunction may occur due to a disease process that is selective for the ANS cells and fibres, as seen in pure autonomic failure, multiple system atrophy (Shy–Drager syndrome), and genetically acquired syndromes such as familial dysautonomia (Riley–Day syndrome). It may also be secondary to other medical conditions, as in Parkinson's disease, diabetes, infectious peripheral neuropathy, alcoholism, multiple sclerosis, and spinal cord damage. The cardinal signs of ANS dysfunction are detailed in Table 1.12.

In peripheral neuropathies such as Guillain–Barré syndrome, these signs are accompanied by distinct signs of peripheral nerve damage. The initial signs are distal paraesthesias, numbness and muscle weakness, muscle

Table 1.10 Comparison of autonomic nervous system divisions

	Sympathetic	*Parasympathetic*
Afferent cell body location	T1–L2 spinal ganglia	Cranial nerve sensory ganglia (V, VII, IX, X)
		Spinal nerve ganglia S2–S4 (splanchnic nerves)
Peripheral innervation	Skin, blood vessels and viscera throughout body	Limited to head (lacrimal, salivary glands and eye muscles) and viscera of chest, abdomen and pelvis
Preganglionic cell body location	Intermediolateral horn of T1–L2 spinal cord	Brainstem and intermediolateral horn of S2–S4 spinal cord
Postganglionic cell body location	Paravertebral and prevertebral chain ganglia	Near or in peripheral target organ
Preganglionic/postganglionic fibre ratio	1 : 17—widespread effects	1 : 2—localized effects
Neurotransmitter	Acetylcholine	Acetylcholine
	Adrenaline	
Neurotransmitter receptors		
Preganglionic	Nicotinic cholinergic	Nicotinic cholinergic
Postganglionic	Adrenergic (α_1, α_2, β_1, β_2, β_3) (muscarinic, cholinergic at sweat glands)	Muscarinic cholinergic
Function	Alarm and arousal system (fight, flight, and fright)	Homeostasis (rest and recuperation or growth, immunity, digestion and energy conservation)

Table 1.11 General effects of blocking cholinergic or adrenergic receptors

Site of action	*Effect of cholinergic receptor blockade*	*Effect of adrenergic receptor blockade*
Heart	Tachycardia	Bradycardia
Eye	Pupil dilatation, paralysis of accommodation	Pupil constriction
Gastrointestinal tract	Decreased tone, secretion and motility constipation	Decreased gluconeogenesis, increased tone and motility
Bladder	Urinary retention	Incontinence
Sweat glands	Decreased sweating and warm skin	Decreased sweating and warm skin
Salivary glands	Dry mouth	Dry mouth
Arterioles	Vasodilatation	Vasoconstriction
Veins	Venodilatation	Venoconstriction

wasting and decreased stretch reflexes, but no fasciculation. The autonomic signs develop more slowly and become prominent as the weakness advances proximally.

Diabetes is the most common cause of peripheral neuropathy with ANS involvement. The early compromise of small-diameter axons leads to distal loss of pain and temperature sensation, which precedes loss of vibration and position sense. Sweating is impaired and blood flow to the affected region is increased due to sympathetic denervation. The latter signs appear before the somatic sensory signs. Gustatory sweating—abnormal sweating of the face, scalp and neck that starts within a few minutes of starting to chew food—is fairly common in diabetic peripheral neuropathies.

Multiple sclerosis and spinal cord lesions disrupt ANS function by disconnecting the preganglionic neurones from their supraspinal control. The effects depend on the level and severity of the lesion. Complete spinal cord transection is devastating to body temperature control, blood pressure regulation, and bowel, bladder and sexual function.

The enteric nervous system is a functionally separate system, which can work independently of the sympathetic and parasympathetic systems, although they provide supplementary control. It innervates the oesophagus, stomach, intestine, pancreas and gallbladder, and is composed of two plexuses, the myenteric and submucosal, which register changes in the tension of the gut wall and chemical composition of the stomach and intestinal contents, to control the process of food digestion and transportation for excretion. Congenital abnormalities in this system lead to Hirschsprung's disease

Table 1.12 Signs of autonomic nervous system dysfunction

Sign	Cause
Postural hypotension	Postural hypotension reflects dysfunction of the baroreflex pathways, either the afferent limb in the vagus nerve or the efferent limb in the splanchnic nerves
Tachycardia	Defective sympathetic nervous system activity
Impotence	Bladder and sexual dysfunction reflect demyelination of preganglionic fibres
Bladder/bowel dysfunction	
Anhydrosis	Diminished or no sweating is most pronounced distally and reflects involvement of postganglionic sympathetic fibres to sweat glands

(megacolon), characterized by an enlarged colon, constipation and an absence of ganglion cells in the myenteric plexus.

Putting it all together: from anatomy to behaviour

To produce behaviour, external sensory inputs have to be conveyed from the periphery to the brain, which then integrates and assesses the information to produce a motor response. This principle can be extended down to lower organizational levels, such as the nucleus (for example, brainstem nuclei provide input to the thalamic nuclei that is then relayed to different cortical nuclei) and the individual neurone (where inputs from individual fibres converge onto a single neurone, which then assimilates the information and passes it to other neurones).

Sensory and motor systems exist at all levels of the nervous system. Peripheral nerves have sensory and motor components, and these separate in the CNS to become specialized grey matter areas and nuclei associated with either sensory or motor functions. Then, these specific functions are relayed to separate areas in the cerebral cortex, where they are separated in two ways: a specific primary area for discrete sensations within cortex lamina 4 always receives sensory input, while laminae 5 and 6 provide motor output (the other cortical layers are integrative in function).

An important but unexplained feature of the organization of the brain is that most pathways are bilaterally symmetrical and they cross from one side of the nervous system to the other. Thus, each cortex receives sensory input from the opposite side of the body and controls the movement of the contralateral side. Different pathways cross at different levels. For example, the pain pathway crosses in the spinal cord, whereas the pathway for voluntary control of movement crosses at the junction of the brainstem and spinal cord. Crossing in the visual system is more complicated (see Chapter 7). One problem posed

by this organization is that information reaching one side of the body has to be integrated with information reaching the other side. This is achieved in the brain by pathways called commissures, which only contain crossing fibres from one side of the brain to the other. The most prominent and largest of these is the corpus callosum, which connects the frontal, parietal and occipital lobes on each side; the anterior commissure connects the temporal lobes on either side.

Although the brain is anatomically symmetrical in some respects, in terms of some functions the brain is asymmetrical. This is certainly true of higher mental functions such as control of speech or spatial navigation of the body.

In order to produce behaviour, neuronal circuits are regulated by coordinated excitation and inhibition. This principle applies to single neurones and also to groups of neurones (nuclei). Neurones pass information to each other by being switched 'on' or 'off' by the appropriate neurotransmitter. For example, consider the role of the basal ganglia in movement. One of its functions is to scale the activity of the thalamic nuclei in regulating the size of the movement. Damage to the basal ganglia affects the activity of the thalamus and results in altered, abnormal movements; damage to one nucleus produces increased movement, while damage to another produces the opposite effect (see Chapter 10). This is analogous to the actions of the sympathetic and parasympathetic nervous systems; that is, one is excitatory and the other inhibitory for a given function (see Table 1.10).

The multiple levels of function seen in the nervous system are a product of evolution. As the brain evolved, new areas were added on top of pre-existing ones. Consider the evolution of movement: fish have no legs and use whole-body movements to swim, controlled by the spinal cord and hindbrain. Amphibians developed legs and control regions in the brainstem. Humans developed the ability to walk on two legs and independent control of limbs and digit movement, requiring further control areas, which are housed in the forebrain. For sensory areas, the newer regions are the association cortex regions, which provide higher mental processing of inputs such as shape, colour and size.

Sensory, motor and motivational (emotional or limbic) systems are organized both in parallel and in series, to produce a unified conscious experience. Each has anatomically and functionally distinct subsystems that perform specialized tasks; for example, there are parallel systems for touch, smell, taste and hearing, and within each system there are specialized subsystems for different aspects of the modality—sensation is broken down into parallel pathways for pain, proprioception and posture and balance. Motor systems likewise have parallel pathways, one to control voluntary fine movements and others to control reflexes and body posture (see Chapter 9). The most striking feature of these pathways is that they are topographically organized so that there is a complete spatial map of the periphery in the brain for each modality. A key feature of the map is that it is distorted, so that regions that are important in sensory discrimination have the largest cortical representation. Another feature of the system is that there are interconnections between the different parallel streams.

An intuitive assumption based on the many different functions of the nervous system is that distinct brain functions are localized to specific areas of the brain, and indeed this is true for many functions. Thus, localized focal brain lesions lead to discrete neurological deficits. Other higher mental functions have a more widespread dispersal throughout the cortex. For example, there is no one area that we can call primary pain cortex; different aspects of pain are processed in widely anatomically separated brain regions. Similarly, language ability (comprehension, production and appreciation) is widely separated across different lobes of the brain, and damage to focal regions may produce subtle deficits, whereas widespread injury, as occurs in stroke, often causes severe language deficits.

Thus, knowing the names of the different parts of the nervous system is just the beginning of understanding how humans behave. It requires the integration of the motivational, sensory and motor systems. Consider this the next time you are hungry and you go out to buy a sandwich. The decision to go to get food arises in the limbic system, which then instructs the somatic motor system to go into action, causing you to walk to the shops and buy food. The processes of eating and tasting your favourite sandwich are provided by the sensory and motor systems. In addition, this influences the ANS, which feeds back to the hypothalamus to tell the brain that the hunger has been satiated (via increases in blood glucose levels).

There are more than 1000 disorders of the nervous system. Neurological disease and mental illness affect millions of people worldwide and cost billions to treat. The following chapters aim to shed light on how knowledge of the functional anatomy, physiology and pharmacology of the nervous system can be used to diagnose and treat some of the more important nervous system disorders.

ELEMENTS OF CELLULAR AND MOLECULAR NEUROSCIENCE

2

Chapter objectives

After studying this chapter you should be able to:

1. Describe the different cells that make up the central nervous system and peripheral nervous system, and their functions.

2. Explain the resting membrane potential of neurones and how an action potential is generated and propagated.

3. Describe how neurotransmitters are released and inactivated at the synapse.

4. Name the major neurotransmitters of the central nervous system and peripheral nervous system.

5. Describe the major types of neurotransmitter receptor and explain how they act.

ELEMENTS OF CELLULAR AND MOLECULAR NEUROSCIENCE

Introduction

The central and peripheral nervous systems are principally made up of two types of cell, neurones and glia. A few other minor types of cell, such as ependymal cells and choroid epithelial cells, are present in the brain, but these will be described elsewhere in the book.

Neurones

Neurones are the cells of the nervous system that receive signals, process them and transmit the appropriate response either to another neurone or to an effector, such as a secretory cell or a muscle. The exact number of neurones in the human nervous system is unknown, but is estimated to be between 300 and 500 billion ($3–5 \times 10^{11}$). The signals may be received directly from the environment, e.g. light falling on the photoreceptor cells of the retina, or in the form of chemicals released from other neurones at junctions between them, or as electrical signals directly transmitted through low-resistance gap junctions between adjacent neurones.

Neurones come in many different shapes and sizes, but in their most basic form consist of three elements:

1. A cell body (soma), which contains the nucleus and other intracellular organelles concerned particularly with protein synthesis and secretory processes. The large numbers of ribosomes, particularly those associated with the rough endoplasmic reticulum or in the form of polyribosomes, appear as darkly staining Nissl bodies.

2. Highly branched processes extending from the cell body, called dendrites, which may be covered with small spines. These receive most of the inputs from other cells.

3. A single axon extending from the cell body to the target cell. Axons may extend just a few millimetres to a nearby cell or, as in the case of the motor neurones supplying muscles distant from the spinal cord, for several metres. At the start of the axon is an area called the axon hillock or trigger zone, where electrical signals called action potentials can be generated. These are then propagated along the axon, which terminates at a synapse.

This basic structure is exemplified by the typical multipolar neurone shown in Figure 2.1.

The cytoskeleton of the neurone, like that of all cells, consists of microtubules (composed of tubulin), microfilaments (made from actin) and intermediate filaments called neurofilaments, which form the core of the axon. Intracellular organelles manufactured in the cell body are transported along the axon by fast axonal transport along microtubules (anterograde transport), and materials for recycling are returned in the same way (retrograde transport), using the motor proteins kinesin and dynein.

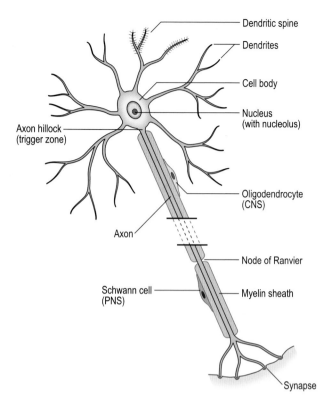

Fig. 2.1 A typical multipolar neurone. CNS, central nervous system; PNS, peripheral nervous system.

Slower axonal transport, which transports proteins to the synapse, may also involve neurofilaments.

The single axon may give off occasional branches called axon collaterals before reaching its target, but the end of every axon is terminated by a large number of branches, each ending with a specialized structure called a synapse. This is where signals are transmitted to other cells. The synapse consists of a presynaptic terminal and a postsynaptic region. Presynaptic terminals contain secretory vesicles and have large numbers of mitochondria. The presynaptic membrane is thickened and has inward projections called active zones. The postsynaptic region may also display a zone of increased density. In some axons there are synapses along the length of the axon without obvious contact zones, which appear as swellings. These vesiculated axons are commonly found in the autonomic nervous system (ANS). Both axons and dendrites are called neurites, but can be distinguished by their morphology, their organelles and the organization of their microtubules.

In general, neurones can be classified into one of three major types, depending largely on the position and number of dendrites and the position of the trigger zone.

Most neurones are multipolar neurones, like the one shown in Figure 2.2A (and Fig. 2.1), and have many processes, which consist of one axon and many dendrites. The trigger zone is at the end of the axon, close to the cell body. These are the most common types of neurone, and examples are the pyramidal cells of the cortex and the Purkinje cells of the cerebellum.

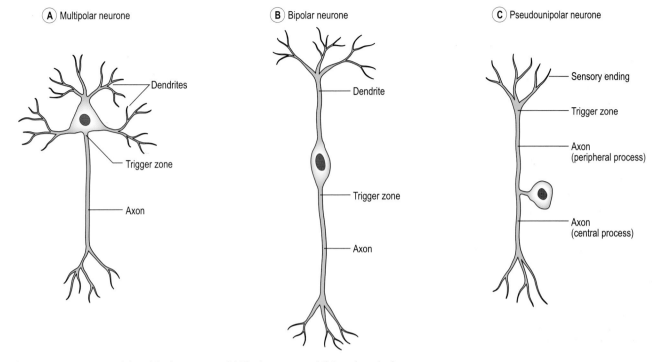

Fig. 2.2 Neurone types. (A) Multipolar neurone. (B) Bipolar neurone. (C) Pseudo-unipolar neurone.

Bipolar neurones (Fig. 2.2B) have a single axon and a single dendrite, which only branches at its end. These are relatively rare, and are almost all found in sensory organs. An example is provided by the bipolar cells found in the retina of the eye. The trigger zone is often found in the same place as in multipolar neurones.

Pseudo-unipolar neurones (Fig. 2.2C) have only a single process extending from the cell body, which is situated part of the way along the axon. This divides the axon into central and peripheral processes. At the end of the peripheral process lies a sensory ending, which may be a bare axon, with the axon hillock very close to the sensory ending. Pseudo-unipolar neurones have no dendrites. The commonest pseudo-unipolar neurones are sensory neurones found in the peripheral nervous system (PNS), which convey signals from the periphery to the spinal cord in the central nervous system (CNS). Their cell bodies are found in the dorsal root ganglion of the spinal cord, and they synapse on neurones in the spinal cord.

Owing to their very active nature, neurones in general have a very high metabolic rate and they need a continuous secure supply of oxygen and glucose. Any interruption of this supply is critical, as deprived neurones will start to die very rapidly. This is particularly problematical because, under most conditions, mature neurones do not divide. During development, epithelial cells lining the neural tube give rise to neuroblasts. These cells divide mitotically to produce amitotic neurones, which then migrate to their final positions in the brain. As this occurs during fetal development and is completed in early childhood, the mature brain does not generally contain neurones that can divide (however, see Box 2.1). Thus, neurones that die cannot usually be replaced. However, one result of this is that brain tumours derived from neurones are very rare, and occur almost exclusively as neuroblastomas in children. Most primary malignant brain tumours (those derived from brain cells and not caused by metastases from elsewhere in the body) are gliomas, which are derived from glial cells (see below).

Box 2.1   Neural stem cells

During the development of the nervous system, cells in the neural tube become multipotent stem cells, which can divide into all the different cells of the brain. Other types of stem cell in other tissues produce other cells; for example, haematopoietic stem cells in the bone marrow can produce all the blood cells. While these blood stem cells remain active throughout life, continually replacing cells, it was thought until recently that stem cells were not present in the nervous system after the initial phase of brain development. However, neural stem cells have now been isolated from both fetal and adult brains. These cells do not normally divide in the adult, but current research is trying to identify the exact conditions under which these cells can be stimulated to divide and grow into mature functioning brain cells.

ELEMENTS OF CELLULAR AND MOLECULAR NEUROSCIENCE

Glial cells

The other main category of cell in the nervous system is represented by glial cells, of which there are three types. They make up about half the brain mass and outnumber neurones about 10-fold. These cells have a number of functions, which include structural and metabolic support, immune functions and electrical insulation of axons.

Astrocytes

In the CNS, the most common glial cells are astrocytes (Fig. 2.3). They can be distinguished from neurones by the presence of a specific protein, glial fibrillary acidic protein. Fibrous astrocytes contain large numbers of filaments and are found in the nerve bundles of the white matter of the brain. Protoplasmic astrocytes have fewer filaments and are found mainly in the grey matter. They have a number of fine processes that surround neurones, capillaries and the ependymal cells lining the ventricles. These astrocytic endfeet do not touch the capillaries, but release factors that induce blood–brain barrier characteristics in the capillary endothelial cells (see Chapter 12). Astrocytes are important in regulating K^+ levels in the extracellular medium around neurones, and in providing a store of glycogen that can be supplied to neurones, in the form of lactate, when required. Astrocytes surrounding neurones have an important role in controlling the distribution of neurotransmitters released by the neurones. They do this in two ways: first, by restricting diffusion; and second, by transporting neurotransmitters into the astrocyte, where they can be metabolized or recycled.

Astrocytes have recently been shown to play a potentially more active role in signalling. Astrocytes are linked to each other by gap junctions, through which small molecules can diffuse. When stimulated by neurotransmitters, they show changes in intracellular levels of Ca^{2+} ions, which spread between astrocytes as waves. Gap junctions also occur between astrocytes and neurones, and could modulate the behaviour of the neurones by allowing the passage of Ca^{2+} between them.

The precursors of astrocytes are radial glial cells which, during early development, span the cerebral cortex, forming a scaffolding for the migration of new nerve cells to their destinations.

Microglial cells

Microglial cells are small cells of the CNS with long spiny processes. During development, they release growth factors and also act as macrophages, removing debris produced by the programmed cell death which occurs on a large scale at this time. In the adult, they are normally relatively inactive. However, in the presence of almost any type of injury or insult to the nervous system, they revert to the role of phagocytotic macrophages, when they are said to be reactive.

Oligodendrocytes and Schwann cells

Oligodendrocytes and Schwann cells are involved in electrically insulating axons in the CNS and PNS, respectively. They are large cells with few processes, which wrap around the axons, forming multiple lipid bilayers,

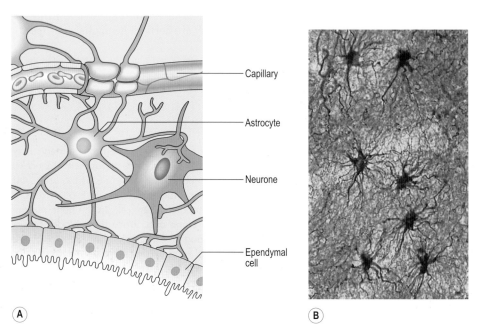

— Capillary

— Astrocyte

— Neurone

— Ependymal cell

(A) (B)

Fig. 2.3 (A) Drawing of an astrocyte. (B) Astrocytes that have been injected with a fluorescent dye so that the processes can be clearly seen. From Young B, Heath JW. Wheater's Functional Histology, 4th edn, 2000, by permission of Harcourt Publishers.

with their plasma membranes forming a myelin sheath (Fig. 2.4). Myelination of nerve fibres is an important process (Box 2.2). These membranes have a high lipid/protein ratio, which makes them excellent insulators (see below). Oligodendrocytes can myelinate more than one axon, and the cell body lies between them. Schwann cells only myelinate a single axon, and the cell body is closely apposed to the myelin sheath.

Schwann cells have a role in the regeneration of peripheral axons following injury. In order for a peripheral nerve to regrow, the tip of the axon must make contact with a Schwann cell. This stimulates mitosis in the Schwann cell, which then extends processes towards the growth cone of the axon. The axon regrows at between 2 and 5 mm per day along the Schwann cells, which remyelinate the new axon. Damaged neurones in the CNS do not seem to regenerate successfully, because CNS glial cells release factors that specifically inhibit axon growth.

Not all axons are myelinated, and this can be seen in the brain and spinal cord as grey matter, which consists of cell bodies and unmyelinated axons, as opposed to white matter, which consists of axons, most of which are myelinated. Dendrites are never myelinated.

Neurone excitability

The basic function of a neurone is to receive signals, either directly from the environment or from other cells. The signals, which may be chemical or electrical, all produce graded electrical changes in the neurone. The input signals mainly occur in the dendrites and cell body of the neurone and may be excitatory or inhibitory. The graded electrical potentials produced are called excitatory postsynaptic potentials (epsps), or inhibitory postsynaptic potentials (ipsps). These graded electrical potentials are added together over time and space (temporal and spatial summation), and, if their total exceeds a threshold value, the trigger zone of the neurone initiates or 'fires' an electrical impulse called an action potential. This impulse is of a fixed size and is propagated unchanged

Box 2.2 Demyelinating diseases

Multiple sclerosis is a progressive disease in which areas of the myelin sheath, mainly in the brain, spinal cord and optic nerve, are damaged, impairing nerve conduction. This is a chronic inflammatory process and there is evidence of both genetic susceptibility and environmental causes, which trigger the immune response. Areas of demyelination, called plaques, evolve into areas of scar tissue that may be partially remyelinated, restoring much of the function, so the disease shows periods of remission. However, other plaques form and eventually there is an accumulation of damage that causes permanent deficits.

Another type of demyelinating disease is Guillain–Barré syndrome, in which infection by a variety of bacteria or viruses triggers an inflammatory demyelination of neurones in the peripheral nervous system. Treatment consists of measures to shorten the course of the disease, and most patients make a good recovery.

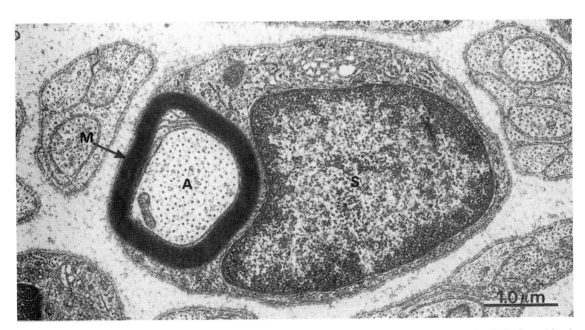

Fig. 2.4 Electron micrograph of a cross-section of a myelinated neurone. From Young B, Heath JW. Wheater's Functional Histology, 4th edn, 2000, by permission of Harcourt Publishers. M, myelin sheath. A, axon.

along the nerve axon to the synapse, where the neurone meets either another neurone or an effector. The synapse releases chemicals, called neurotransmitters, which affect the target cell making it more or less likely to produce a response. In specific cases, such as at the neuromuscular junction, a single action potential in the nerve is sufficient to produce muscle contraction.

Resting membrane potentials

All cells in the body have a voltage difference across the plasma membrane, called the resting membrane potential (RMP). In neurones this is about $-75\,mV$ (inside negative relative to the outside). This is a consequence of the unequal distribution of ions across cell membranes and the different permeabilities of the neurones to these ions.

The two most common cations found in total body water are sodium (Na^+) and potassium (K^+). Their distribution is very different in the intracellular and extracellular fluids. Intracellular fluid (ICF) contains predominantly K^+, while extracellular fluid (ECF) contains predominantly Na^+ (Table 2.1), and it is this difference in ionic concentration between ICF and ECF that, first, allows the generation of the RMP and, second, provides the battery that drives the action potential. The predominant extracellular anion is chloride (Cl^-), whereas the intracellular cations are balanced by the presence of large intracellular anions (A^-), mainly phosphates and the negatively charged side chains of proteins.

The concentration gradients for Na^+ and K^+ are set up by the active transport of Na^+ and K^+ by an Na^+/K^+-ATPase known as the Na^+/K^+ pump (Fig. 2.5). This uses the energy derived from breaking the high-energy phosphoanhydride bond of ATP in order to pump both Na^+ and K^+ against their concentration gradients. Because the ATPase pumps three Na^+ ions out for every two K^+ ions, this produces a small potential of about $5\,mV$. On the extracellular face of the Na^+/K^+ pump is a binding site for the glycoside ouabain, which inhibits the activity of the pump. The Na^+/K^+ pump is essential to all cells, not just excitable cells, as the ion gradients it sets up are used to power many transport processes.

For a voltage to be generated, current must flow, and this occurs due to the presence in the plasma membrane of protein channels that selectively allow ions to diffuse passively down their concentration gradients. At rest, the plasma membrane is slightly permeable to K^+ and almost impermeable to Na^+. This means that K^+ will tend to diffuse out of the cell, but this cannot be electrically balanced by the inward diffusion of Na^+. This means that as K^+ diffuses out, down its concentration gradient, an electrical potential develops, with an excess of negative charge inside the neurone. The neurone also contains negatively charged ions but these cannot leave the cell, as they are too large to cross the plasma membrane. The negative charge inside the neurone creates an electrical gradient, which will tend to pull positively charged ions into the cell. As the membrane at rest is virtually impermeable to Na^+, the only ion that can be attracted into the cell is K^+ (Fig. 2.6).

This means that there is an equilibrium position, whereby the amount of K^+ leaving the cell down its

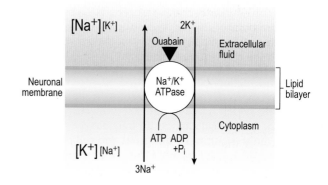

Fig. 2.5 Diagram of an Na^+/K^+ pump. The square brackets represent ionic concentrations, a large symbol indicates a high concentration, and a small symbol indicates a low concentration.

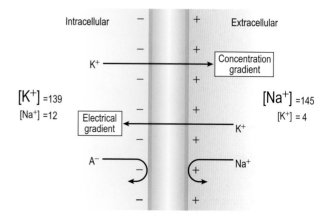

Fig. 2.6 Passive movements of ions across the plasma membrane at rest. Intracellular and extracellular concentration are shown in mmoles per litre.

Table 2.1 Ionic concentrations of intracellular fluid and extracellular fluid

Ions	Intracellular concentration (mM)	Extracellular concentration (mM)
Na^+	12	145
K^+	139	4
Cl^-	4	120
Large anions (A^-)	140	–
Ca^{2+}	<0.0002	1.8

concentration gradient is balanced by the amount being drawn into the cell by the electrical gradient, and there is no net movement of K$^+$ across the cell membrane. However, at this equilibrium position, there is a small excess of negative charge inside the cell and this produces the RMP. Because this potential difference is generated across a very small distance, i.e. the width of the plasma membrane, the actual difference in the number of ions needed on both sides of the membrane to produce the voltage difference is very small and represents a concentration difference of about one part in 10^8. If the membrane is assumed to be permeable only to K$^+$, the predicted RMP can be calculated using the Nernst equation (Box 2.3).

At 37°C, the Nernst equation reduces to:

$$E_m = \frac{61.5}{Z} \log_{10} \frac{[C_o]}{[C_i]}$$

If the values for K$^+$ ($C_o = 4$ mM, $C_i = 139$ mM, $Z = +1$) are inserted in the equation, the value calculated is about −95 mV (inside negative). This is called the K$^+$ equilibrium potential (E_{K+}) and is slightly more negative than the measured RMP, of approximately −75 mV. It is also called the reversal potential, as above and below this potential the current flowing through the channel goes in opposite directions. If the values for Na$^+$ are used instead, the Na$^+$ equilibrium potential (E_{Na+}) is about +66 mV. Thus, it is obviously the movement of K$^+$ that is largely responsible for determining the RMP.

However, if the very slight permeability of the membrane to Na$^+$ (about 1/75th of that of K$^+$) is taken into account, a more complicated equation, called the Goldman–Hodgkin–Katz equation (Box 2.4), is used to calculate the RMP. This allows the relative permeabilities of Na$^+$, K$^+$ and Cl$^-$ to be taken into account. At rest, the

permeability (P) ratios are $P_K/P_{Na}/P_{Cl} = 1.0:0.04:0.45$, which gives an RMP of − 75 mV for the concentrations in Table 2.1.

The membrane permeability to K$^+$ (and Na$^+$) is due to the presence of integral transmembrane proteins that form ion channels. The channels are passive, leak channels, which do not seem to be regulated and are always open. These channels are ion-selective, and the greater permeability of the plasma membrane to K$^+$ is simply due to the fact that there are more K$^+$ leak channels than Na$^+$ channels.

However, present in the membranes of excitable cells, such as neurones and muscles, which can fire action potentials, are other types of ion channel that are voltage-activated and not normally open in the resting state.

Action potentials

All cells have an RMP, but cells that can generate and conduct action potentials are said to be excitable, and this is one of the principal characteristics of neurones. Action potentials are rapid changes in the potential difference across the axonal plasma membrane. During an action potential, the membrane potential first depolarizes very rapidly from −75 mV to about +40 mV (inside positive). It then repolarizes to about −95 mV (a slight hyperpolarization) before returning relatively slowly to its RMP. This is seen in Figure 2.7, which shows a typical action potential as recorded from a neurone. The action potential is an all-or-nothing phenomenon, in that once initiated it has a fixed size. The ability of neurones to generate action potentials is due to the presence in their plasma membrane of ion channels that respond to changes in the membrane potential; that is, they are voltage-sensitive. The different phases of the action potential are due to the opening of two types of voltage-sensitive channel, which are Na$^+$- and K$^+$-selective. The different properties of these two types of channel determine the characteristics of the action potential.

A neurone may be initially at rest (Fig. 2.7, position A). The initial stimulus for the generation of an action potential is depolarization of the neurone at the trigger zone (how this is produced will be explained later).

Box 2.3 The Nernst equation and its components

$$V_m = \frac{RT}{ZF} \log_e \frac{[C_o]}{[C_i]}$$

The components are as follows:

V_m = voltage across the membrane
Z = valency of the ion
R = gas constant
F = Faraday's constant
T = absolute temperature (in Kelvins)
C_o = external concentration
C_i = internal concentration

Box 2.4 Goldman–Hodgkin–Katz equation

$$V_m = RT \log_e \frac{P_K[K^+_o] + P_{Na}[Na^+_o] + P_{Cl}[Cl^-_i]}{P_K[K^+_i] + P_{Na}[Na^+_i] + P_{Cl}[Cl^-_o]}$$

where P_K, P_{Na} and P_{Cl} are the relative permeabilities of the membrane to K$^+$, Na$^+$ and Cl$^-$.

Voltage-sensitive Na$^+$ channels, which have a particularly high density in this part of the axon, will open almost instantaneously, within microseconds, in response to depolarization, a process called activation, and Na$^+$ ions will flow, down their concentration gradient, into the neurone. However, these channels will also close again within about 0.5–1 ms, and will be in a state in which they cannot be reopened; that is, they are inactivated.

If the depolarization of the trigger zone is small, then only a few Na$^+$ channels will open. Unless the total Na$^+$ permeability (gNa$^+$) is greater than the resting K$^+$ permeability (gK$^+$), after they close nothing else will happen. This occurs when the graded input signals to the neurone are weak, and the depolarization is subthreshold.

However, if the depolarization of the trigger zone is larger (Fig. 2.7, position B), usually to about − 55 mV, then a greater number of Na$^+$ channels will be activated, and once the Na$^+$ permeability exceeds the resting K$^+$ permeability, positive feedback occurs, by which depolarization of the membrane will open more Na$^+$ channels, depolarizing the membrane further, until all local Na$^+$ channels are open, allowing Na$^+$ influx.

The voltage then changes rapidly (Fig. 2.7, position C) to a value approaching + 40 mV. The local area of membrane is now effectively permeable only to Na$^+$, the resting K$^+$ permeability being very small compared to the Na$^+$ permeability, and if nothing else were to happen, the cell would develop a new equilibrium position, as predicted by the Nernst equation, at the Na$^+$ equilibrium potential, E_{Na+} = +66 mV.

However, the depolarization of the neurone stops before E_{Na+} is reached (Fig. 2.7, position D), due to three main factors. First, the accumulation of positive ions inside the neurone starts to slow the Na$^+$ influx, through repulsion of positive charges. Second, the inactivation of the Na$^+$ channels stops the continued influx of Na$^+$. Third, the voltage-sensitive K$^+$ channels now open. These channels are activated by the same depolarization that triggered the opening of the Na$^+$ channels but they open

more slowly. The axon now becomes highly permeable to K$^+$ ions, which can now leave the neurone, down their concentration gradient (Fig. 2.7, position E). This process is initially encouraged by the positive charge, which repels K$^+$. The K$^+$ permeability is now higher than at rest and the membrane potential falls to close to the K$^+$ equilibrium potential (−95 mV) (Fig. 2.7, position G). This is called hyperpolarization. When the axon is repolarized below the normal RMP, the K$^+$ channels close and the resting membrane permeability allows the axon to regain its normal RMP (Fig. 2.7, position H). The small number of Na$^+$ and K$^+$ ions that have moved through the voltage-dependent channels are eventually redistributed by the Na$^+$/K$^+$-ATPase in order to maintain the concentration gradients. However, the pump has no active role in action potential generation.

Immediately after an action potential, the Na$^+$ channels remain completely inactivated for a short period, and cannot be opened by depolarization, however large. The Na$^+$ channels only regain their normal resting state once the membrane has repolarized (Fig. 2.7, position F). This is called the absolute refractory period (Fig. 2.7, positions B–F) and ensures that action potentials occur separately and do not propagate in the reverse direction along an excited axon. However, for a short time after this, during the period when some K$^+$ channels are still open and when the membrane is hyperpolarized, it is possible to initiate another action potential if the stimulus is larger than normal—a supra-threshold stimulus—but the action potential is still a fixed size. This second period is called the relative refractory period (Fig. 2.7, positions F–H). Table 2.2 gives a summary of the events during an action potential.

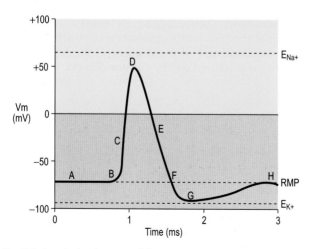

Fig. 2.7 A typical action potential. For events occurring at positions A–H, see text. RMP, resting membrane potential.

Table 2.2 Sequence of events during an action potential (see Fig. 2.7)

Event	Channels	Ion movements	Notes
Initial depolarization to threshold (about − 55 mV)	Na$^+$ channels open (B)	Na$^+$ influx (C)	Absolute refractory period (B–F)
Depolarization to about + 40 mV	Na$^+$ channels close and	K$^+$ efflux (E)	
	K$^+$ channels open (D)		
Repolarization, then hyperpolarization (− 95 mV)	K$^+$ channels close (G)		Relative refractory period (F–H)
Return to resting membrane potential		Movement of K$^+$ through leak channels (G–H)	

The all-or-nothing nature of the action potential, and the enforced time gap between action potentials, means that the action potential is a binary signal. The action potentials are clearly separated one from another, which ensures that the number of action potentials in a given period is clear. This is very important in a system where stimulus strength is coded by frequency. Binary-coded information can be transmitted with less degradation due to noise, an important consideration when the action potentials are transmitted across large distances.

Nerve conduction

So far we have only considered the activity at a given position on the axon, but it is the inactivation of Na^+ channels that also enables the action potential to travel along the axon from the trigger zone to the synapse.

The depolarization caused by the opening of Na^+ channels at any given point will spread passively along the axon equally in both directions. However, any Na^+ channels in the direction from which the action potential has come will still be inactivated, and only those Na^+ channels further down the axon, which have not yet been opened, will be activated by the depolarization. In this way, the wave of depolarization (like a Mexican wave) will propagate from the trigger zone to the synapse, with the depolarization being continually regenerated by newly opening Na^+ channels.

In unmyelinated axons, voltage-gated Na^+ and K^+ channels are spread all along the axon, and the action potential travels continuously along the axon. However, in myelinated axons there is a different mode of propagation. Owing to the tight insulation of the axon by oligodendrocytes or Schwann cells, the axon is effectively separated from the ions that would flow in, except at tiny gaps where the myelin sheath does not cover the surface of the axon. Occurring at regular intervals, these gaps in the myelin are called nodes of Ranvier (see Fig. 2.1) and are zones where the Na^+ and K^+ channels are concentrated. The depolarization at the preceding node spreads passively along the interior of the axon but, as the myelinated axon cannot depolarize, this spread is more rapid than in bare axons. The action potential does not decay as rapidly as in unmyelinated axons, because of the insulation, and at the next node the depolarization is sufficiently large to trigger the opening of large numbers of Na^+ channels. This will regenerate the depolarization to its full voltage. In this way, the action potential jumps rapidly from node to node, a process called saltatory conduction. Failure of saltatory conduction may underlie certain pathologies (Box 2.5).

The advantage of myelination is an increase in the speed of conduction, without a large increase in metabolic cost. Another way of increasing the speed of conduction is by increasing the size of the axon. This reduces the internal electrical resistance and increases the passive depolarization. This strategy is seen in its most exaggerated form in the giant axons of some invertebrates, particularly the giant squid. The large size of these axons means that they are easier to examine experimentally than smaller mammalian axons. Much of the early work on the action potential was done on these axons by Hodgkin and Huxley in the 1950s.

In humans, the fastest axons are both large and myelinated. Table 2.3 shows the Erlanger–Gasser classification of nerve fibres and their conduction velocities. This is presented in more detail in Chapter 1. A difference in conduction velocity can be seen when a mechanical trauma is experienced. The sensory input from the mechanical nociceptors travels along myelinated axons (Aδ fibres) and arrives before the signal carried by unmyelinated axons (C fibres). This gives rise to fast and slow pain. Although the C fibres are smaller, most of the difference in velocity is due to the myelin.

Because myelination allows rapid conduction with a smaller diameter, this allows more axons to be packed into a smaller volume, a significant advantage when wiring something as complex as a brain.

Box 2.5 Conduction failure in multiple sclerosis

The loss of myelin in multiple sclerosis causes the failure of saltatory conduction, as there are no ion channels on the denuded axon. Major symptoms of multiple sclerosis include muscle weakness, lack of coordination and often visual disturbances. These symptoms are due to a slowing or lack of nerve conduction. In many patients, the disease has phases of remission, which vary enormously in their duration. These are thought to be caused by temporary remyelination or by the insertion of new voltage-dependent Na^+ channels in the area lacking myelin.

Table 2.3 Erlanger–Gasser classification of nerve fibres

Type	Example	Average diameter (μm)	Average conduction velocity (m/s)
Aα	Motor neurones	15	100
Aβ	Touch afferents	8	50
Aγ	Muscle spindles	5	20
Aδ	Pain afferents	<3	15
B	Sympathetic preganglionic	3	7
C	Unmyelinated cutaneous pain afferents, sympathetic postganglionic	1	1

Although the electrical polarity of the membrane changes during an action potential, the numbers of Na$^+$ and K$^+$ ions which flow into and out of the neurone in order to bring about this change are relatively small and do not significantly change the internal concentration of either ion. This is because the RMP is only a local charge separation, involving only a very small proportion of the positive charges present, and the main bulk of the intracellular ions is electrically balanced. This can be shown clearly when an axon is poisoned with ouabain. Despite the inhibition of the Na$^+$/K$^+$-ATPase, the axon is able to fire many thousands of action potentials, only stopping eventually when the ion gradients are dissipated.

Synaptic transmission

Where the axon meets the target cell is the synapse. This is where the signal is transmitted either to another neurone or to an effector, such as a muscle or a gland. There are two types of synapse, electrical and chemical.

In an electrical synapse, the two cells are connected by gap junctions. These consist of a cluster of integral membrane proteins around a pore called a connexon. Each connexon is formed from six connexin proteins, and is aligned with a connexon in the opposing cell. This forms a channel between the cells that allows the free passage between them of water, small molecules (up to 1.2 nm in diameter), including some signalling molecules, and ions. Gap junctions are particularly important in coordinating electrical activity in smooth and cardiac muscle. They are also found between astrocytes and between neurones in the retina, where horizontal cells are electrically coupled. Electrical synapses are bidirectional; that is, electrical signalling can flow both ways across the synapses.

In humans, most synapses are chemical synapses; that is, they release chemicals called neurotransmitters into the small gap between the neurone and the subsequent cell. This gap is called the synaptic cleft (Fig. 2.8).

The neurotransmitter diffuses across the gap and interacts with receptor proteins in the target cell. The release of chemical signals involves a third type of voltage-dependent channel. When the depolarization of the action potential reaches the end of the axon, voltage-sensitive channels that are selective for Ca^{2+} are involved in the release of the neurotransmitters, by a process of exocytosis.

The presynaptic terminal contains numerous membrane-bound organelles, such as mitochondria and smooth endoplasmic reticulum. However, their most distinguishing feature is the presence of large numbers of vesicles, which contain the neurotransmitters (Fig. 2.9). Vesicles have a variety of forms, corresponding to the type of neurotransmitter that they contain.

While many of the vesicles are spread throughout the presynaptic terminal, there are some that are anchored close to the synaptic cleft at the presynaptic membrane, ready to be released in areas known as active zones. When an action potential invades the presynaptic terminal,

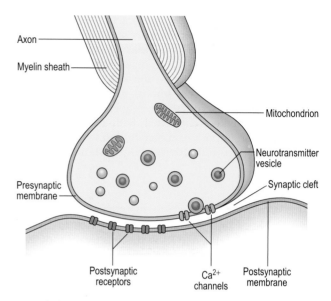

Fig. 2.8 Simplified diagram of a synapse. For clarity, only a few vesicles are shown.

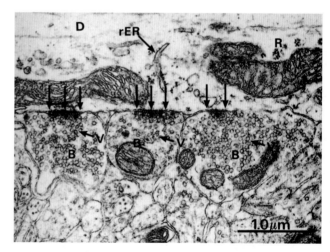

Fig. 2.9 Electronmicrograph of a synapse. Arrows indicate active zones with postsynaptic density; V, neurotransmitter vesicles; rER, rough endoplasmic reticulum; R, ribosomes; B, terminal boutons. From Young B, Heath JW. Wheater's Functional Histology, 4th edn, 2000, by permission of Harcourt Publishers.

the depolarization opens the voltage-sensitive Ca^{2+} channels, which allows Ca^{2+} to flow into the synapse. The concentration of Ca^{2+} is much higher in the ECF than in the ICF (see Table 2.1). Ca^{2+} acts at a number of sites to facilitate exocytosis. First, the vesicle is released from the cytoskeleton. Second, it partially fuses with the presynaptic membrane with the help of proteins in the vesicle and presynaptic membranes. Third, Ca^{2+} activates a protein, called synaptotagmin, which then allows the complete fusion and development of a pore, through which the neurotransmitter can diffuse into the cleft.

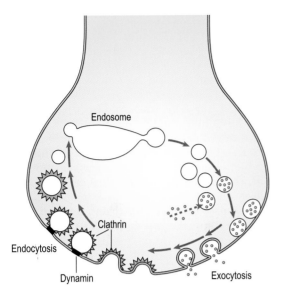

Fig. 2.10 Neurotransmitter is released by exocytosis. The vesicle membrane is coated with clathrin and the vesicle is retrieved by endocytosis. The vesicle then fuses with an endosome. New vesicles are budded from the endosome and filled with neurotransmitter, ready for release.

Exocytosis adds vesicle membrane to the presynaptic membrane, and if this were to remain there, the surface area of the neurone would increase and the plasma membrane would also contain the vesicle membrane proteins. So, in order to retrieve the vesicle for reuse, the vesicle membrane is recycled back into the synapse by endocytosis (Fig. 2.10). The vesicle membrane is first coated with a protein called clathrin, which forms a 'cage' around the vesicle; this is then pulled back into the cell by the cytoskeleton, with the help of a 'collar' of dynamin. The retrieved vesicle is first fused with an endosome, from which new vesicles can bud off. The empty vesicles can then be refilled with neurotransmitter and reused.

Patterns of vesicle release vary enormously. At many synapses in the CNS, not every action potential will release vesicles; that is, the average probability of release is usually less than one. However, at the other extreme, in the PNS, at the synapses between motor nerves and skeletal muscles, the skeletal neuromuscular junction, a single action potential releases about 30 vesicles of neurotransmitter, which is sufficient to produce a twitch of the target muscle.

Neurotransmitters

The first chemical to be identified as a neurotransmitter was acetylcholine (ACh), when its effects on the frog heart were described by Otto Loewi in 1926. Since then, a wide range of chemicals have been identified which act as neurotransmitters (Table 2.4). There are some general patterns of distribution, and in some cases particular neurotransmitters are associated with specific functions in the brain.

Table 2.4 Examples of neurotransmitters

Type	Neurotransmitter
Amino acids	Glutamate
	Aspartate
	γ-Aminobutyrate (GABA)
	Glycine
Amines	Acetylcholine
	Dopamine
	Noradrenaline
	Adrenaline
	Serotonin (5-hydroxytryptamine, 5-HT)
Peptides	Endorphins
	Enkephalins
	Substance P

Peripheral neurotransmitters

In the ANS, the major neurotransmitters are noradrenaline and adrenaline, which are released onto target organs and tissues by the sympathetic nervous system, and ACh, which is released by the parasympathetic nervous system. ACh is also the neurotransmitter released at all skeletal neuromuscular junctions, although the receptor subtypes on the muscle are different from those in the ANS. ACh is also the neurotransmitter that acts at all autonomic ganglia, both sympathetic and parasympathetic.

Central neurotransmitters

In the CNS, the major excitatory and inhibitory neurotransmitters are both amino acids, glutamate and γ-aminobutyric acid (GABA), respectively. These are the main mediators of fast signalling in the brain and spinal cord. Other neurotransmitters include a number of amines, such as noradrenaline, 5-hydroxytryptamine (5-HT/serotonin) and dopamine. These neurotransmitters mainly act in a slower manner, and are often described as modulators of fast neurotransmission. Many neurones release more than one neurotransmitter, although the patterns of excitation required to stimulate their release may differ. One of the neurotransmitters may be, for example, glutamate, whereas the second neurotransmitter may be a peptide. Peptides are released at a higher firing frequency. The slow-acting neurotransmitters frequently have long-lasting modulatory effects on the target neurones.

Histamine, as well as acting as an important neurotransmitter in the brain, is also an inflammatory mediator, released from mast cells and basophils, and promotes vasodilatation and increased capillary permeability.

Following its discovery as a key molecule in the control of blood pressure, nitric oxide (NO), a short-lived gas, is a recent addition to the list of neurotransmitters. While it fulfils the criteria for a neurotransmitter, it does not act on cell surface receptors but binds to an intracellular enzyme, guanylate cyclase, causing changes in intracellular biochemistry. It has been suggested that one role for NO in the CNS may be in the hippocampus, in the formation of new memories.

Postsynaptic events and postsynaptic receptors

The neurotransmitter that is released into the synaptic cleft diffuses passively to the postsynaptic membrane, where it can bind to specific receptors. Typically, this takes less than $5\,\mu s$, as the cleft is very narrow, about 12 nm. Not all the released neurotransmitter reaches the receptors, as diffusion out of the cleft and specific inactivation mechanisms may reduce the amount left for receptor binding.

The action of a given neurotransmitter on a target neurone (or peripherally on a target organ) depends on the identity of the receptors present on the target. Almost all neurotransmitters so far identified have multiple receptor subtypes that they can activate. Receptors for all the classical neurotransmitters (unlike those for some hormones and NO) are integral membrane proteins, which have their neurotransmitter binding sites on or near the extracellular surface. They fall into two major types, depending on their structure and function. The first type comprises ionotropic receptors, which contain an integral ion channel; hence their alternative name, ligand-gated ion channels. The second type comprises metabotropic receptors, which are linked to intracellular biochemical events, via a group of intermediate proteins, called G-proteins (so called because they bind the guanosine phosphates, GTP and GDP, as described later in the text). These are also known as G-protein-coupled receptors (GPCRs). GPCRs, while sharing a common structural motif, are extremely diverse, with hundreds of different types having been identified.

Within each of these major types, there are similarities of structure and function between receptors for different neurotransmitters, suggesting evolution from common precursors.

There is a third group of cell surface receptors, consisting of an extracellular binding site and an intracellular catalytic site which, when the receptor is activated by the ligand, phosphorylates tyrosine residues. These receptors are targets for peptide growth factors and also insulin.

Some ligands, such as the steroid hormones, are lipophilic and can diffuse across the cell membrane. Others, such as thyroid hormone, are internalized by specialized transport mechanisms. These ligands bind to nuclear receptors that affect gene transcription, changing patterns of protein production within cells.

Ionotropic receptors

Ionotropic receptors are integral membrane-spanning proteins, with multiple types of subunit that group together to form an ion channel and its associated ligand-binding sites. An example is the nicotinic ACh receptor (nAChR) (Fig. 2.11; see also Chapter 17). The open nAChR allows the flow of Na^+ and K^+, but other ionotropic receptors have different ion selectivities.

Neurotransmitter binding triggers a conformational change that allows ions to flow selectively through the channel. The subsequent current flow sets up a potential difference called a postsynaptic potential, which may be excitatory (epsp) or inhibitory (ipsp), depending on the ion selectivity and the membrane potential, and makes the neurone more (epsp) or less (ipsp) likely to fire an action potential. If the current flowing through each type of channel is measured at different membrane potentials, there is a voltage at which the net current will be zero. For example, if the channel is only permeable to K^+, this will occur at the Nernst potential for K^+. This is because at this voltage, called the reversal potential, the numbers of ions moving in and out of the neurone are exactly balanced (see earlier). For any given channel, if the membrane potential is higher than the reversal potential, activation of the channel will produce an ipsp, and if it is lower, it will produce an epsp.

In the case of the ACh receptor, the channel is permeable to both Na^+ and K^+ and has a reversal potential of about 0 mV. This can be checked using the Goldman equation, setting the Na^+ and K^+ permeabilities at 1 and the Cl^- permeability to 0. In the resting nerve or muscle, the RMP will be about $-75\,mV$. On activation, current will flow through the ACh receptor, making the membrane potential more positive, until it reaches 0 mV. In skeletal muscle, this depolarization is sufficient to activate the voltage-sensitive Na^+ channels, producing an action potential, and, via the subsequent release of Ca^{2+} from sarcoplasmic reticulum, causes the muscle to contract.

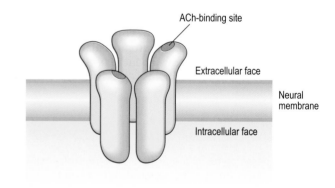

Fig. 2.11 Diagram of the nicotinic acetylcholine (ACh) receptor. The different subunits are labelled α, β, δ and γ. The receptor has two α subunits, each of which has a binding site for ACh on its external face.

In studies on the neuromuscular junction (also called the motor endplate), it was observed that small epsps called mepps (miniature endplate potentials), which occur spontaneously at a rate of about 1 per second, were of similar size (about 0.5 mV) and duration (rising rapidly and decaying more slowly in a total of about 5 ms), and that all epsps were multiples of the mepps. This is because neurotransmitter release occurs in distinct packets called quanta. Each mepp represents the release of a single vesicle of ACh, which is the minimum possible amount that can be released. The amount of ACh in each vesicle is about the same, and the stimulated neurotransmitter release therefore consists of the release from several vesicles, so the response will be multiples of the effect of a single vesicle.

In the CNS, this has been more difficult to establish. This may be due to the variable size and content of the vesicles and the smaller number of vesicles released by each action potential. Also, the amount of neurotransmitter reaching the postsynaptic receptors may be affected by the high-affinity uptake of neurotransmitter into glia and surrounding neurones (see below). Also, in the CNS, the epsp may not be a good measure of neurotransmitter release, as there are limited numbers of postsynaptic receptors, which means that there may be more neurotransmitter molecules than receptors to respond.

Signalling using ionotropic receptors is very rapid and occurs in the major pathways linking brain areas and in the motor pathways of the PNS. Receptors of this type (Table 2.5) can be divided into subtypes. In some cases, the distribution of the subtypes clearly varies, over developmental time and location (see the following chapters for more detail).

Metabotropic receptors

Metabotropic receptors, while having a common mode of action, are extremely varied in their ligands. They are responsible not just for detecting neurotransmitters as diverse as small amino acids and large peptides, but also for the sensory reception of light (where the ligand is a photon), and for detecting some tastes and all smells (Table 2.6).

The common structure of these receptors is a single protein with seven transmembrane segments, with an extracellular ligand-binding site, and an intracellular region that is involved in the interaction with G-proteins (Fig. 2.12). G-proteins are trimers of membrane-associated proteins, which consist of alpha (α), beta (β) and gamma (γ) subunits. The inactive α subunit has guanosine diphosphate (GDP) bound to it. This is exchanged for guanosine triphosphate (GTP) (present in the cytoplasm) upon activation of the G-protein trimer by a receptor, resulting in the α subunit separating from the $\beta\gamma$ subunits. The activated α subunit then alters the activity of an enzyme involved in the synthesis of a second messenger. The α subunits come in different forms, which interact with different intracellular enzymes, and can either stimulate or inhibit these enzymes. However, a few seconds later the GTP is converted to GDP by the intrinsic GTPase activity of the α subunit, which renders the α subunit inactive, whereupon it recombines with the $\beta\gamma$ subunits. The β and γ subunits, which are also released from the receptor, remain bound to each other throughout, and have roles distinct from that of the α subunit. At its simplest, the sequence of events triggered by the binding of a ligand to a metabotropic receptor is as follows (see also Fig. 2.12):

1. The ligand binds to the receptor.

2. The receptor binds the G-protein trimer.

3. The α subunit exchanges GDP for GTP and separates from the $\beta\gamma$ subunits.

4. The activated α subunit binds to its target enzyme.

5. Production of second messengers is either increased or reduced until the GTPase activity of the α subunit dephosphorylates GTP to GDP.

6. The α subunit dissociates from the enzyme and recombines with the $\beta\gamma$ subunit.

Table 2.5 Ionotropic receptors

Neurotransmitter	*Receptor type*
Acetylcholine	Nicotinic acetylcholine
Glutamate	NMDA
	AMPA/Kainate
GABA	GABA$_A$
Glycine	Glycine
Serotonin	5-HT$_3$

NMDA, N-methyl-D-aspartate; AMPA, amino-3-hydroxy-5-methyl-4-isoxazole propionic acid; GABA, γ-aminobutyric acid; 5-HT, 5-hydroxytryptamine.

Table 2.6 A selection of endogenous ligands that have metabotropic receptors

Acetylcholine	Adenosine
Adrenaline	Serum calcium
Noradrenaline	Angiotensin
Serotonin	Bradykinin
Dopamine	Oxytocin
Histamine	Somatostatin
Glutamate	Vasopressin
GABA	

ELEMENTS OF CELLULAR AND MOLECULAR NEUROSCIENCE

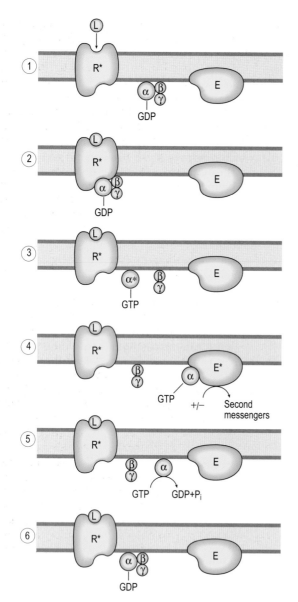

Fig. 2.12 Sequence of events associated with the activation of a G-protein-coupled receptor. R, receptor; E, enzyme; L, ligand; α, β and γ, G-protein subunits; GDP, guanosine diphosphate; GTP, guanosine triphosphate, P_i; phosphate. *Activated state.

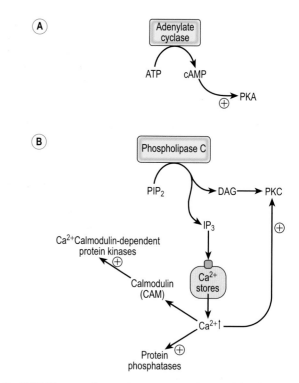

Fig. 2.13 Diagram of second messenger pathways. (A) Pathway generating cyclic AMP (cAMP). PKA, protein kinase A. (B) Pathway generating diacylglycerol (DAG) and inositol 1,4,5-trisphosphate (IP_3). PIP_2, phosphatidylinositol 4,5-bisphosphate; PKC, protein kinase C.

binds to specific IP_3 receptors on intracellular organelles containing Ca^{2+} stores, causing the release of Ca^{2+} into the cytoplasm. Ca^{2+} can activate both protein kinases such as PKC and protein phosphatases (see Fig. 2.13). It can do this either directly or, in some cases, via a Ca^{2+}-binding protein called calmodulin; in this case, the resulting Ca^{2+}–calmodulin complex activates the target protein.

cAMP, DAG, IP_3 and Ca^{2+} are called second messengers, as they act within the cell. In this context, the neurotransmitter can be thought of as the first messenger, although this term is very rarely used.

One of the important points about signalling via GPCRs is that an activated receptor may itself activate multiple G-proteins before the ligand is removed. Additionally, each α subunit can bind to a single enzyme molecule, but for the entire time that the α subunit is bound, the enzyme activity is changed, which can lead to a large change in the concentration of second messengers. This is especially true in the case of PLC-linked systems, as the second messenger IP_3 can itself release large amounts of the Ca^{2+}. This amplification of the neurotransmitter signal can produce significant downstream biochemical changes in the neurone through the levels of phosphorylation of proteins by the activated kinases and phosphatases.

After prolonged activation of the receptors, the response of the receptor to the ligand may be reduced. Two mechanisms of this receptor desensitization are known. One

The target enzymes are commonly either adenylate cyclase or phospholipase C (PLC) (Fig. 2.13). At least 17 genes code for α subunits, and they can be grouped according to whether they activate or inhibit adenylate cyclase (α_s or α_i) or activate PLC (α_q).

Adenylate cyclase catalyses the conversion of ATP to cAMP, which itself activates other intracellular enzymes such as cAMP-dependent protein kinase A. PLC catalyses the breakdown of the membrane lipid phosphatidylinositol 4,5-bisphosphate into two second messengers, diacylglycerol (DAG) and inositol 1,4,5-trisphosphate (IP_3). DAG is an activator of protein kinases, in this case protein kinase C (PKC). IP_3 diffuses into the cytoplasm and involves the phosphorylation of the receptor by a kinase followed by the reversible binding of a protein called arrestin, which inhibits the receptor recognition of the G-protein. The second, which is more long-lasting, is produced when receptors are removed from the membrane by endocytosis.

One of the consequences of GPCR activation is the modulation of neuronal excitability. Many of the ion channels present in neuronal membranes can, like many intracellular proteins, have their properties changed by altering their state of phosphorylation. This can determine the conditions under which they open and for how long they open. Changes in the opening of ion channels then influences whether a neurone fires in response to the stimulus produced by ionotropic receptors and other metabotropic receptors. In this way, GPCRs affect the overall excitability of neurones and thus their firing patterns. In some cases it has been shown that both α and $\beta\gamma$ subunits can interact directly with ion channels to modulate their activity, without the intervention of an enzyme or second messenger.

Neurotransmitter synthesis

The small 'classical' neurotransmitters (amino acids and amines) are manufactured by enzymes present in the presynaptic terminal. For example, the neurotransmitter glutamate is present in large amounts in the cell, and has different metabolic and neurotransmitter pools. In neurones, it is synthesized either from glucose provided by the Krebs cycle or from glutamine produced by glial cells. The neurotransmitters are then concentrated in the vesicles by an antiport system, which transports H^+ out of the vesicle in exchange for the neurotransmitter. The high concentration of H^+ in the vesicle is maintained by an H^+-ATPase in the vesicle membrane.

Peptide transmitters are manufactured in the cell body by ribosomes on the endoplasmic reticulum, and are processed and packaged via the extensive Golgi system into vesicles that are transported down the axon. They appear in the presynaptic terminal in large dense-core vesicles, which are found further away from the synaptic cleft than the small clear vesicles that contain the small molecules. They are released from the synapse when the frequency of action potentials is high and the intracellular Ca^{2+} concentration reaches higher values than under lower-frequency stimulation.

It is possible to trace the neurotransmitter pathways in the brain by immunocytochemistry, using antibodies for the specific enzymes associated with a particular neurotransmitter. For example, ACh is made from acetyl coenzyme A (acetyl-CoA) and choline by the enzyme choline acetyltransferase (CAT), and the presence of CAT can be used to identify neurones that synthesize and release ACh.

Neurotransmitter inactivation

ACh seems to be unique, in that it is inactivated by enzymatic degradation within the cleft itself. This is carried out by acetylcholinesterases (AChEs) in the synaptic cleft at the neuromuscular junction or other cholinergic synapses. These enzymes are found in the folds of the postsynaptic membrane. The esterases cleave ACh into its inactive components, choline and acetate. The choline is then transported back into the presynaptic neurone, by an Na^+-dependent choline transporter, where it can be used to resynthesize ACh in combination with acetyl-CoA derived from glycolysis. As well as the membrane-bound AChEs, there are two soluble esterase enzymes. One of these is another type of AChE, found in the cerebrospinal fluid, and the other, called butyrylcholinesterase or pseudocholinesterase, is found in plasma. It is less substrate-specific than the AChE and can hydrolyse a wide range of esters (Box 2.6). The other small neurotransmitters are taken up into either the presynaptic or postsynaptic neurone by high-affinity transport mechanisms, often by Na^+-linked cotransporters.

Most classical neurotransmitters are inactivated by their removal from the synaptic cleft by high-affinity Na^+-dependent uptake systems. These transporters are found on neurones and, in some cases, on glial cells. The importance of these mechanisms is highlighted by the fact that drugs that inhibit neurotransmitter uptake can have profound effects on brain function. Cocaine inhibits dopamine uptake, which partly accounts for the euphoria and addiction associated with the drug. More usefully, tricyclic antidepressant drugs and selective serotonin uptake inhibitors such as fluoxetine (Prozac) are widely used in the treatment of depression, although the link between reuptake blockade and the therapeutic effect is not clear. Simple diffusion away from the synaptic cleft may also be important in the inactivation of transported molecules, such as glutamate and GABA, and is the main mechanism of inactivation for peptide neurotransmitters. As diffusion may be slow, this may explain why peptide actions are so long-lasting. Peptides may also be removed by non-specific peptidases and receptor-mediated endocytosis.

> **Box 2.6 Butyrylcholinesterase lack and paralysis**
>
> Suxamethonium is a commonly used, short-acting neuromuscular blocking agent that is normally inactivated by butyrylcholinesterase (BChE). However, about 1 in 3000 individuals have an inherited condition in which they have a modified form of BChE that fails to metabolize suxamethonium. These individuals show neuromuscular paralysis that lasts for several hours instead of a few minutes, and hence will need to be ventilated until the suxamethonium is degraded.

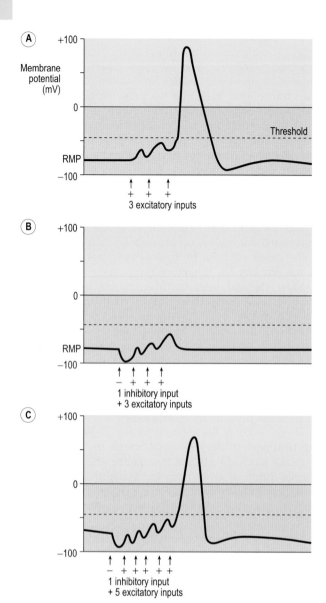

Fig. 2.14 Integration of excitatory and inhibitory inputs. (A) Three closely spaced excitatory inputs cause the neurone to exceed the threshold and fire an action potential. (B) A single inhibitory input prior to the three excitatory inputs prevents the neurone from firing. (C) Increasing the number of excitatory inputs enables threshold to be reached and an action potential to fire.

Summation and neuronal integration

Each neurone in the brain has been estimated to receive (on average) about 10 000 synaptic inputs. If a given input is closer to the trigger zone of the neurone, then it is more likely to affect the firing of that neurone. This is often the case with inhibitory inputs. If the firing frequency of the input is high, then the epsps may summate to produce an action potential (Fig. 2.14A), a process known as temporal

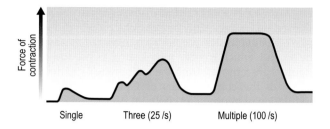

Fig. 2.15 Single twitch and summation of inputs produces tetanus in skeletal muscle. The force of contraction in a skeletal muscle depends on the frequency of firing of the motor nerve.

summation. If another synapse also contributes, then the electrical potentials from all inputs summate in spatial summation. If there is an ipsp, then this may prevent the action potential (Fig. 2.14B). The number of epsps would have to increase to overcome the inhibition (Fig. 2.14C). The density of a given type of receptor at a given synapse (its synaptic strength) will also affect the subsequent behaviour. This spatial and temporal summation, along with the current electrical status of the neurone (i.e. how depolarized or hyperpolarized the neurone is), will all determine whether it fires or not. In most cases, neurones will require the simultaneous activation of a number of excitatory inputs in order to fire, thus ensuring integration of signals. It has been estimated that a minimum of 100 excitatory inputs is required to excite a pyramidal cell in the cortex.

Sometimes, the sum of the inputs will ensure firing of the postsynaptic cell in all cases, but this seems to be relatively rare. At the neuromuscular junction, firing of the motor neurone releases so much neurotransmitter that muscle contraction is always activated, although for a large contraction it requires a high frequency of inputs, as single twitches summate to produce a tetanus (Fig. 2.15). In the cerebellum, inputs from a type of neurone called a climbing fibre always cause the firing of the large Purkinje cell (PC) that it innervates. The cerebellum is involved in the acquisition and refining of motor patterns, and this climbing fibre/PC signal is activated when an error of execution occurs.

CLINICAL EXAMINATION

3

Chapter objectives

After studying this chapter you should be able to:

1. Understand the principles involved in taking a patient's history.

2. Understand the principles involved in performing a mental state examination.

3. Understand the principles involved in performing a neurological examination.

4. Be familiar with the major clinical laboratory techniques that can be used to provide additional or confirmatory information relevant to the clinical examination.

CLINICAL EXAMINATION

Introduction

A clinical examination comprises three components: the history, the examination, and the explanation, where the doctor discusses the nature and implications of the clinical findings. A patient seeks medical help for three main reasons: diagnostic purposes, treatment or reassurance, or a combination of these factors. The foundation of the patient–doctor relationship is largely based on establishing a good rapport during the history-taking and the examination.

Although increasingly sophisticated tests have become available and support the diagnostic process in neurology and psychiatry, the history and clinical examination remain the core of the assessment of a patient who suffers from some form of damage to, or dysfunction of, the nervous system. The important point is to be systematic. The aim of this chapter is to provide a brief overview of the essential points of the clinical examination in neurology, and to describe the main additional laboratory-based investigations that may help in the formulation of a diagnosis.

The clinical examination is preceded by the taking of the patient's history. History-taking provides essential information about the possible aetiology of the disease. It is the most important part of the clinical assessment, during which the following information is obtained about the patient: age, gender, race, occupation, handedness, history of the present complaint, past medical history (including past and/or present drug treatment), family history and social history. For example, the temporal evolution of the problems that the patient is experiencing provides important clues as to their nature. An acute onset is characteristic of trauma or a major vascular accident. A development over days may suggest an inflammatory component. Neoplasms develop in general over months or years. Neurological problems resulting from an immune mechanism, such as multiple sclerosis, also have an evolution over months and years, with a pattern of relapse and remission. Neurodegenerative diseases, such as Parkinson's disease, motor neurone disease or Alzheimer's disease, develop inexorably over years. In some cases, if the patient presents with an impaired state of consciousness, either transient (seizures) or chronic (dementia), a complete history of the patient's problems will require involving others, such as relatives, carers or the general practitioner. Psychiatric histories are often more detailed, as more detail is needed about the patient's personal life, family and social background.

It is also important to first carry out a general physical examination. This is important, as systemic disease may lead to neurological complications (e.g. links between atherosclerosis and stroke, cancer and cerebral metastases, diabetes and peripheral neuropathy, rheumatoid arthritis and cervical cord compression). The whole of the clinical examination must be carried out gently, tactfully and with consideration for the patient, who may be surprised or intimidated by some of the questions or procedures that are part of the examination, or may perceive them as completely unrelated to the complaint. Medical jargon must be avoided and replaced with simple explanations and common language, building the patient's trust and gaining their confidence, thus making the examination as participatory and interactive as possible.

There is no absolute 'gold standard' for the way in which a neurological examination should proceed, and there are variations between clinicians, hospitals and countries. The examination may also vary with the type of complaint that the patient presents with, which may suggest to the experienced clinician a preliminary diagnosis. However, any basic neurological clinical examination of a patient should include an evaluation of: (1) mental state; (2) sensory systems; (3) cranial nerves; (4) motor system and reflexes; (5) coordination; (6) gait; and (7) cortical function. Just as important are observational skills that will help in the detection of physical signs that may give a clue as to the neurological disability.

A first assessment of this type could be carried out by any general practitioner of medicine, before involving a specialist. For diseases in the field of psychiatry, such as depression or schizophrenia, more specialized tests and rating systems may be required, as mentioned in the corresponding case analyses discussed in this book. It is also important to note that the autonomic nervous system is not tested directly during the examination. However, the patient may present with complex indirect signs and symptoms of dysfunction in the sympathetic or parasympathetic systems (e.g. postural hypotension, constipation or faecal incontinence, urinary retention or incontinence, pupillary immobility, disturbances of sweating or erectile failure). If required, the Valsalva manoeuvre is the gold-standard test used to assess the integrity of the autonomic nervous system. It requires the patient to take a deep breath and, while pinching the nose and keeping the mouth closed, to try to exhale against a resistance of 40 mmHg for 15 s. During this test, the heart rate increases and then returns to normal once the subject breaths normally.

After the clinical examination, a series of laboratory-based investigations may be required, in order to obtain information that the clinical examination cannot reveal. Inconsistencies in the history or examination should make one think about the possibility of a functional non-organic disorder.

Parts of the clinical examination

Mental state

Examination of the mental state is the psychiatric equivalent of the physical examination. It is a thorough and systematic evaluation of the emotional and mental state of a patient and is carried out as an interview. Areas that need to be assessed are:

- appearance and behaviour
- speech

- mood
- thought content
- abnormal experiences and beliefs
- cognitive state.

The time devoted to each component depends on the patient's answers and the diagnostic possibilities. Much information can be gathered just through observation and interaction with the patient during the history-taking and the initial general physical examination.

The patient's appearance can often reveal much about an underlying psychiatric disorder. Important points to look for include dress, personal hygiene and general grooming. The general appearance and demeanour of the patient may suggest self-neglect, depression or anxiety. The latter may also be revealed by hyperventilation or sweating. The way in which a patient sits also gives important hints to a possible underlying pathology; are they relaxed and at ease, or sitting tensely and fidgeting? The agitated depressive or the excited manic or schizophrenic may be so agitated that they get up from the seat and pace around the room. A demented or confused patient may leave the chair because they do not understand what is going on. The presence of delusions of persecution may lead the patient to feel threatened by the proceedings and to become angry or to terminate the consultation. Alternatively, patients may appear to drift off to sleep repeatedly, suggesting either a confusional state, with fluctuating levels of consciousness, or over-sedation with existing medication.

The patient's behaviour during the interview may be disinhibited, as in the manic patient who strips; the patient may be manipulative or seductive and may threaten violence if their wishes are not met. Alternatively, the patient may appear unduly submissive or self-critical, or make little or no eye contact with the interviewer. They may appear to be suspicious of questions, due to an underlying personality disorder or paranoid illness. The patient may also seem to be paying little attention to the interviewer or to be listening to someone else when there is no one else in the room; this suggests that they are experiencing auditory hallucinations. Undue terror without any obvious cause, or attempts to touch or shoo away non-existing objects, suggest that the patient is experiencing visual hallucinations.

Gradually, the clinician can also assess whether the patient is confused or, on the contrary, has good insight into their condition. Assessment of drug/alcohol use and social and family circumstances should also be considered. It must be remembered that bizarre behaviour or inability to relate to the interviewer may reflect subnormal intelligence.

Speech is a form of behaviour, and so it is important to assess its form and content. Does the patient speak at all or are they mute, and if so, is this deliberate, organic, or part of a depressive stupor? In a mute patient, it is important to assess all aspects of speech production, including the ability to produce sounds and communicate non-verbally. If the patient does speak, is this spontaneous or only in answer to questions, with monosyllabic or fuller and more elaborate replies, or is the patient vague and evasive? Is speech unduly slow, as in depressive illness, or so quick and continuous that it is impossible to interrupt, as in hypomania and mania? A sudden change in verbal style may indicate an emotionally sensitive subject requiring further questioning.

Mood has both a subjective component, which is reflected in the way the patient describes their emotional state, and an objective component, i.e. what the interviewer sees. The subjective and objective components of mood are usually, but not always, congruent. Facial expression is one of the outward signs of the patient's mood. For example, tearfulness or poverty of expression occurs in depression, elation in mania, tenseness in anxiety, and perplexity in schizophrenia. The emotional expression may be abnormally labile, as in mania or organic brain disease. The patient's mood may also be probed with direct questions, e.g. 'How have you been feeling lately?' Psychiatric symptoms (e.g. paranoid delusions or profound thought disorder) may become apparent during the conversation with the patient.

Abnormal moods include most commonly depression and anxiety, but also elation, irritability, anger and perplexity. When the mood is abnormal, it should be evaluated in detail, in the same way as any other presenting symptom. Some severely depressed patients may see no future, feel despairing and hopeless, and have thoughts of suicide. Suicidal ideation must always be sought for in depressed patients, and very often it is also appropriate to ask about suicidality in those with other disorders such as schizophrenia, alcohol dependence, hypomania, and severe anxiety disorders. Not only is it incorrect to think that discussing suicide with patients encourages them to commit suicide, but failure to discuss it may lead to tragedies that could have been prevented. Intent to commit suicide may be probed with questions such as, 'Is life worth living nowadays? Have you seriously contemplated ending it all?'

The patient should be asked what their main worries are and whether they are preoccupied by any thoughts, e.g. morbid thoughts. Obsessional ruminations are stereotyped thoughts that the patient recognizes as their own, realizes are silly but unsuccessfully tries to resist. They occur in obsessive compulsive neuroses and may be associated with obsessional rituals, acts that the patient feels compelled to carry out, even though they recognize them as being absurd, e.g. compulsive handwashing because they 'feel dirty'. For obsessional rituals, the patient realizes that the compulsion comes from within, unlike delusions of influence, in which the impulse is felt to come from outside forces.

Perceptual abnormalities most often take the form of hallucinations or delusions. Patients suffering delusions have a false and unshakeable belief that is out of keeping with the social milieu from which they come. Hallucinations are apparently normal perceptions that occur in the absence of an appropriate stimulus. In psychiatric illness, hallucinations occur in organic and functional

CLINICAL EXAMINATION

psychoses, e.g. in schizophrenia and affective illnesses, cases of severely raised levels of anxiety due to hyperventilation, grief reactions, and hysterical illnesses. Illusions occur when the object is real but perception is disturbed. They are usually related, in the psychiatric sense, to disorders of the perceptual environment of the object, thereby leading to decreased visual clarity coupled with a state of high emotion in the perceiver. Illusions are common in psychiatric illness, particularly acute confusional states. In affective disorders, the content of any hallucinations or delusions is generally mood-congruent. Depressed patients may think that they are evil, while manic patients may believe that they are God.

Impaired concentration is a characteristic sign of depression; it also occurs in dementia and acute confusional states. Cognitive function can be assessed using the Mini Mental State Examination (see Table 14.3). It includes several components: the level of consciousness, the orientation in time and place, general appearance, mood, interaction with the examiner, attention and memory.

Cranial nerves

Abnormalities in cranial nerves may occur in isolation and involve one nerve only, or may affect several nerves.

Cranial nerve I (olfactory)

The olfactory nerve is tested by exposing the patient to a range of scents (e.g. cinnamon, cloves, vanilla, tobacco and mint). More common odours (e.g. oranges and coffee) could also be used. Each nostril is alternately occluded while the other nostril is tested. Substances that are irritating are avoided (e.g. ammonia). It is also important to note that anosmia (loss of the sense of smell) may not have a neurological cause, but simply be due to a sinus inflammation (catarrh). Hallucinations of an olfactory nature may be associated with epilepsy. Testing of this nerve is not routinely performed, but is done when patients report a decrease in the sense of taste or smell. It is performed in patients with suspected dementia and also in patients with tumours or fractures through the cribriform plate of the skull. The loss of smell may significantly affect the sense of taste.

Cranial nerve II (optic)

Testing of the optic nerve starts with an assessment of the patient's ability to read printed material with each eye separately, i.e. visual acuity. This is tested with a Snellen chart, which consists of a series of letters whose sizes are such that the biggest letter can be seen at 60 m, whereas the smallest can be seen with normal vision only at 5 m. If the patient wears glasses, the type of lens worn is determined, in order to differentiate between myopia and hypermetropia. Acuity at the normal reading distance is also assessed. Then, the visual fields are tested by moving an object (usually the examiner's finger) into

the four visual quadrants. The left and right eyes can be tested together first (binocular vision), and then monocular testing can be done. Any subjective visual sensations are also noted, e.g. visual hallucinations or white flashes in the visual field. Fundoscopic examination of the retina can detect the possible presence of papilloedema, suggesting raised intracranial pressure and also retinal haemorrhages, which may be found in diabetics or hypertensives. Colour blindness, although not regularly tested, is assessed using Ishihara plates, in which a series of coloured spots contain numerical shapes that the patient must identify.

Cranial nerves III (oculomotor), IV (trochlear) and VI (abducens)

This examination assesses the motility of the eye and pupillary function. The examiner first notes the position of the eyes during gazing straight ahead (at this point, a squint or strabismus could become evident), and then assesses any symmetrical or asymmetrical change in the movement of the eyes and specifically asks for the presence of any double vision on looking in particular directions. A lesion to cranial nerve III may lead to deficits of adduction (Fig. 3.1), depression or elevation of the eye, and unilateral ptosis. A lesion of cranial nerve IV will result in deficient abduction and in medial deviation of the eye. A lesion in cranial nerve VI leads to a deficit in the internal rotation of the eye and failure to abduct. Examination of the pupils involves assessment of the size, shape and mobility of the pupils, and the accommodation reflex response. Slight asymmetry between pupillary sizes occurs in up to 20% of people. The pupillary light response (direct and indirect) is also noted. Painful third nerve palsy can be a sign of an intracranial aneurysm pressing on the third nerve. Diabetic neuropathy and atherosclerosis can also cause pupillary dysfunction. A fixed dilated pupil in a person with a mass lesion (e.g. tumour) can occur when the intracranial pressure has reached the point where the brain starts herniating to compress the third nerve. It is a sign of impending death in that situation. Drugs such as morphine and atropine can also alter pupillary size. A small pupil can be part of Horner's syndrome (Fig. 3.2), which may be due, for example, to a carcinoma impinging on the superior cervical ganglion or to damage to the sympathetic pathways anywhere along their craniocervical course.

Cranial nerve V (trigeminal)

Examination of this nerve involves assessment of the normal functioning of each of its three divisions: ophthalmic, maxillary and mandibular. Lesion of the whole nerve leads to a loss of sensation in the skin and mucous membranes of the face and nasopharynx. The sensory testing involves assessing the response to light touch and pin-prick. The presence and symmetry of the corneal reflex are also tested. Motor function is assessed by

Looking to the right

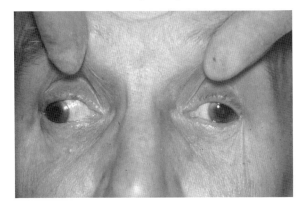

Looking to the left

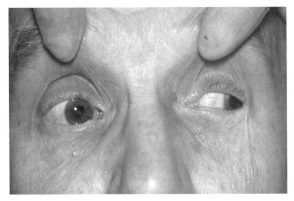

Fig. 3.1 Left oculomotor nerve lesion. Note the inability of the patient's left eye to adduct on command to look right. It deviates laterally due to the unopposed action of the lateral rectus muscle (innervated by cranial nerve six).

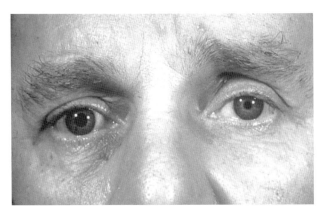

Fig. 3.2 Example of Horner's syndrome (left eye). Note the slight drooping of the patient's left eyelid and asymmetry of the pupils; the left is slightly smaller than the right.

asking the patient to clench their teeth (to check the masseter muscle), as well as testing the strength of the masticator muscles by asking the patient to open the mouth against resistance.

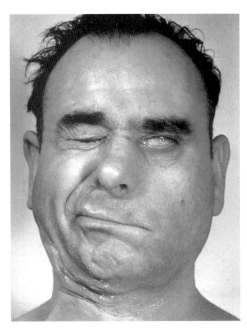

Fig. 3.3 Patient with left facial nerve palsy being asked to shut his eyes and grimace.

Damage to the motor division produces muscle wasting, most easily seen in the temporalis muscle (above the zygomatic arch). Also, the mandible deviates to one side (indicating pterygoid weakness on the side of nerve damage) rather than travelling vertically (normal) on opening and closing of the mouth. The jaw-jerk stretch reflex of the jaw-closing muscles (masseter and temporalis muscles) is weak or absent in normal subjects. Brisk or exaggerated jaw jerks often indicate bilateral lesions of upper motor neurone pathways.

Cranial nerve VII (facial)

Symmetry of facial movement is a key element in the testing of the facial nerve. Several other manipulations can also reveal facial nerve dysfunction; for example, the patient may find it difficult to whistle. The patient may also be asked to smile or show the upper teeth, or inflate the mouth with air and then blow out the cheeks. Lesions above the facial motor nucleus (located in the pons) cause supranuclear palsies, whereas lesions distal to the nucleus cause infranuclear facial palsies. The ability to wrinkle the forehead is used to distinguish between upper and lower motor neurone damage to the facial nerve (Fig. 3.3). Supranuclear paralysis affects mainly the lower part of the face, whereas infranuclear palsies affect both parts of the face. The latter, but not the former, cause atrophy of the facial muscles. This is because the upper part of the face receives bilateral innervation from both the facial nerves, unlike the lower part.

Cranial nerve VIII (auditory and vestibular)

The auditory component of the cranial nerve is assessed by testing hearing. Hearing is tested by blocking one ear while testing the hearing in the other ear by whispering or varying the intensity of speech. This is followed if necessary by Weber's and Rinne's tests, which are tests of hearing involving the use of a tuning fork. Abnormal sensations (e.g. hyperacusis or tinnitus) are also noted by the examiner. Vertigo and nystagmus reflect dysfunction in the vestibular component (although oculokinetic nystagmus can occur physiologically). Vertigo can be associated with the patient's sensation that objects move around them. Nystagmus and vertigo can also be induced by sudden changes in head posture. A vestibular Schwannoma (acoustic neuroma) is a type of VIIIth nerve tumour that presents initially with only mild hearing loss.

Cranial nerves IX (glossopharyngeal) and X (vagus)

The function of these nerves is tested by observing the quality of speech and coughing, and monitoring taste, swallowing and the position of the palate at rest. The movement of the palate is also assessed during voluntary or reflex activity. Damage to the glossopharyngeal nerve can be associated with loss of taste in the posterior part of the tongue. Lesions of the vagus nerve may lead to paralysis of the palate and dysphagia, a hoarse and deep voice, blurred and ineffectual speech, and a displaced uvula. The last of these can be assessed by asking a patient to say 'Ah' and observing the movement of the soft palate and uvula. Damage to either nerve results in loss of the gag reflex.

Cranial nerve XI (spinal part of the accessory nerve)

These nerves are tested by assessing the weakness or wasting of the innervated muscles (upper trapezius and sterno-mastoid) by asking the patient to shrug their shoulders and turn their face to each side against resistance.

Cranial nerve XII (hypoglossal)

If this nerve or its nucleus is damaged, a deviation of the tongue to the side of the lesion can be seen, as well as wasting and fasciculation of the tongue on the same side (Fig. 3.4).

Motor function

The examination of motor function involves the assessment of:

- muscle bulk
- muscle tone
- muscle power
- reflexes

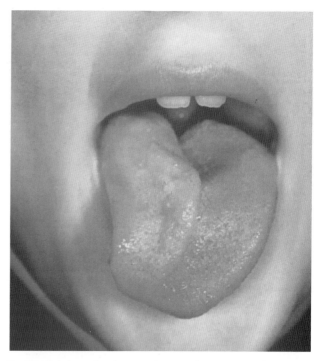

Fig. 3.4 Right hypoglossal nerve palsy; note the atrophy and fasciculation of the right side of the tongue.

- coordination
- presence of any involuntary movements.

Visual inspection to assess the bulk of muscles is very often ignored, and this is an important omission, as wasting of muscles can occasionally give clues to the pathology straight away. Do not say there is no wasting unless you have actually looked at all relevant muscle groups carefully! If necessary, ask the patient to remove or roll up clothing.

Muscle tone is reflected in the intensity of the stretch reflexes. It is also tested by passively flexing and extending the elbows, the wrists, and the hip, knee and ankle joints, and by pronating and supinating the wrists and assessing resistance to these movements. Muscles are hypertonic in Parkinson's disease, whereas hypotonia is seen in lower motor neurone or cerebellar damage. It is important to be able to assess the tone properly, as sometimes it can be the only pointer to pathology in an otherwise normal clinical examination.

The power is tested by assessing the strength of a muscle group across a joint, and is graded from 0 to 5 (Table 3.1). There are several tests for non-organic limb weakness. For example, if it is suspected that weakness of a leg is non-organic in origin, the hands of the examiner can be placed below both the patient's knees and the patient asked to lift the allegedly weak leg. If there is genuine weakness and the patient is really trying to lift that leg, the other leg will press down on the bed. If the weakness is due to hysteria, the other leg will not move.

Table 3.1 MRC scale for assessment of muscle power

0 = No muscle contraction visible (paralysis)

1 = Muscle contraction visible but no movement of joint

2 = Joint movement when effects of gravity are eliminated

3 = Movement sufficient to work against gravity

4 = Movement overcomes gravity and resistance

5 = Normal power

Reflexes

Reflexes can be divided into:

- stretch (deep tendon) reflexes
- superficial reflexes, such as the abdominal reflex and cremasteric reflex (not usually tested)
- brainstem reflexes—pupillary, corneal and gag reflexes (mentioned above)
- primitive reflexes—suck reflex, grasp reflex and palmomental reflex (their presence is often a sign of frontal lobe lesions).

There are several deep tendon reflexes. The standard neurological examination includes the biceps, brachio-radialis, triceps, knee and ankle reflexes. Their intensity can be graded from 0 to 4, where 0 is areflexia, 1 is sluggish, 2 is normal, 3 is hyperactive and 4 indicates the presence of clonus. The patient is examined in the seated or supine position, and the examiner uses a special light hammer to tap on the tendon of the muscle being tested. If reflexes cannot be elicited, reinforcement manoeuvres, such as asking the patient to try pulling apart their clenched hands, may be required. Asymmetrical decrease or loss of reflexes is due to peripheral nerve damage (radiculopathies, plexopathies or mononeuropathies). Hyperreflexia is a sign of upper motor neurone damage and is associated with spasticity and a positive Babinski sign. The latter is evaluated by slow and firm scraping of the sole of the foot on the lateral side. This should elicit a flexor response of the toes. The positive Babinski sign consists of an extension of the big toe, sometimes accompanied by an extension of the other toes. A positive sign is normal in children up to the age of 2 years. In adults, it is indicative of upper motor neurone damage. Occasionally, an equivocal response is obtained, when no movement of the big toe can be elicited at all. This can happen in some people naturally as well as in some pathological conditions, as in the aftermath of spinal cord injury.

Superficial reflexes (e.g. the abdominal reflex) are impaired if there is an upper motor neurone lesion above the spinal level tested. However, they are difficult to elicit in many patients (due to body fat obscuring muscle contraction) and so are less often tested.

Coordination

Good coordination of movement reflects the cooperation of separate groups of muscles. Poor coordination (ataxia) reflects problems with the afferent connections from muscles and joints with the cerebellum. The integrity of cerebellar function as well as that of several other components of the motor system is evaluated using coordination tests such as the finger–nose test and the heel–knee–shin test. When coordination is tested in the upper limbs, the presence of dysdiadochokinesia, i.e. the inability to execute rapidly alternating movements, is a sign of cerebellar ataxia.

Gait

The examination of gait involves an assessment of the patient's ability to rise from a chair, posture and postural stability, and ambulation. The difficulty in rising from a chair may reflect the weakness of muscles or basal ganglia disease. The posture of the patient is also pathognomonic for certain diseases. For example, Parkinson's disease patients have a stooping posture, whereas patients with progressive supranuclear palsy may have a rigid, hyper-erect posture. During assessment of ambulation, the examiner assesses speed, length of stride and ability to turn. Patients with Parkinson's disease have a shuffling, festinating (i.e. rapid and increasingly accelerating) gait, experience difficulty in stopping at will, and also have a decreased arm swing. Patients with progressive supra-nuclear palsy may present with a wide-based stride and slowing of ambulation.

For assessment of postural stability, the patient is asked to stand with the feet next to each other. Patients with cerebellar disease or labyrinthine problems may not be able to stand without separating the feet. The clinician may also perform the Romberg test, during which the patient is asked to stand still and close their eyes. Wide oscillations and a loss of equilibrium may reflect damage to the posterior columns. Ataxia can also be assessed, and is seen as an inability of the patient to walk in a straight line when asked to perform the heel-to-toe task, in which they must place the heel of one foot in direct contact with the toe of the other foot. The gait in cerebellar ataxia is 'drunken'. A waddling gait (like that of a duck) is due to proximal muscular weakness and is seen in muscular dystrophies and myopathies. It is important to remember, however, that the commonest disorders of gait in the general population are due to local pathology in the limbs, e.g. arthritis of hips, and it is important to exclude this.

Involuntary movements include chorea, myoclonus, athetosis, tremor, hemiballismus, dystonia and dyskinesia.

Sensory examination

This part of the examination evaluates the response to painful stimuli, temperature and light touch, and also vibration and joint position sense. It is important to note that sensory changes may be milder and more difficult to detect than motor or reflex changes. As in testing the cranial nerves and doing the motor examination, it is important to compare both sides of the body with each test before you decide whether the results are abnormal or normal. Nociception is tested through the pin-prick sensation. Temperature perception is tested with a cold object (e.g. the side of a tuning fork) but is less often tested than the pin-prick sensation. These are rarely tested together, because if one is present, almost invariably so is the other. Vibration is tested by placing a vibrating tuning fork on the bony prominences of the various joints tested. Light touch is assessed by dabbing a twist of cotton wool onto the skin of the patient (with their eyes closed) and asking them to say when and where they feel the stimulus.

During examination, comparisons of the two sides and proximal to distal are made in order to identify the site of the lesion. When a sensory deficit is suspected or identified, the examiner must determine its modality and map its distribution on a sensory examination chart to see if it matches that found with lesions of the peripheral nerve, spinal nerve, spinal cord, posterior fossa or supratentorial region. For example, decreased response to pin-prick on one half of the body is due to a lesion in the contralateral ascending pathways or the cerebral hemisphere. If the deficit is mainly distal and bilateral (e.g. 'stocking' or 'glove' distribution of a deficit), the cause may be a peripheral neuropathy. It is also important to note that considerable individual variation occurs in the segmental or radicular (dermatome) innervation patterns, and therefore in the anatomical location of dysfunction.

Cortical function

Tests assessing sensory cortical function depend on the integrity of the pathways to the brain; if they are damaged, then these tests should not be performed. Certain sensory and higher mental functions require specific intact cortical lobes. Spatial awareness/perception (parietal lobe) can be assessed by examining sensory input and spatial limb position with a variety of tests. Stereognosis is assessed by asking the patient to identify common objects, such as a key or money, by touch alone. Graphesthesia is the inability to recognize numbers or letters drawn on the skin by touch alone. Assessing the patient's ability to perform simple mathematical calculations such as addition or subtraction examines calculating skills, while asking a patient to copy a drawing of a symmetrical object, such as a clock, examines sensory neglect. All of these tests assess parietal lobe function. Damage to the parietal lobe (in particular to the right parietal lobe) gives rise to apraxias, the inability to grasp relations in space. Constructional apraxia, a failure to comprehend the spatial relationships of objects, can be identified by asking a patient to copy a construction made with building blocks, whereas ideomotor apraxia, a failure to judge limb position, can be identified by asking a patient to mimic getting dressed or copying arm movements made by the examiner.

Higher mental skills, such as reasoning, working memory and the organization and reorganization of information, are functions of the frontal lobes, and damage to these results in characteristic deficits. These abilities can be assessed using the following tests. Reasoning can be assessed by asking the patient to explain the meaning of idioms in their own words, e.g. 'people who live in glass houses shouldn't throw stones' or 'there's no smoke without fire'.

Working (short-term) memory is assessed by examining digit span recall. This involves verbally recalling the order of two series of numbers presented to the patient to view and then removed. If all are correctly recalled, another (longer) series of numbers is used and the test repeated. If these are all correctly recalled, the test is repeated until the subject makes an error on a trial at a given list length. Digit span corresponds to the length of the longest list for which the patient got both trials correct. The normal short-term memory span is between five and nine items. Normally, people show greater recall of numbers at the beginning of the list, as they are rehearsed more often, and good recall of numbers at the end of the list, as they have least time to decay from memory; numbers in the middle of the list are the ones most likely to be forgotten.

The Wisconsin card-sorting test is a sensitive test of executive functions such as rule-changing or set-shifting. The cards given to the patient have symbols on them that differ in number, shape and colour, and the examiner chooses a category for sorting the cards, such as by colour, shape or number. The patient must then sort the pack of cards, by placing each card in turn under an appropriate stimulus card based upon a rule that the examiner has generated (colour, shape or number). After the patient places each card on top of an appropriate stimulus card, the examiner says 'correct' or 'incorrect', depending upon whether their rule is being obeyed. For example, if the rule is shape, e.g. a circle, when the subject places a single cross on top of a single circle (working on a number rule) then they are wrong. The subject should continue placing the cards on top of the appropriate stimulus card until 10 successive correct placings have been scored. When this has been achieved, the sorting rule is changed. Scoring is done in two ways: categories achieved within the number of cards given, and perseverative errors. The former is the number of changes of criterion, and the latter is the number of errors caused by the subject continuing to choose a discontinued criterion. Damage to the frontal cortex gives rise to errors of these types, and the effect is particularly severe if the dorsolateral frontal cortex is damaged.

Abnormalities of speech and language may interfere significantly with history-taking and with the ability of the patient to perform parts of the rest of the examination; therefore, the assessment of any impairments is often performed at the beginning of the clinical examination. The clinician may detect aphasia (i.e. disorders of understanding and expression), dysphonia (disturbance of voice production) or dysarthria (problems with the articulation of words). Damage to Broca's area produces difficulties with verbal output, but not with comprehension, whereas damage to Wernicke's area does not affect verbal output; the subject is normally fluent, but the comprehension of language is impaired and they may talk rapidly, producing a jumble of speech that resembles a 'word salad'.

People with diminished levels of consciousness are assessed using the Glasgow Coma Scale, which is rated from a minimum of 3 to a maximum of 15. The three parameters assessed for this are the verbal, eye-opening and motor responses. A score of <8 indicates coma, 8–12 indicates a severe head injury, and >12 indicates a mild head injury.

The neurologist's approach to the examination of cortical function reflects the attempt to diagnose an organic (physical) disease of the brain that may disrupt mental functions, whereas in psychiatry the clinician may be more interested in dysfunctional brain syndromes that may not be associated with organic disease.

Other investigations

As well as the clinical examination, additional diagnostic techniques may be employed to help identify, or confirm the cause of the problem. Some are outlined below.

Nervous system imaging

Radiography

X-ray contrast images are produced by the differential absorption of X-rays as they pass through air, water, fat and mineral components of the body. Structures like the brain and spinal cord are mostly water and so are largely invisible on the image, whereas bone has high calcium content and so absorbs much X-ray energy. Radiographic analysis can reveal bony fractures (skull or spine) or misalignment, tumours and metastatic processes, general alterations in the skull, inflammatory processes, vascular abnormalities (aneurysms or malformations) or degenerative processes (e.g. calcification of intervertebral discs).

Computed tomography

During CT, a beam of X-rays scans the head or spine in a series of successive planes, and the differential absorption of the rays by the tissue is reflected in an image of the structures scanned. Images are obtained in the coronal or axial plane. CT is used in the diagnosis of brain infarcts and haemorrhages, fractures, hydrocephalus, cerebral atrophy and tumours. For skull analysis, computed tomography (CT) has superseded X-rays for most purposes. It is relatively insensitive to spinal cord pathology, although it can detect herniated discs and bony fractures. An additional injection of contrast medium can help display the vascular system and identify aneurysms and arteriovenous malformations. CT or magnetic resonance imaging (MRI) can be used interchangeably in some indications. However, there are instances when

one or the other technique is preferable. For example, CT is valuable in the evaluation of intracranial abnormalities in patients with craniocerebral trauma. Skull X-ray examination is more accurate for fractures of the cranial vault, whereas CT is preferable for fractures of the base of the skull. In particular, the acutely injured patient may not be amenable to a complex MRI scan. A CT scan (under 10s) is also shorter than an MRI scan (5–10 min), which is an important factor. Acute haemorrhage is also better demonstrated by CT than by MRI analysis. In contrast, MRI is preferable for evaluation of patients in a subacute phase of injury or with chronic injury. For example, 48 h after haemorrhage, even small collections of blood in subdural locations can be imaged by MRI, although they are not visible by CT. Herniation of discs, which ultimately results in compression of nerve roots, can also be rapidly imaged by CT.

Magnetic resonance imaging

MRI generates signals that are due to the interaction of hydrogen ions (essentially components of the water in the nervous tissue) with magnetic fields; it does not involve the use of X-rays. Initially, the protons are oriented in a strong magnetic field, and subsequently they are excited using a lateral magnetic pulse. During relaxation, they emit signals that can be decoded and transformed into an image that reflects the anatomical structures as a function of their water content. Because grey matter contains more water than white matter, a clear difference between the two tissue types is readily seen. Two types of image are obtained: T1-weighted and T2-weighted images (Fig. 3.5). T1-weighted images show details of the anatomy, whereas T2-weighted images highlight areas of increased signal density or pathology.

An easy way to differentiate between MRI and CT scans of the head is that bone appears white with CT and dark with MRI. Areas that are white or bright with CT are called high-density areas, whereas with MRI they are called high-signal areas. Gadolinium can be used as a contrast agent in MRI. Variations in the MRI analysis include fluid-attenuated inversion recovery (FLAIR) and diffusion-weighted imaging (DWI); both are used for detecting small lesion areas in acute ischaemic stroke. Although more cumbersome, MRI analysis has an advantage over the quicker CT scan. It is particularly good for seeing regions of demyelination in the central nervous system. For example, in multiple sclerosis, a normal CT scan may be obtained, whereas the MR image in the same patient will be grossly abnormal (e.g. T2-weighted images would show areas of increased signal intensity corresponding to plaques). MRI also gives better definition and sensitivity in tumour detection. MRI has become a procedure of choice for the evaluation of spinal abnormalities. MRI provides clear images of the spinal cord and roots and disc spaces, and helps in the definitive diagnosis in cases of spinal cord compression, syringomyelia or tumours. A practical limitation of MRI is that, since its strong magnetic field tends to shift any ferromagnetic objects, it can

T1   T2

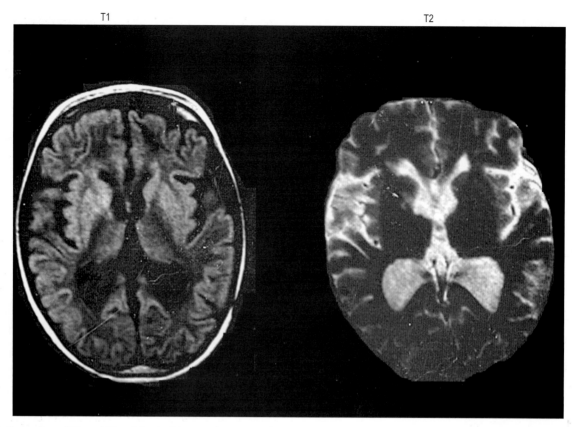

Fig. 3.5 Comparison of T1- and T2-weighted axial magnetic resonance images. The lipid component of the brain is bright in a T1-weighted image, so myelin gives a bright signal. Water (and hence cerebrospinal fluid-filled spaces) appears dark on T1-weighted images but bright on T2-weighted images.

only be used safely in the absence of metal implants (e.g. metal plates), defibrillators and pacemakers. Also, since the MRI machine is like a tube in which the patient has to lie still for long periods for the scan, it is not suitable for claustrophobic patients or people who are not very cooperative, such as children or confused patients, or people in a lot of pain.

Functional MRI (fMRI) is a variation of the technique that is predominantly used as an experimental research technique. It allows the correlation of anatomical location and function without injection of additional substances or tracers. In the brain, blood perfusion is related to neural activity, so fMRI (like positron emission tomography (PET)), can be used to explore the activities of various brain regions when subjects perform specific tasks or are exposed to specific stimuli.

Positron emission tomography and single photon emission tomography

PET is based on the use of compounds labelled with radioisotopes that emit positrons. ^{15}O-labelled compounds can be used to monitor cerebral blood flow and its fluctuations during cerebral activity. PET has a lower spatial and temporal resolution than fMRI. Single photon emission

computed tomography (SPECT) uses a similar principle to PET. The radioisotopes have a longer half-life than those used in PET, and they emit single photons. It is a less costly technique, but the resolution is significantly less.

Angiography and myelography

In analysis by myelography a radio-opaque contrast medium is injected into the lumbar or cisternal subarachnoid space by lumbar puncture (see Chapter 1), to visualize the spinal cord and roots. Myelography can be combined with CT to provide more information on structural changes. It is also possible to take a sample of cerebrospinal fluid (CSF) at the time of injection of the contrast medium. Since the advent of MRI, myelography has been less commonly used.

Angiography consists of the injection of contrast medium into the circulation, usually through a catheter placed in the femoral artery. It helps in the visualization of vascular abnormalities, aneurysms and the blood supply to tumours. This method is now being superseded by magnetic resonance angiography, which provides detailed information on vascular anatomy and blood flow without the need for use of contrast medium, although this can be given intravenously if required.

Doppler/duplex scanning

This technique uses ultrasound imaging of the carotid arteries of the neck. It can reveal arterial stenosis and the characteristics of blood flow through arteries. This is a useful screening method in the investigation of cerebrovascular accidents or transient ischaemic attacks.

Electrical activity

Electroencephalography

Electroencephalography (EEG) recordings are used to characterize globally the electrical activity of the brain. The activity is recorded with scalp electrodes placed equidistantly on the head. A normal EEG recording is characterized by well-defined rhythms that have specific frequencies. EEG is used primarily in the diagnosis of epilepsy, as the analysis of the traces can help identify the seizure locus as well as, in some cases, the type of epilepsy. EEG is also useful in ventilated unconscious patients to detect seizures, as in these patients there may not be any external evidence of seizure activity. It is also used occasionally to confirm brain death, when it can show whether the electrical activity of the brain has ceased or not. EEG can be used in combination with MRI.

Event-related potentials

Changes in EEG recordings can occur in response to stimuli. These are called event-related potentials (ERPs). ERPs are evoked in the primary cortical regions that correspond to the type of stimuli used (e.g. cutaneous stimulation triggers ERPs in somatosensory cortex). As an example, visual ERPs can be used to assess the integrity of the visual system and detect demyelination in the optic pathways. Auditory ERPs are less sensitive than visual ERPs, but can detect the presence of acoustic neuromas. Somatosensory ERPs test the integrity of somatosensory pathways and are sensitive in detecting, for example, the demyelination associated with multiple sclerosis. Evoked potentials can be distinguished from background noise and spontaneous activity with the use of signal-averaging techniques.

Electromyography and nerve conduction tests

These procedures are used in the diagnosis of muscular and peripheral nerve disorders. In electromyography (EMG), spontaneous, voluntary and electrically stimulated muscle activity is recorded, using intramuscular needles or surface electrodes. This technique can detect fibrillations or fasciculations. The latter are due to spontaneous motor unit discharges in degenerating nerve fibres causing irregular flickerings over the surface of the affected muscle, whereas the former arise when muscle fibres are denervated, and are due to the spontaneous and simultaneous discharges of muscle fibres in response

to release of acetylcholine from degenerating motor fibres; they are not visible to the naked eye.

Nerve conduction velocity assessment is based on the use of electrical stimulation of a nerve and measurement of the rate of action potential propagation along the nerve and the amplitude and time of the response. Motor nerve, sensory nerve and mixed nerve conduction studies can be carried out. Conduction studies are carried out in patients with suspected peripheral nerve damage, such as carpal tunnel syndrome (where the median nerve is compressed in the carpal tunnel) or diabetic neuropathy.

Cerebrospinal fluid examination

CSF examination is a procedure commonly used for the diagnosis of infection in the nervous system, multiple sclerosis or other neuroimmunological disorders, as well as to identify bleeding into the subarachnoid space. The CSF is sampled using a lumbar puncture procedure. In general, a CT scan should be performed before a lumbar puncture to rule out raised intracranial pressure. The CSF pressure is measured and fluid is withdrawn for analysis.

The normal volume of CSF is about 150 mL, and this is recycled about every 8 h. Maximum lumbar CSF pressure is 180–190 mm H_2O. An increase indicates infection, increased CSF production or decreased resorption, or the presence of a tumour. The concentration of glucose in the CSF is high in diabetes mellitus. A low glucose concentration may reflect infection or meningeal inflammatory processes. The latter can also be suggested by the presence of polymorphonuclear leukocytes in the CSF. Numbers of mononuclear cells are increased in chronic inflammation. Analysis of the protein types present in the CSF can demonstrate the presence of specific antibodies in multiple sclerosis patients. The CSF can also be analysed serologically in the diagnosis of syphilis. The presence of red blood cells or xanthochromia (a yellow discoloration indicating the presence of bilirubin) in the CSF often indicates subarachnoid haemorrhage.

General comments

In order to make a diagnosis when a lesion or dysfunction in the nervous system occurs, clinicians use certain theoretical constructs. This is particularly the case in neurology, and it is reflected in this overview of how the clinical examination proceeds in a logical and orderly fashion through the complexities of the nervous system. Constructs and models are helpful, even if constructs themselves may be changed by the rapidly advancing pace of knowledge in neuroscience. Examples of such simple constructs include: (1) the hierarchical organization of the nervous system (with higher functions represented rostrally and lower functions represented caudally); (2) the cerebral localization of function; (3) the topographical representation of body parts; and (4) the dominance of one hemisphere. It is important to remember at all times that such constructs are only tools, and the real world of neurology and psychiatry far exceeds any simple models of nervous system function. Neuroscience at the beginning of this millennium is characterized by buoyant and fascinating research findings that are changing many preconceived ideas, but it also remains the area of medicine where many clinical needs are unmet by our current therapeutic strategies.

THE SPINAL CORD

4

Chapter objectives

After studying this chapter you should be able to:

1. Relate the length of the spinal cord to vertebral levels and explain the nature of the cauda equina.

2. Describe the anatomy, organization and blood circulation of the spinal cord.

3. Recognize different segmental features of the spinal cord based on anatomical features.

4. Name the main sensory pathways that convey the sensory modalities of discriminative touch, pain and temperature and proprioception, their course from the periphery to the brain, where they decussate and the clinical signs associated with their damage.

5. Outline the effects of spinal cord trauma.

6. Recognize symptoms associated with distinct spinal cord syndromes.

7. Explain the anatomical basis for performing a lumbar puncture, its main clinical use and associated dangers.

Introduction

Spinal cord injury (SCI), whether through disease or trauma, causes a devastating loss of function below the level of injury and adversely affects several body systems. Moreover, because of the poor regenerative capacity of the central nervous system (CNS), patients suffer from lifelong disability that may range from partial loss of function, to complete quadriplegia and artificial ventilation. In the UK, it is estimated that there are more than 40 000 people suffering from traumatic SCI. This costs over £500 million in support and care. At least one-third to one-half of these patients are readmitted to hospital after the initial trauma.

Neurological assessment of patients with spinal cord damage requires an understanding of several concepts: the basic organization of the spinal cord, the relations between the main nervous pathways that relay sensory and motor information to and from the brain, and the ability to correlate radiological evidence of injury to the vertebral column with different segmental levels of the spinal cord.

The aim of this chapter is to describe the organization of the spinal cord, and the positions and functions of the various relay pathways that reside within it, and then to describe how these are affected in SCI.

Gross anatomy of the spinal cord and vertebral column

The spinal cord connects the brain to the peripheral nervous system (PNS). It is located within the vertebral canal, which provides structural protection, and is held in place by spinal roots, the denticulate ligaments and strands of pia mater (Fig. 4.1). The adult spinal cord is only about 18 inches (46 cm) long and extends from the foramen magnum to the level of the L2 vertebra. This is not so at birth, when it extends much lower (to the L3 vertebral level), but because the vertebral column grows faster than the cord, it leaves the cord positioned progressively higher up in the spinal canal. This means that different spinal cord levels can be related to specific vertebral levels (Table 4.1). The spinal cord tapers off at its caudal end to form the conus medullaris, and beyond this point the spinal canal is filled only with spinal roots descending caudally to find their intervertebral foramen. In the sacral region these fan out, resembling a horse's tail, and this is termed the cauda equina (see Fig. 4.1).

The spinal cord and spinal roots are covered by three layers of meninges—the dura, arachnoid and pia mater—and further protection is provided by the presence of cerebrospinal fluid (CSF), which surrounds the cord in the subarachnoid space. The pia is thin and is difficult to identify as a discrete membrane, except as the denticulate ligaments along the sides of the spinal cord. The denticulate ligaments span the space between the surface of the cord and the dura and have an important protective

mechanical function in relation to the cord. The lowest level at which they are observed is the L1 lumbar root level. The filum terminale is an extension of the pia mater that is attached to the coccygeal segments, whose function is to suspend the cord in the CSF (like the denticulate ligaments). The arachnoid and dura mater extend beyond the L2 level to the level of the S2 vertebra. Thus, if a sample of CSF is needed, a lumbar puncture needle can be inserted below the level of the L2 vertebra without fear of damaging the spinal cord (Box 4.2).

The size of the spinal cord is not uniform along its length. At the cervical and lumbar levels, the spinal cord enlarges to accommodate the increased sensorimotor connections involved with the limbs, via the cervical and lumbar enlargements. The cervical spinal cord is also largest because it carries tract fibres from lower body levels that are ascending to higher levels. Similarly, the size of the vertebral canal changes at different vertebral levels, being greater at the cervical and lumbar levels than at the thoracic levels. The thoracic region is small because the input is only from the ribcage area. As the sacral bones are fused, the canal is reduced to tiny foramina that contain the nerve fibres of the cauda equina. However, this has consequences, for if there is narrowing of the canal

---

Box 4.1	Case history

Humpty Dumpty sat on a wall and Humpty Dumpty had a great fall. He presents 2 weeks later, complaining of weak legs and unsteadiness of gait. He says that he was unable to walk the day after he fell, but progressively recovered movement later that week. Neurological examination reveals that he has muscle weakness and brisk reflexes in his right leg compared to the left leg and there is a Babinski sign in the right foot. Abdominal and cremasteric reflexes are absent on the right side, and there is no voluntary movement of the right leg. There is loss of joint position sense in the right leg, as he has inability to sense movement of his toes either up or down, and there is loss of responses to light touch and vibration on the right leg, extending up as far as the belly button. Also, there is a loss of temperature and pin-prick sensation in the left leg, which extends up the left side to his belly button. He is immediately sent for X-rays and further neurological tests at the local hospital.

This case gives rise to the following questions:

1. What is the location and organization of the sensory tracts in the spinal cord?
2. What is the location and organization of the motor tracts in the spinal cord?
3. What is the clinical significance of a Babinski sign?
4. Why are there dissociated sensory losses in both legs?
5. Where is the lesion?

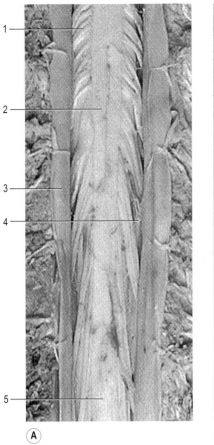

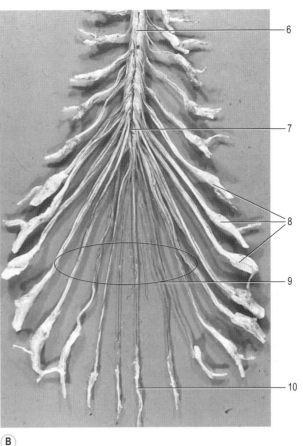

(A)   (B)

1. Cervical dorsal roots.
2. Posterior columns of cervical enlargement.
3. Cut dura mater.
4. Denticulate ligament.
5. Thoracic cord.

6. Spinal cord.
7. Conus medullaris.
8. Spinal ganglia.
9. Cauda equina.
10. Filum terminale.

Fig. 4.1 Gross anatomy of the spinal cord. (A) Dorsal view of the cervicothoracic region showing spinal dorsal roots and meninges. (B) Caudal end of spinal cord showing the cauda equina, conus medullaris, filum terminale and spinal roots.

Table 4.1 Relationship between vertebral level and spinal cord segmental level

Vertebral level	Cord level
Cervical, e.g. C6	Add 1, e.g. C7
Upper thoracic, T1–T6	Add 2 segments
Lower thoracic, T7–T9	Add 3 segments
T10	L1–L2
T11	L3–L4
T12	L5
L1	Conus medullaris
L2–L5	Cauda equina

space, as in spinal stenosis or whiplash injuries that cause vertebral damage (fracture dislocation), subsequent compression of the spinal cord, either directly, or indirectly due to oedema, may occur.

Functional organization of the spinal cord

The spinal cord receives sensory input from the periphery, relays it to the brain and sends motor response signals back to the periphery. The spinal cord is not segmented; rather, the distribution of the spinal roots gives it a functional segregation. The spinal cord is divided into two regions, the grey matter and the white matter. The grey matter is reminiscent of the shape of butterfly wings (Fig. 4.3). The white matter surrounds the grey matter,

Lumbar puncture

Lumbar puncture is performed with the patient lying on their side or leaning forward with their lower back flexed so that the ligamentum flavum is stretched and the vertebral laminae and spinous processes are stretched apart. The skin overlying the lower lumbar vertebrae is anaesthetized with local anaesthetic, and the needle (fitted with a stylet) is inserted in the midline between the L3 and L4 or L4 and L5 vertebrae (Fig. 4.2). After penetrating 4–6cm (more in obese patients), the needle punctures the dura and arachnoid mater to enter the lumbar cistern. This is the subarachnoid, or intrathecal, space (between the subarachnoid and pia mater). When the stylet is removed, cerebrospinal fluid (CSF) normally drips out at the rate of 1 drop/s. If the subarachnoid pressure is high, CSF may spurt out.

There are several reasons for performing lumbar puncture: retrieval of CSF is an important diagnostic tool for evaluating a variety of central nervous system diseases, as its cellular composition may change. Lumbar puncture can be used to introduce contrast media into the subarachnoid space to image the outline of the cord and it can also be used to provide analgesic relief during childbirth by inserting the needle tip into the epidural (extradural) space between the dura mater and vertebral ligaments.

In certain pathological conditions, CSF pressure may be elevated. CSF pressure is normally about 180–200 mmH$_2$O. Lumbar puncture is not performed in patients if examination of the fundus (back) of the interior of the eyeball with an ophthalmoscope reveals raised intracranial pressure. This is because the consequent release of pressure could cause a fatal herniation of the tonsils of the cerebellum through the foramen magnum onto the respiratory centres of the brainstem.

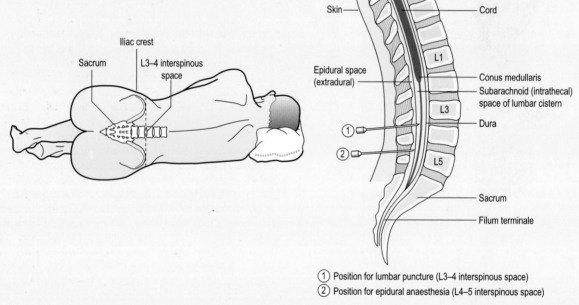

Iliac crest
Sacrum
L3–4 interspinous space

Skin
Cord
Epidural space (extradural)
L1
Conus medullaris
Subarachnoid (intrathecal) space of lumbar cistern
L3
Dura
1
2
L5
Sacrum
Filum terminale

1 Position for lumbar puncture (L3–4 interspinous space)
2 Position for epidural anaesthesia (L4–5 interspinous space)

Fig. 4.2 Procedure for performing lumbar puncture. Adapted from Moore KL, Dalley AF. Clinical Orientated Anatomy, 4th edn. LWW, 1999.

and the amounts of grey and white matter vary at different levels of the spinal cord (Box 4.3).

The spinal cord has two main functions:

1. To specify the characteristics of a stimulus in terms of its modality and position. This is a function of the grey matter.

2. To serve as a relay conduit for impulse propagation to and from the brain. Sensorimotor information is relayed via the dorsal, lateral and ventral funiculi of the white matter.

The grey matter of the spinal cord contains cells and terminals of primary afferents from the periphery. It can be subdivided into different functional regions: the dorsal (posterior) horn, which is associated with sensory perception, and the ventral (anterior) horn, which is associated with motor functions such as reflex movements. The latter contains motor neurones whose axons exit the cord via the ventral root, on their way to the muscles. At thoracic and sacral levels, these two regions are separated by the intermediate zone, which contains the lateral horn, where the cell bodies of the sympathetic and

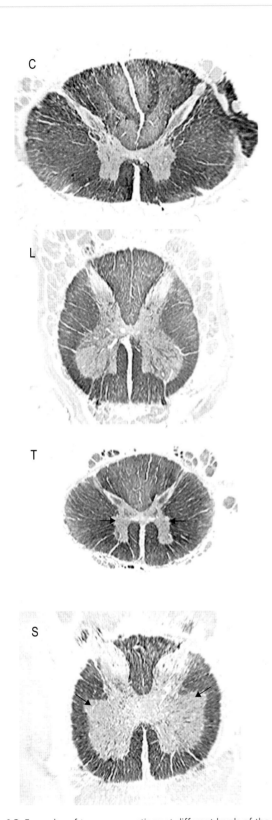

Fig. 4.3 Examples of transverse sections at different levels of the spinal cord showing relative differences in amount of grey and white matter and the shape of the cord. C, cervical; L, lumbar; T, thoracic; S, sacral. Arrows point to the location of the intermediate horn, which houses autonomic preganglionic neurones.

parasympathetic preganglionic fibres (the autonomic system outflow) are found.

The sensations of touch, pressure, pain, temperature and joint and muscle position sense (proprioception) are mediated by specific peripheral receptors. The primary afferents that carry these sensations terminate on cells in different regions (laminae) of the grey matter. The grey matter can be subdivided into 10 laminae (Fig. 4.4A). The dorsal horn is subdivided into six laminae based on cell size. Laminae I and II together constitute the superficial dorsal horn, which receives information from nociceptors. A pale-staining area through which few myelinated fibres pass caps the dorsal horn: this is lamina II, the substantia gelatinosa. This region is involved in the control of pain (see Chapter 5). Laminae III–VI receives input from low-threshold cutaneous receptors. The ventral horn consists of laminae VII–IX and contains cell bodies of motor neurones and interneurones and the terminals of primary afferents from muscle and joints. α-Motor neurone cell bodies are the most prominent cell structures visible in this region. Different muscles have their motor neurones located in discrete cell groups. The motor neurone populations supplying different muscles are differentially organized within the ventral horn (Fig. 4.4B). Distal muscles are represented laterally, while proximal muscles are located more medially. Extensor muscle groups are located more ventrally within the ventral horn, compared to flexor muscle motor neurones.

The grey matter is therefore functionally organized in terms of sensory modality, in the dorsoventral plane. Simplistically, proprioceptive afferents terminate in the ventral horn (to make connections with motor neurones to facilitate reflex activity), low-threshold cutaneous afferents terminate in the deep dorsal horn (laminae III–VI) and nociceptors terminate in the superficial dorsal horn (Fig. 4.4A). Also, within the grey matter at a given segmental level, there is a topographical representation of the periphery in the mediolateral plane. Thus, contiguous skin areas occupy contiguous areas of the spinal cord, and each peripheral nerve has its own terminal area within the spinal cord. Therefore, the site and nature of a peripheral stimulus can be encoded by its rostrocaudal, mediolateral and dorsoventral position within the dorsal horn. This is known as somatotopy, and this feature is faithfully replicated at all levels of the nervous system.

Spinal cord cell types

Spinal cord cells can be classified into two main types according to where their axons project:

- Interneurones represent about 97% of cells in the spinal cord. They are involved in modulating sensory input and motor output and make local connections with other cells in the spinal cord.

- Projection neurones represent the remaining cells. These can be subdivided into cells that give rise

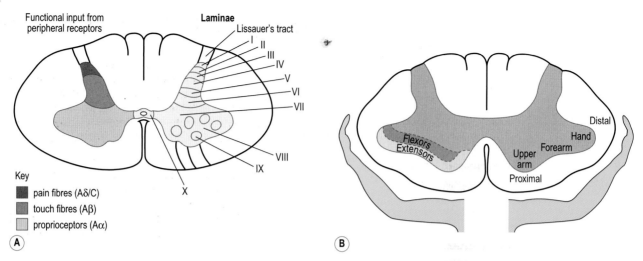

Fig. 4.4 (A) Schematic representation of the functional organization of sensory modality into different laminae of the spinal cord (indicated by Roman numerals). (B) Schematic topographic organization of motor neurones in the cervical ventral horn.

Box 4.3	Identifying segmental features of the spinal cord

From examination of the cross-sections of the spinal cords in Figure 4.3, it is obvious that different levels of the cord are different in shape. It is important to be able to differentiate cervical from thoracic, lumbar and sacral. There are several things to look for:

1. Overall shape. Cervical sections tend to be wide and oval-shaped as compared to, for example, the lumbar section, which appears round.
2. Amount of white matter relative to grey matter. This decreases along the rostrocaudal length of the cord: in the white matter of the cervical cord, there are essentially all the axons going to or from the entire body. In the sacral cord, the white matter contains only those axons going to or from the last few dermatomes; all other axons have 'exited' at higher levels. This is why the sacral cord looks like it has so much grey matter; in reality, it has only lost most of the white matter fibres.
3. Ventral horn enlargement. At segments that control a limb, the motor neurones are large and numerous. This causes enlarged ventral horns at two levels: the lower cervical sections (C5–C8) and the lumbar/sacral sections. If an enlargement is seen, one needs to differentiate cervical from lumbar levels. This can be done by shape or by proportion of white matter.
4. Presence of pointed tips which protrude between the small dorsal and ventral horns. This region is called the intermediate horn, or the intermediolateral cell column, and is the source of all of the sympathetic pre-ganglionic neurones in the body. It occurs only in thoracic sections.

to axons of the ascending pathways, comprising about 1% of the population, and motor neurones, representing the remaining 2% of spinal cord cells, whose axons project from the spinal cord to innervate skeletal muscles.

Spinal cord interneurones can be further classified into two main functional groups with respect to their action on other cells or sensory afferents:

1. Inhibitory neurones, which limit the receptive field (RF) size or activity of other neurones. They use inhibitory neurotransmitters such as γ-aminobutyric acid (GABA), glycine and enkephalin to regulate the activity of other neurones.
2. Excitatory neurones. These cells use glutamate and various neuropeptides as neurotransmitters, and their stimulation evokes action potentials in other cells.

The peripheral RF of excitatory neurones in the dorsal horn can be of three general types:

1. High threshold, which respond only to noxious stimuli.
2. Low threshold, which respond only to innocuous stimuli.
3. Wide dynamic range, which respond to both noxious and innocuous stimuli, i.e. they are multi-receptive neurones.

Receptive fields

An afferent in a peripheral nerve may form several branches when it reaches its peripheral target, and each branch ends in the same type of receptor. The area of skin (or muscle/viscera) where a stimulus can excite the sensory fibre is its RF. Cutaneous RFs measure about 2 cm² on the arm, but only 5 mm² on the fingertips. This gives rise to a

Table 4.2 Main ascending spinal pathways

Pathway	Function
Dorsal column medial lemniscus	Tactile discrimination and conscious proprioception (limb position sense)
Spinothalamic tract	Pain and temperature sensation; crude touch, itch, tickle
Spinocerebellar tract	Unconscious proprioception; assessment and integration of motor performance
Spinoreticular tract	Affective components of pain
Spinotectal tract	Integration of spinal (head/neck) reflexes with visual and auditory stimuli
Spino-olivary tract	Motor learning and modifying motor actions

differential sensory acuity between distal and proximal skin. For example, humans have better sensory acuity (ability to localize a stimu lus) on the fingertips than on the neck skin. The ability to distinguish between two separate simultaneous touches to the skin is called two-point discrimination.

The central branches of primary afferents converge onto cells in the spinal cord. Thus, the RFs of spinal cord cells are larger than those of primary afferents. Consequently, because of convergence, the RFs of higher-order neurones in ascending relay pathways get larger. However, they do not lose the ability to localize stimuli, because their RFs have a sensitivity gradient of excitation and inhibition; they are strongly excited in the middle of the RF and weakly excited at the edge, due to a phenomenon called surround inhibition. Stimulation of the peripheral area causes inhibition of neurones by activation of inhibitory interneurones. This process serves to focus neuronal activity, by opposing the spread of activity due to divergence in ascending pathways, so as to improve the resolution of stimulus localization.

Somatosensory pathways

The somatosensory system includes many types of sensation from the body: touch, pressure, pain, temperature, and joint and muscle position sense (proprioception). These modalities may or may not reach consciousness. They travel in different ascending pathways that are located in specific areas of the spinal cord white matter and terminate in specific areas of the brain. There are several ascending tracts, which travel to varying degrees in the spinal cord. Their names reflect where they originate and terminate in the nervous system. These are detailed in Table 4.2.

There are three important pathways that run the entire length of the spinal cord, and it is essential to know the location and sensory modalities associated with these

pathways, as damage to these pathways results in specific functional deficits.

1. The dorsal column medial lemniscus (DCML) pathway conveys information about discriminative touch. The perception of pressure, vibration and texture is mediated by $A\alpha/\beta$ fibres and enables us to 'read' Braille letters or numbers (graphesthesia), or describe the shape and texture of an object without seeing it.

2. The pain and temperature system uses free nerve endings in skin, muscle, bone and connective tissue to perceive changes in temperature or tissue damage. This is mediated by $A\delta/C$ fibres. These fibres also mediate the sensations of itch, tickle and crude touch. These modalities are conveyed by the spinothalamic tract (STT) pathway.

3. The third modality is called proprioception, and is conveyed by $A\alpha$ fibres, which include receptors for what happens below the body surface: muscle stretch, joint position and tendon tension. This pathway is the spinocerebellar tract (SCBT) pathway and it terminates in the cerebellum, which needs continuous feedback on what the muscles are doing.

Each of these main pathways will be described in turn, but they do share important common features. Each pathway consists of four neurones. Another important feature for conscious sensations is that they decussate (cross) to the contralateral side. Whenever crossing-over occurs, it is always the second-order neurone that decussates. Conceptually, one can consider the transmission of sensory information to consciousness as a 400-m relay team. Runner 1, the peripheral receptor, transfers the information to runner 2 in the spinal cord or brainstem. It is this runner who runs round the bend, or crosses over to the other side of the track (cord or brainstem), to take the information to runner 3, who usually resides in the thalamus (or cerebellum), depending on the pathway involved. This runner takes the information to its final destination in the cortex, where runner 4 receives the information. This relay is the most commonly used, but some afferent pathways, e.g. the spinoreticular tract (SRT), use more neurones, which then activate other areas of the cortex. In other cases, neurone collateral branches pass to motor neurones or interneurones, which then participate in reflex responses.

The discriminative touch system

The DCML system transmits mechanoreceptive sensations from the limbs, trunk and posterior part of the head to the dorsal column nuclei in the medulla. An analogous trigeminal nerve pathway, the trigeminal lemniscus, serving the face, transmits sensory information to the main sensory trigeminal nucleus in the pons. Receptors associated with these pathways have small RFs and do not show much convergence. Thus, this system provides the capacity to accurately define the quality, place, intensity and pattern of a stimulus. The capabilities of this system are:

- fine touch—the ability to recognize the exact location of light touch, and the ability to perform two-point discrimination
- stereognosis—the ability to recognize an object by feeling it
- conscious proprioception—the awareness of body position and awareness of body movements (kinaesthesia)
- weight discrimination
- vibration detection.

The pathway for this system is shown in Figure 4.5. The primary afferents ascend all the way to the medulla, on the same (ipsilateral) side of the cord as they entered, in the dorsal columns. A key feature of this pathway is that it is somatotopically organized, such that afferents from the lower limbs and trunk travel more medially in the gracile funiculus, and afferents from the upper limb travel more laterally, in the cuneate fasciculus, to their respective nuclei in the medulla. Similarly, the trigeminal input from the head is positioned lateral to the input from the body in the medulla. After synapsing in the dorsal column (or the analogous trigeminal) nuclei, the secondary neurones cross in the medulla and ascend as the medial lemniscus to the thalamus, where they synapse in the ventroposterior (VP) nucleus. In the VP nucleus, the head is represented medially and the rest of the body laterally. Finally, information ascends from the thalamus via the posterior limb of the internal capsule, to the primary somatosensory cortex (SI) in the postcentral gyrus.

SI cortex is necessary for the conscious awareness that a stimulus has occurred, and of its quality, location, intensity and duration. SI cortex is not, however, the final station in the somatic sensory pathway. SI cortex sends information to other cortical areas. Further important analysis of somatosensory information occurs in the posterior parietal association cortex. It is these areas that give meaning to the received stimulus. SI cortex is somatotopically organized (Box 4.4).

SI is subdivided into four functionally different zones, Brodmann's areas 1, 2, 3a and 3b, named after the famous German anatomist. Areas 3a and 3b receive about 70% of the input from the VP thalamus, and the other 30% goes to areas 1 and 2. Each area receives input predominantly from one type of somatosensory receptor. Area 3b mostly receives cutaneous input (from slowly and rapidly adapting receptors) and area 3a receives input from proprioceptors in muscles. Area 2 mostly receives input from joints and deep tissues (and is thought to be important for stereognosis), and area 1 receives information from rapidly adapting cutaneous mechanoreceptors. This leads to multiple representations of the body in SI and a rostrocaudal gradient of modality sensitivity in the order of muscle, skin and joint sensation. Within functional areas, cortical neurones are arranged in small vertical

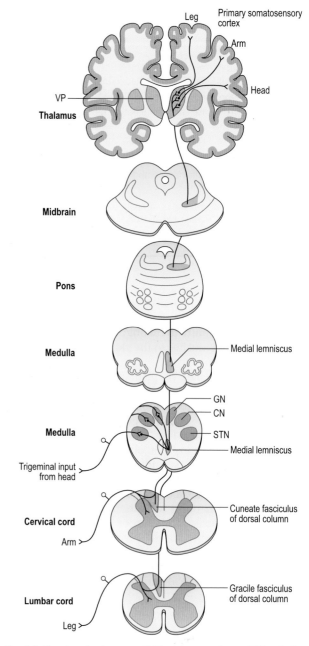

Fig. 4.5 The dorsal column medial lemniscus pathway. STN, spinal trigeminal nucleus; GN, gracile nucleus; CN, cuneate nucleus; VP, ventroposterior nucleus.

columns that have overlapping RFs, respond to the same submodality of stimulation, and have similar response latencies to synchronous afferent inputs.

Cells in the SI subregions also have different functions: area 3b is concerned with texture, shape and stimulus size, information about texture is transmitted to area 1, whilst information on size and shape is sent to area 2. Therefore, discrete lesions in these areas produce predictable deficits. For example, lesions in area 3b cause deficits in texture and shape discrimination, area 1 lesions prevent texture discrimination, and area 2 lesions impair the

Box
4.4 Somatotopic maps in the SI cortex

The dorsal column medial lemniscus (DCML) system is very orderly, in that fibres and cells carrying information from one part of the peripheral receptive surface maintain their positions relative to fibres and cells representing neighbouring parts of the receptive surface. Thus, different parts of the body are represented in an orderly sequence in the tracts and nuclei of the DCML system. This orderly arrangement of cells and fibres is called topographical organization. For the somatosensory system, it is usually called somatotopic organization (cf. retinotopic maps in the visual system and tonotopic maps in the auditory system). The somatotopic organization of SI cortex is shown in Figure 4.6. The extent to which a body part is represented in SI is related to its sensory acuity, not to its size.

The ability to perform point localization and two-point discrimination is best for the face (around the lips), hands (fingertips), and feet (toes). Somatosensory acuity, the ability to distinguish fine detail by touch, is directly related to the amount of neural tissue devoted to the representation of a body part, i.e. to the peripheral innervation density and to the volume of cortex representing the region. In general, the greater the peripheral innervation density, the smaller the receptive fields of the innervating neurones, and the larger the volume of cortex representing that region. Surround (lateral) inhibition also enhances the ability to localize stimuli and perform spatial discriminations by sharpening the profiles of activity within the somatotopically organized neural system.

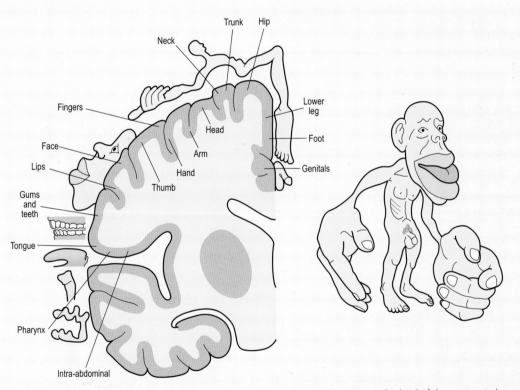

Fig. 4.6 Homuncular organization of the primary somatosensory (SI) cortex in a coronal section at the level of the postcentral gyrus. The body map is not scaled normally but looks like a caricature, with enlarged body parts correlating with areas of highest sensory acuity. Adapted from Penfield W, Rasmussen T. The Cerebral Cortex of Man. New York, Macmillan Press, 1952.

ability to grasp objects, and discriminate size and shape. This has been shown in experiments on monkeys, but in humans such lesions are rare and, in general, combination deficits occur.

These cortical areas have reciprocal connections with each other. Area 3a projects to areas 3b, 2 and the primary motor and premotor cortices, while area 3b projects to areas 1 and 2. All four areas send projections to an area called the secondary somatosensory cortex (SII), located in the parietal cortex, immediately posterior to SI. This area

is necessary for higher-order processing of somatosensory information. The functional importance of the SII cortex is unclear but it is somatotopically organized. One of its roles appears to be in processing aspects of pain; another appears to be tactile learning. For example, it is necessary for stereognosis. SII cannot process sensory information independently of SI. Lesions restricted to the posterior parietal association cortex do not impair the ability to detect a stimulus or even to assess its magnitude. Rather, they interfere with the ability to appreciate the meaning of a stimulus. In fact, in some instances, a lesion to the posterior parietal cortex leads to a loss of body scheme, so that the patient denies a profound left hemiparesis, neglects stimuli to the left side of the body, and even denies that the left side of their body is their own. Such deficits are much more common with right hemisphere lesions than with left hemisphere lesions (Box 4.5).

The ventrolateral system: pain and temperature

This system comprises several pathways that ascend in the ventrolateral part of the spinal cord and relay information to three main sites: the brainstem (via the SRT), hypothalamus (via the spinoparabrachial tract) and thalamus (via the STT). The STT is arguably the most important and conveys information about temperature and pain. These pathways are considered in more detail in Chapter 5. They are evolutionarily old and provide for perceptual capabilities that regulate normal body functions; that is, they are homeostatic in nature and have an emotional or affective component. The STT shares one major principle of organization with the discriminative touch system: primary afferents synapse ipsilaterally, and then the second-order neurones cross. The crossings just occur at different levels; the STT crosses in the spinal cord (usually within one or two segments of entry), whereas the DCML crosses in the brainstem.

Nociceptive afferents enter the spinal cord and ascend one to two segments rostral or caudal in Lissauer's tract (Fig. 4.4A) before entering the grey matter to connect with cells of the STT. The STT ascends the entire length of the cord, as shown in Figure 4.7, and the entire brainstem, staying in about the same location all the way up.

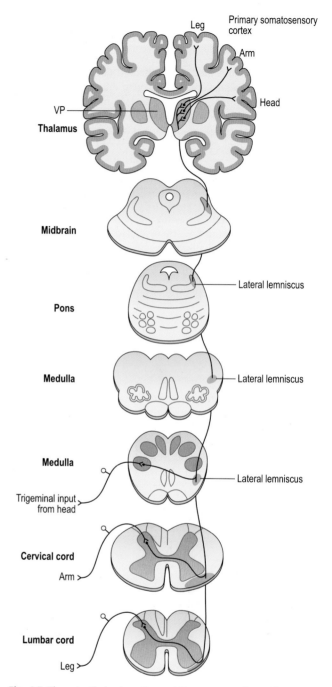

Fig. 4.7 The spinothalamic pathway. VP, ventroposterior nucleus.

As they ascend, new fibres are added to the tract from the anteromedial aspect, so that by the time this tract reaches cervical levels, the sacral fibres are the most lateral and the cervical ones are most medial. Thus, like the DCML tract, the pathway is somatotopically organized. This has clinical implications (Box 4.6). In the midbrain, the STT appears to be continuous with the medial lemniscus. Together, they will enter and synapse in the VP nucleus of the thalamus, and information is finally relayed to SI cortex by the thalamocortical neurones. An analogous pathway exists for the trigeminal nerve. Nociceptors from the face terminate in the spinal trigeminal nucleus of the medulla and then cross to travel in the trigeminal lemniscus to join with the ascending STT fibres running in the spinal lemniscus. These fibres then terminate in the ventroposteromedial thalamic nucleus and from there are relayed to the facial part of the SI cortex.

The STT can be divided into anterior (paleo) and lateral (neo) STT subparts that convey different sensory modalities. The anterior region contains the axons from cells that arise in lamina VII and convey sensations of crude or sensual touch, itch, tickle and pressure from one side of the body to the contralateral cerebral hemisphere. Axons of the lateral STT are more concerned with 'fast pain' from one side of the body to the opposite cerebral hemisphere. This pathway encodes information about stimulus location, intensity and modality.

Other ventrolateral pathways

Spinoreticular tract

This is the oldest ascending pathway in evolutionary terms, and mediates 'slow' pain. The cells originate in laminae V–VII and accompany the STT tract as far as the brainstem reticular formation, to activate the ascending reticular activating system. Stimuli in this pathway are of a general and non-specific nature and act to participate in reflex activity or to relay information to thalamic nuclei. The SRT has two main functions: to arouse the cortex and to stimulate the limbic cortex with regard to the nature of the stimulus. Ascending fibres of this tract are both crossed and uncrossed at segmental levels. Visceral pain is often associated with this pathway.

Spinotectal tract

This pathway runs medially alongside the STT, from the cervical spinal cord to the superior colliculus in the midbrain. It is a crossed pathway that integrates with visual input to mediate visuospinal reflexes in response to tactile stimuli, by turning the eyes/head or body towards a tactile stimulus.

Spino-olivary tract

This crossed pathway runs laterally to the STT and ascends from the spinal cord to the inferior olivary nucleus (ION) in the medulla. The ION is associated with motor learning and relays information from proprioceptors to the contralateral cerebellum. It is thought that this tract may play a role in modifying movements when a moving body part encounters an unexpected obstacle.

Damage to the ventrolateral pathways in the spinal cord through injury, or surgical intervention, results in decreased pain and temperature sensitivity on the contralateral side below the level of the lesion. There is also reduced touch sensation. This is not the case if the lesion

---

Box 4.6 **Clinical relevance of topographical organization of neural pathways**

All the main ascending and descending pathways are topographically organized with respect to the various segmental levels. For the DCML pathway, the sacral and lumbar segments are located medial to the thoracic segments, which are located medial to the cervical segmental input. In contrast, in the spinothalamic tract and corticospinal tract pathways, cervical axons are most medial and sacral most lateral (Fig. 4.8). This is of clinical relevance when an injury or disease affects specific relay pathways. For example, if there is external pressure on the spinal cord, it can explain why there is first a loss of pain and temperature sensation in sacral dermatomes and, if the pressure increases, the loss progresses to lumbar and thoracic levels as higher dermatomes are affected. Similarly, if the problem occurs within the spinal cord, such as in syringomyelia or whiplash injury, then the cervical dermatomes will be affected first, and the lower body is less affected. Often, these patients show sacral sparing, with preservation of all sensations, reflexes and muscle tone in this region.

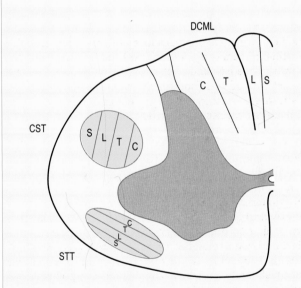

Fig. 4.8 Topographic organizations of the dorsal column medial lemniscus (DCML), spinothalamic (STT) and corticospinal (CST) tracts in a hemi-cross-section of the spinal cord. C, cervical; T, thoracic; L, lumbar; S, sacral.

---

is in the brainstem, because the fast pain fibres that ascend in the STT run laterally, whereas the slow pain fibres running in the SRT ascend more medially. Thus, damage to the STT in the brainstem results in decreased sensitivity and localization of pain and temperature sensation but not the loss of the emotional quality of the sensation.

A surgical procedure called percutaneous chordotomy uses radiofrequency lesioning of the ventrolateral tracts at cervical levels to alleviate the intractable pain associated with some forms of cancer. The relief of pain is not permanent, however, and the induced analgesia subsides after a year or more. The reoccurrence of pain sensations occurs because pain also travels in other uncrossed pathways such as the SRT, and visceral pain travels via the dorsal columns (see Chapter 5).

The proprioceptive system

Proprioception can be divided into conscious and unconscious proprioception. Both are mediated by muscle and joint afferents. The former travels in the DCML and deals with aspects such as judging the weight of an object or where a person's limbs are in space. Unconscious proprioception serves as an important backup to conscious proprioception, and is the sensation of limb and joint position and range and direction of limb movement. It is involved in the acquisition and maintenance of complex, skilled movements such as walking, talking and writing. Unconscious proprioception is mediated by the SCBT, whose primary function is to monitor and modify movements.

The proprioceptive system axons from muscle and joint receptors travel in the dorsal columns. Within a few segments, however, axons responsible for the proprioceptive information concerned with postural adjustments that occur unconsciously, leave the white matter and synapse in Clarke's nucleus (nucleus dorsalis), located at the base of the dorsal horn on the medial side from T1 to L1 of the spinal cord. The second-order neurones then enter the dorsal SCBT on the lateral edge of the cord. This pathway ascends without crossing to the cerebellum and is also somatotopically organized. The SCBT remains at the lateral margin of the brainstem through the medulla, where it enters the cerebellum via the inferior cerebellar peduncle (ICP) to terminate on Purkinje cells. Purkinje cells relay the information to the deep cerebellar nuclei, and from there it is passed to other motor areas of the thalamus, brainstem and basal ganglia. Because Clarke's column only extends from T1 to L1, it only carries information from the lower body and trunk. Information from the upper body is relayed by the cuneocerebellar tract to the accessory cuneate nucleus, and from there to the cerebellum via the ICP. Similarly, information from the face travels in the trigeminocerebellar tract to the cerebellum (Fig. 4.9).

A second spinocerebellar pathway exists and travels in the lateral white matter, just ventral to the dorsal SCBT. The axons of this pathway arise from cells in lamina VII of the spinal cord and receive a diverse input from proprioceptors, nociceptors and descending pathway tracts such as the vestibulospinal and reticulospinal tracts. The ventral SCBT seems to defy the ipsilaterality of the cerebellum, because the fibres cross over in the cord. However, they cross back before entering the cerebellum via the superior cerebellar peduncle. Therefore, the cerebellum still receives information from the ipsilateral side of the body. Ventral SCBT cells have large RFs and

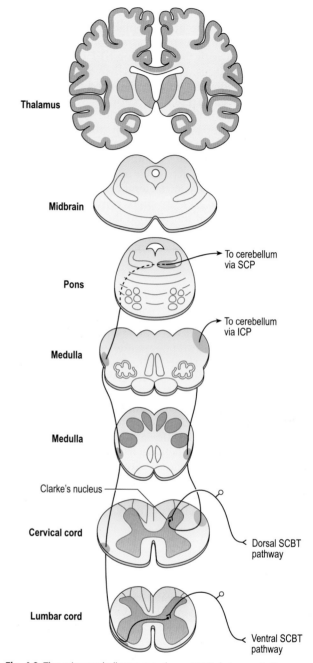

Fig. 4.9 The spinocerebellar tract pathway. ICP, inferior cerebellar peduncle; SCP, superior cerebellar peduncle; SCBT, spinocerebellar tract.

appear to act as comparators of descending inputs and other inputs to motor neurones.

Summary of somatosensory pathways

To summarize, the three main ascending somatosensory pathways each carry a specific modality of sensation associated with specific receptors. Each pathway is somatotopically organized, so that a complete representation of the body is reproduced in each relay nucleus along

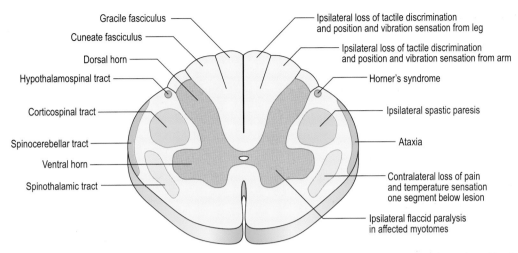

Gracile fasciculus
Cuneate fasciculus
Dorsal horn
Hypothalamospinal tract
Corticospinal tract
Spinocerebellar tract
Ventral horn
Spinothalamic tract

Ipsilateral loss of tactile discrimination and position and vibration sensation from leg
Ipsilateral loss of tactile discrimination and position and vibration sensation from arm
Horner's syndrome
Ipsilateral spastic paresis
Ataxia
Contralateral loss of pain and temperature sensation one segment below lesion
Ipsilateral flaccid paralysis in affected myotomes

Fig. 4.10 Clinical deficits associated with damage to the main ascending and descending pathways at the cervical spinal cord level. Adapted from Fix JD. High Yield Neuroanatomy. Williams and Wilkins, 1995.

the pathway. Any sensory system going to the cerebral cortex will have to cross over at some point, because the cerebral cortex operates on a contralateral basis. The discriminative touch system crosses in the medulla and the pain system crosses in the spinal cord. The proprioceptive system ascends to the cerebellum and does not cross. There is some overlap of modalities between the ascending tracts: some light touch information travels in the STT, so that lesioning the dorsal column does not completely abolish touch and pressure sensation; similarly, visceral pain fibres travel in the dorsal columns and not the STT. Discriminative proprioception also travels in the dorsal columns and follows the medial lemniscus all the way to the cortex, so there is conscious awareness of body position and movement. The pain and temperature system, although it does ascend to the somatosensory cortex, also has multiple targets in the brainstem and other areas. Knowledge of the pathways, point of decussation and cortical areas associated with conscious perception of sensation provides a framework for understanding sensory deficits after damage. This is summarized in Figure 4.10.

As well as conveying sensory information to supraspinal levels, the spinal cord white matter contains many descending pathways (Table 4.3). The main descending pathway is the corticospinal tract (CST), which regulates the control of voluntary movement. Damage to this pathway produces hyperreflexia, hypertonia and a Babinski sign. These descending pathways and their dysfunction are more fully covered in Chapter 9.

The hypothalamospinal tract is clinically important, as damage to this pathway results in Horner's syndrome, which is characterized by miosis, ptosis and anhydrosis. Signs are always ipsilateral. The pathway runs directly from the hypothalamus to the ciliospinal centre, located in the intermediolateral cell column of the T1–T2 spinal cord. It descends through the lateral tegmentum of the brainstem to run in the dorsolateral quadrant of the dorsolateral funiculus.

Table 4.3 Main descending spinal pathways

Pathway	Function
Corticospinal	Control of fine voluntary movement
Rubrospinal	Regulates muscle tone in antigravity (extensor) muscles
Vestibulospinal	Regulates neck muscles involved in head balance reflexes
Raphe spinal	Pain modulation
Coeruleospinal	Autonomic nervous system reflex modulation
Reticulospinal	Postural control via regulation of flexor and extensor reflexes
Tectospinal	Head and neck postural reflex responses to auditory and visual cues
Hypothalamospinal	Sympathetic nervous system control of visceral activity

Blood supply to the spinal cord

Two posterior spinal arteries and a single larger anterior spinal artery supply the spinal cord. These are derived from the vertebral artery. The posterior arteries supply the posterior third of the cord, while the anterior spinal artery supplies the anterior two-thirds of the cord (Fig. 4.11). However, this is not enough to maintain an adequate blood supply to the spinal cord. At each spinal segment, these arteries are reinforced by segmental radiculospinal arteries, which are branches of the body wall arteries. Also, the anterior spinal arteries give rise to smaller penetrating arteries, which anastomose with similar arteries from the posterior spinal arteries within the spinal cord tissue. Radicular arteries supply the dorsal and ventral roots.

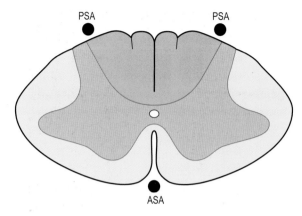

Fig. 4.11 Distribution of main arterial supply to the spinal cord. ASA, anterior spinal artery; PSA, posterior spinal artery. The yellow area demarcates the distribution of the PSA; the remainder demarcates the ASA territory.

These do not connect to the anterior or posterior spinal arteries, and only supply the roots. The venous drainage is by means of three anterior and posterior spinal veins that drain outwards along the nerve roots. They have a similar distribution to the arterial supply and drain into the internal (epidural) and external vertebral venous plexus along the vertebral column, and from this plexus to ascending lumbar veins, the azygos vein and hemiazygos veins.

Damage to the spinal cord

SCI can arise from trauma, degenerative diseases, ischaemia, and infectious, toxic or metabolic disorders (Table 4.4). SCI can either be complete, meaning that there is no voluntary movement or sensation below the level of the lesion on both sides, or incomplete, when there is a variable amount of function below the level of the lesion. The level of the lesion is helpful in predicting the deficits in body function that might occur and how much independence the patient might have after the injury (Table 4.5). The location of the lesion must be at, or above, the level of the highest neurological sign. (For a better understanding of the impact of SCI, see the discussion on the descending pathways in Chapter 9.)

Trauma injuries are often the most common and can be caused directly by penetrating injuries such as gunshot or stab wounds, or indirectly as a result of compression or flexion/extension injuries of structures associated with the vertebral column. This can lead to sensory, motor or sphincter dysfunction or a combination of these, depending on whether the lesion is uni- or bilateral. One of the earliest signs of SCI is pain. Motor dysfunction also occurs early, resulting in hypotonia, muscle wasting and paralysis. Depending on the level of the lesion, there may be deficits in cardiovascular, respiratory and autonomic (bladder, sweating and sexual) function, as well as a loss of protective functions such as pain and temperature sensation (see Table 4.5). These lead to a number of secondary problems, such as urinary infections, pressure sores

Table 4.4 Some common causes of spinal cord injury

Cause of SCI	Example
Trauma	Acts of violence
	Penetrating wounds
	Compression injury (e.g. prolapsed disc)
	Whiplash
	Sports (e.g. diving)
Demyelinating disease	Multiple sclerosis
	Spinal muscular atrophy
	Syringomyelia
	Poliomyelitis
	Spina bifida
Infection	AIDS
	Spinal meningitis
	Tuberculosis
	Syphilis
	Lyme's disease
Metabolic disorder	Subacute combined degeneration (vitamin B_{12} deficiency)
Vascular	Anterior spinal artery occlusion
Tumour	Primary or secondary cancer
	Abscess

and a loss of unconscious control mechanisms, such as regulation of CNS neuronal excitability.

Imaging the spinal cord

In order to assess the possible causes of spinal cord damage, various imaging techniques are used. X-rays can detect vertebral damage due to trauma or cancer, and the radiographs are commonly viewed in the anteroposterior (longitudinal) and lateral directions. X-rays do not visualize the spinal cord but infer damage by changes in the alignment of the vertebral column or reduction of the size of the vertebral canal. Computed tomography (CT) can be used to visualize infarcts and tumours in neural tissue. Magnetic resonance imaging (MRI) can differentiate between grey matter and white matter, so this method is particularly sensitive for distinguishing CNS tissue. It is particularly sensitive for imaging areas of focal demyelination and spinal cord lesions. It can provide axial as well as longitudinal images of the entire spinal cord and is now the method of choice for study of the spinal cord, nerve roots and disc spaces or signs of narrowing (stenosis) or damage (e.g. disc herniation, Fig. 4.12). Myelography requires the introduction of a radio-opaque material into the subarachnoid space by lumbar puncture (see Box 4.2). The fluid travels over the surface of the cord and spinal roots, providing an outline of their structure. This technique is widely used to outline abnormalities of nerve

Table 4.5 Effects of spinal cord injury at different segmental levels in humans*

Segment	Consequence	Patient independence
C1–C2	Quadriplegia	None
	Requires ventilated respiration	Often die at scene of injury
	Acute sympathetic shock syndrome (bradycardia, hypotension, bilateral Horner's syndrome and loss of thermoregulation)	
	Reflex bladder (damage to upper motor neurone control of micturition)	
C4–C5	Quadriplegia	None
	Impaired respiration	Requires constant care
	Reflex bladder (urinary retention and constipation)	
C6–C7	Quadriplegia with impaired arm control	Minimal
C8–T1	Impaired respiration	Requires personal care
	Reflex bladder	Can drive a car with special braces
	Paraplegia	
T2–T3	Impaired respiration	Complete
	Poor trunk control	
	Reflex bladder	
	Paraplegia	
T12–L1	Paraplegia	Complete
	Reflex bladder	
L4–L5	Paraplegia	Complete
	Reflex bladder	
S2–S3	Non-reflex bladder (damage to lower motor neurones, leading to failure to void)	Complete

*Bradycardia, hypotension, bilateral Horner's syndrome and loss of thermoregulation.

roots or to detect localized areas of spinal cord damage due to external compression or penetration (Fig. 4.13).

Pathophysiology of spinal cord injury

Spinal cord damage can be seen as occurring in two phases:

1. Primary damage resulting from cord compression, contusion, laceration or haemorrhage, which occurs immediately on injury.

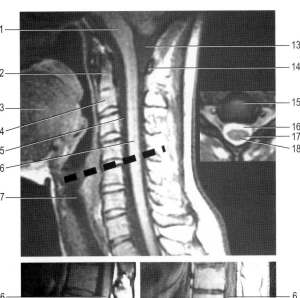
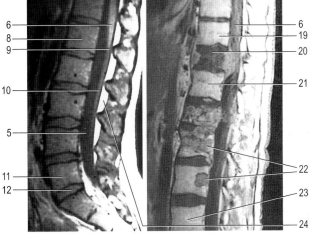

1. Medulla.
2. Dens. of axis.
3. Tongue.
4. C2 vertebra.
5. Subarachnoid space.
6. Spinal cord.
7. Trachea.
8. L1 vertebra.
9. Conus medullaris.
10. Filum terminale.
11. L5 vertebra.
12. Intervertebral disc.
13. Foramen magnum.
14. Atlas.
15. Vertebral body.
16. Cerebrospinal fluid.
17. Grey matter.
18. White matter.
19. T11 vertebra.
20. Herniated cancerous disc.
21. T12 vertebra.
22. Degenerating vertebrae.
23. L4 vertebra.
24. Epidural fat.

Fig. 4.12 Magnetic resonance image of the spinal cord in the sagittal plane. Top: Cervical cord. Inset shows the cord imaged in the transverse plane at the level of the dashed lines. Here (in this T2-weighted image), the grey matter appears paler than the white matter and the cerebrospinal fluid is white. In the remaining images, the cerebrospinal fluid appears black. Bottom left: a normal magnetic resonance image of the thoracolumbar vertebral region, showing the end of the spinal cord. Bottom right: magnetic resonance image showing metastatic intervertebral disc herniation into the spinal canal and compressing the spinal cord.

Normal

Pathological

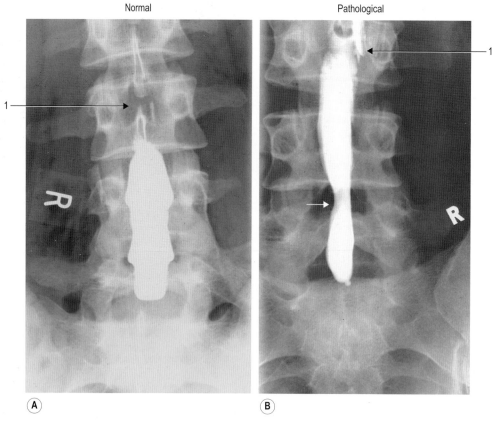

(A)

(B)

Fig. 4.13 Imaging of the spinal cord: Myelography. Anteroposterior view of X-ray images showing contrast outline of the cord. The arrow indicates cord compression by an external structure not visible with X-rays.
1. L3 vertebra.

2. Secondary damage that is initiated by the trauma but occurs over a period of hours, days and months. This mainly involves physiological alterations due to trauma, hypoxia and ischaemia.

Macroscopic damage to the cord

The cord is often swollen and congested even after mild focal indentation, or severe haemorrhagic disruption, usually above and below the level of the lesion (Fig. 4.14). The swollen cord can occupy the entire vertebral canal, causing secondary ischaemia when the swelling exceeds the venous blood pressure. This ischaemia is further exacerbated by loss of autoregulation of blood flow, causing systemic hypotension leading to spinal shock (see Box 4.7) and secondary damage through excitotoxicity.

Microscopic effects of spinal cord injury

In the acute phase of traumatic cord injury, there are variable amounts of oedema, microhaemorrhaging in the grey matter, axonal swelling, ascending/descending tract disruption and foci of infarction. In the first 24h, axons die back from the point of injury and the area of the

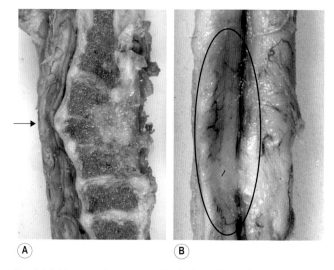

(A)

(B)

Fig. 4.14 Macroscopic anatomy of spinal cord injury. (A) Sagittal section of the spinal cord and vertebral column, showing focal indentation of the ventral spinal cord at the C4 level (arrow). (B) Gross anatomy of the cord following its removal from the vertebral column, showing compression of the ventral horn (oval).

initial injury doubles in size, growing further as the area of hypoperfusion spreads from the grey matter into the white matter. Clearly, this early period presents a period of therapeutic opportunity to limit lesion size if appropriate drugs can be used. Damaged cells, axons and blood vessels release (toxic) chemicals that kill neighbouring tissue. For example, the injury area is flooded with the neurotransmitter glutamate, which then overstimulates adjacent neurones and glial cells, leading to a massive Na^+ and Ca^{2+} influx into cells that cause them to swell and burst and release their cellular contents and free radicals into the extracellular space to continue the process. This excitotoxic cascade also affects the oligodendrocyte cells that myelinate the CNS tracts. This leads to demyelination of surviving fibres and more dysfunction.

Over the following few weeks, there is macrophage infiltration and a gradual removal of degenerative debris (axons, neurones). At the site of injury, the grey matter becomes necrotic and may cavitate. As time progresses, there is infiltration by fibroblasts, and associated collagenous fibrosis occurs, forming scar tissue, providing an impenetrable barrier to regeneration. Frequently, cavitation involves the ventral part of the dorsal columns, which is maximal at the site of injury but may extend a few segments rostral or caudal to the injury. Finally, days or weeks after the initial event, some cells undergo apoptosis, causing another wave of death that may affect up to four spinal segments rostral or caudal to the injury site.

In almost all lesions, even in apparently complete SCI, not all ascending or descending axons are severed, and a peripheral ring at the outer edge of the white matter remains intact (Fig. 4.15). For example, if as few as 10% of the descending CST fibres survive, the patient may be able to walk, whereas if fewer than 4% remain they are unable to do so. However, surviving fibres often do not look normal; they have been stripped of their insulation and so may not conduct nerve impulses properly.

The severity of SCI is graded using the American Spinal Injury Association (ASIA) impairment scale (Table 4.6), which uses neurological and functional assessment of sensory and motor function in 10 muscle groups and 28 dermatomes.

The prognosis for SCI depends on whether the lesion is extrinsic, i.e. outside the substance of the spinal cord (e.g. tumour, in which case it can often be removed surgically, resulting in recovery of function), or intrinsic within the spinal cord. Research has shown that the most important predictor of improved spinal cord outcome is retention of sacral sensation (S4–S5 dermatomes), especially pin-prick sensation, 3–7 days after injury. In general, most SCI patients may regain one level of motor function, and most recovery, if it is to happen at all, occurs within the first 6 months after injury. Ten to 15 per cent of ASIA grade A patients may progress to grade B–D, but very few regain functional strength below the level of the lesion, whereas half of grade B patients will regain functional strength below the lesion and nearly 90% of grade C and D patients recover sufficient strength to walk again.

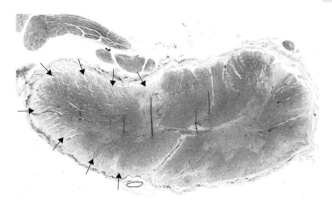

Fig. 4.15 Transverse section showing spinal cord compression; note the distortion of the grey matter on the side of compression and demyelination at the lateral edge of the white matter of the cord on the injured side (arrows).

Table 4.6 ASIA impairment scale

Grade	Description
A	Complete SCI; no preservation of sensory or motor function in S4–S5 cord
B	Incomplete: sensory but not motor function below the neurological level and extending through to S4–S5 cord
C	Incomplete; motor function preserved below the lesion site; most key muscles have strength of <3 (Medical Research Council (MRC) grade score)
D	Incomplete; motor function preserved below the lesion site; most key muscles have strength of <3
E	Normal sensory and motor function

Spinal cord syndromes

Compression of the spinal cord is most often caused by extradural problems, such as disc herniation or primary or secondary vertebral tumours or abscesses (see Figs 4.12 and 4.13). Tumours that arise outside the spinal cord (extramedullary), such as meningiomas or nerve fibromas, may compress the cord; those originating in the cord (intramedullary) are rarer, and include tumours such as gliomas (glial cell carcinomas). Pressure arising from any of these causes may interfere with the arterial or venous blood supply, causing ischaemia or oedema, and conduction blockage in fibres in the white matter, which, if prolonged, may cause focal demyelination. Compression may also cause blockage of CSF flow and changes in the composition of CSF below the level of the lesion. One of the earliest signs of compression injury is pain, which may be restricted to one or more spinal nerves, and the pain is made worse by exercise, coughing or sneezing, or lying down. Motor dysfunction occurs early, resulting in paralysis, spasticity and exaggerated reflexes below the level of the lesion. The degree of sensory loss will depend on the nerve tracts involved. Surgery to remove the extradural

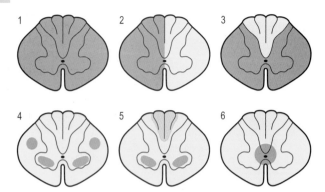

Fig. 4.16 Schematic representations of areas of damage in distinct spinal cord syndromes. 1, complete cord transection; 2, spinal cord hemi-section; 3, anterior cord syndrome; 4, amyotrophic lateral sclerosis; 5, infectious diseases; 6, syringomelia.

Box 4.7 Spinal cord shock

Clinically, there is pain at the level of the injury and a variable amount of sensorimotor loss below the level of the lesion. Severe spinal cord injuries often initially produce spinal shock: a state of temporary loss of function in the spinal cord. All of the functions and muscle reflexes below the level of the lesion are depressed or absent, due to the removal of all descending motor pathways, giving the impression of flaccid paralysis of muscles and loss of sensation. If the lesion is at high cervical levels, severe hypotension may occur as a result of loss of sympathetic vasomotor tone. Spinal shock often lasts about 1 day but may persist for up to a month, after which the spinal cord neurones gradually regain their excitability and the flaccid paralysis gives way to spastic paresis. The first reflexes to reappear are the flexion reflexes. Even after these reappear, limbs are flaccid in the absence of tonic stretch reflex activation. After several months, a return of muscle tone and tendon reflexes may occur.

The presence of spinal shock can be determined by testing the integrity of the anal sphincter reflex (checking for anal sphincter contraction after pulling of the glans penis or clitoris or by pulling on an inserted Foley catheter). However, a sacral cord lesion would nullify this test, as the S2–S4 nerve supply may be damaged.

---

and extramedullary causes is usually successful at reversing the symptoms, provided that irreversible damage due to compromised blood flow has not occurred.

Figure 4.16 details six distinct spinal cord syndromes caused by destructive lesions; the functional losses associated with these syndromes are predictable from knowledge of the anatomy of the spinal cord. The clinical symptoms associated with these syndromes are detailed below. In the first three, the characteristic symptoms appear after an initial period of spinal shock (see Box 4.7) has ended.

Complete cord transection

There is complete loss of all sensory, voluntary movement and autonomic functions below the level of the lesion. Thus, there is bilateral lower motor neurone paralysis and atrophy at the damaged level, bilateral spastic paresis and Babinski sign below the lesion, loss of bladder and bowel function and bilateral loss of all sensation below the level of the lesion. If the injury is a vertebral fracture dislocation at L2–L3 or below, then no cord injury occurs; damage is confined to the cauda equina, and there are no upper motor neurone signs of damage, the only damage being to sensory, motor and autonomic nerve fibres.

Spinal cord hemisection (Brown–Séquard syndrome)

This can be caused by penetrating trauma injuries, e.g. a stab or gunshot wound, or by vertebral damage. A pure hemisection results in ipsilateral loss of all sensations and voluntary muscle movement at the level of the lesion, ipsilateral spastic paresis below the level of the lesion, ipsilateral loss of discriminative (light) touch, vibration sensation and proprioception and a contralateral loss of pain and temperature sensation below the level of the lesion. Damage to the hypothalamospinal (descending sympathetic pathway) tract at T1 or above produces an ipsilateral Horner's syndrome. Such pure lesions are rare, and incomplete hemisections are more common.

Anterior cord syndrome

This can be caused by fracture dislocation of vertebrae, herniation of vertebral discs or occlusion of the anterior spinal artery by a tumour. It results in bilateral motor paralysis at the level of the lesion and bilateral spastic paresis below the level of the lesion. There is a dissociated sensory loss with bilateral loss of temperature and pain below the level of the lesion but no loss of light touch or vibration sensation (supplied by the posterior spinal arteries). Damage to the hypothalamospinal (descending sympathetic pathway) tract at T1 or above produces a bilateral Horner's syndrome, and damage to the parasympathetic centres at S2–S4 results in loss of voluntary control of bladder and bowel function.

Amyotrophic lateral sclerosis (Lou Gehrig's disease)

This is a chronic progressive disease of unknown aetiology that occurs in late middle age, named after the famous US baseball player; it is fatal within 2–6 years of onset. It causes death of the motor neurones and CST axons, resulting in symptoms of lower motor neurone damage, such as muscle atrophy, weakness and fasciculation, superimposed on upper motor neurone disease with paresis, spasticity and Babinski signs. There are no sensory deficits.

Infective diseases: poliomyelitis and syphilis

Polio is an acute viral infection that destroys the lower motor neurones of the spinal cord and brainstem, leading to progressive paralysis and wasting of the muscles. The lower limbs are more often affected than the upper limbs, and in severe cases respiratory function may be threatened. Immunization has greatly reduced the incidence of this disease. In tabes dorsalis (neurosyphilis), the large-diameter myelinated fibres are affected. It results in chronic inflammation of the dorsal roots and spinal ganglia, causing pain and paraesthesia. The cells die, resulting in degeneration of the axons within the dorsal columns. The peak incidence of disease occurs 15–20 years after the initial infection. It is a purely sensory disease and results in bilateral loss of discriminative sensation. If the gracile fasciculus is affected, a positive Romberg sign, indicating sensory ataxia, will also be seen.

Syringomyelia

This is a developmental abnormality that results in central cavitation within the spinal cord originating at the central canal, and is common at the cervical spinal cord level. Thus, it interrupts the STT bilaterally, resulting in loss of pain and temperature sensation below the level of the lesion, particularly in the hands. As the cavity enlarges, there is progressive bilateral flaccid paralysis as the lower motor neurones become affected. Horner's syndrome may become apparent if the descending sympathetic fibres that run in the lateral white matter are affected. Tactile discrimination, vibration and conscious proprioception remain intact.

A similar pattern of damage is seen in the central cord syndrome, which can be caused by whiplash injury (hyperextension of the cervical cord region). The cord is compressed by the vertebral body anteriorly and the ligamentum flavum posteriorly, causing damage to the central part of the cord. There is bilateral muscular atrophy and paralysis at the site of injury, and bilateral spastic paresis with a characteristic sacral sparing, as the sacral fibres of the CST are located furthest laterally and are thus least affected. The lower limbs are less affected than the upper limbs. Similarly, there is bilateral loss of pain and temperature sensation, again with sacral sparing, and a greater effect in the upper than in the lower limbs.

Management of spinal cord injury

It is routine in any patient suspected of having a cervical spinal injury to immobilize the neck to prevent any potential bone fragments from penetrating or compressing the cord and causing further damage. Imaging of the cord and vertebral column is performed using X-rays, CT or MRI. In terms of medical and surgical care of SCI patients, the main aim of treatment is to prevent further damage and to limit the area of secondary injury. Surgically, this can be achieved by removing fragments of damaged bone, disc and ligament to decompress the

Table 4.7 Strategies for spinal cord repair

Level of difficulty	Objective	Technique
Low	Neuroprotection	Pharmacological, e.g. methylprednisolone, glutamate receptor antagonists, ion channel blockers
	Prevention of demyelination	Pharmacological, e.g. 4-aminopyridine
	Preventing scar formation	Targeting glial reaction, e.g. enzyme digestion
	Suppression of CNS inhibitory molecules	Neutralizing antibodies, vaccines, specific receptor antagonists
	Promoting axonal regeneration	Use of growth factors or stimulation of intrinsic growth potential
	Provision of permissive environment	Cellular bridges, e.g. nerve grafts, biodegradable conduits, Schwann cells, glial cell transplants
	Replacement of lost cells	Stem cells
High	Appropriate reconnectivity	Ensure specific target recognition

cord. Pharmacologically, corticosteroids are often administered in an attempt to reduce the inflammatory reaction. Clinical trials have shown that high-dose steroids such as methylprednisolone are effective in preserving motor function if initiated within 8 h of injury and continued for 48 h. They are thought to act by reducing oedema, inflammation, glutamate release and free radical accumulation, but their use remains controversial in some countries. The side effects include increased gastric bleeding and wound infection. Other pharmacological compounds such as GM1 ganglioside and naloxone have been tried, but the results have been equivocal. The other main treatment is rehabilitation medicine, which is used to help the patient make the most of what residual function they have left through functional retraining, and to prevent medical complications from occurring that often lead to re-hospitalization, such as bladder infections, skin lesions and musculoskeletal problems.

The Holy Grail of SCI research is to be able to make the paralysed walk again, but how realistic is this goal? In the past 15 years substantial progress has been made in understanding the molecular consequences of SCI and how axons find their way to appropriate targets during normal development. Successful repair of SCI will involve overcoming (hierarchical) obstacles in four main areas: reducing cell death, promoting axon regeneration in the CNS, remyelination of damaged and regenerating fibres, and appropriate connectivity (Table 4.7). However, we are only at the beginning of applying some of this (pharmacological) knowledge to clinical practice. For example, there is a continual search for drugs that will prevent neuronal cell death and reduce the inflammatory response (see above). Two approaches are in current clinical development to address the issue of conduction failure due to demyelination. The first is pharmacological treatment with fampridine (4-aminopyridine), a K^+ channel blocker that restores action potential conduction in demyelinated fibres. This appears to have beneficial effects in reducing spasticity and sensory and motor functions in some patients, and is undergoing phase 3 trials. The other approach is more controversial and involves transplantation of Schwann cells or oligodendrocytes or stem cells. Major issues with this transplantation approach include the source of the cells, delivery method, immunogenicity and control of growth.

The CNS environment, unlike the PNS, is hostile to regeneration, because CNS neurones have a low intrinsic ability to regenerate, and damage fails to stimulate growth-promoting molecules. More importantly, the damaged CNS is very inhibitory to axonal regeneration, because it produces molecules that cause growth cones to collapse. One major source of the inhibition is myelin. At least three inhibitory proteins are known to exist: Nogo-A, myelin-associated glycoprotein and oligodendrocyte myelin glycoprotein. These molecules bind to a common receptor complex comprising the Nogo receptor and the p75 low-affinity neurotrophic factor receptor, which activates the Rho signalling pathway to mediate growth cone collapse. Antibodies to Nogo-A have been shown in rodents to promote neuronal regeneration of the CST, both of injured and uninjured axons, offering the possibility of creating vaccines against myelin as a future treatment therapy. Pharmaceutical companies are now developing the use of blocking peptides to the Nogo receptor and the nogo protein as therapeutic targets.

Damage to the CNS produces a glial scar within a few weeks of injury; this represents a physical as well as biochemical barrier to regeneration, as it contains inhibitory chondroitin sulphate proteoglycans, which also induce growth cone collapse. Enzymes that digest the glycosaminoglycan side chains have been shown to promote CNS regeneration. Alternatively, bridging of the scar region with biodegradable conduits that can be seeded with various trophic factors or nerve grafts has provided limited regeneration across the injury site.

Cellular transplantation for SCI has been tried for the past 20 years or more, initially with the use of embryonic tissue to bridge the lesion site and act as a relay between disconnected neurones. These studies have shown the feasibility of this method, as the transplants are incorporated into the host tissue and show some functional benefit in rodent models. However, they raise important ethical questions that are likely to preclude their incorporation into clinical practice. More recently, stem cells have been suggested as a more promising therapeutic tool for transplantation. Experiments using this approach are at an early stage, and the main question will be not whether they will survive, but how they will form appropriate connections.

It is highly unlikely that a single therapy will treat SCI; a multiple therapeutic approach will be needed. However, while basic science strives to make people walk again, for many SCI patients walking is not at the top of their wish list for progress. It is the absence of bowel and bladder control and hand use, and the levels of pain, which control the quality of their lives. There are now drugs that can control incontinence and sexual dysfunction, pain and spasticity. For example, in rehabilitation medicine, oral or intrathecal baclofen, a $GABA_B$ receptor agonist, is used to reduce muscle spasticity, presynaptically by increasing inhibition, thus reducing neurotransmitter release, and postsynaptically by reducing the activity of motor neurones. It also has effects on bladder function by decreasing hyperactive contracture of the external urethral sphincter. Thus, we are only on the first few rungs of the clinical ladder to achieving successful spinal cord regeneration. Multiple interventions will be needed in a progressive and coordinated fashion to initiate, maintain and guide appropriate regeneration from the injury site, and to re-establish functional connections. These will provide considerable challenges for basic and clinical scientist alike.

Comments on the case history

Humpty Dumpty suffered spinal cord damage resulting in Brown–Séquard syndrome. The level of the lesion is at T10, the highest level of neurological deficit on the right side. This syndrome results in dissociated sensory loss below the level of the lesion due to damage to the DCML and STT, and the Babinski sign is an indicator of damage to the CST. Humpty Dumpty's cord will not be put back together again!

PAIN AND ANALGESIA

5

Chapter objectives

After studying this chapter you should be able to:

1. Describe the pathways by which nociceptive information is transmitted from the periphery to the cortex.

2. Discuss the role of cells in the spinal cord in the gating of nociceptive transmission.

3. Describe the main mechanisms whereby nociceptive transmission can be modulated at the spinal and supraspinal levels.

4. Define the main principles of pain management and describe the main categories of analgesic drugs.

5. Explain general phenomena such as peripheral sensitization and central sensitization.

Case history

A South-East Asian male, Mr. Un Luc-Kee, was involved in an industrial accident when he was eighteen; his shirtsleeve got caught in a machine dragging his arm into the equipment. Surgeons tried to repair the arm, but the blood supply was severely compromised and eventually the right arm was amputated above the elbow. Since the accident, he has experienced phantom limb pain sensations that radiate up the right arm, and appear to originate from the non-existent right hand. He describes the pain as shooting, burning and stabbing sensations, and it feels worse when it is cold. He rates it as 7 out of 10 on a visual analogue pain rating scale. Intermixed with these are sensations of hyperalgesia and allodynia when the skin over the stump is touched and spontaneous pain that occurs sporadically that feel like electric shocks in the arm. When he is shaving, he feels tingling sensations in the phantom hand. He describes the phantom hand as contorted with the fist closed and the nails digging into the palm skin.

His GP initially prescribed mild analgesics to relieve the pain, but these were largely ineffective. He sought alternative treatments such as TENS (transcutaneous electrical nerve stimulation) and acupuncture, but these have had mixed results; TENS made the pain worse, acupuncture only partially alleviated the pain. Likewise, anticonvulsant and tricyclic antidepressant

drugs such as carbamazepine and amitryptiline had a limited effect, and stronger opiate drug treatment, such as morphine, was initially effective but now much higher doses are required to achieve the same effect.

He is referred to a pain clinic, where the consultant tries a sympathetic nerve blockade that has limited effect. After trying unsuccessfully several new drug combinations, he prescribes the drug gabapentin. After a couple of months of treatment, Un Luc-Kee reports that suddenly the pain in his phantom limb has regressed to a point where he hardly notices it (pain rating{1/10}). The only side effect of this latest treatment was a mild dizziness that occurred during the first few days of treatment.

This case gives rise to the following questions:

1. What pathways transmit pain from the periphery to the brain?
2. Why were TENS and acupuncture ineffective?
3. How does morphine reduce pain and why did it gradually became ineffective in this case?
4. What is the rationale for the other pharmacological and non-pharmacological treatments that were tried?
5. What are the mechanisms that may contribute to phantom limb pain?

Introduction

Pain is one of mankind's oldest and most dreaded fears. Pain is a sensation that evokes an emotional response and involves a complex interaction between the periphery, the spinal cord, the brainstem and higher cortical centres. Intense pain is a penetrating sensation that commands the person's attention and rapidly dominates the mind. To the neuroscientist, pain is a sensory phenomenon registered on perception; to the psychologist it may be a learned or conditioned behaviour but to the doctor, it is a warning sign to be decoded for diagnosis and treatment. People go to see their doctors most often because they are in pain. Thus, it is important that doctors have a sound knowledge of pain, its pathways and of the treatments that are effective in alleviating pain. Pain is a learned experience the perception of which depends on the emotional interpretation of pain, recall of past pain, and social and genetic factors.

Pain is defined by the International Association for the Study of Pain (IASP) as 'an unpleasant sensory or emotional experience that is associated with actual or potential tissue damaging stimuli'. The definition includes the sensory-discriminative and motivational-affective components that make up the complex experience of pain. Among somatovisceral sensations, pain is arguably the

most important. Although pain is used to define all sensations that hurt or are unpleasant, there are actually three distinct types of pain. The first two types of pain are examples of 'good' pain; the third is deemed 'bad' pain.

1. Nociceptive (acute) pain is elicited by a brief noxious stimulus such as pin-prick and induces a flexion withdrawal response to the stimulus. This type of pain is an adaptive sensation whose primary function is to protect the body from injury; it is an early warning alarm system. Loss of this type of pain through disease or injury can lead to life-threatening situations. People who have congenital insensitivity to pain with anhydrosis (CIPA), a rare autosomal-recessive disorder, are characterized by recurrent episodes of unexplained fever, anhydrosis and absence of reaction to noxious stimuli, and mental retardation. Children with this condition often have to have their fingernails and teeth removed to stop self-mutilation (autotomy) behaviour, and many die young. Mutations in the sodium channel subunit $Na_V1.7$ also result in abnormal pain sensations; loss of the subunit results in analgesia, whereas increased expression results in conditions such as paroxymal extreme pain disorder and erythromelalgia (Mitchell's disease). Pain also performs a homeostatic function. A low level of pain is necessary to inform us when

activities put excessive strain on the body such as during certain movements or posture. Even when we sleep, nociceptors work to cause us to toss and turn during the night to prevent bedsores or musculoskeletal strain.

2. In prolonged pain (e.g. sunburn) injury to the body has already occurred and the biological function of pain is to prevent further damage, assist healing and tissue repair. It does this by the development of areas of hypersensitivity in and around the injury site, which are the result of a decreased activation threshold of nociceptors–a phenomenon called peripheral sensitization. The pain recedes once healing has occurred.

3. Chronic (neuropathic) pain is pain that has been present for at least 2–3 months. Chronic pain is defined by the IASP as 'pain resulting from disease or damage to the peripheral or central nervous systems, and from dysfunction of the nervous system'. Thus, it is a ubiquitous term that covers a wide range of conditions such as pain in irritable bowel syndrome, (a visceral pain disorder), through to muscle and joint pain disorders such as fibromyalgia and back pain where there is no obvious nerve damage to nervous system damage and to pain in diseases such as arthritis, diabetes, cancer and AIDS. The quality of pain sensations is distinct from that seen in acute pain (Table 5.1). In neuropathic pain, the pain persists in the absence of the initial injury. Chronic pain often results from abnormal sensitivity of nociceptors and non-nociceptors and pathological changes in the nervous system (Table 5.2) and the pain, rather than the original injury, becomes of greatest concern and is often very difficult to treat. A recent study reported that more than half a million people suffer from neuropathic pain in the UK. Two thirds of chronic pain patients are aged 65 and over.

It is estimated that there are 2 billion chronic pain days yearly worldwide and around one third of the world's population suffers from recurrent or persistent pain, costing billions of pounds in health care, compensation, lost earning potential, personal suffering and litigation.

Despite an explosion in the molecular and cellular fields of nociception, pain therapy continues to be only partially effective and may be accompanied by distressing side effects or have abuse potential. For most acute pain conditions, non-steroidal anti-inflammatory drugs (NSAIDs) or opioids remain the first line of treatment, while these drugs are largely ineffective in neuropathic pain. Chronic pain responds well to drugs whose primary use was not intended for pain, e.g. antidepressants, anticonvulsants and local anaesthetics. It is becoming clear that no one class of drug is effective in treating all forms of pain. Moreover, different types of pain may involve common or dissimilar mechanisms. Therefore treatment, which has for so long been based on empirical measures, such as symptom or temporal properties,

Table 5.1 Clinical features of neuropathic pain
Abnormal pain quality—burning, stabbing, gnawing and sickening
Sensory loss with associated hyperalgesia (increased painful response to a noxious stimulus), allodynia (pain in response to an innocuous stimulus) and hyperpathia (delayed perception, summation and painful after-sensations)
Paroxymal pain (electric-shock like) common
Radiating dysaesthesia (non-painful abnormal sensations)
Pain is poorly localized and diffuse
Pain intensity altered by emotion and fatigue
Onset of pain is immediate or delayed after injury
Sympathetic nervous system dysfunction may be present
Vasomotor (regulation of blood vessels) and sudomotor (stimulation of sweat glands) changes

may be improved by therapies targeting the underlying mechanisms. In the past 20 years rapid progress has been made in uncovering new mechanisms, pathways, brain areas and drugs involved in pain perception and modulation. However, only now are we beginning to put all the pieces of the puzzle of pain together. This chapter aims to provide an overview of some of the pathways and mechanisms of nociception and pain, and the therapies that are involved in pain management.

Nociceptors

Nociceptive afferents do not have specialized receptors; they use free nerve endings and most are polymodal, i.e. they respond to more than one kind of stimulus, such as chemical, thermal or mechanical stimuli. Free nerve endings are found in all parts of the body except the interior of the bones and the brain itself. Acute pain is characterized by activation of nociceptors for a limited duration. Pain sensations can be broadly divided up into bright, sharp, stabbing types of pain, and dull, throbbing, aching types. Aδ fibres mediate the former, or 'fast' pain, whereas C-fibres signal the latter or 'slow pain'. Not all Aδ and C fibres are nociceptors. Some respond to low threshold stimuli such as sensual touching or brushing the skin. Many C fibres are thermoreceptors, and respond to warm or cold, providing homeostatic responses via emotional tagging of sensations. For example, think how pleasant a cool shower feels after sunbathing for a while and conversely how unpleasant a cool shower feels first thing in the morning when the skin is cool! Additionally, there is a population of 'silent' nociceptors that reside in most tissues and are normally insensitive to mechanical and thermal stimuli. They become active under pathological conditions such as inflammation and nerve injury.

Interestingly, most of our knowledge about the neurophysiology of pain comes from the study of cutaneous

Table 5.2 Summary classification of some major characteristics of different types of pain

Type	Duration	Temporal features in relation to cause	Sensation	Nerve fibre class	Adaptive value	Example
Acute	Seconds	Instantaneous Simultaneous	Pain	C/Aδ	Preventative	Pin-prick, muscle ache, visceral distension
Prolonged	Hours to days	Resolves on recovery	Hyperalgesia, allodynia	C/Aδ Aβ	Protective Recovery	Inflamed wound
Chronic	Months to years	Persistent; exceeds repair of injury	Hyperalgesia, allodynia spontaneous pain	C/Aδ Aβ Aβ/δ/C CNS cells	None Maladaptive	Arthritis Neuropathy Central pain

Table 5.3 Comparison of pain characteristics from different target organs

Peripheral target	Sensation	Localization of pain
Skin	Pricking Stabbing Burning	Well localized
Muscle	Aching Soreness/ tenderness Cramping	Poorly localized
Viscera	Dullness Vagueness Fullness Nausea	

nociceptors. Pain from each target organ has its own distinct perceptual quality as shown in Table 5.3.

However, cutaneous pain is clinically less common than muscle and visceral pain. Among the most common reasons for visiting the doctor are chest pain, neck pain, abdominal pain, and headache and back pain. For example, back pain is extremely common, with up to 80% of the population suffering at some point in their life. Visceral pain represents a major clinical challenge as its occurrence is not always correlated with the severity of a disease. For example, bowel cancer produces little or no pain whereas passing a kidney stone, or a stool in a patient with irritable bowel syndrome, can be excruciating.

There are several differences between cutaneous and muscle or visceral nociceptors. The first is that cutaneous sensation is well localized and the pain is usually constant. Visceral and muscle pain is poorly localized, due to the lower innervation densities of these tissues, and is often periodic. Secondly, visceral afferents are insensitive to direct trauma but very sensitive to distension (of hollow-walled muscular

organs) whereas muscle and skin are not. In fact, early 20th century surgeons could perform abdominal surgery using only local anaesthetic of the body wall as healthy organs are largely insensitive to direct mechanical trauma such as cutting or burning. All are sensitive to ischaemia and inflammation. Lastly, as most visceral organs have very few low threshold myelinated fibres and comprise mostly of Aδ and C fibres, their stimulus response properties differ from cutaneous and muscle afferents, which have specialized receptors to detect innocuous stimuli. Visceral afferents encode a stimulus response in an intensity dependent manner, the more painful the stimulus the greater the number of action potentials and frequency of discharge.

Although acute pain results from damage to these free nerve endings, in reality the pain is a result of substances released by damaged tissues: prostaglandins, histamine, bradykinin, cytokines and peptides, H^+ ions. These activate specific receptors located on the free nerve endings. Nociceptors have more than 30 different ion channels or receptors and the list is functionally diverse and still growing! (see Table 5.4). Moreover, the molecular composition of receptors and their relative ratios can change after injury.

Pain pathways

Cutaneous nociceptor afferents terminate mainly in laminae I, II and V of the spinal cord dorsal horn and synapse on second order neurones that carry the signal to either the brainstem or the thalamus. It is only when the nociceptive signal reaches the brainstem that it is translated into a conscious sensory perception. Three ascending pathways are concerned with pain transmission: the spinothalamic tract (STT), the spinoreticular tract (SRT) and the spinoparabrachial tract (SPBT). Each appears to be concerned with a particular aspect of pain processing. Simplistically, the sensory discriminative aspect is signalled by the STT, and the homeostatic and affective (emotional) qualities of pain by the SRT and SPBT

Table 5.4 Function of some of the receptors and ion channels located on nociceptors

Receptor family	Function
P2X = purinergic ATP receptor ASIC = acid sensing ion channel (chemical and mechanical stimuli) TRP = transient response potential receptors (temperature sensitive)	Involved in signal transduction
Voltage-gated Na$^+$ channels (tetrodotoxin resistant or tetrodotoxin sensitive) Voltage-gated Ca^{2+} channels AMPA + NMDA = ionotropic glutamate receptors mGluR = metabotropic glutamate receptors Voltage-gated K$^+$ channels GABA receptors	Involved in membrane excitability
5-HT$_3$ = serotonin receptor CB$_1$ = cannabinoid receptor H$_1$ = histamine receptor EP = prostanoid receptors for prostaglandins IL-1R = receptor for interleukin 1 (cytokine) TrkA = tyrosine kinase A receptor for the neurotrophin nerve growth factor (NGF) BK$_2$ = bradykinin receptor	Involved in peripheral sensitization

(Fig. 5.1). Therefore, fast and slow pain travel by different pathways to different areas of the brain. The fast pathway connects directly to the thalamus, which then relays the information to the primary sensorimotor cortices for analysis and response. Its function is to act as a warning system by signalling the exact location and severity of the injury and the duration of the pain. Fast pain predominantly arises from the STT cells in laminae IV–V of the spinal cord. Slow pain is mediated by C-fibres and signals the emotional aspects of pain. It reaches the thalamus indirectly via connections with the brainstem reticular formation. The slow pain axons innervate the non-specific intralaminar nuclei of the thalamus, and the autonomic centres of the reticular formation in the brainstem. For example, axons of lamina I cells of both the STT and SPBT are more concerned with stimulus intensity than stimulus location. They form part of the forebrain pain pathways associated with the affective quality of pain (unpleasantness and fear of further injury) and involve the prefrontal cortex and amygdala. Slow pain may remind the brain that pain has occurred, that protective attention to the injury site is required and that normal activity may need to be restricted while healing occurs.

The projections to the reticular formation underlie the arousal effects of painful stimuli via activation of the ascending reticular activating system that projects to all areas of the brain. Activation of the reticular formation stimulates noradrenergic neurones in the locus coeruleus, and thus decreases the pain transmission by activating the descending pain modulating systems (see below).

Thalamocortical axons transmit the information from the thalamus to the cortex. There is no one specific cortical region that can be designated as 'pain cortex' (see Box 5.2). Rather, functional brain-imaging studies have revealed several regions that are active when a pain stimulus is sensed and these are associated with different functional components of pain. The discriminative qualities (i.e. 'where and how much it hurts') involve the somatosensory cortex whereas the affective-motivational aspects (e.g. 'I don't like it or stop it!') are associated with the limbic regions (cingulate cortex, insula). Parts of the prefrontal motor cortex are also involved in cognitive evaluative processes, e.g., attention to, anticipation of, memory of or escape from pain.

Visceral and muscular pain pathways

Considering that muscle and visceral pain evoke distinct sensations, it would be logical to expect to find cells in the spinal cord that respond only to muscle or visceral stimulation. Interestingly, no such cells exist in the spinal cord. All cells that have either a visceral or muscle receptive field (RF) also have a separate cutaneous RF. This means that convergence occurs within the spinal cord. It provides an explanation for referred pain. Referred pain is a pain that is localized in one part of the body that is remote from its source. In contrast to cutaneous pain, which is well localized, visceral and muscle pain are poorly localized and are often sensed as somatic pain. This is because of afferent convergence onto spinal cord cells that have a cutaneous receptive field. The area of referral is related to the segmental dermatome and is often to skin or muscle. The classic example is angina in which ischaemic heart muscle causes pain over the skin and radiating down the left arm. Another example is stomach pain which can cause visceral organ spasm, muscle spasm and a skin flare response due to autonomic activity. Referred pain is consistent enough to be of diagnostic value such as lower right quadrant abdominal pain can be used to diagnose appendicitis (Fig. 5.2). Another important feature is that the referral site may show signs of hyperalgesia.

The central terminals of visceral and muscle nociceptors terminate in laminae I and V but not lamina II, unlike skin nociceptor afferents. In lamina I, these fibres converge onto projection neurones of the STT and SPBT, which then project to the brainstem and thalamus and from there to the somatosensory cortex. Visceral afferents also terminate on SRT neurones and onto cells that project to the dorsal column nuclei and recent research suggests that this latter pathway is exclusively involved in visceral pain, whereas the STT and SRT visceral pathways are more concerned with autonomic (visceral) reflex functions than visceral pain. Lesions of the dorsal columns effectively relieve chronic visceral pain and

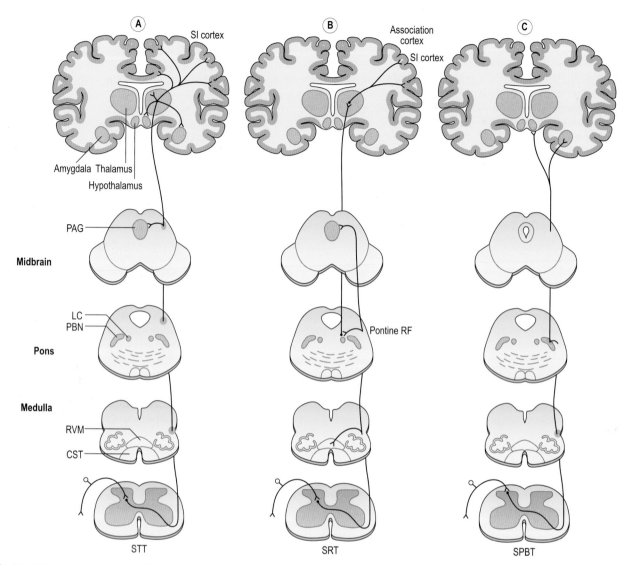

Fig. 5.1 Schematic representation of anterolateral pain pathways: (A) Spinothalamic tract (STT), (B) Spinoreticular tract (SRT) and (C) Spinoparabrachial tract (SPBT). Information is also transmitted to the amygdala and hypothalamic areas of the limbic system. PBN, parabrachial nucleus; SI, primary somatosensory cortex ; PAG, periaquductal grey; RVM, rostroventral medulla; CST, corticospinal tract; LC, locus coeruleus; RF, reticular formation.

have led to new clinical treatments for managing visceral cancer pain.

Given that muscle, viscera and skin converge onto projection neurones that utilize common ascending tracts, how then does the brain know whether the pain is from skin, muscle or viscus? The answer is currently unknown but most likely involves differences in the temporal and spatial coding of inputs onto cells, inducing a differential processing of information by the brain.

How does the central nervous system interpret a stimulus as painful?

As lesion studies have confirmed the role of the STT in pain transmission, it might be expected that STT cells would reveal them as nociceptive specific (NS), i.e. specifically responding to tissue-damaging stimuli. However, it is one of the paradoxes of pain that most of the cells of the STT can be excited by non-noxious stimulation of the skin! Low-threshold sensory skin afferents synapse upon the proximal dendrites of the lamina IV and V neurones. These low-threshold inputs are the only inputs to lamina IV cells (i.e. they have no nociceptive inputs). The same low-threshold afferents also synapse on the dendrites of the lamina V cells. However, cells of lamina V extend some dendrites into laminae I–II where C/Aδ fibres contact the distal dendrites. Thus, the lamina V cells receive convergent inputs from both nociceptor and non-nociceptor afferents (i.e. they are wide dynamic range cells). Therefore, the STT has axons of three different kinds of neurones: those that are nociceptor-specific (lamina I), and those that are

Box
5.2   Pain in the brain

The role of the cortex in pain has been debated for nearly almost 100 years. Based on a careful study of patients with cortical or thalamic lesions, Dr. Henry Head showed that ablation of the thalamus eliminated all pain sensations, whereas cortical lesions did not. However, converging clinical, experimental and, more recently, functional imaging evidence has now altered this view, to show that several brain regions are active, either directly or indirectly, in response to a painful stimulus, but that they process different aspects of the stimulus (Table 5.5). These include the somatosensory SI cortex, SII and the adjacent insula region, the anterior cingulate cortex and the ventromedial prefrontal cortex. Some regions, such as the anterior cingulate cortex and the ventromedial prefrontal cortex, directly feedback to the periaqueductal grey to stimulate anti-nociceptive pathways. Furthermore, pain perception modulation by hypnosis has been shown to alter brain activity in many of these brain areas.

Damage to the prefrontal cortex affects the evaluative cognitive responses to pain. For example, patients with frontal lobe damage disconnecting it from the thalamus rarely complain about the severity of pain. They acknowledge the presence of the pain but state that it does not bother them. Cingulotomy selectively decreases the emotional components of pain perception although it fails to provide significant pain relief in about 25% of patients. It appears that the cingulate cortex may not modulate some forms of chronic pain, e.g. neuropathic pain. Patients with ischaemic damage to SI and SII areas show a loss of pain sensation with preservation of pain affect. Similarly, patients with damage to the insula and SII cortex have elevated pain thresholds to thermal stimuli. Please see Table 5.5 for the presumed functional roles of these cortical areas in pain perception.

Table 5.5 Presumed functional roles of cortical areas in pain perception

Cortical area	Presumed function
SI	Pain localization
SII	Pain intensity; spatially directed attention (touch, visual) to pain
Insula	Regulation of pain-related autonomic activity; pain intensity
Anterior cingulate	Response selection, attention, affect, motor suppression, anticipatory appraisal of pain; pain modulation
Prefrontal cortex	Affect, emotion, memory, anticipatory appraisal of pain; pain modulation

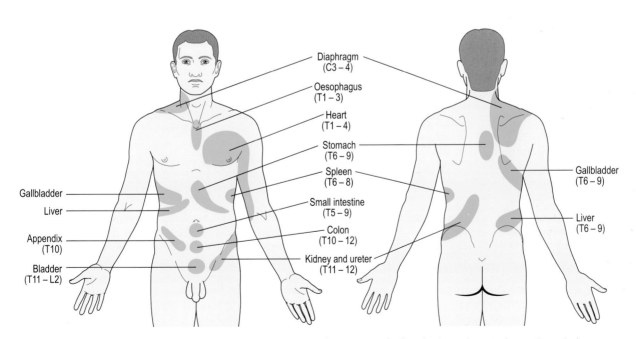

Fig. 5.2 Common cutaneous areas of referred pain from visceral organs; dermatomes of referred pain are in parentheses. C, cervical; T, thoracic; L, lumbar. Adapted from Moore KL, Agur AMR. Essentials of Clinical Anatomy. 2nd edn. Lippincott Williams and Wilkins, 2002.

non-nociceptive (lamina IV) and those that have both nociceptive and non-nociceptive inputs (laminae V). The presence of this convergence of sensory modalities on the lamina V cells presents a problem. The forebrain can only know that action potentials are arriving in the axons of the STT. How can it tell which types of primary afferents are activating the lamina V cells, the nociceptors (C/Aδ) or the low-threshold Aβ afferents?

One theory is that the lamina V cells make up the majority of the STT and have small receptive fields that signal the precise location of stimulus. However, because of the afferent input convergence in lamina V, they are non-specific in the type of stimulus that they register. The lamina I cells unequivocally signal that a noxious stimuli has occurred. However, these cells are fewer in number and have large receptive fields that cannot indicate the precise location of the painful stimulus. It is thought that the pain is signalled by the lamina I and V neurones acting together. If lamina I cells are not active, the detailed information about the type and location of a stimulus provided by the lamina V axons is interpreted as innocuous. If, however, a lamina I cell is active, the stimulation is recognized as painful. Thus, the lamina V cells provide the details about the location of a stimulus and the lamina I cells specify whether it is painful or not. This theory has been confirmed in recent animal studies where lamina I cells have been selectively ablated using a neurotoxin, which led to a significant reduction in the behavioural hyperalgesia associated with tissue injury without affecting the ability to locate the stimulus.

Physiology of pain modulation

The transmission of information from primary afferents to secondary neurones in the spinal cord is not merely a passive process but is a dynamic process involving excitation, inhibition and modulation. The variable nature of pain responses also suggests that modulatory systems must exist in the CNS that regulates pain. Neurones in the superficial dorsal horn are subject to modulation that 'gates' the flow of information to the CNS. Nociceptive sensory information is gated in the substantia gelatinosa of the spinal cord by tonic or phasic inhibitory control mechanisms. Gating is of two kinds:

1. Local—'segmental antinociception' regulated by primary afferent inputs.

2. Widespread—'supraspinal antinociception' which utilizes descending pathways from the brainstem.

In attempting to explain various clinical pain phenomena such as allodynia, referred pain and the variable relationship between tissue injury and pain response, a theory about how pain is perceived called the gate control theory was proposed by Patrick Wall and Ronald Melzack (Fig. 5.3, top). This theory states that pain is a function of the balance between the information traveling into the spinal cord through large (non-nociceptive) nerve fibres and

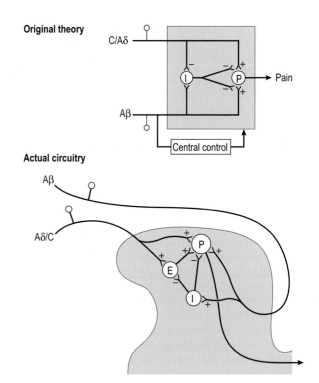

Fig. 5.3 Gate control theory—original circuit shown on the top. P, projection neurone; I, inhibitory neurone. The bottom part of the Figure shows actual circuitry involved. Nociceptors do not have an inhibitory effect on the inhibitory neurone as proposed in the original theory; they activate the P cell either directly or via an excitatory interneurone (E). The Aβ fibres have the connections as proposed in the original theory.

information travelling into the spinal cord through small (nociceptive) nerve fibres. Without any stimulation, both sets of nerve fibres are inactive and the inhibitory neurone (I) blocks the signal in the projection neurone (P) that connects to the brain. The gate is 'closed', and therefore no pain is sensed. With non-painful stimulation, large nerve fibres are activated. This activates P, but it also activates I, which then blocks the signal in P, that connects to the brain. As the gate is 'closed', no stimulation is perceived by the brain. With noxious stimulation, nociceptive fibres become active. They activate P and, according to the original theory, block I (it is now known that this does not occur). Since activity of the inhibitory neurone is blocked, it cannot block the output of the projection neurone that connects with the brain. Therefore, if the relative amount of activity is greater in large nerve fibres, there should be little or no pain. However, if there is more activity in small nerve fibres, then pain ensues, because the gate is 'open'. Wall and Melzack also recognized that the brain could exert descending modulatory influences on the spinal cord. Their theory generated vigorous scientific debate. While the gate control theory can explain some observations seen in pain patients during therapy, it does not explain everything. Over the years, it has undergone some modification (Fig. 5.3, bottom). For example, there is no evidence for an inhibitory connection to interneurones from small fibres. Despite its limitations in the proposed circuitry, its most important contributions to pain research have been the appreciation that the CNS is intimately involved in pain modulation and that the brain has a dynamic role in pain processing. Psychological factors that had been previously thought of as reactions to pain were now considered as integral part of pain processing. Moreover, it offered new sites for pain modulation by pharmacotherapy rather than surgery. Lastly, as a direct result, the theory has led to the production of counter-stimulation devices such as transcutaneous electrical nerve stimulators (TENS) and other techniques that alleviate pain.

Counter-stimulation analgesia

A bump on the head or kick in the shin by accident elicits acute pain. However, if the injury site is rubbed, the pain immediately subsides and it feels better. This reaction can be explained by the gate control theory. Rubbing the head or shin stimulates the non-nociceptive afferents that send impulses into the spinal cord. According to the gate theory, lamina II inhibitory interneurones are activated either directly or indirectly by stimulation of these afferents from the skin that would then block the projection neurone and therefore block the pain. This may explain why 'counter-stimulation' techniques are sometimes effective at relieving pain. For example, this can be done simply by rubbing the skin over a sore muscle or may involve specially designed battery-powered devices designed to electrically stimulate nerves through the skin. The aim of these TENS machines is to stimulate the large (Aβ) sensory fibres in peripheral nerves in the hope that they will in turn activate the inhibitory neurones of lamina II and block pain transmission. Importantly, these devices work best when placed on/near the skin of the injured/painful region. They are commonly used by physiotherapists or midwives during labour and use high-frequency, low-intensity stimuli to activate the low-threshold fibres. They are ineffective if they are positioned far away from the painful site. In practice, most counter-stimulation techniques require the use of 'near noxious' stimulation intensities (felt as a buzzing, or tingling sensation), which recruit both Aβ and Aδ afferents, to be maximally effective. From the spinal cord, the messages go directly to several places in the brain including the thalamus, midbrain and reticular formation. It may be that Aδ fibres rather than Aβ fibres are best at exciting lamina II inhibitory interneurones because the Aδ fibres are able to also recruit the supraspinal control systems (described next). TENS is often used in the treatment of acute pain. It is not always useful in chronic pain, because some forms of chronic pain involve phenotypic changes in the properties of low threshold afferents, so that they behave more like nociceptors. In such cases their activation may actually increase the pain rather than alleviate it.

Supraspinal (descending) analgesia

The gate theory introduced the concept that pain perception could be modulated in the spinal cord. It also became clear that pain could be modulated at each synapse along the pain pathways. Brain regions that are involved in pain perception and emotion project back to the brainstem and spinal cord and these connections can change or modify information that is coming to the brain. This is one way that the brain can reduce pain by a mechanism known as supraspinal (descending) analgesia. It uses feedback loops that involve several different nuclei in the brainstem reticular formation (Fig. 5.4). There are now several lines of evidence to corroborate the involvement of brain mechanisms in analgesia such as the fact that direct deep brain stimulation suppresses nociception, and the discovery of central endogenous opioid and cannabinoid transmission.

Areas of the brainstem that are involved in reducing pain are the periaqueductal gray (PAG), the nucleus raphe magnus (NRM) and the locus coeruleus (LC). The PAG is very important in the control of pain. This region surrounds the cerebral aqueduct in the midbrain. Stimulation of parts of the PAG produces more pronounced analgesia than stimulation of either the NRM or the LC. Neurosurgeons can implant stimulating electrodes near the PAG of intractable pain patients, so that a small electrical shock can be delivered. The patient can control the level of self-stimulation and hence the level of analgesia. This is known as stimulus-induced analgesia. The PAG contains enkephalin-rich neurones that excite the NRM and/or LC neurones by inhibiting GABAergic interneurones in the PAG. This allows PAG neurones to excite the amine-containing cells in NRM and LC that in turn project to the spinal cord to block pain transmission by dorsal horn cells. They can exert this inhibition by different mechanisms:

1. Direct presynaptic inhibition of neurotransmitter release from primary afferent terminals. This works by activating G protein-linked receptors that cause closing of calcium channels, thus reducing transmitter release (Fig. 5.5A).

2. Direct postsynaptic inhibition of projection cells causing hyperpolarization of the membrane due to activation of G protein-linked receptors that cause opening of potassium channels (Fig. 5.5B).

3. Indirect inhibition via activation of local enkephalinergic and/or GABAergic inhibitory interneurones by the descending serotonergic and noradrenergic axons. These interneurones can act both postsynaptically on projection cells by opening potassium channels or presynaptically via closing calcium channels. Enkephalins bind to the same receptors as opiate drugs like morphine and heroin. Therefore, it seems likely that opiate drugs may act by mimicking the activity of the interneurones of lamina II.

Stimulation of NRM causes activation of enkephalin and 5-HT containing neurones. Like the noradrenaline-containing neurones, the majority of NRM axons synapse on lamina II cells. They also synapse on cells in lamina I and III. Stimulation of the raphe nuclei produces a

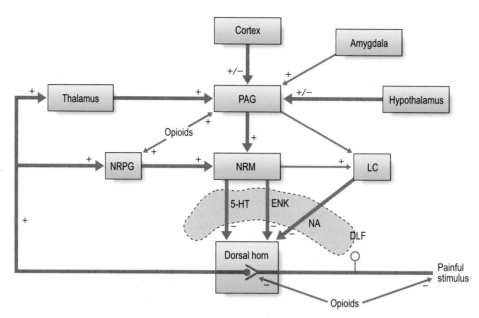

Fig. 5.4 Supraspinal control of pain and its pharmacological modulation by opioids. The periaqueductal grey (PAG) region can be stimulated by input from other regions. In turn, it causes activation of the nucleus raphe magnus (NRM) cells in the rostroventral medulla. Nucleus raphe magnus paragigantocellularis (NRPG) can also stimulate NRM. The NRM sends inhibitory enkephalinergic (ENK) and serotonergic (5-HT) axons via the dorsolateral funiculus (DLF) to the dorsal horn to inhibit substantia gelatinosa cells or nociceptors. Opioids excite cells of the PAG and NRM, as well as having a direct inhibitory effect in the dorsal horn on primary afferents and dorsal horn cells. The locus coeruleus (LC) sends separate noradrenergic (NA) inhibitory inputs to the dorsal horn via the DLF.

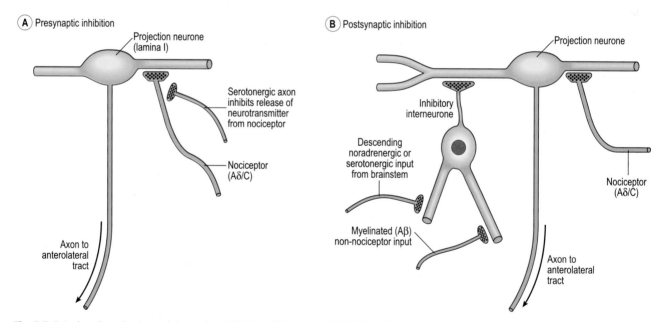

Fig. 5.5 Spinal cord mechanisms of descending inhibition. (A) Presynaptic inhibition; (B) postsynaptic inhibition. See text for details.

powerful analgesia and it is thought that the 5-HT released by this stimulation activates the inhibitory interneurones even more powerfully than noradrenaline and thus blocks pain transmission. However, 5-HT may not be specifically involved in inhibition of pain transmission as serotonergic agonists do not have significant analgesic effects. 5-HT neurones appear to inhibit all somatosensory transmission, and may have a function in the initiation of sleep. A complicating factor is that 5-HT receptors are found in many places in the dorsal horn, including on C fibres, and different 5-HT receptor subtypes mediate different effects of 5-HT.

Arousal analgesia

Recent work has clarified the mechanisms involved in the analgesia seen during intense excitement or arousal. During arousal, the sympathetic nervous system is active in the body. Sympathetic fibres activate the slow pain pathways (STT and SRT) whose axons ascend to activate noradrenergic cells in the locus coeruleus. Noradrenergic axons project back down to the spinal cord (via the dorsolateral fasciculus) and synapse on the cells in lamina I and II forming a feedback loop. Some lamina II cells contain the inhibitory transmitter GABA and they in turn synapse on the cell bodies of large lamina I cells and on the distal dendrites of lamina V cells. Activation of the central noradrenaline system excites the inhibitory interneurones of lamina II and thus inhibits the lamina I STT cells, and blocks pain transmission. Therefore, agents that increase noradrenergic transmission have analgesic potential.

Additionally, activity from autonomic brain areas such as the hypothalamus or the amygdala stimulates the PAG to induce analgesia. This is involved in the fight or flight reaction that produces hypoalgesia in life-threatening situations, e.g. on battlefields.

Psychology of pain

Emotions are central to the experience and expression of pain. Signs of emotional distress are the most frequently recognized evidence that a patient is in pain. The most common emotional aspects associated with pain are anxiety (that the pain will get worse), fear (that it may ultimately kill or severely mutilate them) and depression (that the pain may never go away or get better) that sets up a vicious circle of pain that dominates the patient's life both in acute and chronic pain states (Fig. 5.6). Other emotions may be present such as aggression, anger, guilt or in some individuals, sexual arousal. Emotional distress is thus not only a component of pain, but results from pain and can cause further pain; all these facets require the doctor's attention. In part, it helps to explain why drugs such as antidepressants are effective at relieving pain.

No two people's experience of pain is the same and there are many psychological factors that affect pain. These are summarized in Table 5.6.

There is evidence linking levels of pain perception with the opening or closing of the pain gate in the spinal cord. The gate can be opened or closed depending upon the messages received from the brain. This provides a psycho-physiological basis for factors that modulate chronic pain. This is summarized in Table 5.7.

While relatively little is known about the mechanisms involved, the limbic system and in particular the hypothalamic–pituitary–adrenal axis, which is involved in the stress response, have been implicated. Dysfunction of this pathway has been implicated in some chronic pain conditions such as arthritis and fibromyalgia.

Identification of factors that help reduce pain perception allows psychological management strategies to be

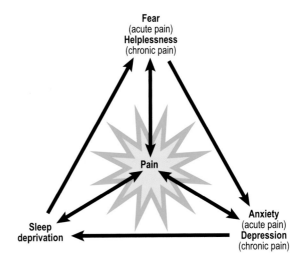

Fig. 5.6 The vicious psychological circle of pain. Untreated pain that persists for any length of time can cause fear and anxiety. If the pain fails to resolve, patients become depressed and lose confidence in themselves and their doctors. Sleeplessness may exacerbate the problem. Adapted from Wall PD, Melzack R. Textbook of Pain. Churchill, 1994.

Table 5.6 Psychological factors influencing pain responses

Prior experience

Cognitive appraisal (meaning of pain)

Mental attitude e.g. fear, anxiety, stress

Cultural beliefs

Personality (neuroticism or extroversion)

Coping strategies (attention, distraction, biofeedback)

Medication

Gender differences

Table 5.7 Factors that regulate spinal gate control

	Gate open	*Gate closed*
Physiological	C/Aδ fibres active	Aβ fibres active
Medical	Extent of injury Insufficient medication	Sufficient medication
Cognitive	Focus on pain	Distraction Reinterpretation of pain
Emotional state	Anxiety Fear Stress Depression	Happy, optimistic Relaxed Rested Prior experience of pain
Behavioural: Personality	Introvert	Extrovert

employed in conjunction with pharmacotherapy. These include cognitive-behavioural therapies that change the patient's beliefs and perceptions of pain, educating the patient about their understanding of pain and addressing pain behaviour rather than the pain perception. One important psychological factor is the placebo effect or the expectation that the doctor will make the patient better (see Box 5.3). Biofeedback (relaxation) techniques can be used to modify biological aspects of pain that produce changes in physiological parameters, e.g. skin temperature or EMG activity has proven beneficial. Similarly, attention and/or distraction strategies that construct a separate image or reinterpret the pain can be very effective at reducing perceived pain levels.

Measuring pain

Several methods can be used to measure pain. The most common is a medical interview when patients are asked to use a rating scale. These scales range from verbal rating scores to visual analogue scales and box scales (Fig. 5.7) and the McGill Pain Questionnaire that consists of 78 adjectives organized into 20 groups based on similarities in pain quality. It offers the patient the opportunity to describe their pain using emotional and sensory descriptors. A pain rating is based on the scale value of the words

and the patient's personal interpretation of the pain is also considered. Non-verbal scales use behavioural assessments based on stereotypical behaviours in response to pain such as grimacing, vocalization, limping, etc. Lastly, there are physiological measures, such as changes in threshold for activation, autonomic activity changes (heart rate, skin temperature), or evoked potentials from reflex activity. Imaging techniques can also be used to measure changes in brain activity in patients in pain.

Pain mechanisms after tissue damage: peripheral and central sensitization

Normally, nociceptors require intense stimuli to activate them. However, the pain sensation does not follow the firing pattern of nociceptors in a simple, predictable fashion. The central processing of this input in terms of summation of afferent input and inhibitory interactions is very important.

Peripheral tissue injury produces two types of change within the nervous system: peripheral sensitization which is manifest as a reduction in the threshold for nociceptor activation and central sensitization, an activity dependent increase in the excitability of CNS neurones. Together they contribute to the post-injury hypersensitivity that is common in chronic pain syndromes.

Peripheral injury induces a decreased pain threshold at the site of injury, coupled with a variable loss of sensory input directly at the site of injury, as well as in the surrounding tissue. The former is the area of primary hyperalgesia and is responsive to both thermal and mechanical stimuli and is mediated by C-fibres, while the latter is the area of secondary hyperalgesia that is only responsive to mechanical stimuli and is mediated by Aβ fibres. Also, a flare response (reddening of the skin) due

---

Box 5.3 The placebo effect

Placebo is Latin for 'I shall please'. Its main use is as a control to test the efficacy of new drugs in clinical conditions. Placebos can be pills, injections or even surgical procedures, and the patient who receives one believes that they have been given the 'good drug' that will alleviate their symptoms. In this regard, the placebo can be a powerful analgesic, but there is great variability in patient responses. The biochemical basis and mechanism of action of placebos remain unclear. Several hypotheses have been suggested to account for its actions. Firstly, that it reduces pain perception by reducing anxiety levels. Secondly, that expectancy can account for the observed changes. Lastly, that the placebo effect is a case of Pavlovian conditioning, whereby association with the drug induces positive emotional responses. The placebo effect does have a physiological basis as its analgesic effect can be antagonized by the opioid antagonist naloxone. Recent research suggests that the placebo effect can activate the dopaminergic reward systems. Thus, the suggestion or belief that a treatment will work is enough to cause the release of endogenous opiates that may activate analgesia systems and other neurotransmitters such as dopamine. The placebo response may also play a role in other alternative medical treatments, such as hypnotherapy and acupuncture.

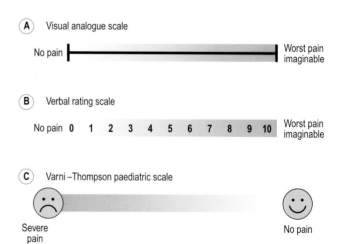

Fig. 5.7 Psychological evaluation of pain using rating scales. (A) Visual analog scale where patient marks a point along a line indicating their pain level. (B) Verbal rating scale where the patient rates the score on a scale of 0–10 where zero is no pain and 10 is the worst pain imaginable. (C) Paediatric pain scale using smiley or sad faces to indicate the level of pain.

to activation of the sympathetic axons occurs, causing release of neuroactive substances that may potentiate the sensitization process (Fig. 5.8).

Much has been learned about the molecular mechanisms of peripheral sensitization after focal nerve or inflammatory injury. This is summarized in Fig. 5.9. Tissue damage leads to the production of an inflammatory chemical soup that activates the various receptors on nociceptors (Table 5.1). This then leads to alterations in signal transduction sensitivity and also a change in the distribution of receptors with down-regulation of some and upregulation of others. Primary hyperalgesia is mediated by a lowering

of the activation threshold of sensitized Aδ and C fibres. It is thought that the major function of non-steroidal anti-inflammatory drugs (NSAIDs) is to prevent peripheral sensitization by inhibiting prostaglandin production, by blocking the action of the enzyme cyclo-oxygenase (COX).

Peripheral sensitization induces a nociceptive afferent barrage that triggers excitability changes in spinal cord neurones, a response that outlasts the stimulus input. These changes are manifest as changes in receptive field size, lowered threshold for activation and increased responsiveness as a direct result of the recruitment of previously subthreshold inputs. Central sensitization is responsible for the secondary hyperalgesia seen after injury. The input from Aβ fibres produces pain by changes in the sensory processing by neurones in the spinal cord and not by changes in the threshold for activation.

The molecular mechanisms of central sensitization are now well understood. Noxious stimuli cause the release of the fast excitatory transmitter glutamate that acts at ionotropic (AMPA, NMDA) and metabotropic glutamate receptors. Co-released are neuropeptides such as substance P, which produce a slow progressive excitatory potential that gives the afferent the opportunity to produce progressively increased response in neurones when repeatedly activated due to summation of these slow potentials. They activate second messenger cascades to produce increased intracellular calcium levels that depolarize the cell resulting in phosphorylation of ion channels and receptors, alter gene expression and upregulation of molecules such as prostaglandins, and COX enzymes (Fig. 5.10). Not surprisingly,

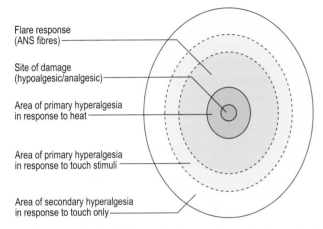

Fig. 5.8 Areas of analgesia flare, and primary and secondary hyperalgesia to different stimuli, after tissue injury. ANS, autonomic nervous system.

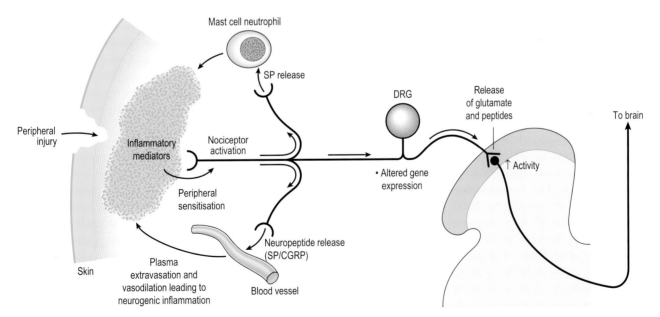

Fig. 5.9 Mechanisms of peripheral sensitization. Peripheral injury results in the creation of an acidic inflammatory 'soup' containing peptides, histamine, bradykinin, protons, adenosine, cytokines, serotonin and prostaglandins. These excite the appropriate receptors on the nociceptors causing activation of protein kinase A and C, leading to phosphorylation of various ion channels and receptors. This results in a lowering of the activation threshold and the excitability of the membrane increases. A secondary consequence of nociceptor activation is the induction of neurogenic inflammation, caused by the release of neuropeptides causing vasodilation and plasma extravasation of proteins from the blood stream, and activation of non-neuronal cells which in turn contribute substances to the inflammatory 'soup'. DRG, dorsal root ganglion; SP, substance P; CGRP, calcitonin gene related peptide.

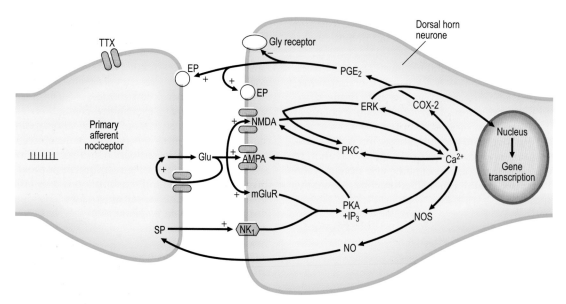

Fig. 5.10 Molecular mechanisms of central sensitization. Prolonged activation of nociceptors results in stimulation of postsynaptic neurones by glutamate and neuropeptides release leading to activation of multiple signaling pathways that result in the phosphorylation of AMPA and NMDA receptors leading to central sensitization by lowering the threshold for activation so that subthreshold inputs become suprathreshold and produce action potentials. Cells can regulate their own activity and that of the primary afferent by release of prostaglandin E2 (PGE2) and nitric oxide (NO). PKA, protein kinase A; PKC, protein kinase C; AMPA and NMDA, ionotropic glutamate receptors; mGluR, metabotropic glutamate receptors; EP, prostaglandin receptor; NOS, nitric oxide synthase; COX 2, inducible isoform 2 of cyclo-oxygenase; Gly, glycine receptor; ERK, extracellular signal-regulated kinases; NK1, neurokinin receptors; TTX, tetrodotoxin-sensitive and tetrodotoxin insensitive sodium channels.

Table 5.8   Causes of neuropathic pain

Cause	Example
Mechanical trauma	Neuropathy, avulsion
Compression	Disk herniation, carpal tunnel syndrome
Inflammation	Arthritis
Infection	Herpes zoster, syphilis
Toxicity	Cisplatin, taxol, vincristine
Disease	Cancer
Ischaemia	Thalamic syndrome, angina
Metabolic	Diabetes
Immune	HIV, multiple sclerosis
Autonomic	Complex regional pain syndrome

Table 5.9   Classification of some common forms of neuropathic pain by site

Peripheral	Spinal	Brain
Neuropathy	Spinal stroke	Stroke
Amputation	Spinal cord injury	Multiple sclerosis
Nerve injury	Multiple sclerosis	Cancer
Avulsion	Cancer	
Radiculopathy	Syringomyelia	
Trigeminal neuralgia	Arachnoiditis	
Cancer	Syphilis	
Herpes zoster		

central sensitization can be prevented by drugs that target the NMDA receptor such as ketamine or by COX2 selective inhibitors such as rofecoxib or by neuropeptide receptor antagonists such as NK1 antagonists.

Neuropathic pain mechanisms

Chronic pain is a common symptom of neurological disease and current pharmacotherapy strategies remain far from satisfactory. Part of this is because the pathophysiological mechanisms of pain remain incompletely understood. Neuropathic pain can be caused by a variety of insults (Table 5.8) and can be classified by site of origin (Table 5.9) or by effective drug treatments. Recently, clinicians and basic scientists have begun to address the mechanisms involved in different types of pain. An example of this is the neuropathic pain that occurs in peripheral neuropathy induced by partial nerve damage. This causes a cascade of changes at different sites along the damaged nerve and at the first synapse in the spinal cord that lead to the generation of spontaneous (stimulus-independent) pain or evoked (stimulus-dependent) pain (Fig. 5.11).

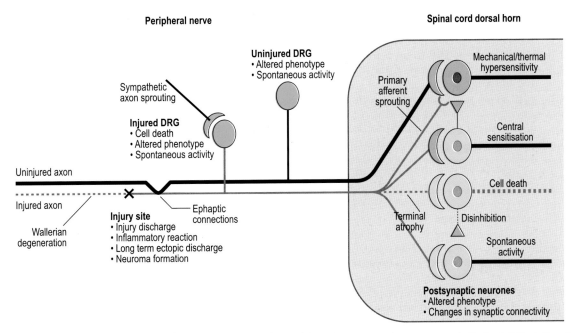

Fig. 5.11 Changes associated with primary afferents after peripheral nerve injury. Axotomy produces a range of effects at distinct sites along the nerve and in the spinal cord that may contribute to pathological pain (see text for further details). DRG, dorsal root ganglion.

Several important peripheral and central nervous system mechanisms have been identified in causing the pain. Peripheral mechanisms include the following:

1. Ectopic impulse generation (spontaneous activity) occurs at the site of injury (neuroma) or the spinal ganglion or the dorsal roots of injured afferents. Abnormal sodium channel expression or redistribution is thought to be responsible for these changes. The pain quality is described as lancinating or shock-like burning pain.

2. Ephaptic connections between injured and uninjured nerve fibres leading to ectopic discharges in injured fibres evoking spontaneous activity in uninjured ones.

3. Abnormal chemical sensitivity develops in primary afferents (phenotypic switching) so that they become sensitive to substances they were not responding to prior to injury, such as catecholamines.

Central mechanisms include:

1. Central sensitization of spinal cord cells due to the injury barrage, ongoing spontaneous activity in uninjured and injured axons, or release of neuroactive substances from glial cells.

2. Disinhibition of spinal cord cells due to afferent cell death, atrophy or decreased supraspinal inhibition or loss of inhibitory neurotransmitters such as GABA.

3. CNS plasticity in the form of degenerative and regenerative events that result in structural rearrangements of neuronal connections leading to permanent aberrant connections.

4. Changes at one level of the nervous system lead to subsequent pathophysiological changes at more rostral levels of the neuraxis, e.g., thalamus and cortex that can lead to altered sensory perceptions such as phantom limb pain (see Box 5.4).

Glial cells and neuropathic pain

Traditionally, the role of glial cells has been thought of primarily in terms of neuronal support functions. However, new findings provide an additional role in the creation and maintenance of neuropathic pain. Glial cells possess many of the same characteristics as neurones such as expressing the same receptors and synthesizing and releasing neurotransmitters. Nerve injury and inflammation induce glial cell activation and recent evidence points to a role for activated glial cells in chronic pain associated with bone cancer and infectious diseases such as AIDS. Once activated, they produce and release proinflammatory cytokines and prostaglandins that activate pain signalling cascades. This may account for the high incidence of pain reported in AIDS patients and in bone cancer patients (see Box 5.5). It also offers another potential avenue for pain control. For example, the drug minocycline, which selectively inhibits activated microglia, is in clinical trials for pain associated with spinal cord injury.

Pharmacology of pain

Pain is a very common symptom, which accompanies a variety of pathological states. Therefore, analgesia, i.e. the relief

Box 5.4 Phantom limb pain

Phantom limb pain occurs in many amputees that suffer a traumatic accident. It also occurs in avulsion (i.e. extrusion of nerve roots) injury patients. The sensations occur when an area of the body which is not damaged is touched and elicits pain sensations that feel as though they originate in the amputated region. For example, stroking the face can elicit phantom pain in arm amputees or stimulating the genitalia can elicit phantom pain in lower limb amputees.

For the brain to perceive a phantom, it must recognize that a body part is no longer present. This raises the intriguing question of whether the brain has an innate map of the body or if body image is generated from peripheral sensory input. One theory suggests that the brain contains an innate body image, a neural network that is genetically determined but modulated by the environment. If this 'neuromatrix' is deprived of modulating input, it produces an abnormal signature pattern that can result in phantom sensations. This theory can account for phantom sensations in congenital amputees and children, although in these cases the phantoms are rarely painful.

The mechanisms behind phantom limb pain remain incompletely understood but involve plasticity at several levels of the nervous system. This is the remapping hypothesis. Damage to the peripheral nerves causes a deafferentation syndrome (i.e. loss of input). The spontaneous pain is thought to arise from either the nerve neuroma or from loss of input to CNS cells causing spontaneous firing in the absence of input. The deafferentation also causes a change in the balance between excitatory and inhibitory inputs to cells. A loss of inhibition leads to an 'unmasking' of pre-existing silent synapses of adjacent uninjured nerves that under normal conditions only provide a sub-threshold input to cells but are not manifest as part of the normal receptive field. Following injury, these sub-threshold inputs become supra-threshold and now evoke action potentials in neurones in response to stimulation of the periphery. The receptive field of such cells in the deafferented spinal cord thus appears to acquire a new receptive field in response to injury. This remapping procedure occurs at subsequent levels of the brainstem, the thalamus and cortex and can be explained in terms of overlap of adjacent afferents from different parts of the body.

The somatosensory and motor cortices contain distorted body maps—the homunculus—for sensory input and motor output, respectively. Due to disinhibition of cells caused by the injury, the area of cortex adjacent to the deafferented cortex gradually 'invades' the silent region and cells become responsive to the new input. In arm amputees, the face somatosensory cortex is adjacent to the arm cortex in the map, and this area now activates the previously arm responsive area of cortex. Thus, a stimulus to the face now produces sensations that are perceived as originating from the face and also from the amputated arm (Fig. 5.12). Increased activity from cells in the deafferented motor cortex may be responsible for the cramping-like pain that many patients experience. This is thought to arise because these cells fire impulses to the amputated region but receive no feedback. The strength of the signal increases in order to try to get a response, making the pain worse. Interestingly, clinical studies using electrical motor cortex stimulation or a mirror box to create the illusion of the missing limb, or the use of a prosthetic limb have all be found to reduce the levels of phantom pain in patients.

To conclude, human pain conditions often involve a collection of different mechanisms, often activated concomitantly. Therefore, it is unlikely that one drug can provide relief in complex cases.

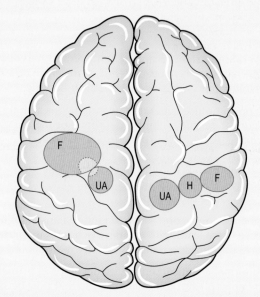

Fig. 5.12 Schematic representation of results from PET studies showing expansion of facial somatosensory cortex and upper arm cortical regions (enlarged F and UA) into the deafferented hand and forearm cortical regions (dotted circle) following upper limb amputation. On the contralateral side, each limb region has its own distinct cortical representation. UA, upper arm; H, hand; F, face regions of the somatosensory homunculus.

of pain, is an essential component of many integrated therapeutic strategies. Pain can be acute or chronic, as described in detail above, and its temporal evolution and severity may be unpredictable and pose a real challenge to the clinician. This is as exemplified by the case history. Unfortunately, at present pain is still managed inadequately in spite of the availability of a wide range of treatments. This inadequacy is due in some instances to the complex nature of pain itself. In other cases, poor pain management is due to misplaced fears as to the long-term effects of analgesics.

Cancer pain

In the UK, the likelihood of developing cancer is now more than one in three and one in four will die from the disease. Cancer affects mainly the elderly, with 65% of cases occurring in those aged over 65.

The symptom that is feared by most cancer patients is severe pain; pain is the first symptom in 25–50% of patients, and two-thirds of cancer patients require pain treatment during the course of their disease, the incidence rising in terminal cancer patients. Clinically used anti-neoplastic drugs such as taxol, vincristine and cisplatin are limited in their use because they cause painful paraesthesias due to toxic damage to the peripheral nerve fibres.

Bone cancer pain is the most common cause of cancer-related pain and represents a major clinical problem. Pain associated with primary cancers originating in the lung, breast, ovary or prostate often spreads to bone. Cancer patients report wide fluctuations in pain intensity varying from ongoing pain that is characterized as constant deep and aching in character, to intermittent episodes of extreme intense pain that occurs spontaneously, or more commonly with movement or weight bearing on a limb.

Treatment for cancer pain has been hampered by the lack of knowledge of the basic neurobiology of mechanisms underlying cancer pain and the lack of suitable models. Treatment has been classically based on the 'WHO analgesic ladder', starting with NSAIDs, followed by weak opioids such as codeine and then strong opioid drugs such as morphine (Table 5.10). However, the efficacy of such drugs is sometimes limited and they have many unwanted effects. Although cancer pain is treated with opioids to provide round-the-clock analgesia, patients often suffer from 'breakthrough' pain whilst taking the analgesic medication. Recently, a new opioid drug formulation called ACTIQ (oral transmucosal fentanyl citrate) has been approved specifically for breakthrough pain. ACTIQ dissolves through the mucous membranes in the mouth and provides rapid pain relief within 5 to 10 minutes. Patients find the drug easy to use, effective, and they tolerate it well.

Breakthroughs in the understanding of cancer pain mechanisms have arisen with the advent of animal models of bone cancer pain that closely model the human condition. In these models, pain severity is directly related to bone degeneration. Pain is thought to be due to tumour cells releasing cytokines and growth factors that activate T cells and osteoclasts. Osteoclast activity can be controlled by a molecule called osteoprotegerin ligand (OPGL), whose receptor is found on osteoclasts. Bone resorption can be blocked by a naturally secreted decoy receptor called osteoprotegerin (OPG), which binds to OPGL, and prevents the activation of osteoclasts. Treatment with OPG prevents bone destruction and the secondary associated spinal cord changes, and most importantly, it significantly reduces the breakthrough pain. Bone degeneration is associated with the release of inflammatory mediators and lowered extracellular pH that lead to the activation and sensitization of bone periosteum primary afferents. This is coupled with neurochemical changes in the spinal cord, particularly increased glial cell activation. Glial cells are known to regulate excitatory amino acid levels, and activated cells are also a source of cytokines and growth factors that will alter the surrounding neuronal microenvironment. Ultimately, all these changes lead to the induction of central sensitization.

Table 5.10 The 1986 WHO Analgesic Ladder suggested for cancer pain management

Non-opioid analgesics if pain persists or increases
Weak opioids and non-opioids if pain persists or increases
Strong opioid and non-opioids

The previous review of the pain pathways and of the local circuits involved in nociception and pain shows that multiple neurotransmitter systems, at various levels of the neuraxis, may constitute therapeutic targets in pain management.

Analgesic drugs may affect different aspects of nociception:

- they may act at the site of injury and decrease the pain associated with inflammatory reactions (e.g. nonsteroidal anti-inflammatory drugs—NSAIDs)
- they may alter nerve conduction (i.e. local anaesthetics)
- they may modify transmission of nociceptive information in the dorsal horn of the spinal cord (e.g. opioids and antidepressant drugs)
- they may activate descending inhibitory controls (e.g. opioids).

A general strategy used to control pain is described in the World Health Organization Analgesic Ladder, which was initially introduced in patients with cancer pain (Box 5.5). The ladder has three levels or 'rungs', as described in Table 5.10. On the first rung (i.e. at the first level), aspirin, paracetamol or other NSAIDs can be given to relieve pain. Next, weak opioid drugs can be introduced (such as codeine, tramadol or dextropropoxyphene). Finally, the third rung is represented by strong opioids such as morphine, hydromorphone, fentanyl, buprenorphine and methadone. The non-opioid drugs can be used in combination with opioids, in order to potentiate the pain-relieving effects. This 3-step gradual approach is based on the use of the two main categories of analgesic drugs: (1) non-opioid and (2) opioid drugs. These categories are described below.

Opium—a trail that goes back to the beginning of medical history

Opium has been known to mankind for millennia. Egyptian papyri mention its medical uses and the Sumerians describe the poppy as 'the plant of joy'. Preparations based on opium extracts have been used to treat cough and diarrhoea. In parallel to this, there has been awareness across cultures of the addictive properties of opium.

The effects of morphine prompted a search for specific receptors, which culminated with the discovery of opiate receptors in 1973. This discovery was followed in 1975 by the identification of the first endogenous opioid peptides, the enkephalins. All the endogenous opioid substances discovered so far are peptides. Opioid peptides are produced following the general pattern of synthesis of neuropeptides. They are synthesized as part of large protein precursors that undergo extensive posttranslational maturation, and after proteolytic cleavage release the bioactive peptides.

The list of opioid peptides continues to increase, and their classification has become very complex. The three main types of peptides, i.e. the enkephalins, dynorphins and β-endorphin derive from three different precursors.

- Proopiomelanocortin is the protein precursor for endorphin. Cells expressing this gene are concentrated

in the arcuate nucleus of the hypothalamus and β-endorphin projections innervate extensively other hypothalamic nuclei, limbic structures and the raphe nuclei.

- Proenkephalin is the precursor for enkephalins. This precursor is expressed predominantly in interneurones.
- Prodynorphin is the precursor for dynorphins and neoendorphins. Cells expressing the precursor are present in several brain areas, particularly areas involved in nociception, and also in the spinal cord.
- Nociceptin and nocistatin are opioid-related peptides which are synthesized as part of the orphanin FQ/nociceptin precursor. As their name suggests, their effects on nociception appear to be mutually antagonistic. Nociceptin binds to the ORL1 receptor, which shows overall 60% homology with the three main opioid receptor types.
- Endomorphin-1 and endomorphin-2 are two recent additions to the large opioid peptide family. These peptides have very high affinity and selectivity for μ opioid receptors. Endomorphin-1 appears to be more widely distributed within the brain than endomorphin-2, whereas the latter is more prevalent in the spinal cord.

Opioid analgesics

The terms 'opioid' and 'opiate' are often used interchangeably, although they have a different meaning. 'Opiate' means that a substance is extracted from opium or is similar in structure to natural substances present in opium. Opium is the dried exudate obtained from unripe seedpods of the poppy *Papaver somniferum*, and contains morphine, codeine, and other alkaloid substances. 'Opioid' is a term that designates substances that are not derived from opium. It refers particularly to opioid peptides, i.e. endogenous compounds that bind to opioid receptors and mimic the effect of morphine-like compounds. This term is now used to designate all agents that act on opioid receptors. Morphine, the prototype opioid drug, has been used for many centuries (Box 5.6).

Opioids and opiates bind to opioid receptors, which are G-protein coupled receptors. Three main receptor types have been identified: mu (μ) receptors—divided into μ_1 and μ_2, delta (δ) receptors—divided into δ_1 and δ_2 and kappa (κ) receptors—divided into κ_1, κ_2 and κ_3.

Opioid substances that act as agonists at opioid receptors, often have limited selectivity for a given receptor type. Opioid agonists reduce neuronal excitability (by increasing potassium conductance) and inhibit neurotransmitter release (by decreasing calcium influx that is required for exocytosis). Administered systemically,

opioid agonists induce a host of effects, which include analgesia. This complex effect profile is a direct consequence of the widespread distribution of opioid receptors in the brain and spinal cord, and also at the periphery. The activation of each main type of opioid receptor can be associated with certain predominant effects as illustrated in Table 5.11. Although opioid agonists, in particular at the mu receptor type, can induce significant analgesia, their use is always associated with unwanted effects, some of which may become life-threatening, such as respiratory depression.

A range of opioid agonists, partial agonists and also opiate antagonists is available in the clinic. These drugs have unique pharmacokinetic and pharmacodynamic characteristics, as described below. The choice of opioid drug used in a patient ideally should take into account these characteristics, but in reality is also influenced by the individual patient response to a particular drug.

Opioid analgesic drugs

Morphine is still the gold standard against which other opioid analgesics are compared. It can be administered via oral, intravenous, intramuscular or subcutaneous routes. Slow-release preparations are also available. The drug undergoes

Table 5.11 Effects associated with the stimulation of opioid receptor subtypes

Effects	Mu receptors	Delta receptors	Kappa receptors
Analgesia			
Supraspinal	+++	+/−	−
Spinal	++	++	+
Respiratory depression	+++	++	+
Pupillary constriction	++	−	−
Reduced GI motility	++	++	+
Sedation	++	−	++
Euphoria	++	−	−
Dysphoria	−	−	+++
Dependence	+++	−	+/−?

+++, strong effect; +, weak effect; −, no effect.

significant first pass metabolism, so only a small fraction reaches systemic circulation after oral administration. One of the metabolites, morphine-6-glucuronide, is biologically active and induces significant analgesia. The administration of morphine leads to pain alleviation, but also to respiratory depression, nausea and vomiting, constipation, sedation, pupillary constriction ('pin-point' pupil) and histamine release. The metabolite morphine 6-glucuronide can accumulate in patients whose renal function is impaired, which increases the risk of respiratory depression.

Heroin (diamorphine) is a prodrug, which is metabolized to morphine (which is ultimately responsible for its effects). Heroin is more lipid soluble than morphine, therefore the effect after intramuscular administration has a more rapid onset. Its properties make it particularly suitable for epidural administration to relieve postoperative pain after major surgery. Its higher solubility also constitutes an advantage for continuous subcutaneous infusion.

Codeine is an analgesic with lower efficacy than morphine (approximately 20% of the potency of morphine potency). Its analgesic effect is due to demethylation in the liver to morphine. It may be used in combination with aspirin or paracetamol and it also has a significant antitussive (suppression of cough) effect. Like morphine, it induces constipation.

Pethidine is a synthetic substance, which is more sedative and has a more rapid onset and a shorter duration of action than morphine. Its metabolite, norpethidine, is active and may accumulate to toxic levels in patients with renal impairment. Its potency is 1/10th of that of morphine.

Methadone is a synthetic compound with a half-life of 24–30 hours. It has significantly higher bioavailability than morphine after oral administration (approximately

80% vs. 25–30% for morphine) and lacks active metabolites. Methadone has activity at the mu opioid receptor, and also inhibits 5-HT reuptake and is an antagonist at NMDA glutamate receptors. It leads to a much milder physical abstinence syndrome than morphine but can induce psychological dependence. Methadone is routinely used in maintenance programs for morphine and heroin addicts. Its interesting profile as an analgesic is still underestimated in the clinic.

Fentanyl is a highly potent compound, with a half-life of 1–2 hours. Fentanyl and related compounds (alfentanil, remifentanil) can be given before or during induction of general anaesthesia. The initial dose can be followed by a prolonged infusion during the surgical procedure. Fentanyl formulations are also used to treat breakthrough cancer pain (Box 5.5).

Buprenorphine is a very lipid soluble compound, which acts as a partial agonist at μ receptors. It is a potent compound (50 times more potent than morphine) but has less efficacy than morphine. Consequently, it may lead to a re-emergence of pain in patients who have received opioids with higher efficacy, such as morphine. It can be used sublingually and it has a longer duration of action than morphine, but is more emetic. It may induce dysphoria and sedation.

Tramadol is an atypical opioid that possesses antinociceptive and anti-hyperalgesic properties. It is an attractive alternative to traditional opioid analgesics because of its improved side effect profile, reduced abuse potential and lack of tolerance and dependence. Tramadol is effective in a broad range of moderate to moderately severe types of pain. It acts weakly at mu receptors but also interacts with monoaminergic systems (but less effectively than tricyclic antidepressants).

Opioid antagonists

The opioid antagonist naloxone is used to reverse the effects of opioid agonists. Naloxone is used in the management of opioid overdose, or to relieve respiratory depression in apnoeic infants after opioids (e.g. pethidine) administered to the mother during labour. The half-life of naloxone is short (<1 hour), therefore repeated injections may be required before reversal of the effect of an agonist (which may have a much longer half-life than naloxone) is achieved.

Important clinical issues in the use of opioid drugs

The use of opioids in the clinic is still fraught in some cases with concerns about tolerance, dependence and addiction, and also the risks posed by the unwanted effects of these compounds.

Tolerance and dependence

Tolerance (i.e. the necessity to increase the dose in order to achieve the same effect) may develop during chronic administration of drugs, and it may be due to both pharmacokinetic and pharmacodynamic changes. Tolerance to opioids can develop rapidly, especially under experimental conditions, when doses are increased steeply. Physical and psychological dependence may also develop. Physical dependence is associated with a withdrawal syndrome when the administration of the drug is stopped abruptly. Psychological dependence leads to craving for the drug. However, it is very important to note that the real risk of tolerance to and dependence on opioids should be assessed during use of opioid drugs in a clinical context. The concept of tolerance can often be misused in pain management, to simply mean the requirement for a higher dose. This only reflects tolerance if the pain has not increased! For example, in pain associated with cancer, the reason for increasing the dose is usually an increase in the pain. Patients can often be maintained on the same oral morphine dosage for months, with no obvious signs of tolerance. Therefore, when opioid analgesics are used in appropriate doses to treat pain that is sensitive to such drugs, tolerance is not a significant and prevalent problem associated with chronic opioid drugs. Similarly, the risk of development of addiction when opioids are used for the relief of pain is extremely low.

Risks associated with the unwanted effects of opioids

The under-use of opioids is sometimes justified by the fear of inducing life-threatening respiratory depression. However, the respiratory depression induced by opioids tends to be short-lived and is often antagonized by the pain. Other unwanted effects of opiates, such as nausea and sedation may dissipate with prolonged use. If strong opioids are required in a patient, the acceptability of the medication and the patient's response may be much improved by the concomitant management of side effects. For example, if tolerance to nausea and vomiting does not develop after a few days, administration of antiemetic compounds is required (sometimes a combination of such drugs). Pharmacological management may become thus more complex but ultimately provide to the patient a pain-free state.

Mode of administration of opioids

Analgesic drugs are available in a variety of formulations, and the versatility of modes of administration is well-illustrated by opioids. As discussed below, each mode of administration has its advantages and drawbacks.

- Oral administration. This is a widely used route and one that most patients prefer. However, it may not always be available (e.g. immediately after surgery), or it can be made difficult by swallowing problems. The occurrence of vomiting will limit the absorption of drugs administered via this route. Furthermore, delays in gastric emptying may also decrease absorption of an orally administered opioid. Even if the drug is absorbed, the metabolism in the gut and the liver (first pass metabolism effect) may lead to reduced bioavailability of the drug using this route.

- Sublingual administration. This avoids the first pass metabolism, as absorption of the drug occurs directly into the circulation.

- Rectal administration. First pass metabolism can also be avoided using the rectal route, if acceptable to the patient. Absorption of the drug is slow, but bioavailability is improved overall. It is a mode of administration that can be considered for maintenance of analgesia.

- Intravenous administration. The administration of a bolus of opioids by this route leads to immediate analgesia. However, this route has a higher risk of over-dosage and the patients must not be left unsupervised for a long time.

- Intramuscular administration. Intermittent intramuscular administration of opioids (e.g. on a 4 hourly basis) is still a standard procedure used worldwide. Pain relief can be achieved satisfactorily, but its maintenance at an optimum level requires regular assessment. Also, repeated injections are painful and the control and adjustment of the doses may not be easy.

- Intrathecal and epidural administration. These techniques allow the use of much lower doses of opioids through spinal catheters. However, side effects do still occur, such as nausea and vomiting and urinary retention, as well as a risk of respiratory depression. Furthermore, local infection or displacement of the catheter may occur.

- Transdermal patch administration. This is a non-invasive mode of administration of the drug and is particularly suitable for lipophilic and potent compounds (e.g. fentanyl).

Clinical experience clearly shows that the patient's response to opioids varies significantly. Ideally, these individual requirements should be taken into account and this is what the procedure called patient controlled analgesia (PCA) is achieving today in many centres. PCA relies on a system whereby the patient can administer their own analgesic according to their needs and to the severity of their pain. The patient can administer intermittent boluses of the drug, which is delivered through a catheter. The placement of the catheter can be intravenous, intramuscular, subcutaneous or even epidural. A minimum time period between doses (the 'lock-out' period) as well as a maximum dose of the opioid chosen can be programmed into the PCA device, thus preventing overdose. Experience shows that patients using PCA titrate their analgesia to the point where they are comfortable, without excess demands. The feeling of control over their pain improves significantly the patient's outlook on their condition. However, for economic reasons, PCA methods are not yet widely available.

Pain sensitivity to opioids

Different types of pain are differentially sensitive to opioid treatments. Some, such as deafferentation pain or muscle spasms are insensitive to opioid drugs; nerve or CNS compression injury or bone cancer are partially sensitive to opioids while acute pain, post surgical pain, and pain associated with myocardial infarction or other types of cancers can be readily treated with opioids. Lastly there are some conditions such as irritable bowel syndrome that are opioid sensitive, but opioid treatment is inadequate.

Non-opioid analgesics

NSAIDs represent the most commonly used group of drugs worldwide, most of which are available without prescription. There is significant variability in patient tolerance and response to these drugs. Examples are: aspirin, paracetamol and ibuprofen. These drugs are mainly used to treat mild or moderate pain, in general associated with inflammatory processes (e.g. rheumatoid arthritis and osteoarthritis). NSAIDs can also be used to treat the severe pain associated with bone metastasis in cancer. The analgesic/antipyretic/anti-inflammatory effects of NSAIDs are largely due to inhibition of cyclo-oxygenase enzymes (COX), and the resulting inhibition of the synthesis of prostaglandins, which are pro-inflammatory. COX has two forms: COX-1 and COX-2. COX-1 is a constitutive enzyme, whereas COX-2 is induced at sites of inflammation. Aspirin, paracetamol, ibuprofen, and diclofenac are non-selective COX inhibitors. In particular, it is the inhibition of COX-1 that underlies the majority of unwanted effects of NSAIDs, such as gastrointestinal irritation and bleeding, dizziness and drowsiness. Nephrotoxicity is due to actions on the constitutively expressed COX-2 enzyme in the kidney. In the stomach, the prostaglandins PGE_2 and PGI_2 inhibit acid secretion and have a gastroprotective action, whereas in the kidney PGE_2 and PGI_2 act as local vasodilators. Therefore, inhibition of their synthesis reduces renal blood flow and may precipitate acute renal failure. In addition, the prolonged use of non-selective NSAIDs is associated with risk of chronic renal failure due to development of interstitial nephritis. All NSAIDs also have antiplatelet activity, leading to increased bleeding time. More recently, selective COX-2 inhibitors have become available, such as rofecoxib and celecoxib. These compounds have similar analgesic efficacy to non-selective COX inhibitors but lack their unwanted effects and are used in the treatment of osteo- and rheumatoid arthritis and dental pain. Although long-term use may lead to nephrotoxicity, their overall improved safety profile makes them suitable for high-risk patients with life-threatening diseases such as cancer.

Commonly used NSAIDs

- Aspirin (acetylsalicyclic acid) is analgesic, anti-inflammatory and anti-pyretic. This is due to the irreversible inhibition of the COX enzyme. COX is required for prostaglandin and thromboxane synthesis, peripherally at the site of injury. Aspirin acts as an acetylating agent, i.e. an acetyl group is covalently attached to a serine residue in the active site of the COX enzyme. This makes aspirin different from other NSAIDs (such as diclofenac and ibuprofen), which are reversible inhibitors. It is unclear whether the effect of aspirin also has a central component. Aspirin-containing preparations should not be given to children under 12 years, because of the risk of development of Reye's syndrome.

- Paracetamol (acetaminophen) is antipyretic and analgesic, but with negligible anti-inflammatory effects. It is well absorbed after oral administration and does not irritate gastric mucosa. It was suggested that paracetamol may act as inhibitor of COX-3, a splice-variant of COX-1, but this is disputed. Paracetamol reduces the levels of prostaglandins but this is not associated with an anti-inflammatory action. Its mode of action remains unclear but recent evidence indicates that paracetamol inhibits prostaglandin synthesis in cells with low levels and production of peroxide. At peripheral sites of inflammation with a high peroxide level, its effect may be inhibited. There is also evidence that paracetamol can modulate the endogenous cannabinoid system, and this may partly underlie its analgesic effects. The prolonged use of paracetamol and the ingestion of high doses are associated with significant risk of hepatotoxicity. Paracetamol overdose is treated with N-acetylcysteine.

- Ibuprofen has analgesic and anti-inflammatory properties. Among the non-selective NSAIDs it is one of the drugs of choice because it is effective and has a relatively low side effect profile. Like other NSAIDs its mechanism of action is principally through COX-2 inhibition. Alternatives to ibuprofen are: diclofenac, naproxen, piroxicam, ketorolac, indomethacin, and mefenamic acid.

Other approaches to pain management

Some types of pain do not respond to either opioid analgesics or NSAIDs, nor can they be managed based only on the principles underlying the World Health Organization Analgesic Ladder. Examples of such types of pain are given below, including their pharmacological management.

Neuropathic pain

Neuropathic pain appears to be relatively insensitive to opioids. It can be significantly relieved with tricyclic antidepressants (e.g. amitryptiline), anticonvulsant agents (e.g. carbamazepine) or local anaesthetics (Box 5.7). The reason for this diversity of treatment is the pathophysiology of neuropathic pain, which is complex and still incompletely defined (see above). It is well-established now that neuropathic pain involves changes in the phenotype of the neurones that are part of nociception pathways, and

Local anaesthetics and sodium channels

Local anaesthetics (e.g. lignocaine, amethocaine, bupivacaine, prilocaine) are agents which block the initiation and propagation of nerve action potentials, by blocking Na$^+$ channels. Their mode of administration varies: surface anaesthesia, infiltration, spinal or epidural anaesthesia. They are generally used for pain associated with localized surgery, childbirth or in dentistry. However, newer drugs, such as tocainide and mexiletine, may be used in future as oral analgesics for neuropathic pain. The main problem associated with local anaesthetics is the risk of systemic toxicity (e.g. hypotension, bradycardia and respiratory depression).

The molecular targets of local anaesthetics are voltage-gated Na$^+$ channels. These channels are present in both nerve and muscle cells. These molecules are also the target of the anticonvulsants phenytoin and carbamazepine and that of some antiarrhythmic drugs. The main component of Na$^+$ channels is the α subunit which forms the ion pore. In mammalian channels, the α subunit is associated with one or two smaller auxiliary subunits designated β_1 and β_2. Na$^+$ channels have three distinct conformational states. The transition between these states is voltage-dependent. When the membrane depolarizes, the channels revert to an open state that conducts ions. This is followed by a non-conducting, inactivated state. When the membrane is in a hyperpolarized state, most Na$^+$ channels are in closed resting states—which represent the third conformational state. The selectivity of local anaesthetics for depolarized Na$^+$ channels is a consequence of the binding of these drugs to the open and inactivated states that predominate at depolarized membrane potentials. These states may be associated with the highest affinity for these drugs. In contrast, the blockade of the channels by tetrodotoxin (TTX), a powerful toxin extracted from the puffer fish, is independent of the conformational state of the channel.

also morphological changes of neurones such as abnormal sprouting of fibres in the superficial dorsal horn.

Two commonly prescribed drugs for chronic neuropathic pain associated with diseases such as peripheral (e.g. diabetic) neuropathy, post herpetic neuralgia, and fibromyalgia are gabapentin and pregabalin. Gabapentin was initially developed as a GABA agonist, but its mechanism of action is still not fully defined. Recent research indicates that it binds with high affinity to the $\alpha_2\delta$-1 subunit of voltage-dependent calcium channels and therefore inhibits calcium influx through L and P/Q channels. It also reduces potassium evoked glutamate release and is an agonist at GABA$_B$ receptors. Pregabalin is related in structure to gabapentin and is more potent. It also binds to the $\alpha_2\delta$ subunit of the voltage-dependent calcium channel. Pregabalin decreases the release of neurotransmitters such as glutamate, noradrenaline and substance

P. Common adverse effects of both include diarrhoea, dizziness, drowsiness, peripheral edema.

Migraine

Migraine is a chronic neurovascular disorder that consists of recurrent attacks of severe headache, autonomic nervous system dysfunction, and in some 20% of patients, an aura involving complex neurological symptoms. The aura symptoms develop over 10–30 min and usually last less than an hour. Symptoms can be visual, sensory or motor, but may also involve language disturbances. When a headache follows, it most often occurs within an hour of the end of the aura. Isolated auras without headache are known as migraine dissociée. The most common aura is visual, and may consist of visual distortions. Sensory disturbances involve one side of the body and are characterized by descriptions of numbness or tingling on the face and in the hand. Premonitory phenomena may also occur, in approximately 60% of migraineurs, often hours to days before the onset of headache. These phenomena include psychological, neurological, constitutional, and autonomic features. Psychological symptoms include depression, euphoria, irritability, restlessness, mental slowness, hyperactivity, fatigue, and drowsiness. Neurological phenomena include photophobia, phonophobia, and hyperosmia. The generalized or constitutional symptoms include a stiff neck, a cold feeling, sluggishness, increased thirst, increased urination, anorexia, diarrhoea, constipation, fluid retention, and food cravings. Some patients just report a poorly characterized feeling that they know a migraine attack is coming.

The typical migraine headache is unilateral and throbbing. It may be bilateral and constant at first, and later become throbbing. Nausea occurs in up to 90% of patients and vomiting occurs in about one-third of migraineurs. During the attack many patients experience intense photophobia, phonophobia, and osmophobia, and seek seclusion in a dark, quiet room. Other symptoms include blurry vision, diarrhoea, abdominal cramps, polyuria (followed by decreased urinary output after the attack), and facial sensations of heat or cold, and sweating. Large population studies have shown that 64% of patients have migraine without aura, 18% have migraine with aura, 13% have both types, whereas the remaining have aura without migraine.

Attacks of migraine may last from 4–72 hours. Different combinations of features may occur between patients or even between attacks in the same patient. It is important to note that tension-type headache (the most common primary headache) may sometimes present as a throbbing pain, but is devoid of the associated features of migraine. This difference is important in terms of treatment of the two conditions.

Migraine attacks can be triggered by a variety of factors: endocrine changes (e.g. during pregnancy or the menstrual cycle), sleep excess or deprivation, physical exercise, stress or tiredness. Paradoxically, migraine may emerge at a time when the patient feels relaxed. Intriguingly, even in

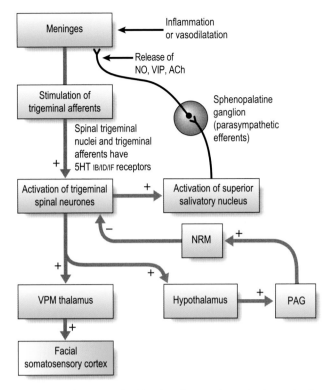

Fig. 5.13 Pathways involved in trigeminovascular activation and pain modulation by serotonin. PAG, periaqueductal grey; NRM, nucleus raphe magnus; SSN, superior salivatory nucleus; VIP, vasoactive intestinal polypeptide; Ach, acetylcholine; VPM, ventroposteromedial thalamic nucleus.

the same patient, it is impossible to predict the sensitivity to common triggers. It is generally recommended that migraineurs should have regular habits and a very smooth lifestyle.

The pathophysiology of migraine is only partly understood. There is a strong genetic component that is polygenic and susceptibility loci have been found on several chromosomes. Imaging studies have detected the activation of the brain stem during migraine attacks. Migraine is associated with a wave of vasoconstriction followed by reactive vasodilatation. The main elements involved in the generation of pain are: the cranial blood vessels, the trigeminal innervation of the vessels and the reflex connections of the trigeminal system with the cranial parasympathetic outflow. Recently, convincing mechanistic explanations have been discovered for some of the symptoms of migraine (see Box 5.8).

As shown in Fig. 5.13, the input from the trigeminal afferents that innervate the meningeal vessels passes through the trigeminal ganglion and synapses with second-order neurones in the trigeminocervical complex. Second-order neurones project to the thalamus. In the pons, there is a connection with neurones in the superior salivatory nucleus, which results in a parasympathetic outflow which is mediated through the pterygopalatine, otic and carotid ganglia. This trigeminal-autonomic reflex exists in normal persons, and is increased in migraine.

Pain is mainly generated at the level of the cranial vessels or in the dura mater. The innervation involved originates from branches of the ophthalmic division of the trigeminal nerve and also branches of the C2 nerve roots (for structures in the posterior fossa). This explains the distribution of pain over the frontal, temporal, parietal, occipital and high cervical (neck) regions. The pain may involve peripheral or central sensitization processes of craniovascular afferents, and the activation of vasodilator mechanism. However, migraine is not primarily caused by a vascular event. It is likely to be due to abnormal neuronal activity in diencephalic or brain stem nuclei (see Box 5.8).

Treatment of migraine attacks

The treatment of migraine consists of non-pharmacological and pharmacological approaches. The non-pharmacological strategy consists of the maintenance of a daily routine which avoids changes in lifestyle and also identifies triggering factors. Pharmacological treatment consists of two strategies: non-specific and migraine-specific treatments.

The non-specific drugs that can be used include aspirin, paracetamol, other NSAIDs, mild opioids or combination analgesics. These analgesic drugs are used to treat other types of pain, including tension-type headache. The administration of drugs that prevent vomiting and increase gastric motility (e.g. metoclopramide) increases the efficacy of these drugs. Many migraineurs report a reasonable relief of pain using a combination of mild analgesics. Such combinations may vary for the same patient, according to the severity of the attack. The migraine-specific drugs include the ergot derivatives and the triptans. Ergotamine and dihydroergotamine are ergot derivatives. They bind to at least two receptor types (adrenergic and 5-HT receptors) and to combinations of different subtypes within these types, and have complex pharmacodynamics. They induce generalized vasoconstriction and their use may lead to ergotism, an overuse syndrome, which may include rebound headaches when attempting to stop the drug.

The triptans are a family of related compounds with a less complex pharmacodynamic profile than the ergot derivatives. Examples of triptans are sumatriptan, almotriptan, eletriptan, frovatriptan, zolmitriptan, naratriptan. All the triptans have a very similar pharmacodynamic profile. They are $5\text{-}HT_{1B/1D}$ receptor agonists. They can be administered non-orally (nasal sprays, suppositories, inhalers, injections). For example, sumatriptan is available in oral, subcutaneous, rectal and intranasal formulations. The oral bioavailability ranges from 14% (sumatriptan) to 69% (almotriptan) or 74% (naratriptan). Triptans have at least three possible sites of action: cranial vasoconstriction (the $5\text{-}HT_{1B}$ component), peripheral neuronal inhibition (the $5\text{-}HT_{1D}$ component) and inhibition of transmission through second-order neurones of the trigeminocervical complex ($5\text{-}HT_{1B}$, $5\text{-}HT_{1D}$ and possibly $5\text{-}HT_{1F}$ component).

Activation of the trigeminovascular system is thought to be responsible for the pain of migraine. The aura symptoms may be due to cortical spreading depression (CSD). CSD can be triggered by focal activation of the cortex and is more readily seen in the occipital cortex than elsewhere. It is characterized by a slowly propagating wave of strong neuronal depolarization that generates intense neuronal activity followed by suppressed activity lasting many minutes. This has been confirmed in migraineurs experiencing aura using blood oxygen level-dependent functional magnetic resonance imaging. CSD produces many changes in the extracellular fluid environment by increasing levels of potassium ions, protons, prostaglandins, arachidonic acid, which can sensitize the meningeal vascular afferents. CSD has also been observed with imaging methods in migraineurs who do not experience aura but the mechanisms for initiation and propagation of the CSD remain incompletely understood. CSD might occur when enhanced activation coincides with precipitating factors.

An alternative view is that migraine occurs due to dysfunction in brainstem nociceptive circuits such that a defect in pain modulation could result in increased activity in trigeminal neurones making them more susceptible to sensitization (Fig. 5.14).

Finally, identification of genes that result in defects in ion channels indicates that migraine may be a channelopathy. Most channelopathies are disorders of neuronal excitability, highlighting the importance of activity in the pathogenesis of migraine. In familial hemiplegic migraine, there is a defect in the α_1 subunit of P/Q type voltage-gated calcium channels. This channel is expressed in all structures that play an important role in the pathogenesis of migraine. They are known to regulate cortical neurone firing and in mutant mice that are deficient in this gene, cortical neurones become hyperactive and may thus contribute to CSD. This channel is also found on cells that regulate the descending inhibitory pain system,

and blocking P/Q channels facilitates pain, adding further evidence to dysfunction of brainstem activity being involved in migraine.

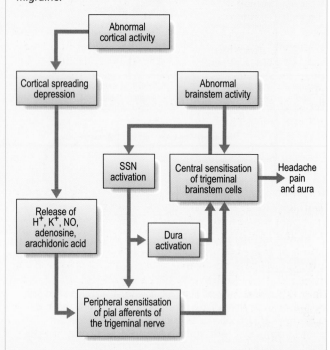

Fig. 5.14 Hypothetical pathophysiological mechanisms involved in migraine. Recent data indicate that abnormal cortical activity leads to cortical spreading depression (CSD) that is the most likely initiating event in stimulating the trigeminal vascular system afferents in migraine. Abnormal activity in trigeminal brainstem neurones involved in the control of facial pain may also contribute to central sensitization of spinal trigeminal neurones (STN) leading to hyperexcitability. When CSD occurs in conjunction with migraine trigger factors, migraine occurs. Adapted from Pietrobon, Striessnig. Nat Rev Neurosci 2003; 4:386.

The side-effects of triptans are tingling, paraesthesias, dizziness, flushing, neck pain or stiffness. They can constrict coronary arteries, leading to symptoms similar to angina pectoris. Contraindications to use are ischaemic heart disease, hypertension and cerebrovascular disease.

Preventative treatment of migraine

If attacks occur at least twice a month, or if there is a clear trend toward an increasing frequency of attacks, preventative treatment may be considered. A variety of drugs, belonging to different pharmacological classes can be used in prophylactic treatment. All such prophylactic therapies are relatively non-specific, have moderate

efficacy and substantial side-effects, as illustrated in the examples given below (unwanted effects in parentheses):

- beta-adrenergic receptor agonists—propranolol, metoprolol (tiredness, postural hypotension)
- tricyclic antidepressants—amitryptiline (drowsiness, dry mouth, postural hypotension)
- anticonvulsants—valproate (weight gain, hair loss, tremor, hepatotoxicity, teratogenic effects)
- calcium-channel blockers—flunarizine (depression, weight gain, tiredness)
- 5-HT receptor antagonists—pizotifen (drowsiness, weight gain), methysergide (drowsiness, leg cramps, retroperitoneal fibrosis).

Novel and better therapeutic targets in the treatment of migraine are likely to emerge from a better understanding of the neural events which lie at the origin of migraine. Promising results have been reported with glutamate ionotropic receptor antagonists and adenosine receptor agonists that target peripheral and central sensitization mechanisms. These are undergoing phase 2 trials and it is hoped that they could be at least as effective as the triptans. Another useful therapy may be to target neuronal hyperexcitability. Drugs that can prevent CSD may be useful anti-migraine drugs, but until the mechanism underlying the neuronal hyperexcitability becomes clearer, treatments may have to be more generalized, in terms of increasing inhibitory or lowering excitatory neurotransmitter levels.

Trigeminal neuralgia

Trigeminal neuralgia is characterized by attacks of excruciating pain in the distribution of the trigeminal nerve. The pain can be initiated by stimulation of 'trigger zones' (e.g. the cheek, chin or lips). It is suggested that the cause of this neuralgia is the vascular compression (by arteries but also occasionally veins) of the axons of the trigeminal root in the pons. This may lead to partial focal demyelination, which may alter the electrical activity of trigeminal neurones through ephaptic connections and spontaneous activity.

The first line of treatment of trigeminal neuralgia is pharmacological. Carbamazepine can be used to treat the paroxysmal pain experienced by patients and effectiveness is reported in 60–80% of cases. Baclofen (a GABA$_B$ receptor agonist) or lamotrigine (an anticonvulsant that inactivates certain sodium channels) could also be considered, as well as NMDA receptor antagonists (e.g. dextromethorphan). If there is no response or gradual loss of efficacy, surgical decompression may be attempted. However, there may be recurrence of the pain several years after surgery. Studies are still needed to optimize treatment choices in trigeminal neuralgia.

Pain in children and in the elderly

A long held misperception claimed that neonates and young children perceive much less pain than adults, because of the immaturity of their central nervous system. This view has now been disproven (see Box 5.9) and it is clear that the management of pain in children can and should follow the same general principles as those used in adult patients. Young children pose a problem in terms of accurate assessment and rating of their pain. Furthermore, children may not be able to articulately ask for pain relief, therefore analgesia maintenance regimes should be considered, in order to provide maximum comfort. Indirect indices of pain relief can be used: the child could look less tense and anxious, cry less and sleep better. The oral administration of drugs is a preferred route,

---

> ### Box 5.9 Development of pain pathways
>
> The question of whether babies, premature or newborn, can feel pain is an important one, as studies show that invasive procedures that would be painful to children or adults are frequently performed on infants admitted to neonatal intensive care units. Premature babies do not 'feel' pain in the truest sense, as pain is a learned experience. However, nociceptive stimuli can have a profound effect on the development of pain pathways.
>
> The newborn nervous system is not a mini-replica of the adult version. Pain-related systems in particular develop during the last trimester and after birth. Much of what we know now about the development of nociceptive systems has been based on rodent models, as the data from the rat and from human post mortems or abortions are very similar. A newborn rat is similar to a 24 week old foetus and a week old rat pup is equivalent to a newborn baby.
>
> Nociceptive afferents are physiologically mature before birth but the nociceptive pathways are not. Thus the neonatal spinal cord is hyperexcitable due to lack of inhibitory control from spinal cord interneurones and descending pathways. Neurotransmitter receptors are also widely distributed throughout the spinal cord and undergo postnatal refinement, so drugs cannot be given simply scaled down to size. Also there are age related differences in various other systems such as the kidneys and the hepatic enzyme systems, so that dosing intervals are not the same as in adults.
>
> Damage to the newborn system causes profound changes that subsequently alter the development of the pain pathways. For example, neonatal skin damage such as repeated heal lancing for blood can induce skin wounding that produces peripheral sensitization. This can cause release of inflammatory mediators and growth factors that cause skin hyperinnervation on healing and changes in the transmitter phenotype of primary afferents. This change leads to central changes in the spinal cord, such as inappropriate growth or cell death, which may have a permanent effect on neural development. Studies have shown that children who underwent traumatic procedures early in life have lowered pain thresholds compared to those that did not.

---

but the use of the rectal route should also be considered, as well as use of local anaesthetic-containing creams. Aspirin should be avoided in children below the age of 12, but all other NSAIDs can be used, as well as mild or strong opioids, after adequate dose adjustment. Children can also be taught how to use PCA devices.

The provision of analgesia in the elderly also presents specific challenges. Elderly patients may have problems of communication, and may under- or over-report pain. Careful assessment using observational techniques may be required. The absorption of drugs and their metabolism in the liver may also change in the elderly, in particular as a consequence of decreased hepatic function.

A decrease in renal function may also be dangerous, as metabolites (e.g. those of morphine and pethidine) may accumulate. Therefore, a reduction in adult doses is often mandatory. Furthermore, the medication taken by the elderly for other diseases may lead to complex drug interactions when analgesics are prescribed. Patients may be particularly vulnerable to side effects such as confusion, sedation and respiratory depression. Smaller, frequently repeated doses of opioids are preferable to larger doses.

General comments on pain management

Mild to moderate pain can be successfully managed with non-opioid analgesics, or opioids with moderate efficacy. Severe pain, acute or chronic, is generally responsive to opioids with higher efficacy. When the latter drugs are used judiciously, they can offer pain relief and improve significantly the quality of life of patients, without significant tolerance or dependence. In the case of pain which is opioid-insensitive, additional drugs can be considered, as well as non-pharmacological strategies. Examples of surgical strategies that can be used to control pain are: cordotomy (i.e. lesion of the spinal pathways that mediate nociception that are located in the anterolateral quadrant of the spinal cord), lesioning of the dorsal root entry zone, spinal cord stimulation and motor cortex stimulation. These are important therapeutic alternatives for intractable pain, resistant to medication.

The complexity of pain management is illustrated by the case presented at the beginning of this chapter. Several new approaches in the management of pain are still at an experimental stage, such as use of antagonists of substance P receptors (i.e. NK_1 receptors), inhibitors of the enzymatic degradation of enkephalins, analogues of adenosine or agonists at nicotinic receptors, agonists or antagonists at excitatory amino acid receptors. Recent research using snail toxins has uncovered conotoxins as new potential drugs for neuropathic pain. α-Conotoxin Vc1.1 targets nicotinic cholinergic receptors and is effective against peripheral neuropathic pain in animal models and accelerates functional recovery of injured neurones. ω-Conotoxins such as ziconotide target N-type calcium channels and have entered clinical trials for peripheral neuropathy. If proved active in the clinic, these new drugs may diversify the management of pain in the future.

CRANIAL NERVES AND THE BRAINSTEM

6

Chapter objectives

After studying this chapter you should be able to:

1. Define the main subregions of the brainstem and state their associated functions.

2. Describe the organization of the cranial nerve nuclei and the main ascending and descending pathways in the brainstem.

3. Describe brainstem reflexes and their clinical importance.

4. Explain the main functions of the reticular formation.

5. List the symptoms associated with damage to cranial nerves.

6. Explain the clinical signs associated with vascular or physical lesions to the different areas of the brainstem.

Introduction

In order to make an accurate diagnosis of the patient's problem, the doctor must carefully evaluate all the neurological findings. To do this, one must have a clear knowledge of the organization and function of the various cranial nerves and tracts within the brainstem. Hence, the purpose of this chapter is to build a three-dimensional picture of the internal workings of the brainstem. By understanding this arrangement, one can assess the signs and symptoms of the patient and precisely locate the level of the lesion.

The brainstem resides in the posterior fossa of the skull and comprises the medulla, pons and midbrain. The medulla is continuous with the spinal cord beyond the foramen magnum, and the midbrain connects to the thalamus and forebrain. The brainstem is essential for life; whilst a human can survive if the cerebral cortex is irreversibly damaged or removed, damage to the brainstem can kill! It is also the origin of conscious perception of different somatic and visceral sensations. The brainstem has three main functions:

1. **Cranial nerve-related functions.** The brainstem contains nuclei associated with 11 of the 12 pairs of cranial nerves, and cranial nerves III–XII emerge from its surface.

2. **Conduit functions.** The brainstem contains ascending and descending pathways that relay sensorimotor information to and from the cortex, cerebellum and spinal cord, as well as other pathways that originate within the brainstem.

3. **Integrative functions.** Cardiorespiratory activities, complex motor patterns, oculomotor functions, consciousness levels, sleep and alertness and autonomic functions occur via the reticular formation and the medial longitudinal fasciculus (MLF) that run throughout the length of the brainstem.

Knowledge of the basic organization and various functions of the brainstem is important in understanding brainstem disorders. Signs of primary brainstem injury (coma, irregular breathing, fixed and dilated pupils, and loss of oculovestibular reflexes or motor flaccidity) usually imply severe brainstem injury and have a poor prognosis.

Anatomical organization of cranial nerves in the brain

An understanding of the functional anatomy of the cranial nerves is of great clinical importance. A part of the physical examination that each patient undergoes is a test of the integrity of the cranial nerves (see Chapter 3). If a sensory or motor deficit is encountered, it is essential to determine if it is a peripheral or a central problem. If it is a peripheral problem, it is important to establish what nerve(s) are involved, or if it is a central problem, to localize where the lesion is and what other systems are affected. To answer these questions, an understanding of the anatomy of the cranial nerves is required.

Box 6.1 Case history

A first-year university student comes into casualty one morning complaining of an inability to see with his left eye. You notice that his left upper eyelid droops. He says that he got very drunk at a Fresher's party last week and on the way home, he fell over and hit his head hard on the pavement, losing consciousness for a short while. Initially, he thought the eye closure was due to swelling, but after a week, the eye had still not opened.

On inspection, his left eyelid was shut and, when the eyelid was lifted, the eyeball deviated down and out. The left pupil was fixed and dilated, whereas the right pupil responded normally to increased light intensity in either eye. When the patient smiled, only minor elevation occurred on the right side of the mouth. Further neurological examination revealed a right-sided Babinski sign, right-sided weakness in the arms and legs and hyperreflexia and hypertonia of the right side limbs. General sensory examination proved normal.

This case gives rise to the following questions:

1. Why is the left eye closed and turned down and out?
2. Why does only the right pupil respond to increased light intensity in the left eye?
3. Why are there facial paralysis and limb motor deficits?

Table 6.1 Classification of cranial nerves

Pure sensory nerves	Pure motor nerves	Mixed nerves
Olfactory (I)	Oculomotor (III) Trochlear (IV)	Trigeminal (V) Facial (VII)
Optic (II)	Abducens (VI)	Glossopharyngeal (IX)
Vestibulochoclear (VIII)	Accessory (XI) Hypoglossal (XII)	Vagus (X)

Cranial nerves have three main functions:

1. to provide the general motor and sensory innervation of the skin, muscles, and joints in the head and neck region

2. to mediate special senses (vision, hearing, taste and olfaction)

3. to regulate autonomic (visceral) functions—via parasympathetic innervation of autonomic ganglia (e.g. breathing, heart rate, blood pressure, coughing and swallowing)

Cranial nerves are either sensory, motor or mixed nerves (containing motor, sensory and autonomic fibres). This is summarized in Table 6.1.

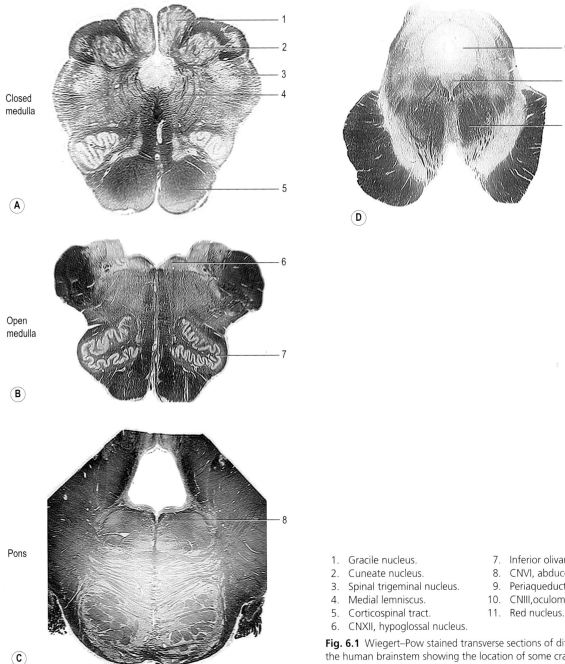

Closed
medulla

Open
medulla

Pons

Midbrain

1. Gracile nucleus.
2. Cuneate nucleus.
3. Spinal trigeminal nucleus.
4. Medial lemniscus.
5. Corticospinal tract.
6. CNXII, hypoglossal nucleus.
7. Inferior olivary nucleus.
8. CNVI, abducens nucleus.
9. Periaqueductal grey.
10. CNIII, oculomotor nucleus.
11. Red nucleus.

Fig. 6.1 Wiegert–Pow stained transverse sections of different levels of the human brainstem showing the location of some cranial nerve and brainstem nuclei.

Internal organization of the brainstem

The anatomy of the brainstem and organization of different cranial nerve nuclei is extremely complicated and has traditionally been taught by recognizing features in histological specimens from different levels of the brainstem (Fig. 6.1). However, with modern imaging methods, it is now not necessary to be able to recognize these internal features, which are seen only in post mortem histological specimens; however, one needs to be able to recognize their shape to be able to identify them in medical images such as MRI. In order to diagnose brainstem lesions, one has to be familiar with its topographical organization, and with the deficits that occur with cranial nerve lesions.

The brainstem is functionally associated with 11 of the 12 pairs of cranial nerves. Cranial nerve I, the olfactory nerve, does not attach to the brainstem but projects directly to the forebrain, and is functionally associated with the limbic system. Similarly, cranial nerve II does not directly attach to the brainstem but it does have afferent nerve branches that terminate in midbrain nuclei. For the other cranial nerves, their inputs are organized sequentially in a rostrocaudal fashion from nerve III to nerve XII (Fig. 6.2A). This gives the different subdivisions of the brainstem functional significance (Table 6.2).

The basic organization of the brainstem is the same for each region. Essentially, it is divided into three sections in the dorsoventral (transverse) axis (Fig. 6.2B). In the

dorsal part are located the cranial nerve nuclei; in the ventral part are located fibres of descending pathways; in the middle (which is called the tegmentum) are located the ascending pathways and various nuclei associated with the reticular formation. This latter structure receives input from all parts of the nervous system and exerts widespread influences on CNS functions (see later).

In the mediolateral plane, the cranial nerve nuclei are organized with respect to function. Cranial nerve nuclei associated with purely sensory nerves are located in the lateral brainstem, while purely motor cranial nerve nuclei are located most medially. Cranial nerve nuclei with mixed sensory and motor fibre input are located in-between. Each of these nerves has more than one nucleus of origin—at least one sensory (afferent) and one motor (efferent). Sometimes, more than one nerve will originate from a single nucleus: for example, the sense of taste is shared by two nerves (VII, IX) but merges into a single nucleus, the solitary nucleus.

Similarly, the ascending tracts are generally organized in a mediolateral fashion within the tegmentum. Tracts associated with motor function such as the MLF or the rubrospinal tract located more medially to those with sensory functions such as the medial lemniscus (touch and vibration), the spinothalamic tract (pain and temperature) or the lateral lemniscus (hearing). Although their exact location may vary at different rostrocaudal levels of the brainstem, the pattern of motor systems being medially located to sensory systems is always preserved.

Figure 6.3 shows a dorsal view of the brainstem to show the relative mediolateral positions of the cranial nerve nuclei in the different parts of the brainstem. This is a schematic to demonstrate the overall picture; in reality, some of these nuclei would overlap. There are up to seven different nuclei columns, corresponding to the different cranial nerve fibre types (see Box 6.2 and Fig. 6.2B), that can be arranged in a mediolateral row. In reality, the only place this occurs is in the open (rostral) medulla, near its junction with the pons. At other levels, fewer columns are present. What is clear is that sensory nuclei are located laterally to motor ones.

In summary, the organization of the brainstem is topographical in the rostrocaudal, dorsoventral and mediolateral planes: Cranial nerve attachments run sequentially

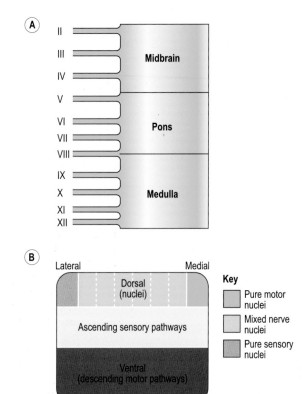

Fig. 6.2 Schematic representations of the brainstem viewed in the rostrocaudal (A) and transverse (B) planes. (A) shows the input of cranial nerves into the different regions of the brainstem. (B) shows the organization of ascending, descending tracts and cranial nerve nuclei within the brainstem.

Table 6.2 Main functions of the brainstem

Brainstem region	Associated cranial nerve input	Main functions
Midbrain	II–IV	Auditory, visual and pupillary reflexes and eye movements Regulates cortical arousal
Pons	V–VIII	Mastication, eye movement, facial expression, blinking, salivation, equilibrium and audition
Medulla	VIII–XII	Equilibrium, audition, deglutition, coughing, vomiting, salivation, tongue movement, respiration and circulation

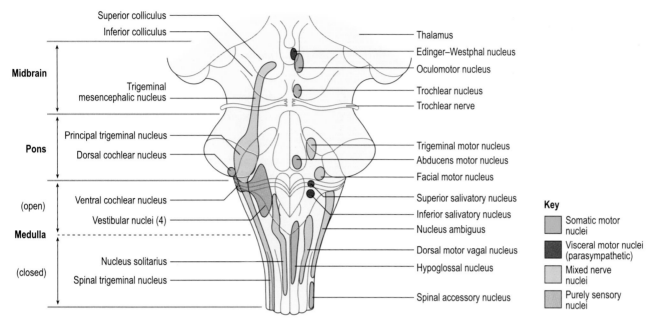

Fig. 6.3 Superior view of the brainstem, showing the schematic organization of cranial nerve nuclei, separated for clarity. Sensory nuclei are shown only on the left and motor nuclei are on the right side.

Labels in figure:
Superior colliculus
Inferior colliculus
Midbrain
Trigeminal mesencephalic nucleus
Pons
Principal trigeminal nucleus
Dorsal cochlear nucleus
(open)
Ventral cochlear nucleus
Vestibular nuclei (4)
Medulla
(closed)
Nucleus solitarius
Spinal trigeminal nucleus

Thalamus
Edinger–Westphal nucleus
Oculomotor nucleus
Trochlear nucleus
Trochlear nerve
Trigeminal motor nucleus
Abducens motor nucleus
Facial motor nucleus
Superior salivatory nucleus
Inferior salivatory nucleus
Nucleus ambiguus
Dorsal motor vagal nucleus
Hypoglossal nucleus
Spinal accessory nucleus

Key
Somatic motor nuclei
Visceral motor nuclei (parasympathetic)
Mixed nerve nuclei
Purely sensory nuclei

Box 6.2 Comparison of spinal and cranial nerves

Functionally, cranial nerves are analogous to spinal nerves in that they contain motor, sensory and visceral afferents, but there are differences between cranial and spinal nerves:

- Cranial nerves do not possess dorsal and ventral roots.
- Cranial motor afferent cell bodies are located in brainstem nuclei (not in external ganglia).
- Cranial nerves possess four types of sensory afferents (spinal nerves contain two). In addition to general somatic and visceral afferents, afferents also innervate specialized sensory organs located only in the head and neck.
- Cranial nerves possess three types of motor fibres, whereas spinal nerves contain two (general motor/ visceral). General somatic efferents innervate the extra-ocular muscles (nerves III, IV, VI) and intrinsic tongue muscles (nerve XII). General visceral efferents (controlling autonomic effectors) innervate the sweat/ tear glands and smooth muscles (nerves III, VII, IX and X). Specialized visceral fibres controlling the striated (skeletal) muscles associated with the facial expression, chewing, neck, larynx and pharynx movements (nerves V, VII, IX, X, XI) that are derived from the branchial arches during development.

from III–XII, nerve nuclei are located dorsally within the brainstem, descending tracts, ventrally with ascending pathways sandwiched in-between. Sensory cranial nerve nuclei are located laterally and motor nuclei medially, mixed ones in-between. The functional significance of this is that neurones with similar functions are in close proximity and that different functional deficits occur depending on whether the lesion is lateral or near the midline. As the location of ascending and descending tracts and the mediolateral position of cranial nuclei are relatively constant along their rostrocaudal distribution in the brainstem, specific combinations of signs can reliably indicate the site of a lesion. Therefore, analysis of brainstem disorders is greatly simplified by the answers to two questions:

1. Is it lateral or medial—delineated by presence/ absence of sensory and motor function?
2. What is the level of the lesion—delineated by specific cranial nerves?

In order to determine this, it is important to know what deficits are associated with each cranial nerve and how to test for them. The specific tests for cranial nerves are described in Chapter 3 and deficits associated with specific branches of the cranial nerves or their nuclei are detailed in Table 6.3.

Reticular formation

Running through the core of the brainstem tegmentum is the RF, which consists of a diffuse network of neurones that exerts a widespread influence on CNS functions.

Table 6.3 Cranial nerves summary

Cranial nerve	Nucleus name	Nucleus location	Function	Symptom/sign of damage
Olfactory (CNI)	Anterior olfactory	Olfactory tract	Smell	Anosmia
Optic (CNII)	Lateral geniculate	Thalamus	Vision	Blindness
Oculomotor (CNIII)	Oculomotor	Midbrain	Eye movement (elevation, adduction)	Eye deviates down and out
	Edinger–Westphal*	Midbrain	Pupil dilation	Loss of pupillary/ accommodation reflexes
Trochlear (CNIV)	Trochlear	Midbrain	Eye movement (depression of adducted eye)	Diplopia, lateral deviation of eye
Trigeminal (CNV)	Principal	Pons	Facial sensation (touch)	Facial anaesthesia
	Spinal	Medulla	Facial sensation (pain)	Loss of facial pain sensation
	Mesencephalic	Pons/midbrain	Proprioception	Clinically insignificant
	Motor	Pons	Mastication	Weakness/loss of mastication
Abducens (CNVI)	Abducens	Pons	Eye movement (abduction)	Medial eye deviation
Facial (CNVII)	Motor	Pons	Facial expression	Paralysis of facial muscles; hyperacusis
	Solitary	Pons	Taste	Aguesia (loss of taste to anterior two-thirds of tongue)
	Superior salivatory*	Pons	Salivation, lacrimation	Dry mouth, loss of lacrimation
Vestibulocochlear (CN VIII)	Vestibular	Medulla	Balance	Vertigo, dysequilibrium, nystagmus
	Cochlear	Medulla	Hearing	Deafness
Glossopharyngeal (CN IX)	Nucleus ambiguus	Medulla	Taste	Aguesia (posterior 1/3rd of tongue)
	Inferior salivatory*	Medulla	Salivation	Insignificant
	Solitary	Medulla	Innervation of pharynx	Loss of gag reflex
Vagus (X)	Nucleus ambiguus	Medulla	Swallowing and talking	Dysphagia and hoarseness of voice
	Dorsal motor vagal*	Medulla	Cardiac, GI tract, respiration	Tachycardia, loss of cough reflex
	Solitary	Medulla	Taste	Aguesia
Cranial accessory (XI)	Nucleus ambiguus	Medulla	Pharynx/larynx muscles	Insignificant
Spinal accessory	Spinal accessory	Cervical cord	Neck and shoulder movement	Head turning/shoulder shrugging weakness
Hypoglossal (XII)	Hypoglossal	Medulla	Tongue movement	Atrophy of tongue muscles, deviation on protrusion, fasciculation

*Nuclei associated with the parasympathetic nervous system.

Within this region, cells aggregate to form nuclei that are associated with regulating various sensorimotor, cortical arousal and autonomic functions (Table 6.4). They help to regulate, or fine tune, complex behaviours such as chewing, swallowing, coughing, sneezing, fighting and copulation, using automated pattern generators.

The RF is functionally divided into three regions: (1) a midline region, containing the raphe nuclei, that has a predominantly inhibitory function; (2) a medial (magnocellular) region that provides the output pathways to the spinal cord and forebrain regions; and (3) a lateral (parvocellular) region that receives input from ascending sensory pathways, and from the cerebellum, basal ganglia, hypothalamus, cranial nerves and the cerebral cortex (Fig. 6.4). This region provides input to the medial region.

The RF contains sets of neurones that utilize specific amines that function as neuromodulators. The serotonergic (5-HT) cells have the largest territorial distribution within the CNS, and project to the forebrain and to the

Table 6.4 Function of different parts of the reticular formation

	Location	Function
Ascending reticular activating system (ARAS)	Midbrain	Arousal
Periaqueductal grey region		REM sleep/pain modulation
Locus coeruleus		Arousal and attention
Raphe nucleus		Wakefulness
Interstitial nucleus of Cajal, nucleus of Darkschewitz, rostral interstitial nucleus of the MLF		Accessory nuclei associated with the vertical gaze centre
Pontine paramedian reticular formation (PPRF)	Pons	Horizontal gaze centre
Micturition centre		Bladder control
Pneumotaxic centre (medial parabrachial nucleus)		Respiration
Salivatory nucleus		Lacrimation/salivation
Supratrigeminal nucleus		Mastication
Pedunculopontine nucleus		Locomotor centre, REM sleep
Dorsal and ventral respiratory nuclei	Medulla	Respiratory centres
Cardiovascular nuclei		Heart rate/blood pressure
Raphe magnus nucleus		Pain modulation
Area postrema		Vomiting
Chemosensitive trigger zone		pCO_2/pH levels
Lateral reticular nucleus		Pattern generators for coughing and swallowing

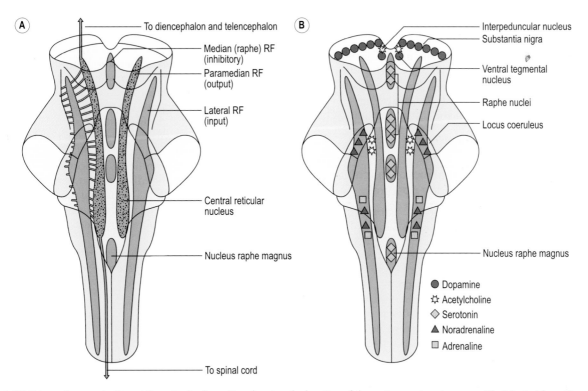

Fig. 6.4 (A) Schematic organization of the reticular formation showing the location of the various aminergic groups (B). Adapted from Fitzgerald. MJT 4th edition. WB Saunders, 2002.

spinal cord. Dopamine cells in the midbrain project to the basal ganglia and limbic cortical areas. Cells of the locus coeruleus contain noradrenaline and project to the spinal cord and forebrain. Adrenaline cells are rare and are confined to the medulla, and project to the hypothalamus and sympathetic preganglionic neurones in the spinal cord. Cholinergic cells of the midbrain project to the thalamus and basal forebrain. An imbalance in aminergic levels is associated with depression, hyperactivity and agitation, or insomnia.

Principal functions of the RF

Mediating behavioural responses: arousal, alertness, and affect

The monoamine cell groups of the upper pons and midbrain form the ascending reticular activating system (ARAS) that projects to the cerebral cortex, hippocampus, amygdala, hypothalamus and thalamus. ARAS regulates sleep and wake cycles, various emotional and behavioural responses, and orientation responses to various stimuli. Clinically, this area is important in regulating levels of consciousness: depletion of serotonin leads to insomnia. Damage to the midbrain reticular formation can lead to coma, stupor or a persistent vegetative state. Certain drugs, anaesthetics or metabolic disturbances also affect consciousness levels through their actions on the RF. Levels of RF activity are reflected on an EEG (electroencephalogram) by characteristic patterns that vary with different states of consciousness.

Modulating pain perception

The raphe and the locus coeruleus nuclei contain neurones that synapse onto interneurones in dorsal horn of the spinal cord where they mediate stimulus-induced analgesia (see Chapter 5). The RF is also involved in stress-induced analgesia and the diffuse noxious inhibitory control of pain.

Modulating spinal and cranial motor functions (muscle tone, reflexes and body posture)

The RF influences motor activities through reciprocal connections with the red nucleus, the basal ganglia nuclei, the vestibular nuclei, the motor cortex and the cerebellum. Activation of the pontine RF and medullary RF has antagonistic roles in the control of body posture via regulation of flexor and extensor reflexes. The pontine RF gives rise to the medial reticulospinal tract (RST) that facilitates extensor reflexes, inhibits flexor reflexes and increases muscle tone in axial and proximal limb muscles. The lateral RST originates in the medullary RF, facilitates flexor reflexes, inhibits extensor reflexes and decreases muscle tone in axial and proximal limb muscles. Damage to the brainstem at different levels can result in specific changes in posture, known as decerebrate or decorticate rigidity (see Chapter 9).

Gaze centres in the midbrain and pons control conjugate eye movements in the horizontal and vertical directions, via connections with the vestibular and ocular motor nerve nuclei in the brainstem and with connections from the frontal and posterior parietal eye fields.

Coordinating motor survival (autonomic) centres

The medulla contains the nuclei that control vital (survival) functions: the respiratory and cardiovascular centres, swallowing, blood pressure and vomiting (Box 6.3). A key nucleus involved in these functions is the nucleus of the solitary tract (NTS). It is involved in the coordination of swallowing and breathing so that one does not swallow air or inhale food or vomit. The NTS also receives afferents from stretch receptors in the lungs and from CSF chemoreceptors on the surface of the medulla. These fibres project onto neurones situated in the respiratory centres located in the medullary RF. NTS also receives information from aortic baroreceptors located in the carotid body in the carotid artery (via cranial nerve IX) and relays this information to the cardiovascular control centres (in the medullary RF) to regulate blood pressure (see Box 6.4).

Blood supply to the brainstem

The entire brainstem derives its blood supply from the posterior (vertebral-basilar) part of the cerebral circulation (Fig. 6.7). The medulla is supplied from the ventral surface by the two vertebral arteries that then join to form the basilar artery, which courses along the ventral surface of the pons. Further rostrally, in the midbrain, the basilar artery diverges to become the posterior cerebral arteries. Branches from the three main arteries, the vertebral, basilar and posterior cerebral, supply both the dorsal and ventral surfaces of the brainstem. These branches subdivide into three groups that supply different regions of each part of the brainstem (see Fig. 6.7).

There is a paramedian region either side of the ventral midline that is supplied by short arteries. Next to this region is an intermediate region, supplied by short circumferential arteries. The lateral zone, which supplies the dorsal aspect of the brainstem, is supplied by branches of long circumferential arteries, such as the posterior cerebral artery.

The paramedian and lateral zones are often involved in vascular accidents that give rise to characteristic clinical deficits (see later).

Brainstem reflexes

The brainstem is home to circuitry involved in several reflexes (Table 6.5). The presence or absence of these reflexes is used to determine brainstem death in a patient (see Box 6.5).

The pupillary light reflex

Normally, shining a light into one eye causes both pupils to constrict. In the stimulated eye, this is the direct light reflex, and in the non-stimulated eye, it is the consensual

Box 6.3 Nausea and vomiting

There is a wide variety of causes for nausea and vomiting: pregnancy, movement (e.g. travel sickness), vestibular disease, injury, migraine. Treatment is based on the use of antiemetics. Nausea is easier to prevent that to stop after it has started. Vomiting (emesis) is coordinated by the vomiting centre located in the lateral medullary reticular formation (Fig. 6.5). This region receives input from the chemoreceptor trigger zone, located in the area postrema of the medulla, which is rich in dopaminergic (D_2) and serotonergic ($5\text{-}HT_3$) receptors. This region is not protected by the blood–brain barrier (BBB) and is sensitive to circulating toxins or drugs. There is also input from the limbic system (that responds to unpleasant smells or sights), the spinoreticular tract (in response to physical trauma), the NTS (involved in the gag reflex), and the stomach, via the vagus nerve and the vestibular system. In motion sickness, nausea is thought to arise due to conflicting signals from the visual and vestibular systems. The output from the vomiting centre is to the spinal motor neurones innervating the abdominal muscles.

Drugs used to fight diseases such as Parkinson's disease and cancer, frequently cause nausea and vomiting because they activate the chemoreceptor trigger zone. Dopamine antagonists such as domperidone and metoclopramide are used to treat nausea. Domperidone does not cross the BBB and has few side effects. Metoclopramide also has an effect on the gut, facilitating the absorption of many drugs, such as analgesics. $5\text{-}HT_3$ antagonists such as ondansteron, inhibit receptors in the gut and the chemoreceptor trigger zone, and reduce nausea, but may result in constipation. D_2 and $5\text{-}HT_3$ antagonists are ineffective in preventing motion sickness. Anticholinergic drugs such as hyoscine (a muscarinic receptor antagonist), or antihistamine drugs such as cinnarizine, act directly on the vomiting centre to reduce sickness.

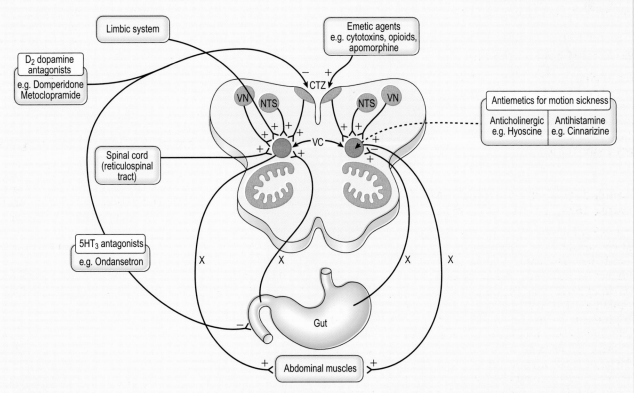

Fig. 6.5 Pathways involved in nausea and their pharmacological modulation. CTZ, chemotrigger zone; NTS, solitary nucleus; VN, vestibular nucleus; VC, vomiting centre; +, excitatory; –, inhibitory; X, Vagus nerve. Adapted from Neal MJ, Medical Pharmacology at a Glance, 3rd edn. Blackwell Science Ltd. 1997.

light reflex. Pupils are constricted by the pupillary sphincter in response to autonomic parasympathetic stimulation by the postganglionic ciliary nerves. This reflex is triggered by stimulation of the part of the optic nerve leading to the pretectal nucleus (in the superior colliculus), which, in turn, stimulates neurones in the Edinger–Westphal nucleus. From here parasympathetic preganglionic fibres travel in the oculomotor nerve (cranial nerve III) to the ciliary ganglion. Dilation of the pupils occurs more indirectly, via sympathetic stimulation. The pupillary dilator

Box
6.4
Brainstem control of respiration and heart rate

The medulla houses the respiratory and cardiovascular nuclei of the RF. These control the respiratory and heart rates in response to peripheral stimuli or changes in the partial pressure of oxygen, carbon dioxide and blood pH (Fig. 6.6).

The medulla houses the dorsal (inspiratory) and ventral (expiratory) respiratory groups in the nucleus of the solitary tract (NTS) and nucleus ambiguus respectively. Their function is to control the basic rhythm of breathing, and they can maintain breathing independently of the rest of the brain, as occurs in a persistent vegetative state.

Other centres in the pons are involved in co-ordinating breathing patterns. The pneumotaxic centre, located in the medial parabrachial nucleus inhibits the inspiratory neurones to prevent the lungs becoming over inflated. It limits inspiration and facilitates expiration. When this area is active, breathing rate is more rapid. The apneustic centre stimulates the dorsal respiratory group, prolonging inspiration and reducing expiration. When the pneumotaxic centre is active, the apneustic region is inhibited.

Damage at different brainstem levels leads to altered patterns of respiration: damage above the pons leads to a normal breathing pattern whereas damage between the pneumotaxic and apneustic centres leads to apneusis (breathing with prolonged inspiratory pauses) or Cheyne–Stokes respiration. Damage between the apneustic centre and the respiratory cell groups leads to irregular breathing patterns, and damage below the respiratory groups eliminates the respiratory drive.

Breathing is also regulated by the blood levels of CO_2 and H^+. Chemosensitive cells located in the ventrolateral part of the medulla, close to where the choroid plexus projects through the lateral aperture of the fourth ventricle, detect local acidity or alkalinity changes in the CSF, and strongly increase or decrease respiratory drive via connections with the medullary respiratory centre.

The cardiovascular (baroreceptor) centre is located in the medial NTS and is activated by the carotid sinus stretch receptors (baroreceptors). Changes in heart rate or blood pressure stimulate these centres resulting in activation of the (autonomic) cardio-inhibitory neurones of the dorsal motor vagal nucleus, to reduce heart rate, or the lateral medullary RF to reduce peripheral arteriole sympathetic tone. These are the barovagal and barosympathetic reflexes that help to lower high blood pressure.

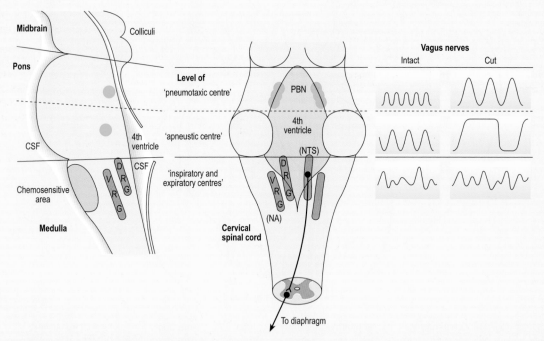

Fig. 6.6 The left and middle diagrams show lateral and dorsal views of the location of brainstem respiratory control neurone groups. The pneumotaxic centre is located in the medial parabrachial nucleus (PBN). The dorsal respiratory group (DRG) located in the solitary nucleus (NTS) and ventral respiratory group (VRG) of neurones located in the nucleus ambiguus (NA) house the inspiratory and expiratory centres, respectively. The right panel shows the breathing patterns seen in decerebrate animals with damage at different brainstem levels. After transection at the upper line, normal breathing can still occur without any influence from above the pons. After transection at the dashed line, the pneumotaxic centre is disconnected from influencing the apneustic centre, so that prolonged inspiration takes place unless inhibition occurs via stimulation of the lung stretch receptors ('vagus intact'). Transection at the lower line removes all influences above the level of the medulla and produces irregular breathing patterns. CSF, cerebrospinal fluid; V, ventricle. Adapted from Jenner S. Human Physiology. Churchill Livingstone, 1989.

is stimulated by postganglionic fibres from the superior cervical ganglion. Damage to the sympathetic nervous system fibres results in Horner's syndrome. This is characterized by pupil constriction (miosis), decreased facial sweating (anhydrosis), and slight ptosis (drooping of the eyelid). As the sympathetic pathway has a complex course from the hypothalamus through the brainstem to the T1 thoracic cord, and then on to the superior cervical ganglion before returning to the head, damage anywhere along this pathway can cause this syndrome.

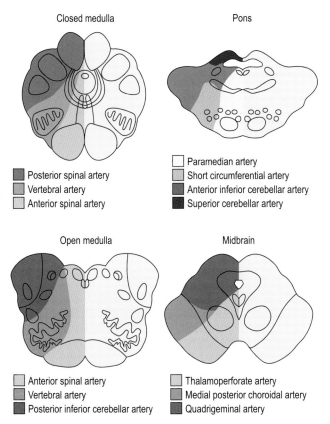

Fig. 6.7 Arterial blood supply to different regions of the brainstem. Only one side is shown for clarity.

Brain cells require an adequate oxygen supply to function normally. Prolonged hypoxia or ischaemia may be fatal to brain cells. Inadequate or incomplete resuscitation may fail to revive brain functions and thus lead to brain death, whereby all cortical function is lost, but brainstem reflexes and spontaneous breathing are still present. This is termed a persistent vegetative state.

In brainstem death, spontaneous breath ceases and there is a loss of reflexes. Cardiovascular function can be artificially maintained for a short while but will eventually deteriorate due to loss of function of the brainstem regulatory centres in the medulla. RF cell death leads to the loss of cortical arousal, and thus the lack of brain activity and hence brain death.

Several criteria must be met in order to diagnose brainstem death. There must be no pupillary, corneal, gag, cough, caloric or doll's eye reflex responses or response to painful stimuli applied to cranial nerve territories. Absence of spontaneous breaths can only be confirmed after hypercapnia tests, where the pCO_2 is >50 mmHg.

Brainstem death tests are performed by two doctors either independently or together, and are then repeated, prior to declaration of brain death. Before testing, any analgesic medications, drugs, neuromuscular blockers, metabolic imbalances or lowered body temperature, should be allowed to clear or reverse as these may account for brainstem inactivity. An EEG is not necessary.

Table 6.5 Location and pathways of brainstem reflexes

Reflex	Afferent arc	Efferent arc	Brainstem area
Pupillary light reflex	CN II	CN III (E-W)	Midbrain
Accommodation reflex	CN II	CN III (E-W)	Midbrain
Vestibulo-ocular reflex	CN VIII	CN III, IV, VI	Pons–midbrain
Jaw jerk	CN V_3	CN V_3	Pons
Blinking—sound (startle), light (e.g. flashing lights), corneal touch	CN VIII CN II CN V_1	CN VII	Pons
Gag reflex	CN IX	CN X	Medulla

CN, cranial nerve; E-W, Edinger–Westphal; V_1, ophthalmic and V_3, mandibular branches of nerve V.

Parasympathetic fibre damage results in dilated pupils (mydriasis), as the fibres are located superficially within the nerve. Ophthalmologists use short-acting parasympathetic blocking drugs that are derivatives of atropine, to dilate the pupil to examine the interior of the eye.

If only the illuminated pupil constricts, then there is damage to the crossing fibres, i.e. damage in the midbrain. If the optic nerve (afferent input) is damaged on one side then both the direct and consensual reflexes will be lost from the blind eye. The unaffected eye will show both reflexes in response to light. If cranial nerve III (efferent output from Edinger–Westphal nucleus) is damaged, then both reflexes will be lost in the ipsilateral eye and pupillary dilation will be observed in that eye. A unilateral fixed and dilated pupil is suggestive of increased intracranial pressure pressing on cranial nerve III.

The pupillary light reflex is a very important reflex and occurs even when someone is unconscious. The circuitry involved in these reflexes is detailed in Chapter 7 (see Fig. 7.6B).

The accommodation reflex

Another reflex associated with the cranial nerve III is the accommodation reflex. At rest, the lens is thin, to allow the eye to focus on far objects. To focus on near objects, the lens must thicken, by a process called accommodation, as described in Chapter 7. Accommodation and convergence of the eyes is mediated by increased tone of the medial rectus muscle and pupil constriction (contraction of the pupillae constrictor muscle), which occur together when a person views a close object. The pathway is as follows: optic nerve afferents travel to the lateral geniculate nucleus and then to the primary visual cortex. For the efferent pathway: occipital lobe fibres project to cells of the accommodation centre in the midbrain, and from here they travel to the Edinger–Westphal nucleus. Parasympathetic fibre activation results in ciliary muscle contraction, which shortens the suspensory ligament, allowing relaxation of the lens and causing passive thickening. The accommodation centre also stimulates the somatic motoneurones of the medial rectus muscles, producing convergence of the eyes to a near object, so that focus is maintained. The circuitry is detailed in Chapter 7 (see Fig. 7.6C).

Doll's eye (vestibulo-ocular) reflex

This involves conjugate eye movements in response to head movement. The normal response is for the patient's eyes to deviate in the opposite direction to head turning, i.e. if the head is briskly extended, the eyes go downwards and if the move is to the right, the eyes move to the left. Normally the cortex inhibits these reflexes, but in a comatose patient, they are disinhibited (see Chapter 8). If present, they show that the pathway (medial longitudinal fasciculus) between the relevant nuclei in the pons and midbrain is intact.

Gag reflex

Stimulation of the uvula (soft palate) or the lateral walls of the oropharynx triggers closing of the trachea. However, under general anaesthesia this reflex does not work, and unconscious patients may vomit. Thus, it is important that no food or drink be consumed for 8–12 hours before an operation, otherwise acidic vomit goes into trachea, which can be very dangerous.

Jaw jerk reflex

This monosynaptic reflex is the head equivalent of the patella reflex in the spinal cord. It is mediated by the trigeminal nerve and in normal people, the reflex is weak or absent. It only becomes prominent if there is damage to the descending corticobulbar fibres.

Blink reflexes

There are several blink reflexes (Table 6.5). Touching the cornea of one eye induces a bilateral blink response. A novel (loud) sound induces a bilateral blink (startle) response. Flashing lights induce a bilateral blink response. Stimulation of sensory afferents from cranial nerves II, V or VII activates RF interneurones that project bilaterally to the facial motor nucleus. Unconscious blinking, in contrast, functions to maintain normal hydration of the eye, and this process is probably mediated by the RF.

Brainstem lesions

Brainstem damage can be caused by vascular accidents, tumors or raised intracranial pressure that, if not treated, ultimately leads to brain tissue herniation. Vascular lesions are the most common and produce characteristic clinical syndromes (Table 6.6). Brainstem lesions are unique in that unilateral lesions produce ipsilateral cranial nerve dysfunction and contralateral dysfunction of the ascending tracts (i.e. ipsilateral facial deficits and contralateral body deficits). Certain common symptoms are associated with brainstem lesions depending on their mediolateral location. Unilateral medial lesions in general damage the corticospinal tract, thus producing contralateral spastic hemiplegia (partial paralysis of muscles, increased muscle tone) and a Babinski sign, and also the medial lemniscal pathway, resulting in contralateral loss of light touch, position and vibration senses. In addition, the level of a medial brainstem lesion can be determined by the involvement of the cranial nerves XII, VI and III.

Table 6.6 Unilateral vascular lesions of the medial brainstem

Brainstem area	Possible vascular cause	Specific symptoms (in addition to common symptoms)
Medulla (Déjerine's syndrome)	Anterior spinal/vertebral artery	CN XII: ipsilateral weakness and wasting of the tongue muscles
Pons	Basilar artery branches—paramedian pontine	CN VI: medial deviation of the eye (adduction paralysis) Pontine RF (gaze centre): ipsilateral gaze paralysis Cerebellar systems (pons): ipsilateral limb ataxia (loss of muscle co-ordination) and nystagmus (rapid oscillation of eyeball)
Midbrain (Weber's syndrome, Benedict's syndrome)	Posterior cerebral artery	CN III: ophthalmoplegia (eye deviates down and out) Red nucleus: contralateral cerebellar ataxia

Table 6.7 Unilateral vascular lesions of the lateral brainstem

Brainstem area	Possible vascular cause	Specific symptoms (in addition to common symptoms)
Medulla (Wallenberg's syndrome)	Posterior inferior cerebellar artery	CN IX–X Dysarthria, dysphagia (difficulty in talking and swallowing), hoarseness, (ipsilateral vocal cord paralysis) Loss of gag reflex Partial loss of taste sensation
Pons	Anterior inferior cerebellar artery	CN V, VII, VIII Deafness or tinnitis Partial loss of taste sensation Ipsilateral facial muscle paralysis, inability to shut eyes Impaired salivation/lacrimation Hyperacusis (abnormally loud sounds) Jaw deviation during opening
Midbrain	Superior cerebellar artery, branches of posterior cerebral artery	Contralateral hemianaesthesia (ascending tract damage) Intentional tremor (damage to superior cerebellar peduncle)

Unilateral lateral lesions, in general, produce five common symptoms that are distinct from medial symptoms:

1. Contralateral loss of pain/thermal sensation (spinothalamic tract damage).
2. Ipsilateral loss of facial skin sensation (trigeminothalamic tract damage).
3. Horner's syndrome: miosis, ptosis (drooping) of eyelid, impaired sweating (descending autonomic fibres injured).
4. Nystagmus, nausea, vomiting (vestibular and dorsal motor vagal nuclei injury).
5. Ipsilateral limb ataxia (cerebellar peduncle damage).

As with medial lesions, the level is determined by the involvement of cranial nerves V–X (see Table 6.7).

Bilateral motor and sensory signs are almost certainly an indication of a brainstem lesion. Vascular occlusion of the basilar artery, which supplies the majority of the ventral part of the brainstem, can be catastrophic, resulting in quadriplegia and often in death, due to respiratory failure. It may result in 'locked-in syndrome' where the patient presents with quadriplegia, muteness and facial paralysis. The symptoms resemble coma, but the patient can communicate through eye/eyelid movement (EEG activity is normal). Damage to the basilar artery in the midbrain region produces complex syndromes that include visual hallucinations, gaze palsies and oculomotor dysfunction.

Damage to the MLF results in a (horizontal) gaze disorder called internuclear ophthalmoplegia. It disconnects the abducens nucleus from the contralateral occulomotor nucleus and is characterized by disconjugate gaze with nystagmus and impaired adduction of the abducting eye (Fig. 6.8). The most common cause in the young, or if damage is bilateral, is multiple sclerosis; in older patients, vascular disease is more likely.

Some brainstem syndromes are more common than others. Wallenberg's syndrome (Fig. 6.9) is the most common brainstem stroke, and many patients show gradual recovery of function after this stroke. Anterior inferior

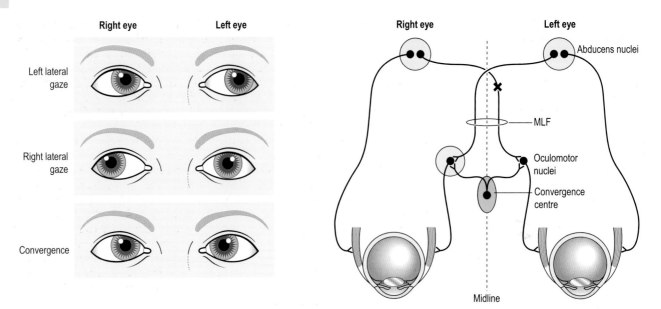

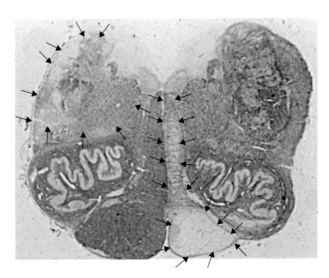

Fig. 6.8 Internuclear ophthalmoplegia results from a lesion in the medial longitudinal fasiculus (MLF) pathway, which connects the abducens nucleus to the contralateral oculomotor nucleus. On the side of the lesion (left MLF, indicated by the 'X'), the person is unable to adduct the eye during contralateral gaze but is able to adduct the eye on convergence, thus distinguishing it from oculomotor nerve palsy. Adapted from Kingsley RE. Concise Text of Neuroscience, 2nd edn. LWW, 2000.

Fig. 6.9 Brainstem lesions resulting from vascular damage. Left side: arrows demarcate damage to the medulla area supplied by the posterior inferior cerebellar artery leading to symptoms associated with Wallenberg's syndrome. Right side: arrows demarcate damage in the territory supplied by the anterior spinal artery.

cerebellar artery infarcts are only a tenth of the prevalence of posterior inferior cerebellar artery strokes, and Déjerine's syndrome is rare, accounting for only 0.5% of all brain strokes. Bilateral occlusions are rarer than unilateral ones and generally have a poorer prognosis.

Compression injuries of the brainstem by cerebellar or cortical herniation are often fatal (see Chapter 9). In addition, hydrocephalus or a pineal gland tumour (pinealoma) may cause Parinaud's syndrome, which is characterized by compression of the dorsal (tectum) midbrain region, encompassing the superior colliculi and midbrain tegmentum. Symptoms include paralysis of upward gaze and accommodation, fixed pupils and nystagmus.

Comments on the case history

This case (see Box 6.1) is an example of Weber's syndrome caused by damage to the posterior cerebral artery that supplies the ventral midbrain. This affected the corticospinal and corticobulbar tracts, the red nucleus and the fibres of the oculomotor nerve.

The oculomotor nerve has somatic fibres that innervate all the extrinsic eye muscles that adduct and elevate the eyeball and upper eyelid, and also parasympathetic fibres of the Edinger–Westphal (E-W) nucleus that innervate the ciliary and pupillary muscles regulating the processes of accommodation and pupil constriction. Damage to this nerve causes the eye to deviate down and out, due to unopposed action of lateral rectus (abductor) and superior oblique (depressor) muscles innervated by the abducens and trochlear nerves, respectively. Paralysis of the superior levator muscle causes severe ptosis due to the unopposed action of orbicularis oculi (innervated by the facial nerve). In this case, the left and right optic nerves and right oculomotor nerve are intact, but the left oculomotor nerve (including its parasympathetic component) is not. A fully dilated, non-reactive pupil is due to the unopposed action of the dilator pupillae muscle (supplied by the sympathetic nervous system). Pupils are always monitored during head injury cases, because rapidly increasing intracranial pressure (often resulting from an acute cranial bleed), compresses the oculomotor nerve against the temporal bone. Autonomic nervous system fibres reside superficially in this nerve, and these are affected first so that the pupil dilates progressively on the affected side. Pupillary dilation is an urgent indication of surgical decompression of the brain.

The oculomotor nerve forms the efferent arc of two important visual reflexes. The first is the pupillary light reflex that results in constriction of the iris muscle of the pupil to bright light. This reflex involves four sets of neurones. Light activates retinal afferents (CN II) that terminate in the midbrain pretectal nuclei. Axons from this area innervate both E-W nuclei; preganglionic parasympathetic fibres from E-W travel in the oculomotor nerve and synapse in the ciliary ganglion and the postganglionic fibres innervate the constrictor muscle of iris (sphincter pupillae). The other reflex that is affected in this patient is the accommodation reflex. In this case, the pupil is fixed and fails to respond to changes in the depth of the visual field; thus, vision is blurred in the affected eye.

The vascular lesion has also damaged the left descending upper motoneurone fibres of the corticobulbar and corticospinal tracts. This results in muscle paralysis/paresis and abnormal reflexes. This is manifest in the inability to smile voluntarily on the right (contralateral) side. There is no direct damage to the facial nerve, because otherwise paralysis would affect all the muscles of facial expression and thus other facial nerve motor tests (Chapter 3), would reveal abnormal responses. An upper motoneurone lesion affecting the corticobulbar tract results in contralateral lower facial muscle paralysis/paresis, since the upper facial muscles are innervated by both the contralateral and ipsilateral corticobulbar tracts, and thus remain innervated by the contralateral side. Similarly, impairment of the left corticospinal tract results in right-sided hyperreflexia (due to disinhibition of lower motoneurones), a Babinski sign and increased muscle tone. The prognosis for this patient is poor and there is unlikely to be any improvement in functional recovery.

THE VISUAL SYSTEM

7

Chapter objectives

After studying this chapter you should be able to:

1. Describe the structure of the eye and the visual pathways.

2. Understand how visual deficits indicate specific defects in the visual pathways.

3. Describe how the eye focuses light and how the retina responds to it.

4. Describe briefly how the brain processes visual information, including colour information.

Introduction

'Beauty is in the eye of the beholder.' Most of our ideas about our surroundings, and our memory of them, are based on sight. But how do we see and assign emotional meaning to what we see? Vision is the process by which the brain receives light from the outside world and converts it into a recognizable percept. This is a complex process, which starts with the focusing of light rays onto the sensory surface of the eye, the retina. This two-dimensional image is then conveyed to regions of the brain that take different properties of the image, such as colour, form, movement and depth perception, and seamlessly convert them into a three-dimensional percept. Furthermore, objects are recognized in many different orientations, under a wide range of lighting conditions and, when they are at different distances from the observer, at a variety of sizes.

Human beings are very visually oriented and visual deficits can have profound effects on daily life. Depending on the cause and where in the visual pathway the lesion occurs, the deficit can be monocular, being restricted to one eye, or binocular, affecting both (Table 7.1). At the beginning of the 21st century, the World Health Organization estimated that there were 180 million people worldwide who are permanently visually impaired, with numbers rising by 2 million per year. Nearly 60% of these are elderly (>60 years old) and 5% are under the age of 14 years. It is estimated that up to 80% of visual deficits could be remedied with a simple visit to the optician, or appropriate drugs.

The three main causes of visual loss in the developed world are cataracts, glaucoma and diabetes; in the less developed world, cataracts and infections such as trachoma and river blindness (onchocerciasis) account for 75% of blindness cases. The latter two diseases cause inflammation of the conjunctiva and scarring of the cornea, which eventually leads to blindness. River blindness affects over 20 million people worldwide, and in parts of Africa produces blindness rates of up to 35%. It can be treated (and prevented for 9 months) with a single dose of ivermectin. Trachoma is also easily treated with antibiotics, such as tetracycline. Together, these diseases account for over 75% of the world's blindness (Box 7.1).

Structure of the eye

The human eye consists of two regions. The anterior segment, which consists of the cornea, anterior chamber, posterior chamber and lens, is concerned with light gathering and focusing. The posterior segment consists of the choroid and, most importantly, the retina, where the light signal is converted into electrical impulses that are transmitted via the optic nerve to the brain. The structure of the eye is shown in Figure 7.1.

The eyeball consists of three layers. The outermost layer of the eyeball is the sclera. This white, opaque, fibrous layer protects the eye and allows attachment of the muscles controlling the movement of the eye, the extraocular muscles. The movement of these muscles is controlled by cranial nerves III, IV and VI (see below).

Table 7.1 Some causes of blindness

Monocular causes	Binocular causes
Vascular	**Trauma to visual pathway (post-chiasm)**
Transient ischaemic attack	Stroke
Amaurosis fugax	Tumour (e.g. pituitary adenoma)
Inflammation	Raised intracranial pressure (papilloedema)
Temporal arteritis	Disease
Optic neuritis	Diabetes
Trauma	Trachoma
Optic nerve damage	Glaucoma
Retina detachment	River blindness
Disease	Macular degeneration (old age)
Cataracts	Cataracts
Multiple sclerosis	

Box 7.1 Case history

Fifty-five-year-old Mr. Magoo visits his optician for a sight test, as he is finding it difficult to read with his old pair of glasses, and thinks that he may need a new pair. When he was younger his eyesight was good, except that he was colour-blind and could not tell red from green. His optician measures his visual acuity and examines his eye with an ophthalmoscope. He also measures the intraocular pressure. He finds that there are no signs of raised intraocular pressure or visual field defects, but that Mr Magoo's myopia has got significantly worse. He prescribes a new pair of glasses.

This case gives rise to the following questions:

1. What is the structure of the eye and what are the pathways that convey visual information?
2. Can defects in vision indicate specific defects in the visual pathways?
3. How does the eye respond to light?
4. What is visual acuity, why does is decline with age, and how can it be remedied?
5. How is colour perceived and processed by the visual system, and what are the causes of colour-blindness?
6. Which areas of the brain are involved in processing visual information, and how is this information coded?

At the anterior pole of the eye, the sclera becomes the conjunctiva (the white of the eye), and this merges with the transparent cornea that allows light into the eye. It is richly innervated with nociceptive fibres, which, in response to irritation, trigger blinking and the secretion of tears from the lacrimal gland, keeping the cornea free of dust.

The middle layer consists of the choroid, the ciliary body and the iris; together, they form the uvea. The choroid lines the whole of the posterior segment, except where the optic nerve leaves the eye. It consists of a highly vascularized brown membrane. The colour pigment is produced by the melanocytes of the retinal epithelium, and this absorbs light that has not been detected by the retina. By absorbing this light, the choroid prevents it from being scattered back onto the retina and confusing the image.

At the junction of the anterior and posterior segments, and continuous with the choroid, is the ciliary body. This consists mainly of three sets of smooth muscle, the ciliary muscles, which are involved in changing the shape of the lens during the process of focusing. On the surface of the ciliary body, the ciliary process continually produces a clear fluid, called the aqueous humour, which is secreted into the small posterior chamber. The fluid then flows through the pupil into the anterior chamber, and provides nutrients to the lens and cornea. It eventually drains into the venous blood through the canal of Schlemm. Blockage of this leads to glaucoma, by raising the intraocular pressure. This reduces blood flow in the retinal capillaries (Fig. 7.2), and the subsequent ischaemia causes damage to the retina and may lead to blindness. Intraocular pressure is normally 13–29 mmHg.

The suspensory ligaments extend from the ciliary body to attach to the lens. Contraction of the ciliary muscles pulls on the suspensory ligaments and can change the shape of the lens. In the relaxed eye, the suspensory ligaments maintain the lens in a stretched, flattened shape.

The iris is the coloured part of the eye, and extends from the ciliary body across the front of the lens, leaving a circular aperture, the pupil, where light can pass from the anterior chamber into the lens. The size of the pupil can control the amount of light entering the lens and posterior segment, and this is determined by the contraction of the muscles of the iris.

The lens sits at the junction of the anterior and posterior segments of the eye, and consists of a transparent biconvex structure. It acts as a fine control for focusing light onto the retina, just like the lens of a camera, and, as in a camera, the image on the retina is reversed and upside down. The lens is surrounded by a flexible capsule and contains concentric layers of lens fibres, which contain transparent proteins, called crystallins. Cataracts occur when the lens of the eye becomes opaque (Fig. 7.2F). The most usual cause of this is old age, when the crystallin proteins become oxidized and aggregate. Cataracts can be treated by removal of the affected lens and its replacement with a synthetic lens. High levels of UV light increase the rate at which the lens becomes opaque; hence the higher prevalence of cataracts in countries at low latitudes.

The posterior segment of the eye is filled with a transparent, thick gelatinous fluid called the vitreous humour. This is composed of fine collagen fibres and contains large amounts of water. This maintains the shape of the eyeball and also contains phagocytic cells, which remove any debris that might accumulate in the posterior segment and interfere with light transmission.

The innermost layer of the eye, the retina, covers the choroid, the ciliary body and the posterior face of the iris.

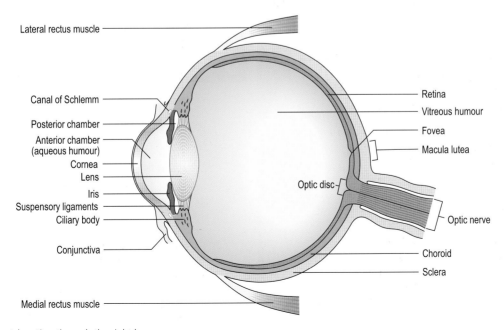

Fig. 7.1 Horizontal section through the right human eye.

The retina can be investigated during examination of the eye (Box 7.2). The retina consists of two layers. The outer pigmented layer, like the choroid, prevents light scattering and also provides a source of vitamin A, which is needed by the light-gathering cells. Vitamin A deficiency leads to night blindness due to a lack of the protein rhodopsin used by some photoreceptors. The inner neural layer of the retina consists of the light-gathering cells, the photoreceptors and associated neurones, as well as glial cells and a dense capillary network. Apart from the photoreceptors, the other neurones are of four types, the bipolar and ganglion cells, which are the first- and second-order neurones of the visual pathway, and the horizontal and amacrine cells, which are interneurones. The centre of the retina, in an area which corresponds to the centre of the visual field, is called the macula lutea (yellow spot), at the centre of which is the fovea. This is the region of the retina where visual acuity is greatest. It lies on a direct line from the centre of the visual field through the centre of the lens.

The output of the retina consists of the axons of the ganglion cells, which form the optic nerve. They leave the

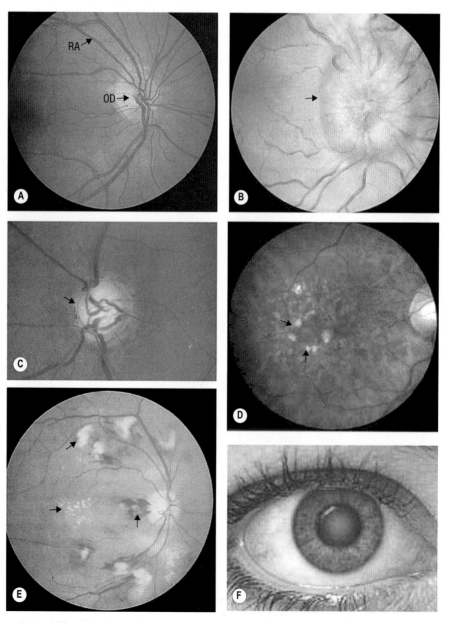

Fig. 7.2 Ophthalmoscope images: (A) a normal eye, showing the optic disc (OD), and the retinal arteries (RA); (B) abnormal fundus, showing papilloedema due to bulging of the optic disc (arrow); (C) glaucoma, where the optic cup is larger and deeper than normal (arrow); (D) macula degeneration, where the macula region is spotty or absent (arrows); (E) cotton wool-like deposits are seen in the eye around blood vessels (arrows) in hypertensive diabetic neuropathy; (F) abnormal lens function—cataract. (A), (B), (C) and (E) from Munro J, Edwards C, eds. Macleod's Clinical Examination, 9th edn. Churchill Livingstone, 1995. (D) taken from www.eyesearch.com.

retina at an area called the optic disc. In this area where the axons converge, there are no photoreceptors, so this part of the visual field corresponds to the blind spot. Objects that are projected onto this area of the retina are invisible, although visual processing tends to fill in the background pattern, so we are unaware of a 'hole' in our vision. Retinal ganglion cell axons become myelinated after the optic disc, and form the optic nerve. This is not a peripheral nerve, because it is myelinated by oligodendrocytes, and is part of the central nervous system. It is an extension of the brain! If damaged, it does not show regeneration in mammals.

Box 7.2 Examination of the eye

An ophthalmoscope is an instrument that enables direct observation of the retina, a technique known as fundoscopy (Fig. 7.2). Because the optic nerve is within the meninges, any changes in pressure in the brain produce a swelling of the optic nerve, called papilloedema, which can be seen in the retina as a swollen optic disc and constricted blood vessels; it is often asymmetrical. Papilloedema does not normally impair vision, but if left untreated it will impair the retinal ganglion cell function, leading to blindness because of ischaemia of the retinal cells.

Changes in the appearance of the blood vessels, and other changes, such as spots, haemorrhages and dark patches, can indicate the development and progression of conditions such as hypertensive and diabetic retinopathy, subdural haemorrhage or hydrocephalus (Fig. 7.2E).

Visual pathways

We view the outside world with two eyes, with each eye seeing it from a slightly different angle. This slight disparity provides clues about the distance of the object of interest and has important consequences for the organization of information in the visual regions of the brain: information can be compared so that distance can be accurately judged. However, we do not see two objects, but only one. The brain fuses the image by a process called stereopsis, and this gives us a three-dimensional appreciation of the object. When the eyes cannot fuse an image, the resultant deficit is called amblyopia.

The visual system has to perform three basic functions: first, to see an object clearly; second, to identify it; and finally, to track it. These roles are carried out by different parts of the visual pathway (Fig. 7.3).

From each eye, the optic nerves, each containing 0.8–1.5 million axons, travel to the optic chiasm, an X-shaped structure at the base of the brain, anterior to the pituitary gland. Here, about 60% of the neurones from each nerve cross and continue in the opposite nerve as the optic tract. These axons are from the ganglion cells situated on the part of the retina on the nasal side. Thus, after the optic chiasm, each optic tract carries the output from the ipsilateral temporal (lateral) retina and the contralateral nasal retina. This means that all of the information from one-half of the visual field is carried in the contralateral optic tract; that is, the left hemifield is 'viewed' by the right hemisphere and vice versa.

Most of the axons in the optic tract travel via the lateral root of the optic tract to terminate in the lateral geniculate nucleus (LGN) of the thalamus. However, about 10% of the axons from the medial root terminate

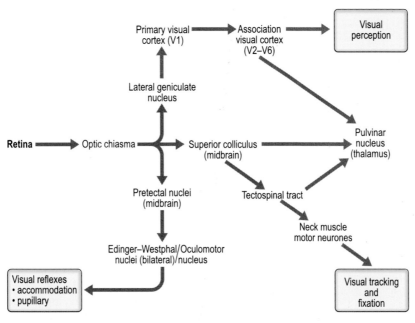

Fig. 7.3 Functions of the visual pathways.

Visual fields and the visual pathways

The visual field corresponds to the visual space seen by each eye. The visual field of each eye is described as being subdivided into four quadrants, left/right and inferior/superior, each of which travels to a different area of the visual cortex (left/right hemispheres, above/below calcarine sulcus) in a highly organized manner. The projection of the visual field onto the retina is inverted both laterally and vertically, so that something in the top left of the visual field falls on the bottom right of the retina (Fig. 7.4). This will then go via the right lateral geniculate nucleus to the right visual cortex, where it will end up in the part of the visual cortex inferior to the calcarine sulcus. This projection of the retina to precise areas of the visual cortex is called retinotopic mapping.

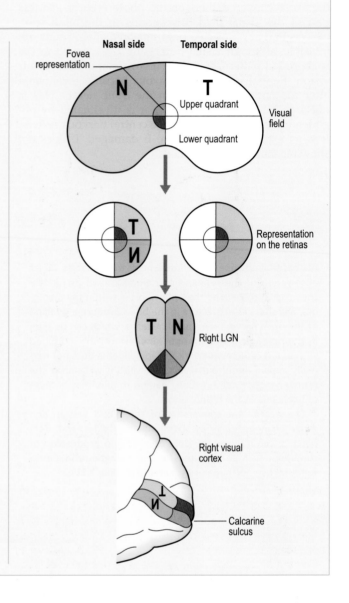

Fig. 7.4 Representation of the visual field projections to the visual cortex. For clarity, only the left visual field is shown. Note that the image is reversed from right to left and from top to bottom in the retina, and this organization continues to the primary visual cortex. In the optic tract, the foveal input is in the middle of the field, but beyond the lateral geniculate nucleus the foveal input moves to the posterior part of the optic radiation and travels through the parietal loop to the posterior part of the visual cortex. The right half of the visual field projects similarly to the left visual cortex. N, nasal side of visual field; T, temporal side of visual field.

Terms used in visual field testing

- Homonymous = matching (i.e. of the same part of the visual field)
- Heteronymous = different (i.e. on opposite sides of the visual field)
- Anopia = loss of vision
- Hemianopia = loss of vision in half of the visual field
- Quadrantanopia = loss of vision in a quadrant of the visual field
- Scotoma = patch of blindness

either in the superior colliculus or the pretectal nucleus of the midbrain. These fibres are involved in controlling the movement of extraocular muscles and the pupillary light reflexes. A few fibres terminate in the suprachiasmatic nucleus of the hypothalamus and the reticular formation, where they are involved in the setting of circadian rhythms and in gaze responses.

From the LGN, axons project along a tract called the optic radiation to the primary visual cortex, which occupies the areas either side of the calcarine sulcus, at the back of the occipital lobe. The fibres in the optic radiation take two different routes to the inferior part of the visual cortex. One passes directly posterior through the parietal lobe, carrying fibres from the fovea and the lower quadrant of the visual field, while the other courses more laterally through the temporal lobe, before

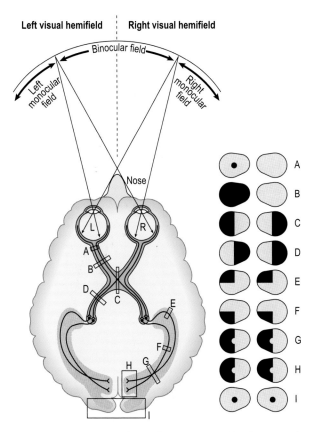

Fig. 7.5 Locations of visual field defects in the visual pathways and the deficits produced by them (see Table 7.2 for a description of each defect). Note the difference in homonymous hemianopsia between lesion D and lesion G, which are on opposite sides of the pathway.

Table 7.2 Visual field defects (see Fig. 7.5)

A	Complete blindness in left eye—complete section of left optic nerve
B	Scotoma in the left visual field—partial lesion of left optic nerve; in young adults this may be due to multiple sclerosis
C	Bitemporal heteronymous hemianopia—usually caused by compression of the chiasm by an adenoma, a benign tumour of the pituitary
D	Right homonymous hemianopia—section of the left optic tract
E	Right homonymous upper quadrantanopia—damage to the right Meyer's loop, possibly caused by a tumour or stroke in the temporal lobe
F	Right homonymous hemianopia—damage to the optic radiation, often due to tumours or stroke. Classically, following a haemorrhage from the middle cerebral artery, this defect occurs for a number of days, due to oedema
G	Right homonymous lower quadrantanopia—parietal lobe lesion
H	Homonymous hemianopia with macula sparing—a lesion above or below the calcarine sulcus, usually due to a stroke in the posterior cerebral artery. The macula sparing is due to sparing of the occipital pole, the most posterior area where the macula is represented
I	Bilateral central scotomas—bilateral lesion in the posterior region of the primary visual cortex, above the calcarine sulcus, often caused by a backward fall or concussion

terminating below the calcarine sulcus. This latter pathway is called Meyer's loop, and these fibres represent the upper part of the visual field. The primary visual cortex (Brodmann area 17) is also called the striate cortex because of the prominent horizontal striations caused by myelinated fibres passing through the cortical layers. The remainder of the occipital lobe forms the visual association areas. This area also receives input about visual tracking via the superior colliculus and pulvinar nucleus (see Fig. 7.3).

Visual field defects

Because of the organization of the visual pathways, specific types of visual field defect are identifiable with specific lesions. This can be examined by covering one eye and assessing the various quadrants using visual field confrontation methods as described in Chapter 3. Lesions to structures anterior to the optic chiasm produce unilateral defects in the visual field of the corresponding eye, whereas lesions occurring posterior to the optic chiasm produce binocular visual deficits (Fig. 7.5 and Table 7.2).

Pupillary light reflexes

The pupils are normally symmetrical (Box 7.5). The pupillary reflex causes the pupil diameter to vary between 1.5 mm in bright light and 8 mm in complete darkness in young people. The range is smaller in the elderly. This is achieved by the contraction (and relaxation) of two sets of smooth muscle in the iris, the pupillary dilator and the sphincter.

If a light is shone into one eye, both pupils constrict. In the stimulated eye, this reflex is called the direct light reflex, and in the non-stimulated eye, the consensual light reflex (Fig. 7.6B). This reflex, and changes due to various pathologies, are described in detail in Chapter 6.

Administration of morphine interferes with pupil responses, and results in pinpoint pupils. Thus, it is not given to head injury patients before primary assessment has been done.

Focusing of light on the retina

As light passes from the air to the retina, it is refracted by the cornea and the lens, in order to produce a focused image

Box
7.5 **Clinical significance of pupil asymmetry**

Pupil asymmetry can indicate damage to the sympathetic or parasympathetic nervous system (Fig. 7.6A). In a clinical context, whether the symmetry occurs in the dark or the light is important. Asymmetry in the dark implies that the sympathetic nervous system is not functioning properly. Conversely, if it occurs in the light, then the parasympathetic nervous system is dysfunctional. Table 7.3 shows the different types of causes of pupil asymmetry.

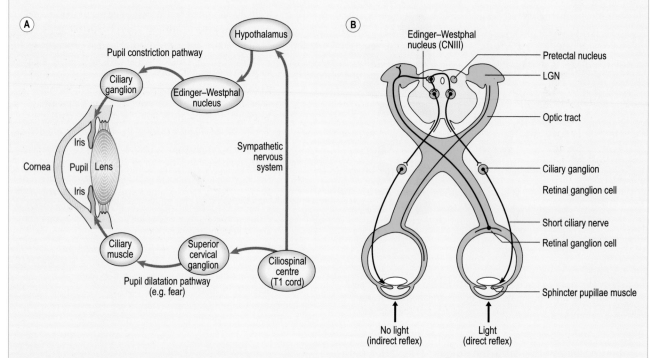

Fig. 7.6 Neural control of pupil size. (A) Autonomic control: hypothalamic stimulation of the sympathetic nervous system causes pupil dilatation. (B) Parasympathetic activation causes the reverse. See text for further details. LGN, lateral geniculate nucleus.

Table 7.3 Causes of pupil asymmetry

Name of deficit	Symptom	Cause
Argyll Robertson	Small pupils that do not react well to light but react equally to accommodation	Pineal tumour Neurosyphilis
Marcus Gunn	Weak direct reflex Strong consensual reflex	Ipsilateral damage to optic nerve
Horner's syndrome	Unilateral asymmetry of pupil (< 0.5–1 mm difference) Normal direct and consensual reflexes Does not dilate in response to cocaine drops	Oculosympathetic damage
Non-reactive	No response to light or accommodation	Cranial nerve compression Iris disease Brain herniation Acute glaucoma

on the retina. This means that light from a point source must be focused onto a single point on the retina, regardless of whether it comes from a distant or a near object.

Accommodation

More than two-thirds of the focusing power of the relaxed eye, which is measured in units called dioptres, is produced by the cornea (42 out of 60 dioptres), with the remainder being produced by the lens (Fig. 7.7A). However, while the cornea has a fixed focusing power, the lens, which is elastic, can change its shape and so can increase the amount by which light is refracted, increasing its focusing power from about 18 to 30 dioptres. The contraction of the ciliary muscles reduces the tension in the suspensory ligaments and allows the lens to contract into a more spherical shape. This thickening of the lens is called accommodation, and allows light from near objects to be correctly focused on the retina (Fig. 7.7B). However, with age, the lens becomes less elastic, a condition known as presbyopia, in which there is failure of the accommodation reflex. This stiffening of the lens occurs throughout life but accelerates at about 40 years of age; hence the need

for 'reading glasses' by most people in later life. By about the age of 60 years, accommodation no longer occurs, as the lens can no longer rebound (Boxes 7.3 and 7.4).

In the accommodation reflex, there is also convergence of the eyes, so that the point of crossing of the visual axes of the eyes becomes closer, and constriction of the pupil occurs to maintain focus. The circuitry for the accommodation reflex is shown in Fig. 7.7C.

Defects in focusing

Normally, the eye is a sphere, and parallel light rays, such as those from a distant object, are focused on the retina when the ciliary muscles are relaxed. This is called emmetropia (Fig. 7.8A). In myopia (near-sightedness), the eye is elongated, so that the focal point, where the light rays converge into a single point, occurs in front of the retina. This can be corrected by a concave lens placed in front of the eye (Fig. 7.8C). Hyperopia (far-sightedness) is due to a shortened eye, so the focal point falls behind the retina. Again, this can be corrected by a lens, this time

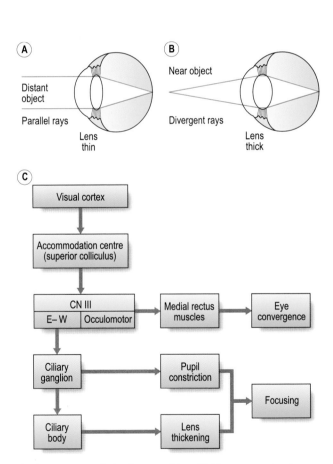

Fig. 7.7 Accommodation for near vision. (A) Unaccommodated eye. (B) Accommodation produces a rounder lens in order to focus on near objects. (C) Neural circuit for accommodation. E–W, Edinger–Westphal.

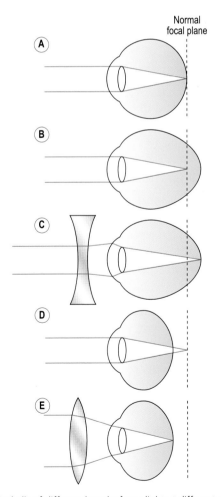

Fig. 7.8 Eyeballs of different lengths focus light at different points. (A) Emmetropia. (B) Myopia. (C) Myopia corrected. (D) Hyperopia. (E) Hyperopia corrected.

a convex one (Fig. 7.8E). These refractive errors can also be caused by the corneal surface being either too curved (myopia) or too flat (hyperopia). In people who have astigmatism, the visual image is distorted due to failure of the light rays to meet at a common focal point. This is because of the irregular shape of the cornea or lens, producing different focal points in the vertical and horizontal planes. It can be corrected by using an artificial lens that is more curved in one plane than the other.

Laser treatment by photorefractive keratectomy is an outpatient corneal surgery procedure that can reduce or correct mild to moderate myopia or hyperopia. This is done by use of a laser that precisely reshapes the cornea.

Control of eye movements

In order to keep the visual image in the centre of the visual field, the eye must move both when the head is moving, i.e. gaze stabilization, and when the object of interest is moving, i.e. gaze shifting. Three sets of muscles (Fig. 7.9) control the movement of the eye in three axes, and these extraocular muscles are controlled by the oculomotor, trochlear and abducens cranial nerves. In order for both eyes to move in parallel, i.e. have conjugate eye movements, different muscles are contracted in each eye (Box 7.6). For example, contraction of the lateral rectus in one eye is accompanied by contraction of the medial rectus in the other.

Testing of eye movements can identify damage to the cranial nerves. Damage to the oculomotor nerve causes the eye to deviate down and out because of unopposed action of the lateral rectus and superior oblique muscles, while damage to the other nerves produces different effects (Table 7.4).

The oculomotor nerve also controls the superior levator muscle, which opens the eyelid. Oculomotor nerve damage causes severe drooping of the eyelid (ptosis), due to the unopposed action of the orbicularis oculi, which is controlled by the facial nerve.

Rapid rotation of the head is detected by the semicircular canals and triggers an equal and opposite rotation of both eyes. This is the vestibulo-ocular reflex, which is described in Chapter 8.

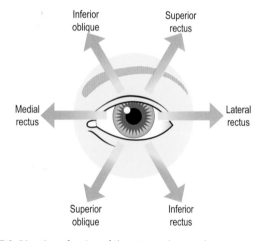

Fig. 7.9 Direction of action of the extraocular muscles.

Box 7.6   Double vision

The eyes are normally parallel in all positions of gaze except convergence. When they are not, a squint is present and double vision (diplopia) ensues. This is where the patient is aware of two images of the same object simultaneously. It is usually due to the limited movement of one eye, a 'lazy eye'. This may be due to either nerve or muscle damage, or a restriction in the mechanical movement of the eye. A weakness in a particular muscle produces diplopia in the direction of movement of that muscle, with an image that is further out from the affected eye.

Table 7.4   Functions of extraocular muscles

Muscle	Normal action	Nerve supply	Eye position after nerve injury
Medial rectus	Adduction (in)	Oculomotor	
Superior rectus	Elevation after abduction (up and out)	Oculomotor	Depressed after abduction (down and out)
Inferior rectus	Depression after abduction (down and out)	Oculomotor	
Inferior oblique	Elevation after adduction (up and in)	Oculomotor	
Superior oblique	Depression after adduction (down and in)	Trochlear	Elevation after abduction (up and out)
Lateral rectus	Abduction (out)	Abducens	Adducted (in)

As well as voluntary control of conjugate eye movements, there are two other types of eye movement that are under voluntary control: saccades and pursuit movements. Saccades are the quick flicks that the eyes make when they jump from one fixation point to another. The perception of an object is entirely built up from repeated scanning of areas of interest in the object. For example, when looking at a portrait painting of a face, the eyes scan across many features of the image to build a picture. The saccades are not random, but are controlled by what a person wants or expects to see. In the brain, saccades are controlled by the frontal eye field regions in the frontal lobe. Stimulation of the right frontal eye field causes eye movement to the contralateral side; damage causes drifting to the ipsilateral side. The frontal eye fields connect to the gaze centres in the pons and midbrain, and to other pursuit centres in the brain. The parieto-occipital centre is part of the visual association cortex, and is responsible for involuntary visual pursuit. It is responsible for keeping the eyes fixed on an object after it has been located, and bringing it into the fovea by generating a new saccade (Box 7.5).

Structure and function of the retina

The retina contains five types of neurone arranged in three layers, and is part of the central nervous system (Fig. 7.10). The different neurones process the signal from the photoreceptors before it is transmitted to the brain via the optic nerve. The retina also contains two types of glial cell, Müller cells and astrocytes, which provide structural and metabolic support. The five types of neurone and their functions are shown in Table 7.5.

The layers of the retina are arranged with the photoreceptors lying closest to the pigment epithelium, and the capillaries and nerve axons lying on the inner (choroid) surface, so light has to pass through these other layers before it is detected by the photoreceptors. A detached retina is said to occur when the pigment epithelial cell

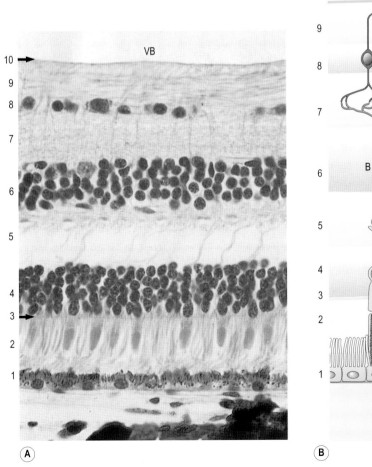

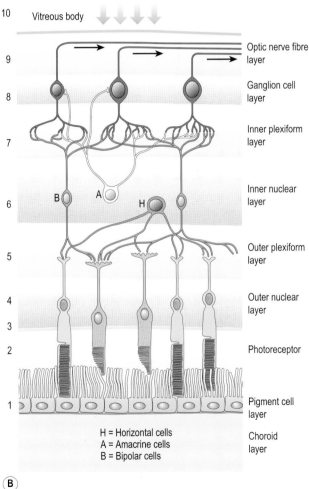

Fig. 7.10 Layers of the retina. (A) Haematoxylin and eosin-stained section of the retina, ×640. (B) Diagrammatic representation. For clarity, Müller cells and astrocytes are not shown. From Young, B., Lowe, J.S., Stevens, A. and Heath, J.W., Wheater's Function Histology 5th edition. 2006, Elsevier, Churchill Livingstone.

Table 7.5 Functions of retinal visual cells

Cell type	Function
Photoreceptors (rods and cones)	Signal transducers—scotopic and photopic vision
Bipolar cells	Relay cell
Retinal ganglion cells	Output cell
Horizontal cells	Interneurone—contrast detection via lateral inhibition
Amacrine cells	Interneurone—signal modulation

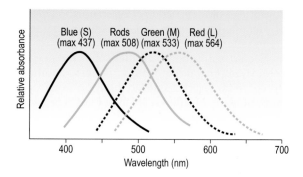

Fig. 7.11 Spectral sensitivities of rods and cones. S, short-wavelength cones; M, medium-wavelength cones; L, long-wavelength cones. Adapted from Longstaff A. Instant Notes in Neuroscience. 2nd edition. 2005, Taylor and Francis Group.

layer comes away from the photoreceptor layer, which is mechanically unstable. This causes the photoreceptors to stop working and die, resulting in blurred vision (Box 7.6).

The photoreceptors make synaptic connections with bipolar cells, which make connections with ganglion cells, whose axons form the optic nerve. Horizontal cells receive inputs from photoreceptors and synapse with bipolar cells. Amacrine cells make many different types of connection between bipolar and ganglion cells.

Light falling on the retina produces changes in membrane potential in the retinal cells, but only ganglion cells, the output cells, fire action potentials. All the other retinal cells respond with graded potentials, which release graded amounts of neurotransmitter. Mechanisms exist within the retina to increase contrast and increase colour detection, but the graded potentials allow subtle changes in light levels falling on the retina to be detected.

Photoreceptors and the detection of light

There are two types of photoreceptor, the rods and the cones, which have a broadly similar structure but different functions. Rods are very sensitive to light, and can detect light at very low levels, over a wide range of wavelengths. They are effective in dim light, but can only 'see' shades of grey. This is called scotopic vision. Nocturnal animals have mostly or entirely rods. Their high sensitivity is due to the fact that they collect light over a longer period and from a larger area than cones, but this also means that they cannot detect very fast-flickering light.

Cones are less sensitive to light than are rods, and so can only work in relatively high light levels; this is photopic vision. There are three different types of cone, each sensitive to a pattern of wavelengths, due to the different types of opsin (cone pigments). Humans are trichromats, because they use a three-cone system to absorb light of different wavelengths. These correspond approximately to red, green and blue (violet), so that between them cones are able to detect colour (Fig. 7.11). The peak wavelengths of the cones do not correspond exactly to red, green and blue, so cones are better described as long-wavelength (L), medium-wavelength (M) and short-wavelength (S) cones. Colour vision depends on the

Box 7.7 Colour blindness

Most colour blindness, assessed using Ishihara plates, is genetically inherited and is due to either a lack of, or the abnormal function, of one or more types of cone cell. However, most colour-blind people can see colour, but they confuse the wavelength and brightness of light over certain parts of the spectrum.

Anomalous trichromats have all three cone populations, but have an abnormal opsin, so that the wavelengths absorbed are slightly different.

Dichromats lack one of the cone populations:

- protanopes—lack L cones, so are red blind
- deuteranopes—lack M cones, so are green blind
- tritanopes—lack S cones, so are blue blind.

Problems with S cones lead to blue–yellow colour blindness (both appear grey), whereas problems with either M or L cones result in red–green colour blindness, where both red and green are indistinguishable from each other (and appear grey). This red–green colour blindness is X-linked, as the genes for both M and L opsins are on the X chromosome. Therefore, this type of colour blindness is more common in men than in women. The S cone defect is located on chromosome 7.

Rare individuals who lack two types of cone have no colour vision, and those who lack cones completely have no photopic vision, and are blind in daylight, when their rods are completely saturated. People who lack rod cells have no peripheral vision and are blind at low light levels—night blindness.

difference between different signals from different cone populations. Deficits in different cone combinations lead to colour blindness (Box 7.7).

Apart from these deficits, photoreceptors can also degenerate (Box 7.8).

Macular degeneration

Macular degeneration (MD) accounts for over 45% of visual impairment in patients over 65 years of age. It causes a progressive loss of central vision, critically limiting the ability to perform visual tasks. Central to the disease is the loss of photoreceptors.

There are two main types of MD. In about 10% of cases the blood vessels become leaky, damaging the retina (see Fig. 7.2). Progression is rapid, but this type of MD can be treated with laser therapy, to destroy the leaky vessels. However, in the remaining 90% of cases, there is a gradual loss of the retinal pigment epithelium, which is followed by a loss of the associated photoreceptors. This loss is much more gradual, but at present there is no treatment for this form of MD. It has been suggested that one of the roles of the yellow macular pigment, which consists of two carotenoids, lutein and zeaxanthin, may be as an antioxidant, protecting the centre of the visual field, which receives most light, from the harmful effects of UV and blue light.

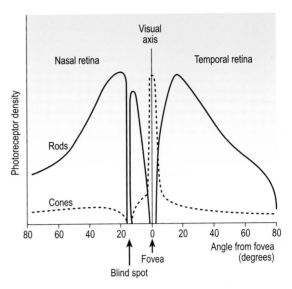

Fig. 7.12 Distribution of rods (solid lines) and cones (dashed lines) across the retina. Adapted from Longstaff A. Instant Notes in Neuroscience. 2nd edition, 2005, Taylor and Francis Group.

The rods and the cones are differently distributed across the retina, with cones being concentrated in the fovea (Fig. 7.12). In this area, they are packed at the highest possible density, giving high-acuity colour vision. Furthermore, in this area the overlying capillaries and nerve axons are displaced, so the cones receive the maximum amount of light. The rods are distributed more peripherally, and are preferentially sensitive to movement. Overall, there are fewer S cones (with none in the fovea), and L and M cones are distributed in patches across the retina, so colour vision is grainy.

Rod cells are much more sensitive to light than are cone cells, to the point where they are saturated and unresponsive in normal daylight. Upon transition from light to dark, vision is initially reduced for 10–15 min, but is then restored, as the rod cells become unsaturated and more sensitive over a period of about 30 min. This is called dark adaptation, and is due to chemical changes in the rods. The light stimulates the regeneration of rhodopsin, and as rhodopsin regenerates in the rod, the eye becomes adapted to the lower light level. In reverse, light adaptation is much faster. Rod cells are much less sensitive to red light than L cones, as shown by the distance between the curves in Figure 7.11. This property is used by people who work in low light conditions, such as astronomers, who wish to retain the maximum dark adaptation of their scotopic vision.

In each retina, the rods outnumber the cones by approximately 20 to 1. There are many more rods and cones (100 million) than bipolar cells, which are more numerous than ganglion cells (1 million). This means that, on average, ganglion cells must receive convergent input from more than one photoreceptor. The pattern of connection varies between rods and cones. A group of rods projects to a smaller number of bipolar cells, which projects to a smaller number of ganglion cells. This enables the collected light from many rods to be integrated, in order to affect a single ganglion cell, allowing scotopic vision to have low acuity but high sensitivity. In contrast, cones are linked to fewer bipolar cells and input from cones is much less integrated. This non-convergence is highest in the fovea, where single cones connect to single bipolar and single ganglion cells, increasing the acuity of this region. Additionally, in the fovea the cone photoreceptors are narrower, allowing even more cones to pack together.

Mechanism of phototransduction by photoreceptors

Both rods and cones consist of outer and inner segments (Fig. 7.13). The outer segments of cones have multiple invaginations of the plasma membrane, while rods contain layer upon layer of flattened discs. These discs are continually shed from the outer segments and are removed by the pigment epithelium, while new ones are generated from the base. The outer segments are specialized for phototransduction, while the inner segment contains the nucleus and biosynthetic machinery.

The outer segment membranes are packed with the proteins that detect light, and rods contain more pigment than cones, enabling them to capture more light. Rod cells contain rhodopsin, and there are three different opsins in the cone cells. Rhodopsin and cone opsins are G-protein-coupled (GPCR) receptors (see Chapter 2).

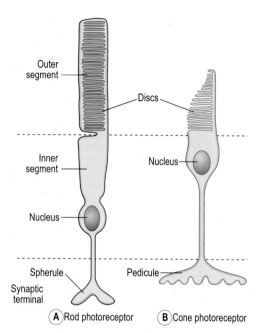

Fig. 7.13 Structure of rod photoreceptor (left) and cone photoreceptor (right).

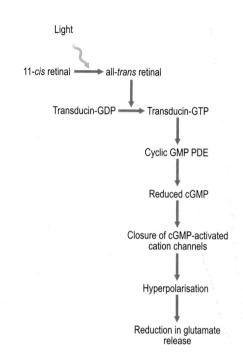

GMP PDE = Guanosine monophosphate phosphodiesterase
GTP = Guanosine triphosphate

Fig. 7.14 The sequence of events in the response to light in a rod cell. PDE, phosphodiesterase.

Each receptor contains a molecule of retinal (which is derived from retinol, vitamin A), which is in the 11-*cis* form in the dark but is converted to the all-*trans* isomer by light. This then allows transducin, a G-protein, to be activated by the opsin and to bind GTP in place of GDP. The α subunit of transducin then dissociates from the βγ subunits and activates the enzyme cyclic GMP phosphodiesterase (cGMP PDE). The effect of light is thus to decrease the concentration of cGMP in the photoreceptors (Fig. 7.14). Deficits in these processes can lead to visual defects (Box 7.9).

In the dark, the photoreceptor membranes are 'leaky' and are depolarized to about $-40\,mV$ by the movement of current that is actively pumped out from the inner segment and enters through open cation channels in the outer segment. This allows the continual influx of small amounts of Na^+, called the dark current. As a result of this depolarization, glutamate is constantly released in the dark to activate bipolar cells. However, these channels are kept open by cGMP, so, in the presence of light, when the cGMP concentration falls, these channels close and the photoreceptor hyperpolarizes; under these conditions, glutamate release is reduced. Because of the amplification inherent in the GPCR system, a single photon can produce a potential change of about $1\,mV$ (by blocking the entry of about a million Na^+ ions). Thus, the overall response of the photoreceptor depends on the light intensity.

The cascade is stopped by a number of mechanisms:

- The intrinsic GTPase activity of transducin converts the bound GTP to GDP. The inactive transducin then recombines with the βγ subunits.

Retinitis pigmentosa is an inherited visual defect that starts with night blindness and a loss of peripheral vision, and can develop into complete loss of vision. There is narrowing of the retinal blood vessels, and clumps of disrupted retinal pigment are seen, often associated with the vessels. It is a heterogeneous disorder, whose different forms may be inherited as an autosomal-dominant, autosomal-recessive or X-linked disease. Some of the forms are due to defects in the rhodopsin molecule, while others are due to defects in the cGMP phosphodiesterase or ion channels in the photoreceptors. The loss of night and peripheral vision is due to the initial loss of rods, after which patients are completely dependent on cones (photopic vision). However, the cones also progressively degenerate, leading to eventual blindness. In many patients, the mutation responsible is in the rod (e.g. in rhodopsin), but why this should lead to a loss of cones as well as rods is a mystery.

- The rhodopsin molecules are inactivated by phosphorylation by rhodopsin kinase and the binding of visual arrestin (see Chapter 2).

After prolonged exposure to light (a few seconds), the link between rhodopsin and retinal is hydrolysed, and the all-*trans*-retinal dissociates. This is called bleaching. In the dark, the rhodopsin is regenerated. This increases the sensitivity of the photoreceptor, and underlies dark adaptation.

Contrast detection in the retina: 'on' and 'off' channels

One of the crucial elements in the recognition of objects by the visual system involves identifying the edges of objects, which can usually be detected by changes in light levels. Connections between bipolar cells, horizontal cells and ganglion cells act to increase contrast between light and dark areas.

There are two populations of cone bipolar cells, called 'on' and 'off' bipolar cells. These respond to input from cone cells in different ways: 'on' cells depolarize and 'off' cells hyperpolarize. Along with the horizontal cells, they enhance contrast.

The two types of bipolar cell can be distinguished by their structure and response:

- Invaginating bipolar cells form specialized synapses, called triad ribbon synapses, which are invaginated into the base of the photoreceptors. The triad consists of the dendrites of the bipolar cell and two horizontal cells. In response to light and the subsequent reduction in glutamate release from the photoreceptor, these 'on' bipolar cells depolarize.

- Flat bipolar cells form basal synapses with photoreceptors. In response to light, these 'off' bipolar cells are hyperpolarized.

Rod photoreceptors are all connected to 'on' rod bipolar cells, which are larger than the cone bipolar cells; the latter are termed midget bipolar cells, and depolarize in response to light. All of the bipolar cells respond to a reduction in glutamate release, but their different responses are due to the different types of glutamate receptor present in their cell membranes.

Both types of cone bipolar cell release glutamate, and synapse with ganglion cells that have the same response pattern. That is, 'on' bipolar cells produce an increase in action potential firing rate in their ganglion cells, and 'off' bipolar cells reduce the firing rate in their ganglion cells.

This leads to two channels. In response to light, the 'on' channel leads to an increase in ganglion cell firing rate, and the 'off' channel leads to reduced ganglion firing. So, in the dark, glutamate release inhibits the 'on' channel and excites the 'off' channel. In the light, the reverse happens; a reduction in glutamate excites the 'on' channel and inhibits the 'off' channel.

Each retinal ganglion cell is affected by the light falling on its circular receptive field. The ganglion cells show different responses, depending on whether light falls in the centre of the field or in the surrounding ring (Fig. 7.15). An 'on' ganglion cell increases its firing rate in response

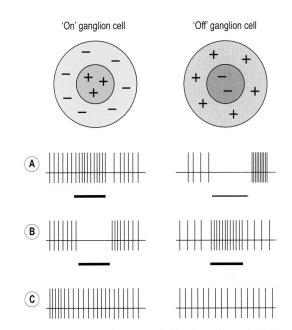

Fig. 7.15 Centre–surround receptive fields of ganglion cells. (A) Centre illumination. (B) Surround illumination. (C) Diffuse illumination.

to illumination of the centre of its field and decreases it in response to illumination of its periphery. In diffuse illumination of both the centre and surround, there is no change in the firing rate. For an 'off' ganglion cell, firing increases with surround illumination, stops with light on the centre, and is unaffected by diffuse lighting. This property of ganglion cells is shared by their bipolar cells, but because bipolar cells do not fire action potentials, it is their graded potentials that vary. This surround–centre antagonism is mediated in part by horizontal cells, which, although they do not synapse directly on bipolar cells, affect the glutamate release from photoreceptors onto bipolar cells.

Horizontal cells increase the contrast in the retina by a mechanism called lateral inhibition. Horizontal cells connect the outputs from neighbouring photoreceptors. In the dark, they are excited by glutamate released from the photoreceptors, which stimulates γ-aminobutyric acid (GABA) release onto neighbouring photoreceptors. GABA inhibits photoreceptors, reducing their glutamate release (Fig. 7.16). This means that in response to centre illumination, a neighbouring photoreceptor, which will continue to release glutamate, will excite the horizontal cell. This inhibits glutamate release from the centre photoreceptor, allowing bipolar cells to depolarize further than they would without the horizontal cell effect. When the surround is illuminated, the reduction in glutamate release from the surround photoreceptors reduces the GABA release from the horizontal cell, and so the centre photoreceptor releases more glutamate, causing the centre bipolar cell to be inhibited. The function of centre–surround inhibition is to exaggerate contrast at borders.

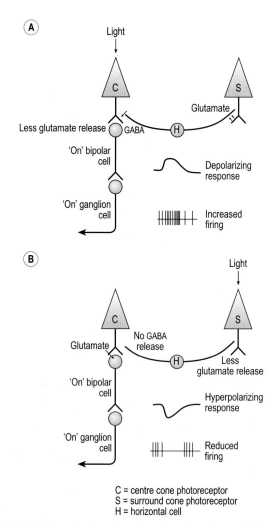

Fig. 7.16 Horizontal cells reduce glutamate release from neighbouring photoreceptors. (A) Centre illumination: GABAergic inhibition by horizontal cells enhances the bipolar and ganglion cell responses; (B) Surround illumination: no GABA is released from the horizontal cell, so the 'on' channel is suppressed.

Rod cell signalling via amacrine cells

Rods are connected to depolarizing 'on' bipolar cells that are connected to ganglion cells via amacrine cells. These are a very diverse population of cells that have no axons but many neurites, have properties of both axons and dendrites, and use a wide variety of neurotransmitters to modify synaptic transmission. They have been implicated in the detection of the direction of motion, particularly in peripheral vision.

At high light levels, rods are saturated and all signalling occurs through the cone cells and 'on' and 'off' channels. In lower light levels, such as at dusk, in the dark-adapted eye, changes in membrane potential are transferred to neighbouring cone cells through gap junctions. This increases the signals occurring in cone pathways and maintains colour vision and visual acuity at low light levels. However, at very low light levels, this boosting

of cone cells is insufficient to maintain colour vision, and all vision occurs via rod–amacrine cell pathways.

Colour responses of ganglion cells

Like bipolar cells, ganglion cells show 'on' and 'off' surround inhibition, but they differ from bipolar cells in producing action potentials, and thus their responses are described in terms of action potential rate, not graded depolarization. They are also spontaneously active. Therefore, inhibition of these cells can be seen as a decrease in the resting rate of action potentials, and their centre–surround organization makes these cells extremely sensitive to moving stimuli.

Ganglion cells can also be distinguished by their responses to colour. Studies in monkeys (which have a similar visual system to humans) have shown that there are two major populations of ganglion cells, which can be distinguished easily by their size and their destination (see below), as well as by their response characteristics.

The most numerous ganglion cells (90%, about 1 million per retina) are parvocellular (P) cells; these are found near the fovea. Magnocellular (M) cells are larger and less common (5%). There are also non-M, non-P cells, but these are less well characterized and make up the remaining 5% of cells. The receptive fields of P cells are smaller than those of M cells, and they often show sustained responses. However, the most striking difference is that they respond differently to coloured light. This is because P cells obtain their input from single cones (or a group of cones with the same wavelength sensitivity, S, M or L), while M cells receive their input from rod cells. M cells are more sensitive than P cells to low-contrast stimuli and are used for retinal control of eye movement and object fixation, while P cells can distinguish fine detail and are important for spatial discrimination. This separation of functional detection of different features of the image at the first stage in the visual pathway is maintained throughout the visual pathway.

Some non-M, non-P cells receive their input from M and L cones together (but not S), and have larger receptive fields, so they are good at measuring the brightness. The centre–surround inhibition lets 'on' M cells respond best to green (M cones) and red (L cones) light in the centre, while 'off' M cells fire when the light illuminates the surround.

The output of P ganglion cells shows colour opponency; that is, they are excited by one cone population and inhibited by another (Fig. 7.17). There are two populations of colour opponent P cells. The most common are single red–green opponent.

There are four different possible responses, depending on whether the ganglion cell is an 'on' or 'off' cell (Fig. 7.17A):

- red 'on' centre, green 'off' surround
- green 'on' centre, red 'off' surround
- red 'off' centre, green 'on' surround
- green 'off' centre, red 'on' surround.

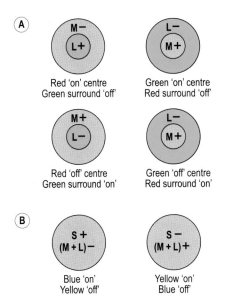

Fig. 7.17 Colour opponency in ganglion cells. (A) Red–green single opponent cells. (B) Blue–yellow opponent cells.

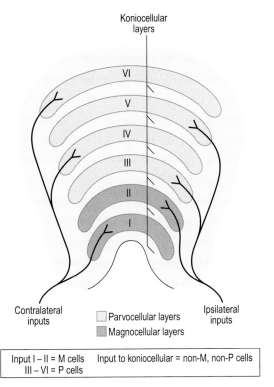

Fig. 7.18 Layers in the lateral geniculate nucleus. Magnocellular layers (1 and 2) are shown shaded. Inputs I and II: M cells. Inputs III–VI: P cells. Input to Koniocellular layer: non-M, non-P cells.

The other type of colour opponency compares input from S cones with that of M and L combined. This is called blue–yellow opponency, as the combination of input from M and L cones gives the perception of yellow. These cells do not show a centre–surround response, but are either excited by blue light and inhibited by yellow or vice versa (Fig. 7.17B).

Perceived colour is based on the relative activities in different ganglion cells, whose receptive fields' centres receive input from the three different cones. This can be demonstrated, for example, by staring at a red, green or blue square for 30–60 s, to fatigue the appropriate cone. Then, if one stares at a white box, something strange happens. Staring at this white box leaves the opponent colour unopposed, and so the white background becomes that colour. For blue, the white background becomes yellow, for red it becomes green, and vice versa.

Processing of visual information

Retinal ganglion cells are not mere relay cells for visual information, but they extract different aspects of the image. What we 'see' depends on the features extracted in the retina, and how this information is integrated and interpreted by the brain. In the retina, the visual information is split into two streams, one for colour and one for form and motion. This is parallel processing, and is important because we view the world with two eyes, providing two parallel streams of information, albeit from slightly different angles. In the central visual pathways, these streams are compared to give information about object depth, contrast and movement as well as image resolution. Because we use two eyes, there are two

separate images in the brain, and somewhere in the visual cortex they are merged together.

Visual processing in the lateral geniculate nucleus

The LGN has six layers (Fig. 7.18), which receive inputs from the M and P ganglion cells. The two ventral layers called the magnocellular layers are composed of large cells and are innervated by M ganglion cells (layer 1 from the contralateral eye and layer 2 from the ipsilateral eye). The more dorsal parvocellular layers are composed of small cells and receive input from the P ganglion cells, with layers 3 and 5 ipsilateral and 4 and 6 contralateral. In between these layers are even smaller cells, which make up the koniocellular layers. These receive input from ganglion cells that signal average illumination (non-M, non-P cells).

Just like the retinal ganglion cells, the LGN cells have circular receptive fields and show the same centre–surround inhibition and colour opponency as the ganglion cells to which they connect. Each layer shows precise topographical mapping of the retina, with a large part of each layer being occupied with input from the fovea. The maps are in register, so at any vertical point through the LGN the same receptive field is represented. As only input from one half of the visual field goes to each layer of the LGN, there are no binocular responses.

There are two types of neurone in the LGN: geniculostriate neurones, which project to the visual cortex, and a population of small interneurones. As well as receiving input from the retinal ganglion cells, the geniculostriate neurones receive input from the visual cortex and the reticular formation. This is suggested to play a role in visual attention, ensuring that only significant retinal input passes to the visual cortex.

Organization and response properties of cells in the visual cortex

The primary visual cortex (V1 or Brodmann's area 17) is divided into six layers, with inputs from parallel streams, deriving from the magnocellular, parvocellular and koniocellular layers of the LGN. The different pathways carry different types of information regarding form, movement, colour and visual attention. The mapping is retinotopic, whereby neighbouring retinal ganglion cells pass information to neighbouring areas further along the visual pathway. In this map, the fovea is disproportionately represented, and peripheral vision has little representation.

Unlike neurones in the retina and the LGN, those of the visual cortex do not have circular receptive fields, but respond to lines of a particular orientation. Like many other regions of the brain, the visual cortex is arranged in functional columns. In a given column, which is 30–100 μm across, all the neurones spanning layers 1–6 respond to bars of light of a particular orientation; hence the name orientation column.

In each orientation column (Fig. 7.19), there are two types of cell. Simple cells are found in layers 4 and 6 and respond to stationary bars of a certain orientation from a single visual field; that is, they are monocular. In the other layers of each orientation column, mainly 2, 3 and 5, there are complex cells, which are not direction sensitive but respond preferentially to bars of light of the same orientation as the simple cells, but moving across the receptive field, parallel to the preferred orientation. However, these cells are binocular, as they respond to input from both eyes, although they show a preference for the visual field of the simple cells. Moving across the cortex, each successive column has a preferred orientation, which changes by about 15°. Across a distance of about 1 mm, there are columns for each possible orientation for a single eye, from a given part of the visual field. This set of orientation columns is called an ocular dominance column. Parallel to this are a similar set of columns representing input from the same part of the visual field of the other eye. The area of the cortex consisting of two ocular dominance columns, one from each eye, which is about 1 mm², is called a hypercolumn and represents all of the input from a part of the visual field to the primary visual cortex.

Arranged within the ocular dominance columns are columns of complex cells, which are wavelength-sensitive. These colour-sensitive cells are arranged in cylindrical regions called blobs; they receive convergent input from the parvocellular and koniocellular LGN layers. They can be detected using staining methods, as they contain high levels of the mitochondrial enzyme cytochrome oxidase. The areas between the blobs are called the interblob regions. The receptive fields of most of the blob neurones are circular, and show varying types of colour opponency. The most complex of these are the double opponent cells, which signal colour contrast. There are four types, depending on the preferred stimulus. For example, one type has a maximal 'on' response to a red spot on a green background, and an 'off' response to a green spot on a red background. The other red–green type is the reverse, and a similar combination occurs for blue and yellow.

Parallel processing in the visual cortex

The different streams of input from the LGN—motion, form and colour—are processed simultaneously in different layers of the visual cortex. Inputs from the M cells of the LGN, which synapse in a different sublayer of layer 4 to P cells, concern motion, but not colour. Inputs from P cells of the LGN are processed in two streams. One stream in the parvocellular–blob pathway mediates colour vision, while the other, the parvocellular–interblob pathway, performs high-resolution analysis of form. These complex cells are binocular but not wavelength sensitive. They are also important for depth perception.

Outputs from the primary visual cortex

Visual perception is not carried out in just one area, but involves many different association regions of the cerebral

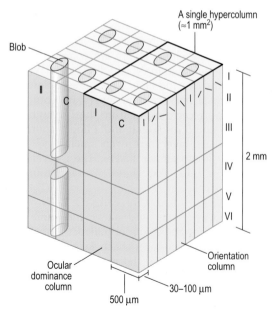

Fig. 7.19 Simple and complex cells are arranged in orientation columns, and these columns are arranged to ocular dominance columns and hypercolumns in the visual cortex. I, ipsilateral; C, contralateral.

cortex that receive output from the V1 area. In monkeys (and by inference, humans), there are 32 different areas known to be involved in further processing of visual input (Fig. 7.20). Many of these areas have some form of retinotopic map, and there are complex interconnections between these regions.

The parallel processing of different information streams continues beyond V1. Many outputs go to the secondary visual cortex (V2, Brodmann area 18), which, on staining for cytochrome oxidase, a metabolic activity marker, shows a pattern of thick and thin stripes. V2 thick stripes receive inputs from the M pathway (via V1 layer 4) and analyse motion. This information is then further processed in other regions, V3 and then V5, the medial temporal (MT) visual cortex and medial superior temporal (MST) cortex, before moving to other visual association areas such as the posterior parietal cortex. V5 also plays a key role in depth perception.

The thin stripes of V2 receive inputs from blobs and analyse colour. Output from this area goes to V4. Interblob neurones project to interstripe regions, which also project to V3 and V4. Eventually, visual information seems to be divided into two streams (Table 7.6). The 'where' stream is carried dorsally, to the MT and posterior parietal cortices, and carries information about an object's location and motion, including one's own body and its spatial relationship to an object (visual guidance and reaching movements). The ventral 'what' stream projects to the inferotemporal cortex, which can identify or recognize an object or a pattern or a specific face. V4 projects to V6 and activates cells that respond to complex shapes and have a role in object shape recognition.

The existence of these two streams is confirmed by the effects of selective lesions to the different areas. Damage to the posterior parietal cortex causes optic ataxia, where patients can recognize objects but cannot grasp them. Damage to MST cortex and MT visual cortex results in loss of visual motion perception (akinetopsia) in different directions. This has obvious lifestyle implications: think how difficult it might be to cross a busy road or even to pour a drink without the cup overflowing.

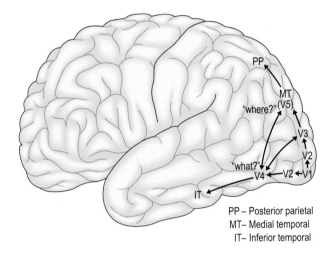

PP – Posterior parietal
MT– Medial temporal
IT– Inferior temporal

Fig. 7.20 Extrastriate visual cortex. Visual information from the primary visual cortex is processed as two streams.

Table 7.6 Separation of visual information

	Pathway	
	Dorsal stream: 'Where things are or how they move'	**Ventral stream: 'What things are or are like'**
Function	Motion perception and spatial location	Colour and shape perception
	Visual guidance of hand and eye movements	Object recognition
Retinal ganglion cell type	M cells (non-macular)	P cells (fovea)
LGN cells	M1–M2	P3–P6
Cortical input area	V1	V1
Visual association areas	V2, V3, V5, MST cortex, posterior parietal cortex	V2, V4, V6, anterior inferior temporal lobe
Other cortical area involvement	Dorsolateral prefrontal cortex	Ventrolateral prefrontal cortex
	Frontal eye fields	Medial temporal lobe
Effect of lesion	Optic ataxia	Visual agnosia
	Ocular apraxia	Prosopagnosia
	Akinetopsia	Achromatopsia
		Alexia

MST, medial superior temporal.

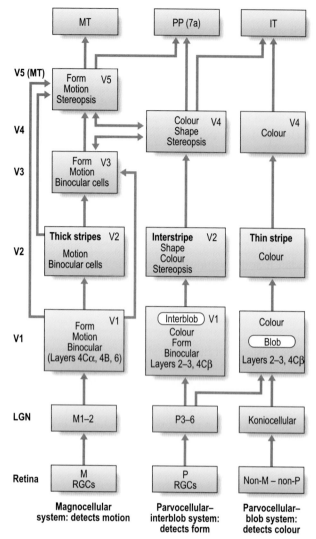

Fig. 7.21 A model of how we see. Integration of parallel processing of the different streams of information. MT, medial temporal cortex; PP, posterior parietal cortex; IT, inferior temporal cortex. RGC, retinal ganglion cell. Adapted from DeYoe, Van Essen. TINS. 1988;11:219–226.

damage to V6 causes an inability to distinguish two-dimensional patterns.

In a particular condition called blindsight (cortical blindness), patients who are totally blind due to the bilateral loss of V1 can still navigate to some extent through space without colliding with objects that they reportedly cannot see. This occurs due to a pathway which goes from the magnocellular neurones of the LGN directly to the thick stripes of V2, providing input to the 'where' pathway.

However, eventually the different streams (Table 7.6) are integrated to produce a coherent image of a three-dimensional world. This processing of information in parallel streams can explain how some visual illusory effects are produced. For example, depth perception is much reduced in computer-generated pictures if the shading is produced by colour contrast as opposed to luminance. This seems to indicate that depth information is processed by the colour-blind magnocellular pathways.

Summary

In summary, the visual system is a highly complex system, designed to pick out different features of an image: its colour, motion and shape (Fig. 7.21). To do this requires a variety of neuronal equipment. Some of this separation occurs early in the pathway, and information is processed in parallel throughout the rest of the pathway. For example, colour is detected by cones, which activate P cells that project via parvocellular LGN layers to blob regions of the visual cortex, and onwards to V4. Cones, on the other hand, see only in black and white, work best at low light levels and are excellent motion detectors. Information travels via the M layers of the LGN to interblob regions of the visual cortex, and are forwarded to the V5 and the posterior parietal cortex. The parvocellular–interblob pathway is specialized for shape perception, as cells in this pathway are sensitive to the orientation of edges. Within the cortex there are many complex interactions between the many different visual association regions. We get visual input from two eyes, and the visual image is upside-down in the visual cortex. Somehow, somewhere in the cortex, through the interactions between the various visual centres, the image is inverted again to appear the 'right way up', and binocular input is transformed into one seamless three-dimensional percept of the outside world. While we have discovered much about the visual system, there is still more to learn.

In contrast, patients with damage to the inferotemporal cortex have visual agnosia, where the position of an object is recognized but it cannot be named or a copy drawn (except from memory). In a particular form of this condition, called prosopagnosia, patients cannot recognize individual faces, however familiar. For example, a married person with this condition would not recognize their spouse visually, but would recognize the sound of their voice. Alexia is the inability to read written words. Damage to V4 results in loss of colour vision, achromatopsia, while

HEARING AND BALANCE:
THE AUDITORY AND VESTIBULAR SYSTEMS

8

Chapter objectives

After studying this chapter you should be able to:

1. Describe the auditory pathways.

2. Describe how the organ of Corti contributes to the analysis of sound frequency.

3. Describe the mechanisms by which pitch, loudness and sound location are discriminated in the central auditory system.

4. Distinguish between conduction deafness and sensorineural deafness.

5. List the functional roles of the vestibular apparatus.

6. Describe how the vestibular system detects angular and linear acceleration.

7. Describe the vestibulo-ocular reflex and how nystagmus can occur.

8. List clinical signs of auditory and vestibular system dysfunction.

9. Outline the management of hearing and balance disorders.

Introduction

Hearing is one of our most important senses, because of its role in the perception of speech and the ability to communicate. Hearing deficits are common, particularly in the young and the elderly. The symptoms of hearing loss, earache, tinnitus (ringing in the ears), vertigo and otorrhea are associated with ear problems. About one in seven of the UK population have some form of hearing impairment, ranging from profound deafness to mild difficulties in understanding speech. Hearing loss is hardest for young children. They are deprived of the normal acquisition of speech and consequently other forms of communication. Acute deafness in adolescents can have a significant psychological impact, as it deprives them of social contact with their peers. In the elderly, deafness causes increased isolation and estrangement from family and friends.

The vestibular system is intimately involved in maintaining balance, and the most frequently reported symptoms of vestibular disorders are dizziness, unsteadiness when walking, vertigo and nausea. These symptoms can range from mild, lasting minutes, to severe, resulting in total disability. As the vestibular system interacts with many other parts of the nervous system, symptoms may manifest as problems with vision, movement, thinking, and memory. Vestibular disorders occur frequently and can affect people of all ages. Balance disorders increase in frequency in the elderly, and by the age of 75 years become one of the most common reasons for visiting the doctor. In many cases, the cause lies in the inner ear.

The impact of deafness and balance disorders in society is significant in terms of financial and emotional costs: the cost of diagnosis and treatment, hearing aids, speech therapy or vestibular rehabilitation, and lost work potential.

This chapter reviews the anatomy and physiology of the auditory and vestibular systems and describes clinical signs and symptoms associated with their dysfunction (Box 8.1).

The auditory system

The auditory system is a specialized sensory system that has two main functions: to detect and localize sound, and to decode sounds into meaningful language. It comprises the cochlea, the afferent auditory pathways and the auditory cortex in the temporal lobe, and can detect frequencies from 20 Hz to 20 kHz. The auditory pathway is more elaborate than the visual or somatosensory pathways, in that both ears detect and signal the location of the sound. Complex inhibitory circuitry is used to magnify the differences in the timing and intensity of sounds that occur between the two sides during normal hearing.

Anatomy of the ear

The ear apparatus comprises three main regions: the outer, middle and inner ear (Fig. 8.1) each of which has specific functions (Table 8.1).

The outer ear (auricle) collects sound waves with the help of the pinna, and channels them through the external auditory canal to the middle ear. The tympanic membrane (eardrum) separates the middle ear from the outer ear. The tympanic membrane is shaped like the diaphragm of a loudspeaker, with an area of about 18 mm². Normally it is translucent, and the handle (manubrium) of the malleus, the first bone of the ossicular chain of the middle ear, is visible. Sound waves collected by the external ear are transmitted to the inner ear via vibration

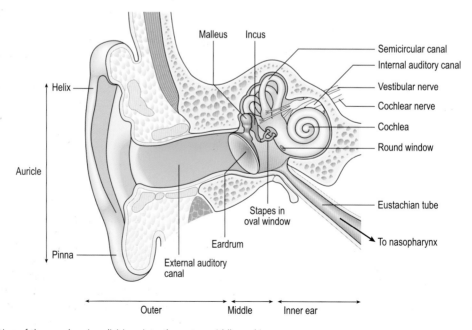

Fig. 8.1 Cross-section of the ear showing divisions into the outer, middle and inner ears.

Table 8.1 Characteristics of the auditory system

Division	Mode of operation	Function
Outer ear	Air vibration	Protection, localization, amplification
Middle ear	Mechanical vibration	Impedance matching, pressure equalization, inner ear stimulation
Inner ear	Mechanical, hydrodynamic and electrochemical	Sound filtering, signal transduction
Central auditory nervous system	Electrochemical	Information processing

Box 8.1 Case history

A 63-year-old retired road construction labourer has had progressively worsening tinnitus for the past several years, and also had episodes of feeling unwell. On several occasions, he reported that the room span around like a merry-go-round. In the last 6 months, he has begun to stagger to the right when walking, and has had difficulty in coordinating his right hand. A month ago, he noticed muscle weakness on the right side of his face. On examination, the doctor detected a right-sided hearing deficit. The patient also had no ability to wrinkle his forehead or retract the right side of his face when asked to smile. There was no corneal reflex on the right side. He had trouble coordinating his right hand, and had intentional tremor on finger-to-nose testing and heel-to-shin testing of the right upper and lower limbs. The doctor immediately referred the patient to an ear, nose and throat (ENT) specialist at the local hospital for further tests. Audiometry tests revealed a high-tone hearing loss of 20 decibels on the right. The examination also showed that the patient had a wide-based gait, and inability to tandem walk. There was no nystagmus on caloric stimulation of the right ear. The ENT specialist sent the patient for a magnetic resonance imaging (MRI) scan, which revealed a tumour in the right posterior fossa at the cerebellopontine angle.

This case gives rise to the following questions:

1. What are the possible causes of deafness?
2. What are the causes of this patient's symptoms?
3. What is the rationale underlying the different tests for deafness?
4. What are the links between hearing and balance disorders?

of the tympanic membrane and the middle ear ossicles. In order for pressure differences not to impede the vibrations produced by the sound, the middle ear atmospheric pressure needs to be the same as that in the outer ear. This is achieved by the eustachian tubes, which open automatically during swallowing, linking the middle ears to the atmosphere via the nasopharynx (see Fig. 8.1).

The middle ear converts the sound pressure waves into vibration of the fluid in the inner ear by movement of the oval window, an elastic membrane separating the inner ear from the middle ear. Three small bones accomplish this: the malleus, incus and stapes. These transfer the sound vibrations from the tympanic membrane to the oval window. The oval window is only one-sixth of the area of the tympanic membrane. The bones are moved by two muscles, the tensor tympani and tensor stapedius, innervated by branches of the trigeminal and facial nerves respectively.

The inner ear houses the cochlea (hearing) and vestibular apparatus (balance), which are contained within the bony labyrinth of the temporal bone (see Fig. 8.1). Movement of the liquid (endolymph) in the inner ear activates these receptors. The hearing receptors are located within the cochlea, while the balance receptors are located in the semicircular canals and vestibule. A delicate continuous membrane is suspended within the bony labyrinth, creating a second chamber within the first in the cochlea. This is the membranous labyrinth or cochlear duct (Fig. 8.2).

The cochlea is shaped like a snail's shell and consists of three fluid-filled spaces (Fig. 8.2A) enclosed in a bony core called the modiolus:

1. scala vestibuli, which runs from the oval window
2. scala tympani, which ends at the round window
3. scala media (cochlear duct).

The scala vestibuli and scala tympani contain perilymph (similar to cerebrospinal fluid), and are continuous with each other at the apex (also called the helicotrema) of the cochlea. The cochlear duct contains endolymph (similar to the intracellular cytoplasm of cells), which is necessary for auditory and vestibular hair cells to function normally; it is unique to the vestibulocochlear system. The cochlea contains a delicate vestibular (Reissner) membrane, which separates the scala vestibuli from the cochlear duct, and the basilar membrane, which separates the scala tympani from the cochlear duct. The scala media houses the auditory receptor organ, the organ of Corti (Fig. 8.2B).

Auditory receptors

The organ of Corti consists of inner and outer hair cells and supporting cells. At birth, there are about 16 000 hair cells in each ear, and these are solely responsible for how we perceive sound. Hair cells have stereocilia that form bundles that act like antennae. These project into the surrounding endolymph or insert into the tectorial membrane, and move in response to fluid displacements caused by sound waves. This generates an electrical signal by opening specific ion channels in the cells.

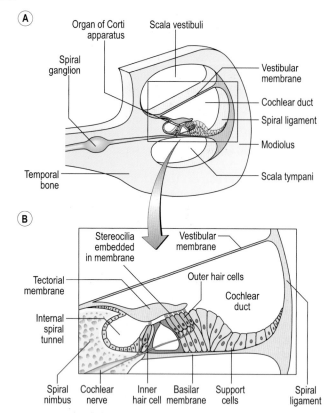

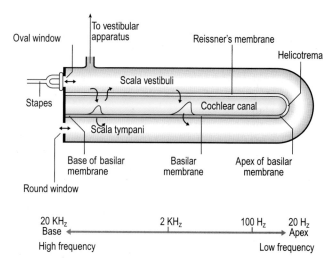

Fig. 8.2 Anatomy of the cochlea. (A) Transverse section through one turn of the cochlea helix. (B) Magnified view of box region in (A), showing the organ of Corti.

Fig. 8.3 Tonotopic organization of the 'unwound' basilar membrane. Vibration of the stapes causes displacement of the scala vestibule perilymph that is transmitted through Reissner's membrane to cause endolymph movement within the cochlear canal. This causes the basilar membrane to resonate at different positions along its length according to frequency. High-frequency sounds travel along the basilar membrane and dissipate energy at the narrow, taut end, whereas low-frequency sounds propagate towards the apex of the membrane before dissipating their energy. This sets up a frequency map along the length of the membrane.

Inner hair cells are arranged in a single row. They have a 1 : 1 relationship with auditory neurones and play a major role in auditory discrimination. Their stereocilia are not embedded in the tectorial membrane; rather, they lie just underneath, swaying in the endolymph. Each hair cell is innervated by 20 afferent fibres.

Outer hair cells increase from three rows at the base to five rows at the apex of the basilar membrane. They receive synapses from a larger number of auditory afferents. It is thought that they help to sharpen the frequency tuning of the cochlea. The tips of their stereocilia are embedded in the overlying tectorial membrane.

Sound transduction

Sound waves collected by the outer ear are channelled to the tympanic membrane. Sound waves are then transmitted from the eardrum along the ossicular chain, causing the stapes to induce vibrations of the oval window. These vibrations set the perilymph fluid of the scala vestibuli in motion. The round window serves as a pressure valve, bulging outwards as pressure rises in the inner ear. As of the size differential between the tympanic membrane and oval window, sound is amplified four-fold in the middle ear. Sound waves are converted into perilymphatic pressure, which is transmitted through the vestibular membrane to

the basilar membrane. Because the tectorial membrane sits on the basilar membrane, it too is set in motion by displacement of endolymph fluid, stimulating hair cells embedded in this membrane. When the basilar membrane is in motion, the stereocilia bend, causing changes in the membrane potential and evoking action potential firing due to opening of voltage-gated Ca^{2+} channels.

The width of the basilar membrane increases from the base to the apex, allowing different parts to resonate at different frequencies along its course. Also, the base is taut, while the apex end is more flexible, making it differentially sensitive to vibration. Consequently, the highest frequencies (and pitch) set the narrow (base) end resonating, while lower frequencies set the apex in motion. This means that the properties of the basilar membrane result in a frequency gradient along its length (Fig. 8.3). This produces a tonotopic map of sound frequency. This map is faithfully repeated at several relay stations along the auditory pathway. The loudness of the sound is determined by the intensity of the sound waves: greater intensity causes greater vibration of the basilar membrane, and hence greater activation of spiral ganglion cells.

Auditory pathways

The central circuitry of the auditory pathways is among the most complex of any of the sensory systems. It is organized in such a way as to discriminate three important parameters of hearing: location, intensity and timing. The ascending pathways are organized as two main systems: one is tonotopically 'hard-wired' according to frequency, providing a fast, secure pathway to the cortex; the other surrounds this system and is less precisely organized with respect to frequency, but is additionally sensitive to the timing and intensity of the sound. This pattern is maintained all the way to the cortex. Parts of this surrounding system are organized to preserve binaural hearing.

The cell bodies of the cochlear nerve afferents are located in the spiral ganglion. Their peripheral processes synapse with the hair cells and their central processes converge with the central processes of the vestibular nerve, to form the vestibulo-cochlear nerve in the internal auditory canal (see Fig. 8.1). The cochlear nerve afferents terminate in the cochlear nucleus, located at the border of the medulla and pons. The cochlear nucleus comprises two subnuclei, dorsal and ventral, which have cell types that are able to extract different features from incoming sound. In these nuclei, the sound is split into two streams with different functions: one for location and one for quality (similar to the visual system, in which motion and form processing are separated). The ventral cochlear nucleus (VCN) has two main types of cell, which are specialized for encoding intensity (stellate cells) and timing (bushy cells), thus providing information about sound location, while the dorsal cochlear nucleus (DCN) encodes pitch information and analyses the quality of sound. The DCN dissects the tiny frequency differences that make words like 'hat' sound different from 'hot', 'hut' and 'hit'. Each cochlear nucleus gives rise to a separate, 'parallel' ascending pathway that conveys specific attributes of the sound to higher centres.

The majority of axon collaterals of neurones in the DCN cross the midline to form the contralateral lateral lemniscus (LL), which ascends to the contralateral inferior colliculus (IC) in the midbrain. Other axon collaterals ascend ipsilaterally in the LL to the IC. Similarly, ventral nucleus fibres enter both the LL via the superior olivary nucleus (SON) and the trapezoid body. Axons from the SON go to the LL nuclei and to the IC. From the IC, auditory fibres travel to synapse in the main auditory nucleus of the thalamus, the medial geniculate nucleus (MGN). From there, thalamocortical axons travel to the primary auditory cortex (AI or Heschl's gyrus) in the temporal lobe via the auditory radiation of the internal capsule (Fig. 8.4). Auditory cortical cells receive input from both ears but preferentially respond to input from the contralateral ear. Surrounding AI are the association areas of hearing, which are involved in decoding sound into language.

Like the basilar membrane, the IC, MGN and AI are all tonotopically organized. For example, in AI high tones are represented posteromedially and low tones anterolaterally. Additionally, cells in AI are organized into separate columns based on whether sound from the ipsilateral ear excites or inhibits them (similar to ocular dominance columns in the visual system). These columns are perpendicular to the tonotopic frequency columns in AI. Tonotopic maps are not immutable; they can be modified by experience or damage (Box 8.2).

The central auditory pathways are unlike other ascending pathways, because of the presence of three pairs of

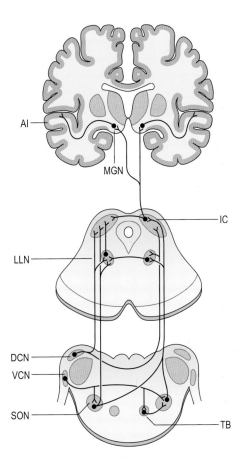

Fig. 8.4 The auditory pathways. DCN, dorsal cochlear nucleus; VCN, ventral cochlear nucleus; TB, trapezoid body; SON, superior olivary nucleus; LLN, lateral lemniscus nucleus; IC, inferior colliculus; MGN, medial geniculate nucleus; AI, primary auditory cortex. Connections of one side are shown for clarity.

accessory nuclei (between the cochlear nuclei and the inferior colliculus) that modulate the input and the bilateral representation of auditory impulses.

The superior olivary nucleus

The SON receives bilateral sound input (via the VCN) and gives rise to fibres that travel in both the ipsilateral and contralateral LL. The ipsilateral inputs are excitatory, whereas the contralateral ones are inhibitory (an effect mediated by the trapezoid body). The SON plays a key role in the localization of sounds in space, because it is responsive to differences in intensity and timing between sounds entering the ears simultaneously (Fig. 8.5).

The trapezoid body

Axons from the VCN that decussate run through the trapezoid body (TB). This structure helps locate the spatial direction of the sound by exaggerating differences, through crossed inhibition of SON cells. Some collaterals from the TB enter the facial and trigeminal nerves to form part of the efferent pathways of the acoustic reflexes.

Auditory cortex plasticity

The brain is not a 'hard-wired', immutable structure but is, in fact, a highly plastic organ. The cortex contains many maps of the body's image for different perceptual functions: for vision, for touch, for movement and for hearing. These maps can be changed by experience and by damage.

Located in the supratemporal gyrus of the temporal lobe are the structures involved in hearing and language comprehension. They consist of the primary auditory cortex (AI) and its association areas. Studies have shown that AI is the region that is responsible for sound localization, whereas the association areas are more important in language functions (See Box 8.3).

AI cortical cells are tonotopically organized on the basis of sound frequency, but the organization of this map can be changed by experience or activity. For example, in auditory learning tasks there is an increased representation for those frequencies that are used during training. In patients with chronic tinnitus, magnetic resonance imaging analysis has shown that there is a change in the map in the auditory cortex as compared to healthy subjects, in that the tinnitus frequency expands into adjacent frequency regions. This has been likened to an auditory phantom, and may involve mechanisms akin to those proposed for phantom limb pain (see Box 5.4).

Deaf patients also show considerable plasticity in the auditory cortex. Recent functional imaging studies have shown that a significant amount of cross-modality plasticity occurs in the temporal lobe. For example, in congenitally deaf people, the auditory cortical regions do not respond to sound but instead to visual cues in response to sign language. Tactile sensitivity can also activate this region, reflecting increased attention to a stimulus.

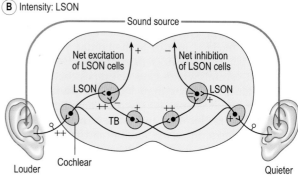

Fig. 8.5 Sound localization: the role of the superior olivary nuclei. (A) The medial SON (MSON) participates in coincidence detection via timing differences. Sound travels different distances to reach the right and left ears. The MSON neurones are maximally excited when action potentials from both ears activate the cells simultaneously. Different neurones are sensitive to different interaural time delays, created by receiving input from cochlear axons of different lengths, and so create a spatial map based on sound location. The MSON cells can detect delays as short as $10\,\mu s$. (B) The lateral SON (LSON) participates in localization via interaural intensity differences. A sound reaching the nearer of the two ears is perceived to be loudest because of stronger excitation of the ipsilateral LSON cells as compared to the contralateral LSON (++ vs +) from the cochlear nuclei. Input to the contralateral LSON is relayed via inhibitory cells of the trapezoid body (TB) and so inhibits cells of the contralateral SON. The LSON cells only encode sounds arising from the ipsilateral side, and both nuclei are needed to represent the full range of positions in the horizontal plane. Sounds emanating near the midline produce lower firing rates on the ipsilateral side because of enhanced inhibition from the contralateral side, so that at or beyond the midline the contralateral TB input can completely silence the LSON neurones.

The lateral lemniscus nuclei

The lateral lemniscus nuclei (LLN) are located in and adjacent to the LL, and send axons to both the ipsilateral and contralateral LL. They receive input from collaterals of the SON. There are reciprocal connections between the nuclei on the two sides. They are thought to participate in acoustic reflexes.

The inferior colliculus

The IC is an important auditory centre, and receives input from three main sources: the LL, the contralateral IC and descending axons from AI. Its efferents project to the MGN and to the contralateral IC (inhibitory function), the superior colliculus and the reticular formation. Functionally, the IC integrates spatial information from the SON, intensity information from the ventral cochlear nucleus, and

pitch information from the dorsal cochlear nucleus. It participates in acoustic reflexes.

Brainstem acoustic reflexes

There are reciprocal connections between all of the relay nuclei in the auditory pathways that allow for auditory modulation. Brainstem reflexes function mainly (1) to prevent damage to the auditory system; and (2) to distinguish selective sounds from background noise. Fibre collaterals emerge from the LL and connect to interneurones of the reticular formation and to cranial nerve motor nuclei to produce reflex arcs: The efferent fibres from these regions innervate the middle ear muscles.

1. Fibres enter the Vth and VIIth motor nuclei to link with motor neurones supplying tensor tympani (V) and stapedius (VII) muscles in the middle ear. The muscles exert a damping action on the middle ear ossicles. The tensor tympani is activated by one's own voice, and the stapedius by external sounds. Damage to these nerve branches may lead to hyperacusis (abnormally loud sounds).

2. Loud, unexpected sounds such as the noise from an unexpected explosion cause flinching. This is a startle reflex, a type of arousal reflex, and is mediated by reticulospinal fibres that connect to the motor nucleus of cranial nerve VII and the spinal cord.

3. Cholinergic efferent fibres originating from cells located near the SON form the olivocochlear bundle, which preferentially innervates outer hair cells. When activated, the outer hair cells contract, pulling the tectorial membrane down towards the organ of Corti. This may produce an increase in the amplitude and frequency sensitivity of the inner hair cells. This provides a feedback mechanism for regulating selective attention to certain sounds, i.e. being able to extract sound from the surrounding noise.

Auditory perception

The sounds that a person hears are produced by the brain; sound waves make no noise. As well as being very sensitive to air pressure changes, the auditory system is adept at perceiving many different sounds at once. For example, when listening to music, one is able to pick out all the different instruments contributing to the song, and the singers. But certain sounds convey meaning, and the analysis of sounds that convey meaning is more complex than the detection of sound. Detecting sounds is performed in AI, while assigning meaning is the function of the association auditory cortex (AII). This higher mental function is asymmetrical in the brain. Decoding sounds into language is the main function of Wernicke's area, which is predominantly found on the left side of the brain in humans. The right side of the brain deals with non-verbal tasks, such as musical appreciation and comprehension.

As in the visual system, where information is split into a dorsal 'where' stream for where things are and a ventral 'what' stream for what things are, auditory sounds are split into dorsal and ventral streams, so that we can identify objects by sound. For example, sirens are associated with fire engines, police cars and ambulances, and ring tones with mobile phones. These patterns of activity are relayed from the AI and AII areas and further processed via the 'what' pathway in the inferior temporal lobe, sending information to the prefrontal cortex. Information about spatial tuning and sound-guided movement is relayed from AI and AII via the 'where' pathway to the posterior parietal cortex and then to the motor cortex, in order that responses can be made to the sound. For example, when the telephone rings during the middle of the night, we automatically know where the phone is and reach to pick it up without thinking. In fact, the hand automatically makes the appropriate shape to pick up the receiver on the basis of the sound heard.

Functional imaging studies have shown that auditory information is also processed in other parts of the brain, such as the nucleus accumbens, amygdala and medial prefrontal cortex, which are associated with putting emotional labels on sounds or tunes.

Physiology of hearing

Sound intensity and frequency

Sound loudness is measured in terms of intensity or pressure, both representing the extent to which air molecules are condensed with each phase of the sound wave. The amplitude of the waves determines the intensity of the sound; the louder the sound, the greater the amplitude. A log scale, called the decibel (dB) scale, is used to specify intensity, because of the wide range of amplitudes to which the ear is sensitive. A 10-dB increase in sound represents a 10-fold increase in intensity. Sound becomes uncomfortable to the ear at around 120 dB, and frankly painful above 140 dB. Jet engines have an intensity of around 140 dB, whispering 20 dB, talking 50 dB, and factory noise 100 dB. Prolonged exposure to loud sounds kills the hair cells and causes deafness or a hearing deficit. The louder the sound, the quicker the loss, with higher frequencies being lost first. Most people fail to notice the deficit until they cannot hear someone else's speech.

Sounds are recognized as tones when the pressure waves have a single frequency, or noise when many irregular waves of different frequencies interfere with each other. Sound frequency specifies the rate at which the alternate phases of condensation occur. It determines the pitch of the perceived sound. Most sounds are mixtures of frequencies (and are called complex tones), and the particular mixture determines the timbre. Timbre gives characteristic information about the nature of the sound. For example, it allows us to distinguish the sounds of two different musical instruments playing the same note.

Sound discrimination

The range over which a sound excites an auditory neurone determines its receptive field (RF). The frequency at which the neurone is excited with the lowest-intensity sound is its 'characteristic frequency'. However, with suprathreshold stimulation, the auditory neurones respond to a wider range of frequencies. Many auditory afferents respond to sounds at frequencies below their best frequency when the sounds are loud, and thus the RFs overlap. The discreteness of tuning of single primary afferents is greater than can be accounted for if the basilar membrane acts simply as a linear frequency analyser. This has led to the idea that the ear is an active biomechanical sensory organ. Thus, the non-linear properties of the cochlea, active control of hair cell excitability, and intrinsic properties of hair cells, provide for their very precise frequency tuning.

Central neural codes

Pitch, loudness and the localization of sound in space are represented in different ways by neurones of the auditory system.

Pitch is encoded in the firing of specific populations of spiral ganglion neurones. The most important factor is where along the basilar membrane the fibres end. This mechanism, which contributes to perception of sounds over much of the auditory spectrum, is referred to as the place theory. According to this theory, the frequency spectrum of a complex sound is encoded in the pattern of firing of a population of afferent fibres that originate from different parts of the cochlea.

Loudness is signalled by two mechanisms. The louder the tone, the greater the firing frequency of the hair cell along the basilar membrane. However, the dynamic range of most primary afferents is only 20–30 dB, not nearly enough to account for the 120-dB range for loudness discrimination. The existence of a subpopulation (about 20%) of high-threshold primary afferents, which innervate the inner hair cells with a widely distributed range of thresholds, accounts for the latter. In this subpopulation, the number of active neurones and their firing frequency signal loudness.

Accurate sound localization requires bilaterally intact auditory pathways, including the auditory cortex. Sounds from anywhere in the horizontal acoustic plane reaches the two ears asymmetrically, due to differential shielding of the noise from its source by the head, resulting in the creation of a sound shadow. This results in a difference in sound intensity, and hence loudness detected by the auditory neurones. Similarly, when sounds arrive in the sagittal plane of the head, the intensity of sound arriving at both ears will be the same, but we can still tell whether the sound originates from in front or behind the head, and above or below the ear level. This ability is due to the site and shape of the pinna and the plane of the tympana. These factors result in different patterns of deflection and impingement of sound waves, according to their direction. Centrally, the initial localization processing seems to occur in the SON (see Fig. 8.5A), where individual cells are sensitive to time and phase differences in the sound arriving at the two ears. The ability to perceive speech is critically dependent on the timing and pattern discrimination (Box 8.3).

Clinical signs associated with damage to the cochlear nerve

The clinical signs of damage to the auditory nerve are deafness and tinnitus. Lesions to the auditory pathway within the brainstem, thalamus or cortex do not produce significant hearing loss; rather, they produce difficulty in locating or discriminating the sound, especially with difficult auditory tasks. Hearing problems that are associated with lesions central to the cochlear nucleus are: poor speech discrimination, poor sound localization, poor selective attention and poor auditory short-term memory. Unilateral hearing loss indicates damage to the ipsilateral ear or nerve. Deafness can be of two types:

- Conduction deafness results from any interference with the passage of sound waves through the external or middle ear that prevents sound waves from reaching the cochlea (e.g. wax build-up in outer ear, or middle ear infections such as otitis media). Sound wave propagation still occurs via bone conduction. Conduction deafness is never complete or total.

- Nerve (perception or sensorineural) deafness results from damage to the receptor cells of the organ of Corti, the cochlear nerve or nucleus. The defect is in the segment of the auditory mechanism common to both air and bone conduction, and thus hearing failure in both routes occurs. The amount of loss depends on degree of damage to the organ or nerve.

Clinical tests

There are two simple tuning fork tests, the Rinne and Weber tests, which together can distinguish conduction from perception deafness. Both depend on the differences between air conduction and bone conduction of sound. Sound transmitted by air conduction depends on the integrity of the middle ear, while bone conduction can bypass the middle ear and activate the basilar membrane of the inner ear directly. These two tests are described in Table 8.2.

Other hearing tests

Audiometry

An audiometer that produces pure tone sounds at specific volumes is used to test each ear separately. The auditory threshold for a range of tones is determined by decreasing the volume of each tone until a person can no longer hear it. Audiometric tests can identify the frequencies lost: in middle ear disease, low-frequency loss is common, whereas cochlear nerve damage is associated with high-frequency impairment.

Tympanometry

This procedure measures the impedance (resistance to pressure) of the middle ear. It is used to help determine the cause of conductive hearing loss. It does not require the active participation of the person being tested, and is commonly used in children. A device is placed in the ear canal and it detects how much sound passes through the middle ear and how much is reflected back as pressure changes in the ear canal. The results indicate whether the problem is a blocked eustachian tube, fluid in the middle ear, or a disruption in the ossicular chain. Tympanometry

Box
8.3   Relationship between hearing and speaking

The language areas in the brain are located in the dominant hemisphere. When the language areas are damaged, the resultant clinical syndrome is called aphasia. Thus, there is a clear neuroanatomical basis for language.

The basic unit of speech is the phoneme, i.e. the smallest speech sound. For example, pin has three phonemes: p, i and n. Morphemes are combinations of phonemes that provide meaning (words). Syntax represents the rules governing word sequences (grammatical structure), and semantics is the way in which language governs meaning.

Basic circuit for understanding spoken language (Fig. 8.6)

1. When a person hears a sentence, this is transmitted via the auditory apparatus to the primary auditory cortex in the temporal lobe.
2. This then connects to Wernicke's area (in the temporal lobe), which decodes the language into meaning.
3. If the sentence is to be repeated, or replied to, the information has to be transmitted forwards to Broca's area (expressive speech) in the frontal lobe (via the arcuate fasciculus).
4. Broca's area then produces speech via the motor programmes of the motor cortex, which activate the tongue and laryngeal muscles.

Basic circuit for understanding written speech

1. Visual input is transmitted to the visual cortex (areas 17–19) in the occipital lobe.
2. Input from the visual association area is sent to the left angular gyrus, where the objects are recognized and named.
3. Input then goes to Wernicke's area, where words are assembled into sentences, and the appropriate messages are sent via the arcuate and superior longitudinal fasciculi to Broca's area.
4. Broca's area activates motor programmes in the primary motor cortex that elicit speech via appropriate brainstem centres and muscles of the tongue and larynx.

Effects of damage to specific cortical areas

*   Wernicke's area: receptive aphasia—fluent meaningless speech with severely impaired speech understanding.
*   Broca's area: expressive aphasia—abbreviated, ungrammatical but meaningful speech, but speech understanding impaired where syntax conveys meaning.
*   Arcuate fasciculus: conduction aphasia—speech deficiencies are similar to those in receptive aphasia, but because comprehension remains intact, the patient makes attempts to say the right words.
*   Angular gyrus: alexia (inability to read) with agraphia (inability to write), but the patient can comprehend speech and speak normally.

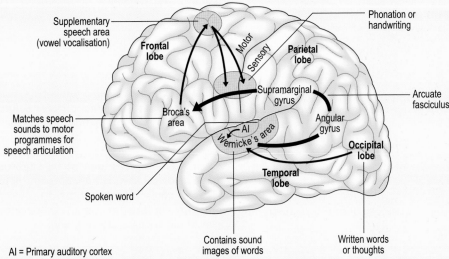

AI = Primary auditory cortex

Fig. 8.6 Cortical pathways for understanding language. See text for details. AI, primary auditory cortex.

also detects changes in the contraction of the stapedius muscle, which is attached to the stapes. This muscle normally contracts in response to loud noises; this is a protective acoustic reflex, protecting the inner ear. The acoustic reflex changes if the hearing loss is neural. When the acoustic reflex is decreased, the stapedius muscle cannot remain contracted during continuous exposure to loud noise.

Table 8.2 Comparison of the Rinne and Weber hearing tests

Test	Method	Normal response	Conduction deafness	Sensorineural deafness
Rinne	Place a vibrating tuning fork in contact with the mastoid process, and then close to the pinna. Compares air conduction with bone conduction and determines their relative sensitivities in each ear separately	Sound is heard louder and longer by air conduction because sound energy travelling through bone dissipates more quickly	Bone conduction is better than air conduction on the affected side	Air conduction is better than bone conduction in the affected ear. Sound is loudest in the unaffected ear
Weber	Place a vibrating tuning fork in the middle of the forehead and ask the patient in which ear the tone is heard. It detects relative hearing loss differences between the two ears	Sound is heard equally well on both sides	Sound is louder in the affected ear	Sound is louder in the unaffected ear

Electrocochleography

Electrocochleography measures the activity of the cochlea and the auditory nerve. This and the auditory brainstem response test can be used to measure hearing in people who cannot or will not respond voluntarily to sound. For example, these tests are used to find out whether infants and children have profound hearing loss, and whether a person is faking or exaggerating hearing loss (psychogenic hypoacusis). Sometimes the tests can help determine the cause of sensorineural hearing loss.

Auditory brainstem response

This is another test that can distinguish between sensory and neural hearing loss. It measures nerve impulses in the brain resulting from stimulation of the auditory nerves by calibrated clicks presented to the ear. Computer averaging of scalp-evoked potentials produces an image of the wave pattern of the nerve impulses. This technique is used to evaluate deficits due to trauma or disease involving the brainstem, especially in children. Children who have been thought to be 'slow learners' have been shown to actually have hearing deficits rather than being mentally retarded. The auditory brainstem response can also be used to monitor certain brain functions in people who are comatose or in those undergoing brain surgery.

Main causes of hearing loss

Infection

Prenatal causes

Viruses, e.g. German measles (rubella) during pregnancy, can cause complete destruction of the cochlear nerve in the fetus. Meningitis also leads to deafness by destroying the inner ear cells.

Perinatal causes

These are middle ear infections, e.g. otitis media, a bacterial infection causing swelling and outward bulging of the tympanic membrane, pain and pus collection in middle ear. These are most common in children, as the eustachian tubes are not fully formed and thus do not drain well into the nasopharynx. 'Glue ear'—otitis media with effusion—is the biggest single cause of hearing loss in children, affecting more than 20% of 2-year-olds and 15% of 5-year-olds in winter, often as a complication of acute ear infections and respiratory illnesses. Ear infections are often easily treated with antibiotics such as amoxycillin or analgesic drugs such as paracetamol and ibuprofen.

Ototoxic agents

Prolonged use of certain drugs (see Table 8.3), in particular the aminoglycoside antibiotics, can be ototoxic and can affect both divisions of the vestibulocochlear nerve. Antibiotics predominantly affect the organ of Corti by accumulating at high concentrations in the endolymph. Hair cell damage is accompanied by subsequent retrograde degeneration of the auditory neurones. The risk of ototoxicity is enhanced by persistently elevated plasma concentrations of the drugs. Repeated courses of therapy continue to damage more cells, leading to more vestibulo-cochlear dysfunction.

Hereditary diseases

More than 100 genetic diseases cause deafness. Genetic causes are responsible for more than half of all cases of congenital deafness. Genes for about 20 hereditary forms of deafness have been cloned: they are involved in making hair cell bundles, transforming sound energy into electrical activity, and the connections between hair cells. Otosclerosis is the most common adult cause of hearing loss, and is an autosomal-dominant genetic disorder.

Table 8.3 Common ototoxic drugs

Neomycin	Most potent of all antibiotics in destroying the organ of Corti.
Streptomycin or Gentamycin	Affects the vestibular part of nerve more than cochlear part.
Salicylates (e.g. aspirin metabolites)	Reversible hearing loss and tinnitus
Quinine and its synthetic substitutes	Produce permanent deafness
Anti-cancer drugs	e.g. Cisplatin or vincristine

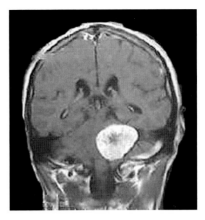

Fig. 8.7 Magnetic resonance image showing an acoustic neuroma compressing the cerebellopontine angle. From British Acoustic Neuroma Association.

It is characterized by fusion of stapes to the oval window, causing difficulty in movement, followed by eventual cessation of ear ossicle movement. It is amenable to microsurgery (stapes replacement).

Gradual hearing deterioration

This is a commonly associated with the work environment. Persistent loud sounds, such as aircraft or pneumatic drills, cause deterioration of hearing by destroying auditory cells (frequency- and intensity-dependent). Any noise > 85 dB is potentially damaging. The perception of higher frequencies is affected first, and then that of lower ones. The amount of damage depends on exposure time, so reducing the intensity and length of exposure to loud sounds limits the damage. Presbyacusis is the progressive hearing loss that occurs with normal ageing. High frequencies (18–20 kHz) are lost first, and lower frequencies (4–8 kHz) later.

Trauma and tumours

Head injuries that fracture the temporal bone may cause hearing damage. Bleeding from the ear and Battle's sign (postauricular haematoma) are common symptoms associated with temporal bone fractures. Slow-growing acoustic tumours usually arise in the vestibular division of cranial nerve VIII (Fig. 8.7). They affect both divisions of the vestibulocochlear nerve. Tinnitus, vertigo, deafness and symptoms of damage to cranial nerves VII and V are associated with these tumours (see Box 8.3) as they emerge from the internal auditory meatus at the cerebellopontine angle, to impinge on the brainstem.

Treatment for hearing deficits

Treatment depends on the cause. For example, if fluid or wax blocks the outer or middle ear, the fluid can be drained or the wax removed. For sensorineural deafness, often no cure is available, and in these situations treatment involves compensating for the hearing loss. Most affected people use a hearing aid. Rarely, a cochlear implant is used.

Hearing aids

Sound amplification with a hearing aid helps people who have conductive or sensorineural hearing loss, particularly if they have trouble hearing the frequencies of normal speech. It can also help people who have predominantly high-frequency sensorineural hearing loss and those who have hearing loss in only one ear. Hearing aids use a microphone to pick up sounds, an amplifier to magnify the volume and a speaker to transmit the amplified sounds. Air conduction hearing aids, which are generally superior to bone conduction hearing aids, are most commonly used.

Cochlear implants

This is a type of hearing aid for profoundly deaf people, and consists of an internal coil, electrodes, an external coil, a speech processor and a microphone. The internal coil is surgically implanted in the skull behind and above the ear, and the electrodes are implanted in the cochlea. The external coil is held in place by magnets on the skin over the internal coil. The speech processor, connected to the external coil by a wire, may be worn in a pocket or special holster. The microphone is placed in a hearing aid worn behind the ear.

Tympanostomy tubes (grommets)

Grommets are indicated for recurrent (5–6 episodes/year) infections such as chronic otitis media with effusion (glue ear), recurrent acute otitis media, and complications of acute otitis media in children. These infections are caused by blockages of ventilation in the inner ear canal, leading to bacterial infection or fluid build-up. The tubes are usually left in place for 8–12 months. They profoundly improve hearing and language-learning abilities in young children, and reduce the frequency of infection.

Surgery

The type of surgery used depends on the cause of the hearing deficit. It is indicated for removal of acoustic tumours or insertion of grommets.

The vestibular system

The functions of the vestibular system are maintaining balance (posture and equilibrium) and coordinating movements of the eyeball. These functions are related to the positioning of the head. The main processes involved are:

1. detection and conscious perception of head position and movement

2. compensatory eye movements during head movement, providing stabilization of the visual image and target fixation

3. compensatory postural adjustments of the trunk and limb muscles following head movement

In order to accomplish this, the vestibular system is connected with the spinal cord (via the medial and lateral vestibulospinal tracts (VSTs)), the cerebellum (via the flocculonodular lobe and fastigial nucleus) and the cranial nerve nuclei (III, IV and VI) associated with ocular movements.

Anatomy

The vestibular apparatus, like the cochlea, is contained within the membranous labyrinth of the inner ear and comprises three distinct regions: the semicircular canals, the utricle, which lies at the base of the semicircular canals, and the saccule, which resides between the utricle and the cochlea (Fig. 8.8). There are five sense organs: the utricle, the saccule and, at the base of each semicircular canal, an ampulla. These house the sensory hair receptors, the maculae (for the utricle and saccule) and the cristae (for the ampullae). They are innervated by the peripheral axons of vestibular ganglion cells, whose central axons run in the vestibulocochlear nerve that projects to the vestibular nuclei in the brainstem. Some vestibular afferents bypass the vestibular nucleus and terminate directly in the flocculo-nodular lobe of the cerebellum.

These vestibular system receptor organs monitor two components of motion: (1) angular acceleration, i.e. the detection of rotational movements, e.g. shaking or nodding the head; and (2) linear acceleration, the detection of motion with respect to gravity, e.g. the sensation when a lift suddenly goes into freefall, or what happens when the body begins to lean to one side.

The semicircular canals

The semicircular canals are activated by circular motion and are filled with endolymph. The motion of the fluid informs the brain whether one is moving. The semicircular canals, and the visual and skeletal systems, have specific functions that determine an individual's orientation in space. The vestibule is the region of the inner ear where the semicircular canals converge, close to the cochlea.

The semicircular canals detect angular acceleration/deceleration of the head. There are three canals, corresponding to the three directions of movement, so that each canal detects motion in a single plane. They lie in orthogonal planes, meaning that there is an angle of about 90°

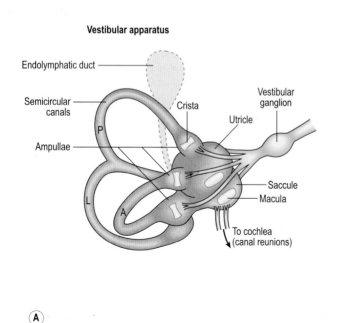

Vestibular apparatus

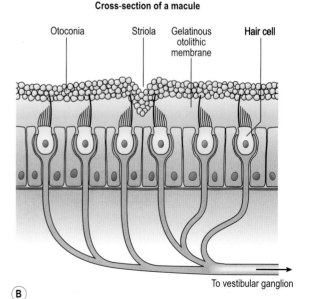

Cross-section of a macule

Fig. 8.8 (A) Anatomy of the vestibular apparatus. (B) Cross-section of a macule.

between any one pair. Horizontal canals are in the same plane and function synergistically. Similarly, the anterior canal on one side and the posterior canal on the other side (and vice versa) are in the same plane and form a synergistic pair. The orientation of the synergistic pairs of canals is important. With the line of sight in the horizontal plane, the horizontal canals are tilted upwards by 25–30°. Each pair of vertical canals is orthogonal to the other and oriented approximately 45° to the right and to the left, respectively. The semicircular canals signal the brain about the direction and speed of rotation of the head, e.g. when nodding the head up and down or looking from right to left. Each canal is a continuous endolymph-filled hoop (Fig. 8.9). The sensory hair cells are located in a small swelling at the base, near the confluence of the canals called the ampulla. The lateral ampulla is activated by turning the head to the left or right, head flexion activates the superior ampulla, and the inferior ampulla is active during head extension.

The hair cells are arranged as a single tuft that projects up into a gelatinous mass, the cupula. Together, these form the crista. When the head rotates in the plane of the canal, the inertia of the endolymph causes it to wash over the cupula, deflecting the hair cells. The same arrangement is mirrored on both sides of the head. Each tuft of hair cells is polarized. If deflected one way, it will be excited; if deflected the other way, it will be inhibited (Fig. 8.9). Thus, the canals on either side of the head operate in a push–pull rhythm; when one is excited, the other is inhibited. Specifically, it is the canal towards the direction of rotation that is excited. However, if, for example, both sides push at once, then debilitating vertigo and nausea ensue. This is why infections of the endolymph or damage to the inner ear can cause vertigo. In cases of severe intractable vertigo, this can be relieved by cutting one vestibular nerve so that the brain gradually gets used to receiving input from one side only.

The utricle and saccule

The utricle and saccule detect linear acceleration and the pull of gravity. Each organ has a sheet of hair cells, the macula, whose cilia are embedded in a gelatinous mass, just like the semicircular canals. Unlike the canals, however, this gel has small crystals of calcium carbonate embedded in it, called otoliths. The otoliths provide the inertia, so that when movement to one side occurs, the otolith–gel mass causes the hair cells to deviate (Fig. 8.10). The hair cells are excited (or inhibited) by bending of the stereocilia towards (or away from) the kinocilium, just as for hair cells of the semicircular canals. Once movement reaches a constant speed, the otoliths come to equilibrium and the motion is no longer perceived.

Hair cells of the utricle and saccule are polarized towards a central shallow groove, the striola (see Fig. 8.8B), which divides each into medial and lateral halves. The kinocilia are arranged in different directions on either side of the striola, so that a single sheet of hair cells can detect motion forwards and back, and side to side. In the utricle, the deflection of kinocilia towards the striola excites the hair cells, while in the saccule, deflection away from the striola excites the hair cells. Each macula can therefore cover two dimensions of movement. The utricle lies horizontally in the ear and detects motion in the horizontal plane. The saccule is oriented vertically, so it detects motion in the sagittal plane (up and down, forwards and back). The saccular and utricular maculae are functionally antagonistic on the two sides of the head, so that, for example, tilting the head laterally to one side has opposite effects on the corresponding hair cells of the two utricular maculae.

A major role of the saccule and utricle is to keep the head vertically oriented with respect to gravity. If the head and body start to tilt, such as when a student falls asleep in a lecture, the vestibular nuclei will automatically compensate

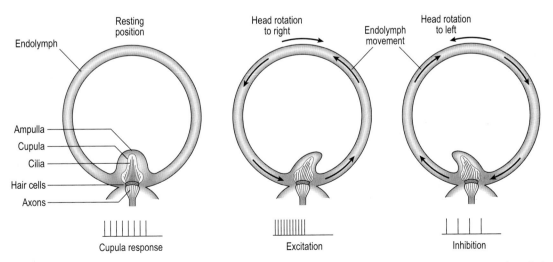

Fig. 8.9 Anatomy of a semicircular canal. Head rotation causes endolymph movement, which causes cupula displacement and vestibular afferent discharge on head rotation. Hair cells are normally spontaneously active, and rotation in one direction causes an increased discharge, while rotation in the opposite direction causes decreased firing.

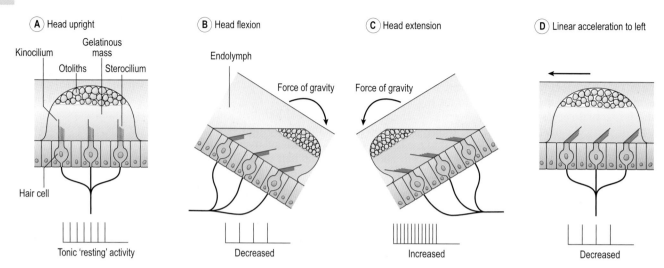

Fig. 8.10 Effects of different head movements on activity of the macula. (A) Head in an upright 'resting' position. (B) Head flexion. (C) Head extension. (D) Linear acceleration.

with the correct postural adjustments via activation of the VSTs. This is the head-righting reflex.

The vestibulo-ocular reflex

An important role of the semicircular canal system is to keep the eyes still while the head moves. When the head is nodded, shaken or swivelled, there is no difficulty in staying focused on an image, but if the image is moving rapidly and the head is still, then the eyes are unable to keep pace with the quick movements. This is because the semicircular canals exert direct control over the eyes, so that they can directly compensate for head movements, but not vice versa. The entire compensatory reflex is called the vestibulo-ocular reflex (VOR). This reflex keeps the eyes fixed on a particular object when the rest of the body is in motion. It works automatically by sensing head rotations and elicits a compensatory adjustment in the opposite direction. As it is a reflex, it also works in the dark or if the eyes are shut. It can be used to assess brainstem integrity in comatose patients (Box 8.4).

The VOR moves the eyes in response to head movements, and involves the three pairs of extraocular eye muscles: the medial–lateral rectus pair (adduction/abduction), the inferior rectus–superior oblique (depression and extorsion, elevation and intorsion) and the superior rectus–inferior oblique (elevation and intorsion, depression and extorsion). These pairs of muscles are aligned closely to the planes of orientation of the semicircular canals. It is easiest to explain how the VOR works by using the medial–lateral rectus pair coupled to the horizontal canal as an example (Fig. 8.12).

When the head rotates to the left, the left horizontal canal is excited, and the right is inhibited. To keep the eyes fixed on an object of interest, the right lateral rectus and the left medial rectus muscles must contract in order to move the eyes to the right. On the other side, the right horizontal canal is wired to the complementary set of muscles. Since it is inhibited, it will not excite its target muscles (the right medial rectus and the left lateral rectus), and nor will it inhibit the muscles that must be used (the right lateral rectus and the left medial rectus). Eventually, as the eyes track to the right, they will end up on the limit of right lateral gaze, and then, under the influence of a signal arising from the lateral gaze centre in the cortex, they rapidly flick back to the centre of the visual field as they lose contact with the object of interest, ready to track another object of interest. This slow drift to one side and rapid re-centreing of the eye is called nystagmus and is a normal physiological event.

The axonal connections between the vestibular and oculomotor nuclei that mediate the VOR travel in a tract called the medial longitudinal fasciculus (MLF), which runs throughout the length of the brainstem. The integrity of this tract is crucial for the normal functioning of the VOR (Box 8.4). It is occasionally damaged by medial brainstem strokes.

Nystagmus can be artificially induced by rapidly spinning someone around in a barber's (Bárány) chair for a brief period, thereby evoking the VOR. For example, consider spinning to the right. At onset, the head and labyrinths accelerate to the right, causing the endolymph to flow to the left, and the cupulae of both horizontal semicircular canals are deflected to the left. The hair cells of the right horizontal canal are excited and so increase their rate of firing, while those of the left canal are inhibited. A VOR occurs, leading to a rhythmic back and forth movement of the eyes, slow to the left and fast to the right. This (rotatory) nystagmus is the attempt by the vestibular system to provide for continued visual fixation on a target during a rotatory movement of the head and body. The direction of nystagmus is specified by the direction of the fast phase. Thus, rotation to the right produces a right lateral nystagmus.

Box 8.4 Clinical applications of the vestibulo-ocular reflex

The vestibulo-ocular reflex (VOR) can be used to assess the level of brainstem damage in a comatose patient. While the unconscious patient is lying in the supine position, the head is rotated from side to side or tilted up and down. Normally, the eyes will rotate in the opposite direction, giving the impression that the gaze is fixed straight ahead, much like the eyes in a toy doll. This is known as the doll's eye reflex.

This reflex can also be elicited using the caloric test (Fig. 8.11). In a normal patient, cool water decreases the temperature of the endolymph and inhibits the hair cell activity on that side. This produces nystagmus of the eyes with the slow phase (S) towards the side of irrigation and the fast phase (F) away from the irrigation. With warm water irrigation, the opposite happens. This can be remembered by the pneumonic 'COWS'—cold opposite, warm same. In unconscious patients whose cortex is non-functional but whose brainstem is intact, there is no F phase (due to lack of signal from the gaze centres), so now cold irrigation leads only to a slow deviation to the side of irrigation—'cold same'—whereas warm irrigation produces the opposite response. Bilateral irrigation of the ears with cold water produces downward eye movements, while the opposite occurs with bilateral warm water irrigation.

If the medial longitudinal fasciculus (MLF) is damaged, irrigation results in lateral deviation of the eye only on the less active side. Pons or low midbrain brainstem damage or vestibular nerve damage produces no eye movement.

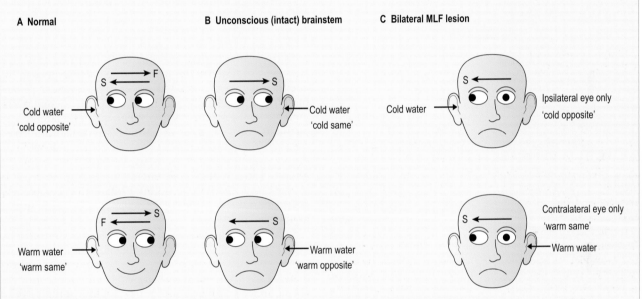

Fig. 8.11 Ocular responses to caloric stimulation of the semicircular canals. Caloric testing involves the patient laying supine with the head tilted backwards at an angle of 30° so that the horizontal canal is vertically orientated. Water is flushed into the ear, and this sets up convection currents in the semicircular canal endolymph that cause movements of the eyes. (A) Normal patient (conscious). (B) Unconscious patient (brainstem intact). (C) Unconscious patient with a bilateral medial longitudinal fasciculus lesion.

When the spinning abruptly stops, the endolymph does not stop as quickly as the horizontal canals. This equates to a flow of endolymph and cupula displacement in the direction of the previous rotation, i.e. to the right. For the left horizontal canal, endolymph flow is towards the utricle, and for the right horizontal canal, it is away from the utricle. Thus, the firing frequency of vestibular nerve afferents is increased on the left and decreased on the right. This is the pattern of excitation and inhibition that would occur if the subject were being rotated to the left, and the brain interprets this signal as such. Consequently, for a short period of time after stopping rotation, a post-rotatory nystagmus occurs in the opposite direction: the eyes move slowly to the right and, when they reach the limit of lateral gaze, quickly to the left. This effect lasts for 20–30s after cessation of rotation. Many will be familiar with the disorientating effects when getting off a merry-go-round at the funfair.

If the subject tries to reach out and touch an object during the period of post-rotatory nystagmus, the movement will miss the target in the direction of the slow phase of nystagmus, i.e. to the right in this case. This

THE AUDITORY AND VESTIBULAR SYSTEMS

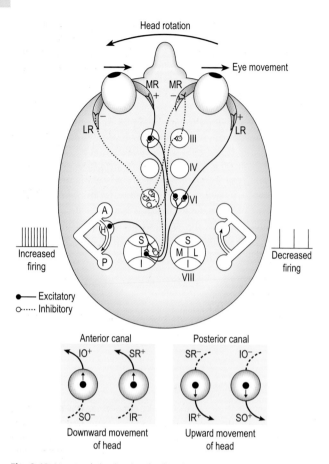

Fig. 8.12 Neuronal circuitry involved in the vestibulo-ocular reflex. When the head turns to the left, the eyes move to the right, causing increased firing in the left horizontal canal and decreased response in the right. Cells that receive information from the left horizontal canal are excited relative to the right canal and stimulate cells in the vestibular nuclei of the brainstem. Neurones from the left medial vestibular nucleus project to the abducens nucleus (VI) on the right side, to stimulate the right lateral rectus muscle. They also project to the oculomotor nucleus (III) on the left side, to stimulate the left medial rectus muscle. The same vestibular cells also inhibit the opposing muscles (the right medial rectus and the left lateral rectus via connections with the left abducens and right oculomotor nuclei; if eye movement was in the vertical direction, then the trochlear nucleus (IV) would also be involved, in place of the abducens nucleus). Actions of the various extraocular eye muscles resulting from stimulation of the semicircular canals are shown. A, anterior canal; P, posterior canal; H, horizontal canal. Muscles: MR, medial rectus; LR, lateral rectus; IO, inferior oblique; SR, superior rectus; SO, superior oblique; IR, inferior rectus.

inaccuracy is called past pointing and occurs because the brain perceives that a leftward rotation is occurring, due to the inputs from the semicircular canals. Therefore, to take this into account, it automatically compensates for the movement by adding a few degrees of motion to the right. This causes the object to be missed to the right. In terms of the muscles of posture and balance, the direct effect is also to compensate for the perceived rotation.

During post-rotatory nystagmus, there is a perception of spinning or falling in the direction of the nystagmus,

i.e. to the left. This sensation is called vertigo. Any attempt to walk during the perception of vertigo can lead to a fall. Since the perception is one of falling to the left, there will be an attempt to compensate with a fast, voluntary contraction of the extensor muscles on the left. This can lead to an abrupt fall to the right. Therefore, the consequences of suddenly stopping rotation to the right are nystagmus and vertigo to the left, and past pointing and falling to the right.

Central pathways of the vestibular system

Primary afferent fibres from the vestibular apparatus terminate mainly in the vestibular nuclei. A small number of fibres project directly into the vestibulocerebellum (flocculo-nodular lobe and uvula). Vestibular afferents terminate in four subnuclei, the superior, inferior, lateral and medial nuclei, and axons from these subnuclei project to five areas (Figs 8.13 and 8.14) to participate in reflexes.

The superior and medial nuclei receive input from the cristae and are involved in the VOR via connections with the ocular nuclei and reticular formation, gaze centres and tectal nuclei. Input from the maculae goes to the lateral, inferior and medial nuclei. These nuclei project to spinal motor nuclei via the lateral and medial VSTs, which are involved in postural balance. The lateral VST facilitates the action of the antigravity (extensor) muscles, while the medial VST mainly influences the activity of the axial muscles of the head and neck (head-righting reflex). The superior and lateral vestibular nuclei also interact with the flocculonodular lobe of the cerebellum. Damage to the vestibular nerve or its nuclei often results in balance disorders.

Other second-order axons project to the contralateral ventral posterior nucleus of the thalamus, and from there to the somatosensory cortex (area 3a) and the posterior parietal cortex (area 5). These connections account for our conscious appreciation of our equilibrium and head position. The precise location of the cortical area (primary vestibular cortex) for the conscious perception of vestibular function is unknown, but is thought to be just caudal to the facial somatosensory area, as electrical stimulation of this area elicits sensations of vertigo. Functional imaging in caloric testing in volunteers also shows that the insula and temporoparietal areas are involved.

Vestibular system damage: balance disorders

Vestibular dysfunction produces rather distinct signs and symptoms (Table 8.4). However, these signs may not be very useful for precise localization of the lesion or for identification of the exact disease process.

Causes of balance disorders

Infections, head injury, ischaemia affecting the inner ear or the brain, certain medications and ageing may change

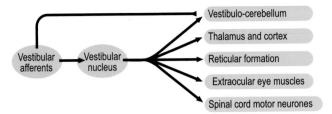

Fig. 8.13 Central projections of the vestibular apparatus.

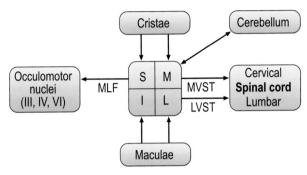

Fig. 8.14 Connections of the vestibular nuclei. MLF, medial longitudinal fasciculus; MVST, medial vestibulospinal tract; LVST, lateral vestibulospinal tract; S, superior vestibular nucleus; I, inferior vestibular nucleus; M, medial vestibular nucleus; L, lateral vestibular nucleus.

Table 8.4 Symptoms of balance disorders
A sensation of dizziness or vertigo
Falling or a feeling of falling (towards the dysfunctional side)
Lightheadedness or feeling woozy (syncope)
Visual blurring
Disorientation
Spontaneous nystagmus
Ataxia

our balance system and result in dysequilibrium. A conflict of signals to the brain about the sensation of movement can cause motion sickness (e.g. when an individual tries to read while riding in a car). Some symptoms of motion sickness are dizziness, sweating, nausea, vomiting and generalized discomfort.

Examples of balance disorders

Seventy percent of cases of vertigo are caused by common syndromes:

1. Benign paroxysmal positional vertigo (BPPV) is a brief (60s), intense sensation of vertigo that occurs because of a specific positional change of the head, e.g. when getting out of bed in the morning. The exact cause of BPPV is unknown, although it is thought to be due to a dislodged otolith from the utricle, which then gets stuck in the ampulla, making it sensitive to gravity.

In certain positions, it stimulates the cupula, causing abnormal sensations. These persist until the crystals relocate elsewhere or disperse. BPPV may be triggered by an inner ear infection, head injury, ageing or drugs.

2. Ménière's disease is an inner ear fluid balance disorder that causes episodes of vertigo, fluctuating hearing loss, tinnitus, and the sensation of fullness in the ear. It is probably caused by an imbalance between the production and reabsorption of endolymph, which eventually ruptures the membranes, causing changes in ion concentrations of the solute; these lead to depolarization of the endolymph fluid, ultimately killing the hair cells.

3. Labyrinthitis is an infection or inflammation of the semicircular canals causing dizziness and loss of balance.

4. Vestibular neuritis is a (viral) infection of the vestibular nerve.

5. Perilymph fistula is a leakage of inner ear fluid into the middle ear. It can occur after head injury or physical exertion, or is idiopathic.

Diagnosis of balance disorders

The diagnosis of a balance disorder is complicated, because there are many types of balance disorder and because other medical conditions, including ear infections, blood pressure changes and vision problems, or some medications may contribute to the problem. Examples of diagnostic tests are:

1. Hallpike's manoeuvre—with the patient lying in the supine position, the head is lowered quickly below the horizontal plane of the table and turned to one side. The patient then sits up and the test is repeated, turning the head to the other side. If there is vestibular dysfunction, the patient will develop nystagmus and complain of vertigo within 10s of head movement.

2. Audiometry.

3. The caloric test—weak nystagmus or the absence of nystagmus may indicate an inner ear disorder.

4. Imaging of the head and brain.

5. Posturography—this requires the individual to stand on a 'tilt table' capable of movement within a controlled visual environment; body sway is recorded in response to movement of the platform and/or the visual environment.

Treatment of balance disorders

There are various treatments for balance disorders. If the balance disorder is secondary to another disorder, the primary cause is addressed (e.g. ear infection, stroke or multiple sclerosis). Vestibular rehabilitation may also be attempted, whereby exercises include movements of the head and body specifically developed for the patient. This form of therapy is thought to promote compensation for the disorder. For people with Ménière's disease, dietary changes, such as reducing the intake of sodium, alcohol and caffeine, and/or avoiding nicotine may be helpful. Some aminoglycoside antibiotics, such as gentamicin and streptomycin, are specifically used to treat Ménière's disease to kill hair cells to disable the vestibular apparatus. However, these also affect the cochlear hair cells and cause hearing loss. In cases that do not respond to medical management, surgery may be indicated, e.g. insertion of a shunt in Ménière's disease, to drain the excess fluid, or section of the vestibular nerve to relieve chronic vertigo.

Comments on the case history

This case history (Box 8.1) describes a large acoustic neuroma that has emerged from the internal auditory canal into the skull cavity, and is compressing cranial nerves V and VII, the nerves of facial sensation and expression. This accounts for the loss of facial sensation and corneal reflex, and the inability to smile or wrinkle the forehead. Acoustic tumours are benign and develop slowly over a period of years. They expand in size at their site of origin, and, when large, displace normal brain tissue. The tumour does not invade the brain, but compresses the hindbrain as it enlarges. The tumour assumes a pear shape, with the small end in the internal auditory canal. Large tumours (>2.5 cm) can be life-threatening when they cause severe pressure on the brainstem and cerebellum, which may manifest as severe headaches, clumsy gait and mental confusion. This is a life-threatening complication requiring urgent treatment. In the worst case, it may cause severe raised intracranial pressure leading to tonsillar herniation. Unless the tumour is removed, the prognosis for this patient is poor.

Early symptoms are easily overlooked, making diagnosis more difficult. However, there are symptoms pointing to the possibility of an acoustic neuroma. The first symptom in 90% of patients with a tumour is a hearing deficit in one ear, often accompanied by tinnitus. The loss of hearing is usually subtle and worsens slowly, and there may be a feeling of fullness in the affected ear. These early symptoms are sometimes mistaken for normal hearing changes that occur with ageing. The patient may compensate by talking more loudly.

Since the balance (vestibular) portion of cranial nerve VIII is most commonly where the tumour arises, unsteadiness and balance problems may occur during growth of the neuroma. The heel-to-shin and finger-to-nose tests assess motor coordination and are associated with the cerebellum. A wide-based gait indicates some cerebellar dysfunction, and absence of nystagmus on caloric stimulation indicates damage of the vestibular connection to the oculomotor nuclei.

Treatment options for this patient include radiotherapy and surgery. Radiotherapy usually arrests growth of the tumour, and some tumours shrink, but they rarely disappear. Follow-up of these patients is important, because approximately 20% of tumours continue to grow after radiosurgery or at some time in the future.

Only surgical removal of the tumour can cure the patient. Removal can be either partial or total, depending on its size and the risk of complications in the patient. Preservation of the facial nerve is the primary task if there is to be a successful outcome to the surgical procedure when hearing is already lost. In this patient, if the tumour is removed, the facial nerve symptoms may resolve, but the deafness is likely to be permanent.

MOTOR SYSTEMS I: DESCENDING PATHWAYS AND CEREBELLUM

9

Chapter objectives

After studying this chapter you should be able to:

1. Define the terms upper motor neurone and lower motor neurone.

2. Describe the interconnections between the lower motor neurones, cerebellum, basal ganglia and upper motor neurones.

3. Describe the neural pathways for monosynaptic reflexes.

4. Describe the neural pathways for polysynaptic reflexes.

5. Name and describe the locations of the main descending motor pathways.

6. Describe the clinical signs associated with upper and lower motor neurone lesions.

7. Describe the anatomy of the cerebellum and its role in movement control.

8. List five signs of cerebellar damage.

9. Describe the mechanisms underlying decorticate and decerebrate rigidity posturing.

Introduction

Movements, whether involuntary or voluntary, are elicited by coordinated and graded patterns of muscular contractions, orchestrated by the motor neurones of the spinal cord and brainstem. A major function of the brain is to control motor behaviour, which is manifested as coordinated movements of the eyes, the mouth, the limbs and the body. For example, consider a person playing tennis. In order to serve an ace to an opponent, the player must first assess where the opponent is standing, and then throw the ball up into the air and coordinate the arm to use the racket to hit the ball in a particular predetermined direction, so that the opponent cannot return the serve. Coupled to this are the postural adjustments required to maintain appropriate balance, so as not to foot fault while serving, and to coordinate the movements of the various muscles of the body to produce sufficient power and racket speed to hit the ball at the top of the throw.

To perform all these different functions concomitantly would not be possible without the coordinated efforts of four distinct but interactive systems, which are hierarchically ordered (Fig. 9.1). The first of these systems comprises the lower motor neurones (LMNs) of the spinal

cord ventral horn and the brainstem, whose axons innervate the striated muscles (via neuromuscular junctions) of the body and head, respectively. LMNs receive sensory input from proprioceptors, which, together with other spinal cord and brainstem interneurones, act to modulate lower motor neurone activity and to coordinate the movement of different muscle groups.

The activity of LMNs is modulated by the second system, which consists of upper motor neurones (UMNs), whose cell bodies lie in the cortex and brainstem. The axons of UMNs form the descending motor pathways that synapse on the cell bodies of interneurones or LMNs in the brainstem or spinal cord; they never innervate muscles directly. Traditionally, UMN axons are divided into two descending systems: the pyramidal and extrapyramidal tracts. The pyramidal tract arises from the motor cortex and is essential for planning, initiating and directing voluntary movements and complex spatiotemporal sequences of movements. The extrapyramidal tracts, which are evolutionarily older, arise from the brainstem. They play an important role in postural control, usually involving many muscle groups, particularly antigravity muscles, and navigation movements.

The third and fourth systems are arranged in parallel with the hierarchical organization of LMNs and UMNs.

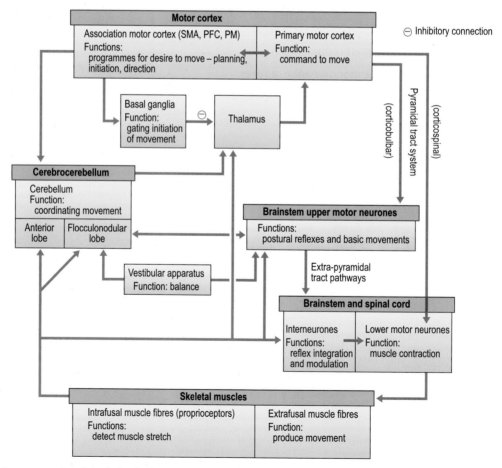

Fig. 9.1 Schematic representation of circuits involved in motor function. SMA, supplementary motor area; PFC, prefrontal cortex; PM, pre-motor cortex.

These are the cerebellum and basal ganglia; they are large collections of nuclei that modify movement on a minute-to-minute basis. They do not project directly to LMNs, but are important for successful motor performance. Their output regulates the activity of the UMNs. The basal ganglia and cerebellum receive information from the motor cortex, and both structures send information back to it via the thalamus. The output of the cerebellum to the motor cortex is excitatory, while the basal ganglia are inhibitory. The balance between these two systems allows for smooth, coordinated movement. The cerebellum acts as a motor performance error detector, whereas the basal ganglia function to suppress unwanted movements, as well as to prepare the motor cortex for the initiation of movements (see Chapter 10). All levels of the motor hierarchy, except the basal ganglia, receive information from somatic proprioceptors that continually inform the motor system about the position and movement of the body and limbs. Disturbances to any of these structures lead to paresis (weakness), paralysis or spasticity of movement, as demonstrated in the case history in Box 9.1.

Involuntary motor control of smooth muscle is performed by the autonomic nervous system (ANS). The LMNs of this system reside outside the spinal cord, in the paravertebral and prevertebral sympathetic chain ganglia, in the parasympathetic postganglionic ganglia near the target organ, or in the gut wall itself in the case of the enteric system. Their function is controlled by the hypothalamus, the brainstem reticular formation and spinal cord autonomic centres. The importance of the autonomic control of organs such as the heart, bladder and sexual organs, and the pharmacological means of modulating its function, makes visceral motor control systems an important topic in clinical medicine. These issues are addressed in Chapter 1, and will not be discussed further here.

In order to understand how voluntary motor behaviour is produced, it is necessary to begin by considering the interaction between the LMNs and the skeletal muscles.

Skeletal muscle contraction

Voluntary movements are carried out by the active contraction of skeletal muscle. Striated muscles make up about 40% of the mass of an adult human, and are attached to the skeleton by tendons. They act in pairs, with the contraction of one muscle being associated with the relaxation of the opposing (antagonistic) muscle. Each muscle is made up of muscle fibres, each muscle fibre receives input from a single LMN.

When the LMN axon reaches the muscle, it branches, and each branch forms a specialized synapse on the striated muscle fibre, called the neuromuscular junction (NMJ). Upon stimulation, the LMN axon releases acetylcholine (ACh) into the synaptic cleft. The region of the muscle that lies under the synapse is the motor endplate, and contains a high density of nicotinic acetylcholine receptors (nAChRs).

The NMJ is an unusual synapse compared to other synapses in the vertebrate central nervous system (CNS). It releases only a single type of neurotransmitter onto a single type of postsynaptic receptor (in invertebrates and in ANS there is release of more than one neurotransmitter), and each action potential releases a large number (200–300) of vesicles into the synaptic cleft.

The release of so many vesicles leads to a rapid rise (within $200\,\mu s$) in the concentration of ACh to about $1\,mM$. The postsynaptic membrane of the endplate is highly folded and contains abundant nAChRs, and an enzyme, acetylcholinesterase (AChE). This enzyme is responsible for the breakdown of ACh released into the cleft. It is present as both soluble and membrane-associated forms and, by hydrolysing ACh into choline and acetate, reduces the concentration of ACh back to baseline levels, within $1\,ms$. The choline is then transported back into the motor axon, where it is recycled to produce ACh.

The binding of two molecules of ACh to each nAChR opens this ligand-gated ion channel, to allow the movement of Na^+ and K^+. The subsequent depolarization of the endplate is sufficiently large to exceed the threshold for firing an action potential in the muscle plasma membrane, and this triggers Ca^{2+} release from intracellular stores, in sufficient amounts to cause muscle contraction. In some diseases, autoantibodies bind to the nAChR to prevent activation (Box 9.2).

Box 9.1 Case history

David N., a 63-year-old retired actor, sought help because of progressive weakness of his arms and legs, along with slurred speech. He complained of frequent muscle cramps in his legs. Neurological examination showed bilateral loss of strength in his arms, shoulders and feet. There was some wasting of the muscles of the hands and of the feet, and fasciculations were observed in the tongue. Stretch reflexes were hyperactive in his arms and legs, and a Babinski sign was present bilaterally. There was increased resistance to passive flexion of the elbow and the knee, which was strong at the beginning of the movement but collapsed towards the end of the movement. Clonus was present in response to Achilles' tendon reflex stimulation. All sensations and mental status were normal. David was prescribed the drug riluzole. He became progressively weaker during the next 3 years, with increasing atrophy and fasciculations in the limb and trunk muscles, as well as difficulty in breathing. He became confined to a wheelchair and died 4 years after the initial examination.

This case gives rise to the following questions:

1. What are the causes of the various symptoms?
2. What nervous system regions are affected?
3. Why was David given riluzole?

Diseases of the neuromuscular junction

Normally, large amounts of acetylcholine (ACh) are released from motor neurones with each action potential, more than enough to ensure excitation of the motor unit. However, there are certain conditions in which this does not occur, and muscle weakness ensues. In myasthenia gravis, autoantibodies are produced that destroy the nicotinic ACh receptors, so the muscle cannot respond to the ACh released. The cardinal sign is variable muscle weakness, with the head, eyes and proximal muscles being more commonly involved than distal limb muscles. Muscle tone, reflexes, bulk and sensations are normal. Treatment consists of using acetylcholinesterase inhibitors such as neostigmine and pyridostigmine, and immune suppression. In Lambert–Eaton syndrome, autoantibodies are directed against the presynaptic voltage-dependent Ca^{2+} channels, which allow the influx of Ca^{2+}, triggering exocytosis of ACh. This reduces the amount of ACh released. Patients present with proximal weakness, and sensory and autonomic disturbances.

Suxamethonium and genetic variability

Suxamethonium has been used as a neuromuscular blocking agent in clinical anaesthesia for the past 60 years, despite adverse effects like anaphylaxis, hyperkalaemia and malignant hyperthermia. It is still the gold standard neuromuscular blocking agent due to its rapid onset of effect (30–60 s) when injected intravenously, and short duration of action (2–6 min). It is rapidly hydrolysed by non-specific cholinesterase enzymes, called pseudocholinesterases, present in plasma, and normally its effect wears off within 5–10 min as the drug is metabolized. However, in about 1 in 3000 individuals, the effects are more long-lasting and may continue for many hours. This is due to an autosomal-recessive genetic variation that causes the production of a form of plasma cholinesterase that cannot metabolize suxamethonium. In this case, the patient requires ventilatory support. Suxamethonium should be used with caution in patients with atypical plasma cholinesterase, or with muscle diseases. The recent approval of sugammadex may soon render suxamethonium obsolete. Sugammadex can instantly reverse neuromuscular blockade of the longer lasting paralysing agents, especially roncuronium and vercuronium. This means that roncuronium can be given is sufficiently high doses to work quickly and reliably without the adverse effects of suxamethonium.

Blocking activity at the neuromuscular junction

Activation of the NMJ can be affected by ACh antagonists that act either presynaptically or postsynaptically. Presynaptic ACh release can be prevented by certain toxins such as botulinum toxin, from the bacterium *Clostridium botulinum*. It prevents the exocytosis of ACh vesicles, by destroying the proteins that allow fusion of the vesicle to the presynaptic membrane, thus paralysing the muscle. Severe botulism can be fatal, and recovery is slow, taking several weeks. Today, local injections of the toxin (known as Botox) are used by cosmetic surgeons to paralyse facial muscles, reducing wrinkles, and are also used to treat enduring muscle spasms.

The poison curare, used by indigenous South American hunters, is a mixture of plant alkaloids that act by inhibiting the postsynaptic nAChRs of the NMJ. A similar mechanism of action occurs in cobra snake bites. Here, one of the peptides in the venom, α-bungarotoxin, binds tightly to the nAChRs, taking days to be removed from the receptor. Both produce muscle weakness and respiratory arrest. Prey caught in this way can be safely eaten. Neither poison is absorbed in the gut. One of the alkaloids in curare, tubocurarine, was first used to produce blockade of skeletal muscle during surgery. It is now obsolete in the clinic and has been replaced by other, similar drugs (e.g. gallamine, pancuronium, vercuronium, atracurium or rocuronium), which vary in their duration of action (15–60 min). All are competitive antagonists of ACh. Therefore, they prevent the depolarization of the muscle membrane, and so are called non-depolarizing blocking agents. They also act on presynaptic receptors, interfering with the entry of Ca^{2+}, which causes inhibition of the release of ACh. These agents do not cross the blood–brain barrier. Their action can be rapidly reversed by the administration of AChE inhibitors, such as neostigmine. This prevents breakdown of ACh released into the cleft, effectively increasing the local concentration of ACh, which can then compete with the blocking agent.

Another class of drugs used to induce neuromuscular blockade are agonists of nAChR. These drugs, which have some structural similarity to ACh, act by producing a sustained depolarization of the endplate, and so are called depolarizing blocking agents. This makes the muscle non-responsive to stimulation, as the voltage-sensitive Na^+ channels that produce the muscle action potential are all inactivated. The only clinically relevant member of this group is suxamethonium (Box 9.3). Its blocking action occurs in two phases. In phase 1, there is an initial brief depolarization of the skeletal muscle fibres, causing small contractions (fasciculations), and repolarization is inhibited. In phase 2, desensitization blockade occurs. After the drug has been present for a period of time, the motor endplate loses its sensitivity, and depolarization cannot occur. Desensitization continues for several minutes, even after drug is no longer present. Therefore, this dual block effect delays recovery.

The motor unit

The smallest functional component of the motor system is the motor unit. This consists of the LMN and the muscle fibres that it innervates. Although each muscle fibre is supplied by only one motor neurone, each motor neurone innervates between three and a few thousand muscle fibres. This is the innervation ratio, which determines the precision with which a muscle can be controlled. Muscles with a low innervation ratio, such as the extraocular muscles (ratio of three fibres per motor neurone), which control eye movements, are very finely regulated, whereas muscles with a high ratio, such as the gastrocnemius (ratio of 1000–2000 fibres per motor neurone), are less precisely regulated. Additionally, this organization reduces the chance that damage to one or a few motor neurones will significantly affect the muscle action. If a single LMN dies, some of the muscle fibres that were innervated by the motor axon become innervated by an adjacent motor neurone, which sprouts new connections and takes over the control of the denervated muscle fibres. Thus, the average size of the motor units in the muscle increases, but with functional consequences: instead of smaller motor units, with finer control, there are now fewer, but larger, units and the muscle precision decreases.

The types of motor unit can be distinguished by the properties of the muscle fibre and the firing characteristics of its LMN. The most numerous are slow muscle units, which innervate muscle fibres rich in haemoglobin. They are found in muscles that are important for activities requiring sustained contractions, such as postural control (antigravity muscles). Prolonged activation of these units produces little reduction in muscle force even after an hour or more. Fast muscles have less haemoglobin, appear paler, and fatigue more quickly. These contain fast fatigue units, whose activity is important for muscle contractions that require large forces, such as occur in activities like jumping and sprinting. Repetitive activation of these units causes a rapid decline in force of contraction after about 30 s. In addition, there are some motor units that are fast fatigue resistant and can sustain activity for about 5 min before declining. These different motor units allow the nervous system to produce movements appropriate to the circumstances and also help to explain the different types of structural composition of muscles. For example, the muscle of a 100-m sprinter contains more fast fatigue muscle fibres, essential for producing power, than those of a marathon runner, whose muscles are conditioned for endurance, and therefore have more slow muscle fibres.

Slow muscle fibres are innervated by small α-motor neurones, while fast fibres are innervated by large α-motor neurones. This relationship is important, as soma size determines the order in which motor units are recruited during a voluntary movement: smallest ones first, then fast fatigue resistant and finally fast fatigue. This is known as the size principle. Motor neurones are deactivated in reverse order as the voluntary movement is terminated. Recruiting an increased number of motor units generates

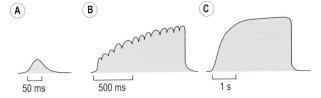

Fig. 9.2 Summation of muscle contraction. (A) Single twitch. (B) Unfused tetanus (12 Hz). (C) Fused tetanus (30 Hz).

the increased force of contraction. During a submaximal contraction of each muscle, each motor unit fires a small burst of action potentials and then rests. Greater force is generated by having more motor units active and reducing the pause time. For finely controlled movements, such as hand movements, small motor units are used; for more powerful ones, such as quadriceps activation, larger motor units are recruited.

A single impulse in the motor neurone causes a single contraction in the muscle, a twitch (Fig. 9.2). This lasts much longer than the refractory period of the action potential, so if a second impulse arrives before the muscle relaxes, then the second twitch is superimposed on the first. This generates more force in the muscle. Trains of action potentials will cause twitches to summate. At low frequencies (12 Hz), this will produce a force that oscillates about a plateau value (unfused tetanus), but as the frequency increases (30 Hz), the force becomes smooth and reaches a plateau that is the maximum force attainable by that motor unit. This is called a fused tetanus, and there are no longer peaks and troughs corresponding to individual twitches evoked by the motor neurone action potential. Asynchronous firing of different motor neurones produces a steady-state input to muscles, causing the contraction of a relatively constant number of motor units, and averages out the changes in muscle tension due to contractions and relaxations of different motor units. This allows movements to be executed smoothly. The firing frequency of motor neurones also regulates the muscle tension produced by motor units.

Motor pools

The motor neurones that innervate the same muscle are called a motor pool, and the various motor neurone pools are topographically organized: LMNs innervating flexors are separate from extensors, and LMNs innervating distal muscles are spatially separate from those innervating proximal muscles (see Fig. 4.4B). The force of contraction of a whole muscle depends on the frequency of firing of the individual motor neurones but also on the proportion of the motor pool that is active. Initially, increases in force are brought about by increases in firing rate, but larger increases in force are provided by increasing the number of active motor units. This is called recruitment. All the neurones within a motor pool are excited by common inputs in the spinal cord. Which neurones fire first will depend on both their size and the specific arrangement of synaptic inputs. Smaller neurones are more easily excited than larger ones, and neurones with more inputs are excited more easily than more sparsely innervated ones.

There are two types of LMN found in the same pool: α- and γ-motor neurones. α-Motor neurones are larger and innervate the striated (extrafusal) muscles that generate the forces needed for movement and postural balance. γ-Motor neurones are smaller and only innervate the muscle spindle sensory receptors embedded within capsules in the muscle, called intrafusal fibres. Their function is to regulate the tension of the muscle spindle by setting the muscle fibres to a set length (see later).

Reflexes

A reflex is the simplest motor response to sensory input. The reflex directly couples the sensory signal to a motor output, and produces simple stereotyped responses to particular sensory inputs. Reflexes occur in both the autonomic and somatic nervous systems. The neural pathways involved are called reflex arcs, and in their simplest form consist of a sensory neurone and a motor neurone. This is called a monosynaptic reflex. The sensory receptors have their cell bodies in the dorsal root ganglion of the peripheral nervous system (PNS) and synapse on the cell bodies of LMNs in the spinal cord or brainstem. The axons of the LMNs travel in the spinal nerve of the same spinal segment, and axon collaterals may travel up and down the spinal cord to affect motor neurones in adjacent segments.

Monosynaptic reflexes

In humans there is only one type of monosynaptic reflex, called the stretch reflex, also known as the myotatic (or deep tendon) reflex (Fig. 9.3). It occurs when the tendon of a muscle is hit with a reflex hammer (see Chapter 3) with adequate force to cause stretching of the muscle. This elicits a brief contraction of that muscle via activation of the intrafusal and extrafusal muscle fibres. The reflex acts to prevent rapid muscle stretch when the force on it increases rapidly, and returns the muscle back to its original length. This reflex is most prominent in extensor (antigravity and postural) muscles and is most easily seen in the knee-jerk reflex. When the patellar ligament is tapped just below the knee, there is a rapid contraction of the quadriceps muscles of the upper thigh, which swings the lower leg forward. The contraction is stimulated by input from sensory organs called muscle spindles, which are embedded in the muscle, and act directly on the large α-motor neurones supplying the muscle. As there are no other synapses between the sensory neurone and the motor neurone, the reflex is very rapid. Tendon reflexes are used to assess the functional integrity of the spinal cord at specific levels (Table 9.1). All stretch reflexes are

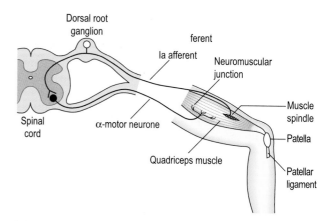

Fig. 9.3 The stretch reflex arc. Stimulation of the patellar ligament stretches the quadriceps muscle, exciting the muscle spindle, which fires action potentials to stimulate the α-motor neurone in the lumbar spinal cord. The motor axon releases acetylcholine at the neuromuscular junction, causing the homonymous muscle to contract.

Table 9.1 Main deep tendon reflexes

Muscle (joint) assessed	Spinal level assessed
Supinator (wrist)	C5–C6
Biceps (elbow)	C5–C6
Triceps (elbow)	C7
Quadriceps (knee)	L3–L4
Gastrocnemius (ankle)	S1

ipsilateral, so any reflex testing must be performed on both sides to determine if there is a difference.

Muscle spindles

The muscle fibres that form most of the muscle bulk and produce the contraction are called extrafusal fibres. In parallel with these are specialized sensory receptors called muscle spindles (Fig. 9.4). These sense the force acting on the muscle and provide sensory input to the spinal cord about the length and the rate of change of length (velocity) of the muscle.

Muscle spindles consist of a small capsule containing a small number (about 8–10) of modified muscle fibres called intrafusal fibres, which have a central region that is non-contractile, and around which are wrapped the ends of sensory nerves. Intrafusal fibres are arranged in parallel with the extrafusal muscle fibres. There are two types of intrafusal fibre: nuclear bag fibres and nuclear chain fibres.

Nuclear bag fibres are modified multinucleated muscle fibres, swollen in the middle to form a non-contractile bag-like structure. They are innervated by myelinated afferent nerves. There are two types of nuclear bag fibre: dynamic primary Ia afferents, which are large in diameter (~16 μm), and static secondary (II) afferents, which are smaller in

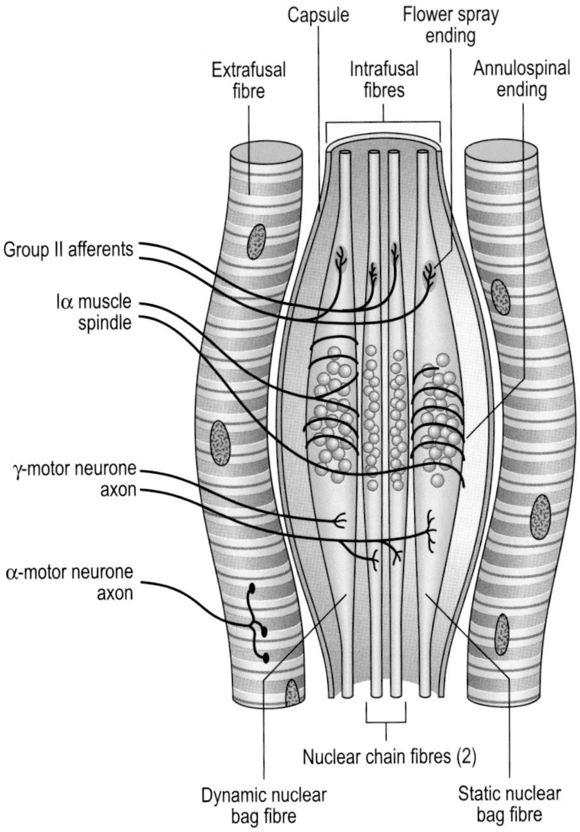

Fig. 9.4 Anatomy of a muscle spindle (simplified). A muscle spindle contains two types of intrafusal fibre, nuclear bag fibres and nuclear chain fibres. Bag fibres are innervated by Ia spindle afferents while chain fibres are innervated by group II muscle afferents. Intrafusal fibres have their own motor innervation from γ-motor neurones. α-Motor neurones synapse on extrafusal fibres.

diameter (8 μm). These differ in their responses to muscle stretch: static fibres are stiffer than dynamic ones, and so signal muscle length rather than velocity. The Ia fibres are rapidly adapting, whereas the group II fibres are non-adapting and so fire even though the muscle has stopped moving. The peripheral endings of Ia afferents are called annulo-spiral endings, while those of the group II muscle spindle afferents are called flower spray endings.

Nuclear chain fibres are slender and have nuclei arranged along their length in a chain-like fashion. They are innervated by both Ia and II afferents. They are stiff, like the static fibres, and respond to length.

Each muscle spindle contains at least one dynamic and one static fibre, and a variable number (3–5) of chain fibres, and the distal portion consists of striate muscle with contractile properties. It is the group II static afferents that allow the brain to know the position of the muscle when it is still, such as when you are holding your arms outstretched with your eyes shut.

When the tendon is tapped, the rapid, phasic component of the monosynaptic reflex is triggered by the stretching of the dynamic Ia afferents in the central non-contractile part of the muscle spindle, so that they fire action potentials, which are relayed to the spinal cord. Subsequently, as the non-contractile pole ends of the intrafusal fibres are also stretched, they elongate slowly, which reduces the firing of the Ia neurones. The remaining tension produces static responses in both the Ia and II afferents. The longer-lasting tonic component is maintained by the static responses of the muscle spindles. This is very important in maintaining posture.

Gamma (γ) motor neurones

The muscle spindle is the only sensory receptor to have its own motor supply. γ-Motor neurones innervate the striated portions of the intrafusal fibres. Therefore, they are also called fusimotor neurones. Stimulation of γ-motor neurones does not cause movement of the joint to which the extrafusal muscles are attached. It only places tension on the central portion of the intrafusal fibres. Therefore, although they are not part of the stretch reflex *per se*, they set the sensitivity of the muscle to stretch by regulating the tension of the intrafusal fibres; that is, they keep the muscle spindle taut. γ-Motor neurones receive little peripheral afferent input; most of their input is from supraspinal descending pathways such as the reticulospinal and vestibulospinal pathways.

Appreciating the relationship between the extrafusal and intrafusal fibres is important in understanding motor function. As the extrafusal fibres of the muscle contract, the stretch on the muscle spindles is reduced, and sensory information from the muscle spindles would stop unless the muscle spindles themselves also shortened. During intentional activity, at the same time as the α-motor neurones fire to produce shortening of the extrafusal fibres, the γ-motor neurones are stimulated to shorten the intrafusal fibres. This α–γ co-activation ensures that the muscle spindle is shortened at the same rate as the muscle and the sensitivity of the muscle spindles is maintained despite the shortening of the muscle. The γ-motor neurones conduct action potentials more slowly than the α-motor neurones. This means that the intrafusal fibres will contract fractionally later than the extrafusal fibres, giving time for the sensory systems to respond.

Reciprocal and synergistic innervation

Skeletal muscles act in antagonist pairs. Contraction of one muscle is prevented by the tone of the opposing muscle, unless that muscle is simultaneously relaxed. During the knee-jerk reflex, as well as stimulation of the α-motor neurones supplying the quadriceps muscles, there is reciprocal inhibition of the hamstring muscles at the back of the thigh. This occurs via an inhibitory interneurone in the spinal cord, which is stimulated by the sensory input from the muscle spindles of the quadriceps. This is a polysynaptic reflex.

The quadriceps muscle group comprises four leg extensor muscles that function synergistically to extend the lower leg about the knee joint. The majority of the muscle spindle input is to the motor neurones in the same motor pool (the homonymous muscle). However, about 40% of the synapses occur with motor neurones going to all the other leg extensors. Thus, activation of the muscle spindles in one extensor muscle will produce synergistic contractions in all four muscles.

Supraspinal control of stretch reflexes

Stretch reflexes are subject to descending modulation via direct or indirect connections between UMNs and the α- and γ-motor neurones. Alterations in the activity of these pathways may affect the size or threshold for activation of the reflex. For example, the amplitude of the reflex can be reinforced by various measures, including clenching of the teeth, pulling interlocked fingers (Jendrassic manoeuvre) and general distraction of attention. These measures only work when the reinforcement is at a higher level than the reflex being tested, and the reinforcement is thought to be due to the removal of tonic inhibition from the LMNs.

Polysynaptic reflexes

In monosynaptic reflexes, the α-motor neurone receives input directly from the Ia afferents. However, most inputs to α-motor neurones arise from spinal cord interneurones. Most of the axons from descending pathways do not form synapses directly with α-motor neurones, but terminate on these interneurones. When there are more than two synapses involved in a reflex arc, this constitutes a polysynaptic reflex.

Golgi tendon organs

As well as muscle spindles, muscles have a second type of sensory organ called the Golgi tendon organ (GTO), which is found in the tendons. This is placed in series with the muscle fibres, and measures muscle tension. An increase in muscle tension activates a negative (autogenic) feedback reflex of the homonymous muscle called the inverse myotactic reflex (Fig. 9.5), which prevents further increases in tension. This reflex protects the tendon from being injured by too much tension. It also plays a role in mechanisms related to muscle fatigue and joint hyperextension/flexion.

GTOs consist of collagen fibres that contain the endings of Ib afferent neurones at the tendon–muscle interface. GTOs are relatively insensitive to passive stretch but are sensitive to active contraction, when most of the force acts directly on the tendon. When the muscle tension increases, the collagen fibres are stretched, causing the Ib afferents to fire. The frequency of firing is proportional to the level of tension. These afferents synapse onto interneurones, which, in turn, synapse onto the α-motor neurones of both the homonymous (inhibitory action) and antagonistic (facilitatory action) muscles. Thus, the function of this reflex is to 'switch off movement' and allow the muscle to relax.

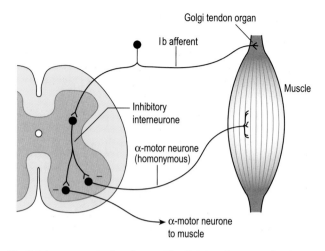

Fig. 9.5 Inverse myotactic reflex arc. The Golgi tendon organ fires in response to an increase in tension and activates spinal cord interneurones that inhibit the α-motor neurones innervating the homonymous and synergistic muscles, thereby relieving excess muscle tension and relaxing the muscle. At the same time, connections with other sets of interneurones allow excitation of α-motor neurones innervating the antagonistic muscles, causing their contraction (not shown).

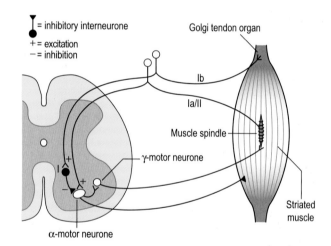

Fig. 9.6 Cooperation of myotactic reflexes. Activity of the Ia and group II fibres produces α- and γ-motor neurone co-activation, which produces muscle contraction while maintaining its sensitivity during contraction. Stimulation of the Golgi tendon organ (Ib) fibre inhibits the α-motor neurones (and γ-motor neurones), producing relaxation. Differences in the conduction velocity (Ib fibres are slower than Ia/II fibres) and the presence of inhibitory interneurones allow the contraction and relaxation to occur. +, excitation; −, inhibition.

The sensory inputs involved in the myotactic and inverse myotactic reflexes affect the same motor neurones, but with opposite effects (Fig. 9.6). Sometimes, in pathological situations, these two systems get trapped in a loop where they alternatively trigger each other. This causes the muscle to alternately contract and relax several times a second. This is termed clonus. It can be seen in the ankle stretch reflexes, where the foot oscillates about the ankle.

Control of muscle tone (stiffness)

All muscles are under some degree of stretch, and this is responsible for a resting tension in the muscle called muscle tone. The stretch reflex, which maintains muscle length in response to increased load, and the inverse myotactic reflex, which maintains a constant tension, work in opposition. When the load on a muscle is increased, either the muscle must lengthen or the tension must increase. Working together, these reflexes control the tone of the muscle. If the load on a muscle increases but the length is maintained, the contraction is isometric. This is normally the case for postural muscles. Alternatively, if the load is moved by shortening the muscle, this isotonic contraction maintains a constant tension. Damage to LMNs or descending pathways will change the level of tone within muscles.

Flexor and crossed extensor reflexes

These two linked reflexes are stimulated by noxious stimuli, both actual (such as a sharp object) and perceived (such as threatening behaviour). These polysynaptic reflexes trigger a complex set of actions (Fig. 9.7).

The flexion reflex is an important protective reflex. Stimulation produces a withdrawal of the entire threatened limb from the harmful stimulus on the ipsilateral side, with a compensatory extension of the opposite side. These reflexes may be important in maintaining balance as the centre of gravity changes. For example, treading on a sharp object produces a withdrawal of the foot with an extension of the other leg in order to support the extra weight (Fig. 9.7).

Flexion reflexes differ from myotactic reflexes in that they involve several interneurones between the afferent axons and the motor neurones. This gives the brain opportunities to override, modulate or control these reflexes via activity in descending pathways. This is impossible for the monosynaptic and synaptic reflexes from proprioceptors. Damage to the descending pathways can alter flexion reflexes.

Spinal motor function

A considerable amount of local processing of sensory information occurs in the spinal cord, and this influences motor output. Motor reflexes are simple patterns generated in the spinal cord, but the spinal cord is also involved in producing the complex patterns involved in locomotion. During locomotion, networks of neurones produce cycles of activity in order to contract groups of muscles in a carefully timed sequence. These networks, which are called central pattern generators, are initiated by descending input and are modified by reflexes. They are more prominent in quadrupeds than in bipeds, as is evidenced by the observation that when the spinal cord is transected in animals such as cats and rats, there is greater recovery of locomotion than in humans.

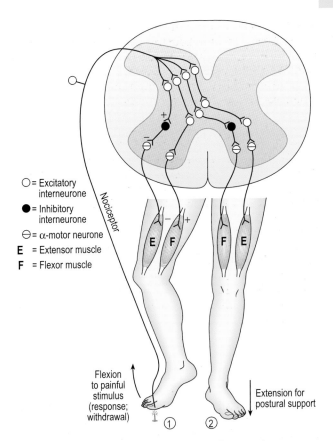

Fig. 9.7 The flexor (1) and crossed extensor (2) reflex arcs. These are polysynaptic reflexes. The flexor withdrawal reflex has a protective function. A noxious stimulus activates nociceptors that stimulate spinal cord interneurones in several spinal segments to excite the ipsilateral flexor α-motor neurones, which withdraw the limb from the stimulus. At the same time, the antagonistic extensor muscles are inhibited. The crossed extensor reflex is a contralateral response to an ipsilateral stimulus, to maintain balance. Here the nociceptors activate interneurones that excite the α-motor neurones of the extensor muscles of the contralateral leg, while inhibiting the flexors of that leg.

Descending pathways

As outlined in Chapter 4, there are several descending motor pathways that originate in the brain and brainstem, and modulate LMN function (Table 9.2). Unlike LMNs, they use glutamate as their neurotransmitter. There are three functionally distinct pathways. The pyramidal pathway arises in the motor cortex and is essential for planning, initiating and directing voluntary movements and complex spatiotemporal sequences of movements. It provides for fine, precise movement and voluntary control of distal muscle groups. The other functionally distinct pathways are termed extrapyramidal, because they arise from the brainstem. They are responsible for orientating the body, head and eyes in response to somatic, auditory, visual or vestibular stimuli and for regulating muscle tone. The medial brainstem pathways arise from cells in the reticular formation, the vestibular nuclei and the tectum. These motor

Table 9.2 Summary of the main functions of the descending tracts

Motor system	Tract	Origin	Distribution	Main action on lower motor neurones (LMNs)		Function
				Excitatory to	Inhibitory to	
Pyramidal	Corticospinal	Motor cortex	Crossed	Hand and finger flexors	Hand and finger extensors	Control of fine voluntary movement
	Corticobulbar	Motor cortex	Bilateral	Cranial flexor LMNs	Cranial extensor LMNs	
Extrapyramidal: lateral	Rubrospinal	Red nucleus of midbrain	Crossed	Limb flexors	Limb extensors	Control of gross limb movements
Extrapyramidal: medial	Medial reticulospinal	Pons	Ipsilateral	Axial and proximal limb extensors	Proximal limb flexors	Postural control of the head and body
	Lateral reticulospinal	Medulla	Bilateral	Proximal limb flexors	Axial and proximal limb extensors	Body and head righting reflexes in response to abnormal positions
	Lateral vestibulospinal	Lateral vestibular nucleus	Ipsilateral	Axial and proximal limb extensors	Axial and proximal limb flexors	
	Medial vestibulospinal	Medial and inferior vestibular nuclei	Bilateral	Axial ipsilateral	Axial contralateral	
	Tectospinal	Superior colliculus	Crossed	Neck extensors	Neck flexors	Postural reflex responses to auditory, visual and somatic cues

pathways provide for reflex movements related to posture and balance, usually involving many muscle groups, particularly antigravity muscles, to prevent the body or head from being destabilized. A lateral brainstem pathway originates in the red nucleus, and provides for voluntary movements of the arms but not the individual digits.

Each of these main motor pathways terminates in the spinal cord in a different pattern, which reflects the modality of movement controlled by that motor pathway (Fig. 9.8).

The pyramidal system comprises the corticospinal and corticobulbar tracts. About 60% of the neurones are in the primary, supplementary and premotor areas of the frontal lobe. The rest are in the somatosensory cortex (30%) and the posterior parietal cortex (10%). They pass through the internal capsule and descend in the ventral part of the brainstem, but they differ in their termination sites. Corticobulbar fibres terminate on LMNs in the brainstem and control facial movements. Corticospinal axons bypass the brainstem LMNs and terminate in the spinal cord, to control limb movements. Corticospinal tract (CST) axons are commonly called pyramidal tract axons (after the area in the medulla where the axons cross the midline, the spinomedullary junction, Fig. 9.9). The CST is concerned with generating voluntary movements of the hands (see Table 9.2) that require precision, speed and agility. It has very little effect on the lower limbs.

At the spinomedullary junction, 85% of the corticospinal axons decussate to form the lateral CST. The 15% of uncrossed fibres form the anterior CST. These decussate in the spinal cord at the same segmental level as the first synapse. Both tracts are excitatory, and most of these axons synapse with spinal cord interneurones; some synapse directly with α-motor neurones, especially those involved in movement of the fingers. The terminal distribution of the corticospinal motor pathway partly overlaps with those of the other lateral and medial extrapyramidal pathways.

The rubrospinal tract is a small contralateral pathway that ends on interneurones in the spinal cord; these convey motor commands to cervical motor neurones for control of limb muscles (Table 9.2). In humans, the rubrospinal axons are intermingled with those of the lateral CST, so that the function of the rubrospinal tract has largely been taken over by the latter. The majority of red nucleus axons do not project to the spinal cord but relay information to the motor cortex from the cerebellum.

The medial brainstem motor pathways are represented by the reticulospinal, vestibulospinal and tectospinal tracts. They are associated with balance and postural control, via the temporal and spatial coordination of movements. Their axons are located in the ventral funiculus (see Fig. 9.8) and end mainly on interneurones in the medial third of the spinal cord grey matter. These interneurones carry the motor commands to α- and

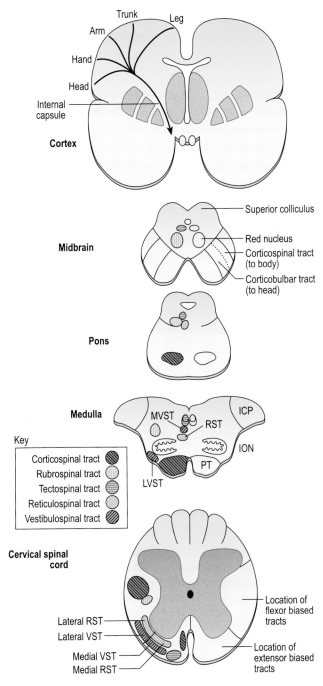

Fig. 9.8 Location of the descending pathways along the neuraxis. The locations of the main descending pathways in the spinal cord are shown schematically. Pathways that act mainly on extensor motor neurones are located in the ventral funiculus, while those acting on flexor motor neurones run in the lateral funiculus. The schematic positions of these pathways at higher levels of the neuraxis are shown. LVST, lateral vestibulospinal tract; MVST, medial vestibulospinal tract; RST, reticulospinal tract; ICP, inferior cerebellar peduncle; ION, inferior olivary nucleus.

γ-motor neurones that innervate proximal limb, trunk and axial muscles (Table 9.2).

The reticulospinal tract (RST) has lateral and medial components (Fig. 9.8). They function in postural control via the regulation of flexor and extensor reflexes, through antagonist mechanisms (Table 9.2). The lateral RST has a predominantly inhibitory effect on segmental reflexes, while the medial RST has a facilitatory effect on extensor motor neurones.

The vestibulospinal tract (VST) is also divided into medial and lateral tracts (Fig. 9.8). The medial VST descends to the cervical and upper thoracic spinal cord, and acts on interneurones that facilitate activity in neck muscles, keeping the head steady to provide a platform for eye movements. It is involved in postural reflexes in response to gravity, or to changes in acceleration of the head. For example, the head-righting reflex occurs when the head droops towards one side. The change in head position is sensed by the vestibular system semicircular canals, which then stimulate the medial pathway to activate motor neurones to lift the head back to the correct position by increasing muscle tone in the appropriate antigravity muscles. The ascending components of the medial pathway coordinate activity of the vestibular and oculomotor nuclei.

The lateral VST arises from the lateral vestibular (Dieter's) nucleus in the medulla and descends in the ventral funiculus to all levels of the spinal cord. Its function is to maintain balance by acting on the extensor motor neurones (Table 9.2), so as to keep the centre of gravity between the feet. It also has important connections with the cerebellum, to regulate posture.

Both the RST and the VST provide information to the spinal cord for the maintenance of posture in response to changes in stability or body position. This involves both feedforward and feedback mechanisms (Fig. 9.10). Postural control involves an element of anticipation in some muscle groups when a movement is to be made. Prior to an intended movement, its effect on postural stability is evaluated and used to generate a change in the activity of muscles that may not necessarily be involved in the movement. For example, consider reaching forwards to open a door. This shifts the centre of gravity and destabilizes the body. Increased compensatory activity occurs in the calf muscles to counter-balance the intended arm movement and re-establish body stabilization. This occurs prior to reaching for the doorknob and is a preprogrammed action carried out by the RST. On the other hand, once postural instability has occurred, a corrective feedback system acting via the VST returns the system to normal.

The tectospinal tract (see Fig. 9.8) originates in the superior colliculus and descends to the contralateral cervical spinal cord, to act upon the axial motor neurones of the neck on both sides of the cord. This pathway is important in generating orientating movements of the head and eyes in response to visual, auditory or somatic stimuli (see Table 9.2).

The motor cortex

The motor cortex consists of three reciprocally interconnected regions: the primary motor cortex (MI), the premotor

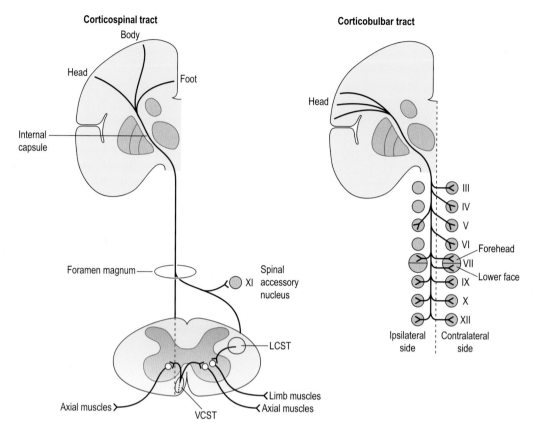

Fig. 9.9 Course and termination sites of the corticospinal and corticobulbar tracts. Both tracts pass through the posterior limb of the internal capsule. The non-ocular brainstem lower motor neurones (LMNs) are supplied bilaterally by the head area of the primary motor cortex, except for the lower facial muscles of the facial motor nucleus, which are supplied only by the contralateral motor cortex. The contralateral input is greater than the ipsilateral input. The ocular motor neurones receive only a contralateral input. The corticospinal tract bypasses the brainstem cranial LMNs. It decussates at the spinomedullary junction to form the lateral and ventral corticospinal tracts that innervate the LMNs of the spinal cord. VCST, ventral corticospinal tract; LCST, lateral corticospinal tract.

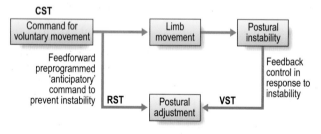

Fig. 9.10 Circuitry involved in the control of postural stability. CST, corticospinal tract; RST, reticulospinal tract; VST, vestibulospinal tract.

(PM) area and the supplementary motor area (medial premotor, or SMA) (Fig. 9.11A, B). The latter two form the secondary (association) motor cortex, and all contribute axons to the pyramidal tract. The areas are functionally distinct. The MI cortex, located in the precentral gyrus, has a topographical representation of the body surface, with the head, lips and hands represented laterally, and the legs and feet medially (Fig. 9.11C), similar to the homunculus that exists in the primary somatosensory cortex (see Fig 4.6). In this

region, the more complex the movement of a particular body part, the more motor cortex is devoted to it. Thus, the lips, tongue and hands, which we use to explore and communicate, have distorted representations due to the variety and complexity of the movements. This topographical representation is also found in the association motor areas.

The MI cortex is involved in the voluntary control of movements, by carrying the motor command to the LMNs. The PM area is involved in planning movements that involve external sensory cues. Activity in PM cells is temporally linked to movements. Here, cells are active when there is an intention to make a movement rather than during the movement. The PM area is about six times larger than MI, and receives a rich sensory input (tactile and visuospatial) from the parietal lobe. It deals with learned motor activities of a complex and sequential nature, by coordinating contractions of specific groups of muscles; for example, it is active during writing. The SMA is also involved in planning movements, but is concerned with internally generated commands or cues. Its cells are active while an intended movement is being thought about. The SMA is crucial for the performance of

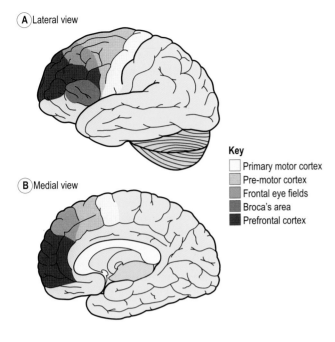

(A) Lateral view

(B) Medial view

Key
- ☐ Primary motor cortex
- ☐ Pre-motor cortex
- ☐ Frontal eye fields
- ☐ Broca's area
- ☐ Prefrontal cortex

(C) Motor homunculus

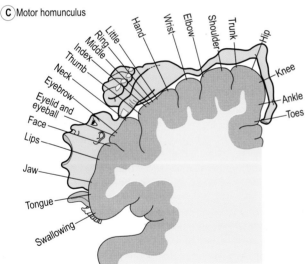

Fig. 9.11 Functional areas of the motor cortex viewed from the lateral (A) and medial (B) surfaces. (C) Homuncular map of the body surface in the primary motor cortex. Note the distorted representation of the cortex for the lips and hands, which require fine control.

complicated tasks involving both sides of the body, e.g. two-handed tasks such as typing. Damage to the PM or SMA results in apraxia (Box 9.4).

The frontal eye field region of the motor cortex controls voluntary scanning movements of the eyes, such as during reading. This region has connections with the superior colliculus and the gaze centres located in the paramedian pontine reticular formation. Stimulation of this region causes conjugate deviation of the eyes towards the opposite side to the stimulation, whereas damage to this region induces a transient conjugate deviation of the eyes towards the side of the lesion.

Apraxia is the loss of ability to carry out familiar learned purposeful movements, in the absence of sensory or motor impairment. Patients with apraxia have normal reflexes and tone, and no muscle weakness, but they have difficulty in performing complex motor tasks such as brushing their hair, cleaning their teeth or dressing themselves.

There are several different sites for initiation of movement in behavioural contexts. The premotor cortex has links with the homologous area on the contralateral side, and the ipsilateral posterior parietal cortex, via commissural pathways. Damage to these pathways results in different types of apraxia. Ideomotor apraxia occurs when a person cannot perform a previously learned movement, or mimic movements of a limb when shown by another person. It is a transient phenomenon, as the contralateral side takes over the role of the damaged side. Constructional apraxia is a failure to comprehend the spatial relationships of objects in space, and may be identified by asking a patient to reconstruct a three-dimensional object using building blocks. It is often due to a lesion in the superior longitudinal fasciculus, which connects the parietal and frontal lobes.

The prefrontal cortex relays input from the limbic system to the motor cortex, about the desired goal of the movement. The MI cortex is involved in a motor loop with the cerebellum, while the SMA forms a loop with the basal ganglia. These loops allow the cortex to recruit and coordinate specific motor programmes.

Limb movements are controlled by the contralateral MI cortex, but LMNs controlling muscles in the trunk or head that normally act in unison, such as those involved in chewing, swallowing and talking, have a bilateral innervation. All the non-ocular brainstem LMNs, except those of the lower facial muscles, have a bilateral corticobulbar innervation (Fig 9.9B). Lesions of the internal capsule, which damage the corticobulbar and corticospinal tracts, produce a pronounced contralateral lower facial weakness but only a transient impairment of the function of other brainstem LMNs.

Actions of upper motor neurones

UMNs have several regulatory functions. They can modulate the activity of α- and γ-LMNs either directly (monosynaptically) or indirectly (via interneurones). This activity can be either excitatory (monosynaptically) or inhibitory (via inhibitory interneurones). In this way, the magnitude of the reflex can be gated. Thus, damage to descending pathways can alter the strength of a reflex. Another important function is efference copy. UMN signals are conveyed to other motor areas of the brain to inform them that an active movement is happening. Cells in the pontine nuclei, for example, receive a copy from the pyramidal tract neurones and relay it to the cerebellum to keep it informed of the intended movement. UMNs can activate the intrinsic pattern generators that produce stereotyped movements. Finally, UMNs terminate not only on LMNs and interneurones, but also on other UMNs. For example, corticobulbar axons terminate on neurones of the extrapyramidal system and the reticulospinal, vestibulospinal and rubrospinal tracts. The cells of the medial brainstem descending pathways are also richly interconnected. This is important because the brain must be able to switch off selective postural systems to accomplish some types of movement. Disconnection of the cerebral cortex from the brainstem motor centres controlling postural pathways affects the postural responses of the limbs to stimuli and can be used as an indicator of the level of brainstem damage in comatose patients (Box 9.5).

Clinical importance of reflexes

Reflexes are extremely important, and tell the doctor about the segmental functioning of the nervous system. The stretch reflex is most important and is routinely tested in the neurological examination. Flexion reflexes are rarely tested, except in unconscious patients, or where a UMN lesion may be suspected.

If the axons of LMNs are severed, then the muscle contraction becomes weakened to the point of paralysis, depending on how many axons are damaged. The strength of the reflex therefore decreases (hyporeflexia). Complete absence of a reflex is called flaccid (floppy) paralysis of a muscle. Within 3 weeks of denervation, the muscle undergoes atrophy (wasting), due to lack of use. In response to denervation, the muscle synthesizes large numbers of ACh receptors, which are distributed over the whole surface of the muscle, rather than being restricted to the NMJ. This means that the muscle becomes hypersensitive, and in response to circulating levels of ACh will show fasciculation (small contractions of muscle fibres). If the damaged nerve can be repaired surgically, then the LMN axons can regrow, at the rate of a few millimetres a day, to eventually reinnervate the muscle. Physiotherapy of muscles artificially moves the muscle, thereby preventing atrophy.

The absence of a limb reflex indicates either a failure of afferent input to reach the LMN, or failure of the efferent output from the LMN to reach the muscle. Most often, decreased reflexes reflect damage to the PNS (nerves or roots) or the muscles. In other cases, it may reflect NMJ disease (Box 9.2). Loss or reduction of the stretch reflex is the only clinical sign needed to localize a lesion involving the LMNs. Damage to LMNs also results in other signs and symptoms (Table 9.3).

While damage to LMNs leads to flaccid paralysis, damage to UMNs results in spasticity, and can be caused by

Box 9.5 Decorticate and decerebrate rigidity

When physical or vascular damage to the brainstem produces functional disconnection between the red nucleus (midbrain) and the vestibular nuclei (pons), patients show an increase in extensor muscle tone, called decerebrate rigidity. It is caused by tonic activity in the lateral vestibulo-spinal and reticulospinal tracts that act on the extensor motor neurones, and the loss of rubrospinal inhibition of extensor motor neurones. This leads to the appearance of the positive neurological signs of increased muscle tone and hyperactive stretch reflexes. In response to a startling or painful stimulus, both the arms and legs extend and pronate. The cerebellum also plays a role in decerebrate rigidity, because ablation of the anterior cerebellar lobe enhances decerebrate posturing, due to the loss of inhibitory input to the lateral vestibulospinal tract. Lesioning the lateral vestibular nucleus or stimulating the anterior cerebellum inhibits this rigidity.

If damage to the brainstem occurs above the level of the red nucleus, decorticate rigidity may ensue due to the loss of corticobulbospinal control. Here, the arms flex and the legs extend in response to the stimulus. This posturing occurs as a result of activity in the brainstem flexor facilitation pathways. The red nucleus now controls posture, and this pathway counteracts the activity of the lateral vestibulospinal and reticulospinal tracts that activate extensor muscles. As, the rubrospinal tract only extends to the cervical spinal cord, it most strongly influences the arms (excites flexors, inhibits extensors) and therefore counteracts the extension of the arms (by the lateral vestibulospinal and reticulospinal tracts) but not the legs.

Damage to the medulla below the level of the vestibular nuclei disconnects the motor neurones from tonic vestibulospinal and reticulospinal tract activity, resulting in flaccid paralysis, hypotonia, loss of respiratory drive and quadriplegia. Essentially, there are no reflexes, and this state resembles the early stages of spinal shock, as there is a complete loss of activity in the motor neurones. Subsequently, over time, some segmental reflexes may recover, but these will be hyperactive, due to loss of descending motor control.

damage to the spinal cord, brainstem or motor cortex, or the tracts connecting them. The spasticity is more marked when the lesion is in the brain, as opposed to the spinal cord.

UMN damage leads to either positive or negative neurological signs (Table 9.3). Negative UMN signs are the loss or absence of function caused by the loss of monosynaptic connections to LMNs. A major negative sign of UMN damage is weakness in the limbs. Weakness in both limbs on one side is called hemiparesis (hemiplegia) and can indicate a brain lesion, most often in the internal capsule, where the descending fibres are grouped close together. Here, a relatively small lesion can have a

Table 9.3 Comparison of symptoms associated with upper motor neurone (UMN) and lower motor neurone (LMN) lesions

	UMN lesion	LMN lesion
Location	CNS	PNS or CNS
Common cause	Stroke, trauma, infectious disease, multiple sclerosis, amyotrophic lateral sclerosis	Trauma, stroke, tumour, diabetes, polio, alcoholism, amyotrophic lateral sclerosis
Classical description	Spastic paralysis/paresis	Flaccid paralysis
Structures involved	Motor cortex, internal capsule, pyramidal tract	Brainstem or spinal cord LMNs or their axons
Distribution	Groups of muscles, never individual muscles	Segmental, limited to muscles innervated by damaged motor neurones or their axons
Effect on voluntary movement	Paralysis or paresis, especially of skilled movements	Paralysis
Effect on muscle tone	**Increased (hypertonia)**	Decreased (hypotonia)
Effect on stretch reflex	**Hyperactive**	Hypoactive to point of absence
	Clonus	
Effect on cutaneous reflexes	Decreased	Decreased
Effect on muscle	No (or slight) atrophy	Pronounced atrophy
		Fasciculation and fibrillation
Muscle strength	Decreased	Decreased

Positive neurological signs are in bold type.
CNS, central nervous system; PNS, peripheral nervous system.

widespread effect. Cerebral strokes affecting the middle or anterior cerebral arteries rarely cause hemiplegia, because of the somatotopic organization of the motor homunculus (Fig. 9.11C). If the weakness occurs in both lower limbs, it is termed paraparesis and usually indicates a spinal cord lesion (often anterior spinal artery occlusion). This weakness has a characteristic pattern, because in the upper limb the flexors are stronger than the extensors, and in the lower limb the reverse is true. This means that the greatest weakness will be shown in the arm extensors and the leg flexors. Some muscle groups, such as the axial trunk muscles and brainstem motor nuclei, receive bilateral descending innervation and so are protected from complete loss of function by stroke.

In contrast, some lesions cause the appearance of signs not normally present, or cause an increase in function; these are referred to as positive neurological signs and are most often due to disinhibition. Hyperreflexia or spasticity (hypertonia) are typical examples of positive neurological signs that usually accompany UMN lesions (Table 9.3). Patients complain of stiffness, inability to relax and jerky movements. Loss of descending inhibition results in the development, after an initial flaccid paralysis, of spastic paralysis. The spinal reflexes remain intact but are no longer subject to control from the motor cortex. Owing to the muscle activity triggered by reflexes, the muscles do not atrophy, there is no fasciculation, and there is a general increase in tone, which is most easily seen in the stronger muscles. This leads to a clasp-knife effect; in response to passive movement of a joint against a background of increased extensor muscle tone, there is

a sudden collapse in the resistance to movement, due to inhibition of the extensor motor neurones by the GTOs and free nerve endings in the muscles and tendons.

The Babinski (extensor plantar) response is a pathological polysynaptic reflex. It is evoked by noxious cutaneous stimulation of the sole of the foot, and normally consists of a flexion withdrawal response. The stimulus causes the toes to curl down, adduct together and withdraw from the stimulus. This reflex tests the integrity of spinal cord segments L4–S2. In cases when the descending input from the cortex is disrupted, either through damage to the motor areas of the cortex or through damage to the CSTs, the plantar reflex changes to an extensor reflex, with dorsiflexion of the big toe and fanning of the other toes. This is a Babinski's sign. This abnormal response is normal in children under the age of 2 years, before they learn to walk, and reflects the immaturity of the CST connections with the LMNs. This cardinal sign indicates reliably the loss of descending control from the CST, and reflects UMN damage.

A common misconception is that all the signs and symptoms of a UMN lesion equate with damage to the pyramidal system and result in spasticity. Pure pyramidal tract lesions in humans are rare. Studies in primates have shown that selective CST lesions produce weakness, hypotonia, loss of fine distal hand movements, a Babinski sign and loss of the cremasteric and abdominal reflexes. The other signs of UMN damage—hypertonia, hyperreflexia and clonus—must reflect damage to the medial brainstem descending pathways. Spasticity probably occurs through the loss of inhibitory control in the VST and RST.

Genetics of amyotrophic lateral sclerosis

Familial amyotrophic lateral sclerosis (ALS) is associated with mutations in the gene that encodes the superoxide dismutase type 1 enzyme (SOD1). The gene is located on chromosome 21, and this enzyme acts as a free radical ion scavenger. There are more than 90 mutations in SOD1 associated with familial ALS. Recent evidence indicates that mutant SOD1 promotes apoptosis by binding to the anti-apoptotic protein bcl-2, and by sequestering the heat shock proteins HSP27 and HSP70, which have neuroprotective roles in motor neurones. Mutant SOD1 is recruited into the mitochondria, and this leads to their death. However, mutations in SOD1 account for only 15–20% of familial cases. SOD mutations are not seen in ALS sufferers with the sporadic form. More recently, two loci on chromosomes 16q and 18q have also been identified in familial ALS patients.

Several pathogenic pathways may be involved in the death of neurones seen in ALS: (1) autoimmunity to some forms of Ca^{2+} channel (e.g. L-type); (2) increased oxidative stress; (3) excitotoxicity due to the loss of glutamate transporters, and overstimulation of glutamate receptors due to reduced reuptake; and (4) excessive neurofilament accumulation within the motor neurone. Abnormal editing of the glutamate AMPA receptor GluR2 has been found in ALS patients, whereby a change in the second transmembrane domain drastically alters the Ca^{2+} permeability of the receptor, from impermeable to permeable.

Polio and post-polio syndrome

Infection with the polio virus results in several different body responses. The most common form (90%) is asymptomatic or evokes only minor malaise. There are two other forms, non-paralytic and paralytic polio, which produce transient (2–10 days with complete recovery) or permanent muscle weakness and paralysis, respectively. In the latter, patients suffer flaccid paralysis of muscles and painful spasms in non-paralysed muscles. The amount of paralysis is inversely proportional to the motor neurone loss. The virus enters through the mouth and travels in the bloodstream to various central nervous system motor targets, such as the cerebellum, vestibular system, motor cortex and reticular formation. It can travel along peripheral nerves to infect lower motor neurones. Polio occurs most often in children. The affected muscles become atrophied and the limb is flaccid and small.

In about one-third of patients who have suffered previously from polio, a late-onset post-polio syndrome occurs 30–40 years after the initial illness. This post-polio syndrome is characterized by muscle weakness, muscle pain and increasing muscle fatigue. The disease is not caused by reactivation of the polio virus (as is the case for shingles) or by re-infection. Rather, it appears to be due to deterioration of the remaining motor units due to their overuse.

Nowadays, in the western hemisphere, polio has been eradicated by a WHO vaccination programme. Children receive three oral polio vaccinations of a live attenuated version of the virus to enable them to develop antibodies to the virus. The first is administered at 2 months (with the DPT vaccination), and there are further vaccinations at 4, 6 and 18 months of age. Paralytic polio is still endemic throughout the Indian subcontinent and in Africa and Asia.

Experimental evidence shows that lesioning the lateral vestibular nucleus reduces spasticity, as does sectioning the dorsal roots, implying that spasticity represents an increase in the gain of the stretch reflexes due to loss of descending inhibition. A similar explanation is proposed to explain clonus.

There are several degenerative diseases that affect motor neurones such as is motor neurone disease, or amyotrophic lateral sclerosis, (ALS, see Box 9.6), poliomyelitis (Box 9.7), spinal muscular atrophy, progressive muscular atrophy, or progressive bulbar palsy.

ALS (also known as Lou Gehrig's disease in the USA) is the most common disease affecting motor systems. ALS is characterized by the progressive degeneration of LMNs and UMNs, particularly in the pyramidal tract. It results in spastic paraparesis or tetraparesis with stiffness and weakness of the hands, muscle cramps and discomfort. As the disease progresses, the hand muscles atrophy, reflexes increase, and the weakness spreads to the trunk and head muscles (except for the extraocular muscles). Onset is around the age of 50 years, and the disease affects 1/100 000 of the population. It is fatal, and most patients die within 6 years of onset. ALS can be divided into sporadic cases, which represent the majority of cases, and familial ALS (around 10%; Box 9.6).

ALS is the disease described in the case history in Box 9.1. David shows the classic positive signs of UMN damage: spasticity, hyperactive stretch reflexes and a Babinski sign. He shows the clasp-knife effect and clonus, which are further indications of damage to UMN pathways. Negative signs of muscle weakness—muscle atrophy and fasciculation—indicate damage to LMNs. As the UMN and LMNs continue to die, David's symptoms get worse. He is prescribed riluzole, which is currently the only drug approved for treating ALS. Riluzole has a complex pharmacology, but one of its effects is to block glutamate activity. However, it prolongs the life of the patient only marginally. Another drug, gabapentin, is sometimes also given to slow the progression of muscle weakness.

Spinal muscular atrophies are hereditary diseases that are also associated with motor neurone death. There is a mutation in the survival motor neurone (SMN1) gene that results in spasticity and muscle weakness. The incidence is 8 cases per 100 000 live births, with a high mortality rate

Table 9.4 Input pathways to the cerebellum

Pathway	Origin	Peduncle	Fibre type	Function
Spinocerebellar	Clarke's nucleus	ICP	Mossy	Proprioceptive and cutaneous sensation from trunk and legs
Cuneocerebellar	Accessory cuneate nucleus	ICP	Mossy	Proprioceptive and cutaneous sensation from arms and neck
Trigeminocerebellar	Trigeminal nuclei	ICP	Mossy	Proprioceptive and cutaneous sensation from face and jaw
Olivocerebellar	Inferior olivary nucleus	ICP	Climbing	Motor skills learning
Vestibulocerebellar	Vestibular nuclei	ICP	Mossy	Balance
Pontocerebellar	Pontine nuclei	MCP	Mossy	Cognitive, visual and motor input from cortex

ICP, inferior cerebellar peduncle; MCP, middle cerebellar peduncle.

during infancy and no known treatment. Death is caused by severe and progressive restrictive lung function.

The cerebellum

We have seen above that the ultimate executors of movements are the LMNs, and they are under the command of the UMNs. Yet it is not enough simply to command the muscles to contract, in order to produce smooth, coordinated movements. This requires additional control mechanisms to order the correct sequence of muscle contractions. This important task is performed by the cerebellum. In order to accomplish this task, the cerebellum receives sensory information about balance, posture and limb position from the ascending tracts (Table 9.4), and compares it with information from the premotor and supplementary motor areas. In effect, it acts as a comparator of movement, and if there is a mismatch between what the muscles should be doing and what the signals from the muscles show them actually doing, then it sends signals (via the motor thalamus) to the primary motor cortex to correct the movement, so that it is performed in a smooth, coordinated fashion. Different parts of the cerebellum coordinate movement in different parts of the body. Movements are not initiated in the cerebellum. It can be thought of as a subordinate to the motor systems of the motor cortex and basal ganglia.

General anatomical organization

The cerebellum lies above the fourth ventricle, in the posterior fossa of the skull. The cerebellum consists of a deeply convoluted cortex composed of numerous small gyri called folia and a core of white matter, within which are embedded the deep nuclei of the cerebellum (Fig. 9.12). The cerebellum has three lobes, the anterior, posterior and flocculonodular lobes (Fig. 9.12A,B), which are further subdivided into lobules. In the horizontal plane, there are three regions: the midline vermis separates the two lateral hemispheres. In the sagittal plane, the cerebellum can be subdivided into three functional areas, the vestibulocerebellum, spinocerebellum and cerebrocerebellum (Fig. 9.12D), based on their source of afferent input. Each subdivision is associated with a pair of deep cerebellar nuclei. The input and output to the cerebellum are via three pairs of peduncles: the inferior, middle and superior cerebellar peduncles (Table 9.4). The inferior and middle cerebellar peduncles are predominantly input pathways, while the superior peduncle is the predominant output pathway from the deep cerebellar nuclei. The inferior cerebellar peduncle arises from the medulla and provides the predominant input to the anterior lobe, from different body regions. The middle cerebellar peduncle is the largest and projects to the posterior lobe from the pontine nuclei of the pons, carrying information from the motor cortex commissural fibres from one side of the cerebellum to the other. The superior cerebellar peduncle connects the posterior lobe to the midbrain and is predominantly an output pathway from the deep cerebellar nuclei, especially the dentate nucleus.

Also present on the inferior surface are the cerebellar tonsils, which lie lateral to the vermis of the cerebellum (Fig. 9.12B). They stand out because their sulci are oriented at right angles to the general direction of the other sulci of the cerebellum. They are anatomically important because they may herniate through the foramen magnum in severe cases of raised intracranial pressure (see Chapter 11). They then press onto the respiratory centres of the medulla and may kill the patient.

Microanatomy of the cerebellar cortex

The cerebellar cortex has a regular structure, and so neural processing is thought to be the same in all parts.

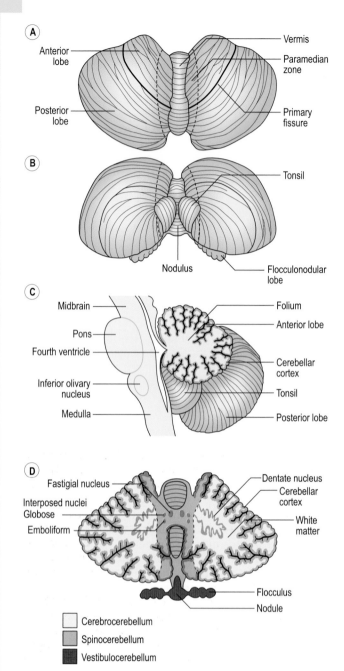

Ⓐ
Anterior lobe
Posterior lobe
Vermis
Paramedian zone
Primary fissure

Ⓑ
Tonsil
Nodulus
Flocculonodular lobe

Ⓒ
Midbrain
Pons
Fourth ventricle
Inferior olivary nucleus
Medulla
Folium
Anterior lobe
Cerebellar cortex
Tonsil
Posterior lobe

Ⓓ
Fastigial nucleus
Interposed nuclei
Globose
Emboliform
Dentate nucleus
Cerebellar cortex
White matter
Flocculus
Nodule

☐ Cerebrocerebellum
☐ Spinocerebellum
■ Vestibulocerebellum

Fig. 9.12 Anatomy of the cerebellum: (A) superior view, (B) inferior view, (C) sagittal view and (D) horizontal view. (D) shows the functional subdivisions and their associated deep cerebellar nuclei.

The cortex has three layers and contains five cell types that form a simple circuit that is repeated many times. The outer layer is the molecular layer, and is almost cell-free. It consists mainly of the axons and dendrites of various cerebellar neurones. The middle layer is a single layer of large neurones called Purkinje cells, the main output cells of the cerebellar cortex. Below this layer is the granular layer, which is densely populated with small neurones called granule cells. Its organization can be described in terms of Purkinje cells, granule cells, and the afferents to the cortex (Fig. 9.13).

There are two sets of afferent fibres that provide input to the cerebellar cortex: mossy fibres and climbing fibres (see Table 9.4). Mossy fibres form the main input to the cerebellum, and are axons of second-order neurones from the spinal cord, brainstem and cerebral cortex that convey proprioceptive information. These inputs are topographically organized, producing somatotopic maps in the cerebellar cortex that are retained in the deep cerebellar nuclei. A whole-body representation is found in the anterior lobe, and two half-body representations, one from each side, are found in the posterior lobe. The head regions of these maps overlap and receive visual and auditory information as well. The presence of these maps has been confirmed with the use of PET scanning.

Collateral branches from mossy fibres make excitatory connections with granule cells, which, in turn, excite Purkinje cells. Each mossy fibre innervates about 600 granule cells and each granule cell receives input from up to four mossy fibres. The axons of the granule cells, the only excitatory cells in the cerebellar cortex, ascend into the molecular layer, bifurcate to form a T-shape, and run parallel to the surface. For this reason, they are called parallel fibres, and each fibre synapses only once with 2000–3000 Purkinje cells. Thus, the input from granule cells to Purkinje cells is very weak, but each Purkinje cell receives input from about 20 000 parallel fibres. Mossy fibres synapse on the dendrites of granule cells, so this is an indirect pathway to Purkinje cells.

A climbing fibre synapses directly on each Purkinje cell body, winding around it and the proximal portions of its dendrites, like ivy climbing a trellis, to make many (~300) connections. All climbing fibres arise from the contralateral inferior olivary nucleus (ION). Purkinje cells become inactivated after stimulation by climbing fibres (postsynaptic depression). This process is involved in motor learning behaviour (see later).

The Purkinje cells are the output cells of the cerebellar cortex. They are inhibitory GABAergic neurones whose axons project to the deep nuclei, which give rise to the cerebellar output to other brain regions. Each Purkinje cell has an intricate, extensive dendritic tree.

There are three types of inhibitory interneurone: stellate, basket and Golgi cells. Axons of stellate and basket cells run perpendicular to the parallel fibres (see Fig. 9.13). When stimulated by granule cells, the stellate and basket cells function by focusing the excitatory input from mossy fibres onto strongly excited 'on-line' Purkinje cells, through inhibiting the weak responses (from other parallel fibres) to adjacent 'off-line' Purkinje cells. This is a form of surround inhibition that produces spatial focusing of cerebellar cortical output. The activation of the on-line Purkinje cells results in the selective inhibition of neurones within the corresponding deep cerebellar nucleus. Golgi cells inhibit the granule cells by way of feedback inhibition from the Purkinje cells that terminates the mossy fibre input, so that the net effect of mossy fibre activation is a brief firing of Purkinje cells. Together,

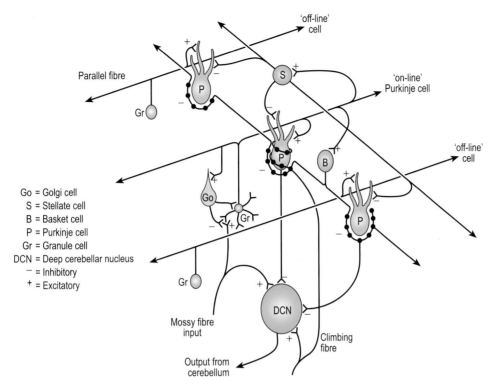

Fig. 9.13 Micro-circuitry of the cerebellar cortex.

Go = Golgi cell
S = Stellate cell
B = Basket cell
P = Purkinje cell
Gr = Granule cell
DCN = Deep cerebellar nucleus
− = Inhibitory
+ = Excitatory

these inhibitory neurones restrict Purkinje cell output in time and space, allowing them to fire only transiently.

Deep cerebellar nuclei

The deep nuclei of the cerebellum receive inhibitory input from Purkinje cell axons. They also receive excitatory collateral input from mossy and climbing fibres. The net output is excitatory and goes to different regions of the brainstem, the reticular formation, red nucleus, spinal cord and motor thalamus.

The most prominent of the deep nuclei is the dentate nucleus (see Fig. 9.12D). It lies most laterally in the white matter core and is functionally associated with the posterior lobe. Most medially are the fastigial nuclei; they are functionally associated with the flocculonodular lobe. Between the fastigial and dentate nuclei are the interposed nuclei, comprising the more medial globose and more lateral emboliform nuclei; they are functionally associated with the anterior lobe.

Functional organization of the cerebellum

The paired flocculus and midline nodulus form the flocculonodular lobe or vestibulocerebellum. They receive input from the vestibular nuclei and the muscle spindles, GTOs and joint afferents in neck muscles (via the cuneocerebellar tract). The vestibulocerebellum functions to maintain the stability of the head on the body. It acts on the neck muscles via the lateral VST, to maintain a steady head position despite movements of the body, and thereby maintains visual fixation on distant objects, such as when a person is running or in a moving vehicle.

The midline cerebellar cortex is called the vermis. This region of cortex coordinates the balance and posture of the body as a whole. Its posterior part is also associated with eye movements in response to vestibular input via the vestibulo-ocular reflex. Damage to the flocculonodular lobe results in nystagmus.

The vestibulocerebellum receives ipsilateral input from the postural muscles of the legs via the dorsal spinocerebellar tract (SCBT) of the spinal cord. These axons synapse in the fastigial nucleus and the vermis. The fastigial nucleus receives the output of the vermis Purkinje cell fibres and sends axons to the reticular formation and also to Dieter's nucleus. Thus, the output to the postural muscles is via the spinal projection of the VST (bilaterally) and RST (Fig. 9.14; Table 9.3) to control muscle tone. Head balance and body balance are interrelated, so there are many cross-connections between the flocculonodular lobe and the vermis.

The spinocerebellum coordinates locomotor and other voluntary movements of the arms and legs. Anatomically, it corresponds to the anterior lobe, the vermis and the area immediately lateral to it, the paramedian region of the posterior lobe. The latter region is not anatomically differentiated from the vermis, but is functionally different because it is interconnected with the interposed deep cerebellar nuclei.

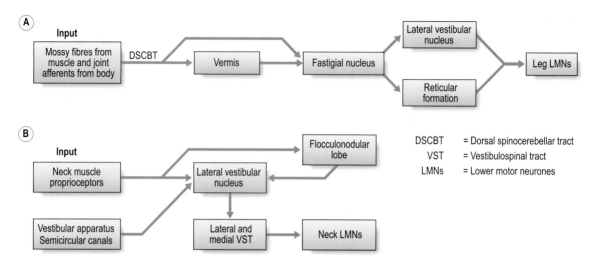

Fig. 9.14 Circuitry of the vestibulocerebellum involved in (A) posture control and (B) head balance.

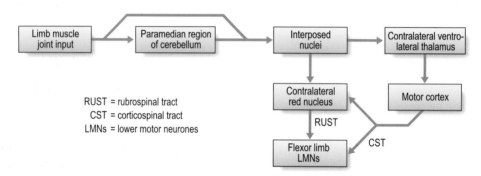

Fig. 9.15 Circuitry of the spinocerebellum involved in the voluntary control of limb movement.

The paramedian region coordinates locomotor and other voluntary movements of the distal limbs. It is the only part of the cerebellum that receives direct input from the spinal cord via the dorsal and ventral SCBTs that monitor the muscle spindles, tendon and joint afferents, and the state of spinal reflexes. The output from the interposed nuclei is to the contralateral red nucleus, which gives rise to the contralateral rubrospinal tract, thereby functionally activating mainly ipsilateral flexor motor neurones (Fig. 9.15).

The largest part of the cerebellum is the cerebrocerebellum, which corresponds to the lateral parts of the posterior lobe. These regions control motor skills associated with speech, hand–eye coordination, independent limb movements and cognitive eye movements. Cognitive eye movements are those in which the eyes move actively, to scan an object of interest. For example, while you are reading this, your eyes are jumping from one fixation point on the line to another, under the control of the cerebral cortex. The cerebellar hemispheres are connected to the dentate nucleus, whose efferent axons project to the contralateral ventro-lateral thalamus and from there to the motor cortex (Fig. 9.16). There are also reciprocal connections with

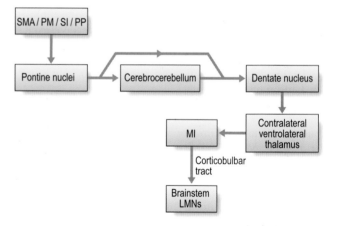

Fig. 9.16 Circuitry of the cerebrocerebellum involved in speech and cognitive movements. SMA, supplementary motor cortex; PM, premotor cortex; PP, posterior parietal cortex; SI, primary somatosensory cortex; MI, primary motor cortex; LMNs, lower motor neurones.

the red nucleus. The hemispheres receive input from the premotor, supplementary, primary motor somatosensory, posterior parietal and visual cortices, via the pontocerebellar tracts from the pontine nuclei.

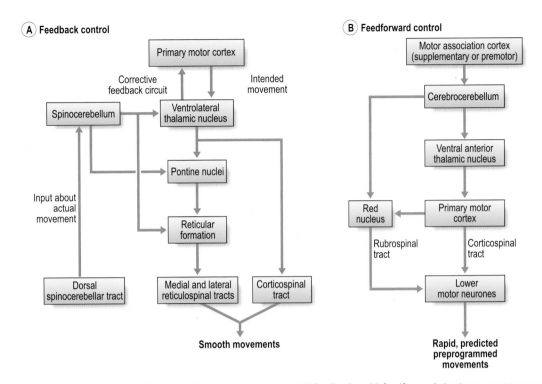

Fig. 9.17 Cerebellar control of movement. The cerebellum can operate using (A) feedback or (B) feedforward circuits to correct errors or predict movement respectively.

Cerebellar function in the control of movement

The cerebellum coordinates complicated multi-joint movements, and is involved in learning new motor tasks (Fig. 9.17). In terms of circuitry, the cerebellum operates in both feedback and feedforward modes. The feedback mode is a corrective error mode, in that the cerebellum compares the motor intention with the actual motor performance. Any mismatch between the two signals generates a signal to make the error smaller. A motor error occurs when the position of a limb is not the intended one, causing an unpredicted muscle stretch that activates the muscle afferents. This unexpected proprioceptive activity is relayed to the cerebellum by the spinocerebellar mossy fibres activated by the movement error, to excite Purkinje cells, which then inhibit the deep cerebellar nuclei that drive the red nucleus and ventrolateral thalamus. This feeds back to the motor cortex to prevent the erroneous movement.

For the execution of well-rehearsed, ballistic (rapid) movements, such as a tennis serve, there is not enough time for feedback correction of errors. In this situation, the cerebellum operates in a feedforward mode, running a programme that predicts the consequences of the motor action. Any unexpected disruptions that occur when the cerebellum is in feedforward mode cannot be corrected for, and so impair the motor performance (resulting in a foul serve in this case).

The predictions inherent in feedforward operation must be learnt during attempts to perform the task. This is motor learning and involves the climbing fibres of the ION. For example, consider learning to juggle with three balls. The idea is to throw the balls in the air, and catch one while the other two are in the air. This requires good hand–eye coordination. During the early attempts, many balls will be dropped. As you get better, fewer balls are dropped, and eventually you learn to juggle. During the learning phase, the climbing fibres are very active and send motor error signals via the olivocerebellar tract to the cerebellum. Climbing fibres, unlike mossy fibres, strongly excite Purkinje cells, overriding the mossy fibre input. Gradually, as the new task is learnt, the error rate is reduced, the activity of climbing fibres is reduced and performance is enhanced. This mechanism is probably used for all acquired voluntary movements, such as learning to walk, skip or ride a bicycle.

Cerebellar diseases

Cerebellar syndromes have a variety of causes (Table 9.5). Some are genetic. Seven genes have been linked to spinocerebellar ataxias. In mutant mice, these gene deletions lead to loss or disturbed migration of granule and Purkinje cells in the cerebellum. Lesions of the cerebellum must be quite large before obvious symptoms appear, as there is much functional redundancy within the cerebellum, due to the multiple somatotopic maps present.

Damage to the cerebellum does not produce paralysis or muscle weakness, or affect the ability to start or stop

Table 9.5 Causes of cerebellar diseases

Stroke

Primary (e.g. medulloblastoma) or secondary tumours

Trauma

Degeneration

Toxicity and metabolic disturbances (e.g. alcoholism, anticonvulsant drugs and hypothyroidism)

Genetic

Miscellaneous (e.g. multiple sclerosis in young people, hydrocephalus)

Developmental (e.g. cerebral palsy)

movements, but does affect the precision and coordination of movements. This is termed ataxia. Focal lesions of the cerebellum produce deficits on the same side of the body as the lesion. The signs of cerebellar damage are:

- asynergia—loss or decomposition of coordinated movement

- dysarthria and dysphonia—speech deficits such as slurring due to errors in the timing of impulses to the muscles controlling speech; articulation problems—words become broken down into individual syllables, and flow becomes 'explosive' or 'scanning'

- intention tremor—swaying to and fro of the limb perpendicular to the direction of movement; this is present only during reaching movements, and not at rest

- nystagmus—horizontal oscillating eye movements

- dysmetria—alteration in the rate and force of movement, e.g. over- or under-reaching for an object

- dysdiadochokinesis—the inability to perform rapid alternating movements such as pronation and supination of the hand

- hypotonia—loss of muscle tone due to decreased activity in γ-motor neurones.

Other signs may include titubation, a rhythmic tremor of the head in an up-and-down ('yes–yes') or side-to-side ('no–no') motion. Pendular (slow) reflexes may also occur, but they are of little use as localizing signs.

The cerebellum is particularly susceptible to the effects of alcohol. Drunkenness is associated with many of the symptoms of mild cerebellar damage! For example, slurred or incoherent speech, incoordination, ataxic gait, clumsiness and double vision are all signs of cerebellar damage. These disorders reflect the role of the cerebellum in the coordination of skilled movements.

Lesions of the vermis lead to truncal ataxia. This is most commonly seen in children, and is due to a tumour called a medulloblastoma, which grows from the granule cell layer to invade (and block) the fourth ventricle. Morning headache, dizziness, vomiting (due to raised intracranial pressure affecting cranial nerve function) and lethargy are common symptoms, and on physical examination, a dramatic feature is the inability to stand upright without support. Attempts to walk result in a wide-based gait, with reeling and swaying from side to side. Truncal ataxia affects the flocculonodular lobe, which regulates balance and the coordination of the para-axial muscles. Symptoms are often absent when the child is lying down. These tumours are highly malignant and can spread to other parts of the nervous system. They are treated surgically, and adjuvant chemotherapy and radiotherapy (except when the child is less than 5 years old, because of adverse effects on brain development) are used to prevent reoccurrence. Survival rates are 60–85% at 5 years after diagnosis, depending on how aggressive the postradiation chemotherapy is. Prognosis is poorer for surgery only, as the tumour re-emerges.

Lesions of the anterior lobe result in gait ataxia. This is most commonly seen in chronic alcoholics, where alcohol abuse has caused neuronal degeneration of granule and Purkinje cells, resulting in cortical atrophy of the anterior lobe. This affects the coordination of the lower limbs, resulting in a staggering, drunken gait, even when the person is sober. As the degeneration progresses, loss of control in trunk and arms and eventually speech may ensue. The person also suffers from dysdiadochokinesis, and the heel-to-shin test is almost impossible to perform, as the patient will have sensory ataxia (positive Romberg sign) due to peripheral neuropathy.

Damage to the posterior lobe commonly results from stroke, tumours, degenerative disease or traumas that affect a cerebellar hemisphere, peduncle, or the midbrain or pons. Symptoms manifest as incoordination of voluntary movement and loss of muscle tone. The patient presents with tremor of the limbs, dysmetria and dysdiadochokinesia, resulting in clumsiness of movements. There are often speech impediments with regard to phonation and articulation.

MOTOR SYSTEMS II:
THE BASAL GANGLIA

10

Chapter objectives

After studying this chapter you should be able to:

1. Describe the organization of the basal ganglia and their connections with other central nervous system regions.

2. Describe the main symptoms and diseases associated with dysfunction of the basal ganglia, and their pathophysiology.

3. Outline the therapeutic management and prognosis of Parkinson's disease and Huntington's disease.

4. Treat the complications of treatment in Parkinson's disease.

5. Define the factors that may contribute to neurodegeneration.

6. Discuss the potential of cell replacement therapies in neurodegenerative diseases.

Introduction

The smooth execution of movements involving the trunk and the limbs, and the maintenance of posture, balance and normal gait, would not be possible without the coordinated activity of supraspinal centres, in particular the cortico-spinal neurones (the 'upper motor neurones', UMNs), the motor neurones in the ventral horn of the spinal cord (the 'lower motor neurones', LMNs) and an intact neuromuscular junction and muscle. Disturbances in the function of the major descending motor pathways are associated with paresis, paralysis or spasticity. Several other structures provide irreplaceable central input required for normal motor activity and are involved in its continuous control and coordination. The basal ganglia and the cerebellum are the main structures fulfilling these roles. They are at the interface between the intention and the execution of the movement. Neuronal activity in these structures is correlated temporally in a complex manner with motor activity. This chapter is dedicated to the basal ganglia, and illustrates how their dysfunction leads to specific alterations in motor performance, which can be severely debilitating (Box 10.1). Disorders of the basal ganglia can lead to either hyperkinetic or hypokinetic manifestations.

Box 10.1 Case history

Gavin Porter, a 57-year-old recently retired businessman, came to the doctor with his wife because of 'trembling', which affected his hands, in particular the right hand. Over the last year, the trembling had become worse, and he sometimes felt that his legs trembled very slightly too. He had also become rather slow in his movements, and sometimes sat for hours in an armchair, with a rather expressionless face. His wife found this irritating, and thought that his general mood had changed and he had become more withdrawn. He was finding it increasingly difficult to button and unbutton his shirt or tie his shoelaces. He had recently suffered two falls, one of which had resulted in a serious skin laceration on his head. When asked, he could not pinpoint a specific cause for these falls. The patient was otherwise in good health. He had taken early retirement in order to enjoy other activities, such as gardening and voluntary work. He seemed to be deeply worried about his progressive physical incapacity. In his moments of anxiety about the future, the trembling was much worse.

This case gives rise to the following questions:

1. What is the cause of the symptoms (i.e. tremor, rigidity, slow movements, altered gait and balance)?
2. Would the confirmation of the diagnosis require additional tests?
3. Are there any risk factors for developing this disease?

The basal ganglia: structure and organization

General organization

The basal ganglia consist of several subcortical interconnected nuclei that are involved in the initiation and execution of movement. They are the caudate nucleus, the putamen and the globus pallidus (in the telencephalon), the subthalamic nucleus (in the diencephalon) and the substantia nigra (in the mesencephalon). The relative locations of these structures are given in Chapter 1.

The caudate nucleus and the putamen are two nuclei that are interconnected and form the striatum. The globus pallidus has an internal (or medial) and an external (or lateral) division. The striatum receives afferents from the neocortex, the thalamus and the substantia nigra. The globus pallidus receives projections from the striatum and the subthalamic nucleus. The major output of the basal ganglia, which represents mainly projections from the globus pallidus (internal division) and substantia nigra, is directed to thalamic nuclei (in particular, the ventral anterior, ventral lateral and centromedian nuclei), which project to motor and prefrontal cortical areas. A smaller contingent of efferent fibres project to the pedunculopontine nucleus in the brainstem tegmentum, and to the superior colliculus. The substantia nigra can be subdivided into substantia nigra pars compacta and substantia nigra pars reticulata. The pars compacta contains neurones that project to the striatum, whereas the pars reticulata receives striatal input and provides the nigral output.

Circuits and neurotransmitters

The basal ganglia form a network of parallel loops and circuits that integrate the neuronal activity in cerebral regions (motor, oculomotor, limbic and associative), the basal ganglia nuclei and thalamic nuclei. Lesion or degeneration in the basal ganglia leads to diseases that present with a range of characteristic motor symptoms. Figure 10.1 summarizes the functional organization of the basal ganglia, and shows the major neurotransmitters present in afferent and efferent pathways.

The striatum is heterogeneous in structure, and consists of two main compartments: the matrix and the striosomes. These two compartments can be identified using the differential distribution of various neurochemical markers, such as the various subtypes of opioid receptors (mu (μ), delta (δ) and kappa (κ)) or acetylcholinesterase. A majority of neurones in the matrix and the striosomes are medium-sized projection neurones, which have highly collateralized axons, and dendrites endowed with dense spines. These cells are called 'medium spiny neurones'.

The cortex provides glutamatergic excitatory input to all striatal projection neurones. The cortical projections are organized somatotopically, innervating both the matrix and the striosomes. The striatum is connected with the globus pallidus and the substantia nigra through two distinct pathways (see Fig. 10.1).

1. The projection of the striatum to the globus pallidus (internal division) and substantia nigra pars reticulata is known as *the direct pathway*. The main neurotransmitter in this projection is γ-aminobutyric acid (GABA), which is co-localized with peptides such as substance P and dynorphins. The globus pallidus (internal division) or substantia nigra pars reticulata neurones project to the thalamus and are also GABAergic. The thalamic neurones, which contain glutamate, project to the cortex, thus closing the loop.

2. In the case of *the indirect pathway*, striatal GABAergic neurones (which also contain enkephalins) project to the globus pallidus (external division). The pallidal neurones are GABAergic and project to the subthalamic nucleus. The subthalamic nucleus glutamatergic neurones project to the globus pallidus (internal segment) and the substantia nigra pars reticulata. The circuit is ultimately completed through the GABAergic nigrothalamic projection, and then the glutamatergic thalamocortical projections, as in the case of the direct pathway. Another link between the direct and the indirect pathways is provided by neurones in the globus pallidus (external division), which establish contact with the globus pallidus (internal division) and substantia nigra pars reticulata through axon collaterals.

In summary, through these two pathways, the cortex can either increase (direct pathway) or decrease (indirect pathway) the excitatory thalamocortical projections. The presence of GABA as a main transmitter in the striatal efferents indicates that the striatal projection neurones will have an inhibitory effect on target cells in the substantia nigra and the globus pallidus. In contrast, the subthalamic nucleus is a source of excitation. Thus, through parallel loops and the balance between excitation and inhibition, the basal ganglia are involved in the transfer of information from the neocortex to the motor areas, in particular involving the premotor and supplementary motor areas. This results in facilitation or inhibition of the major descending motor pathways (e.g. corticospinal projection).

The substantia nigra pars compacta contains neurones that produce dopamine and project to the striatum, exerting a modulatory influence on the activity of striatal projection neurones that are involved in both the direct and the indirect pathways. Cortical input to medium spiny neurones can be controlled by dopaminergic fibres at the level of their dendrites and the dendritic spines. Dopamine appears to facilitate the activity of medium spiny neurones involved in the direct pathway, and to inhibit the activity of the medium spiny neurones involved in the indirect pathway. The striatum also contains several types of interneurone, e.g. cholinergic neurones. Nigral dopaminergic cells provide inhibitory input to striatal cholinergic interneurones. Although the latter represent less than 10% of striatal cells, they exert important integrative functions in the striatum.

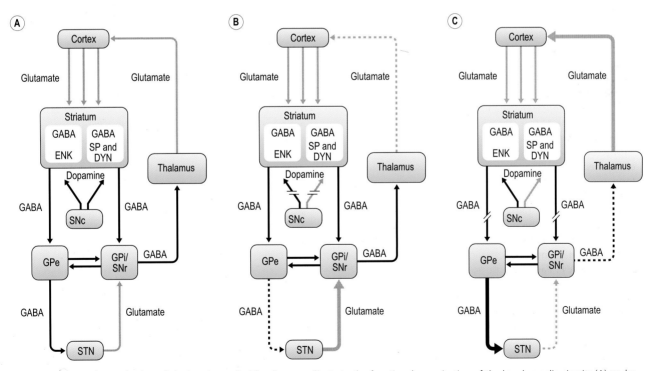

Fig. 10.1 Functional organization of the basal ganglia. The diagrams illustrate the functional organization of the basal ganglia circuits (A) under normal conditions; (B) in Parkinson's disease; and (C) in Huntington's disease. Broken lines indicate pathways that are hypoactive, and thick lines indicate pathways that are hyperactive. DYN, dynorphins; ENK, enkephalins; GABA, γ-aminobutyric acid; GPe, external globus pallidum; GPi, internal globus pallidum; SNc, substantia nigra compacta; SNr, substantia nigra reticulata; SP, substance P; STN, subthalamic nucleus.

Symptoms

Parkinson's disease (PD) was first described in 1817 by James Parkinson, a doctor with encyclopaedic interests, who was practising in the East End of London (Box 10.2). He based his monograph, 'An Essay on the Shaking Palsy', on the analysis of six cases. The cardinal features of this disease are motor: tremor (unilateral or bilateral), bradykinesia and rigidity. They may occur in isolation or in any combination (Box 10.3).

Tremor

The most prominent symptom is the resting tremor of the extremities that almost always accompanies the disease. The tremor has a characteristic frequency of 4–6 Hz and may begin in only one extremity and spread to the others. The distal joints of the limbs are preferentially affected. In the hand, the tremor is characteristic and involves the thumb and fingers rolling together. This is called a 'pill-rolling'

tremor. The tremor is seen at rest and disappears during an intentional movement and during sleep. However, in the late stages of the disease, an 'active' tremor may emerge, with a frequency of 6–8 Hz. Tremor is exacerbated by anxiety. It primarily affects the hands, but it can also affect the lower limbs, jaw and lips.

Bradykinesia/akinesia

Bradykinesia is a slowing of normal movement. In the advanced stages of the disease, the patient becomes akinetic and shows almost no motor initiative. There is reduced arm-swinging when walking, reduced blinking, and various daily simple or complex tasks (e.g. washing, brushing the teeth, dressing and writing) can be affected. There is a gradual loss of normal facial movement and expression (Fig. 10.2). The speech is poorly articulated, and the voice is quiet and monotonous. Eating and swallowing become increasingly difficult. This may result in a tendency to drool (sialorrhoea). It is estimated that up to 70% of patients ultimately experience drooling, which may lead to dermatitis and aspiration.

Rigidity

Parkinsonian patients have increased muscle tone in flexor and extensor muscles and typically present resistance to passive movement of the limbs. This rigidity is due to inappropriate sensitivity of the muscles to stretching and an inability to obtain complete relaxation. The

---

Box 10.2 James Parkinson (1755–1824): a physician and a radical thinker

James Parkinson was a general practitioner whose medical writings attest to his busy medical career. However, his intellectual interests were much wider. He was a respected palaeontologist and his two books 'Organic Remains of a Former World' and 'Outlines of Oryctology' were considered to be reference works by his contemporaries. He also had an interest in politics and in social issues, as a member of several 'reform societies' and 'revolutionary clubs'.

In 'An Essay on the Shaking Palsy', Parkinson gives a short definition of the disease, for which he also provides a Latin synonym—paralysis agitans: 'Involuntary tremulous motion, with lessened muscular power, in parts not in action and even when supported; with a propensity to bend the trunk forwards, and to pass from a walking to a running pace: the senses and intellect being uninjured.' He believed that the disease had 'escaped particular notice', and he hoped that other colleagues in the medical community would 'extend their searches' so that in the end they could 'point out the most appropriate means of relieving a tedious and most distressing malady'. Parkinson provided a graphic depiction of most of the symptoms of the disease, but apparently failed to appreciate features such as the significant muscular rigidity and the bradykinesia.

In the 19th century, important contributions to the description of this disease were made by the French neurologists Trousseau and Charcot, and their pupils. In recognition of James Parkinson's first incisive insight into this pathology, it is the eminent neurologist Jean-Martin Charcot who gave the disease the name of 'Parkinson's disease'.

Box 10.3 Case history

Gavin Porter was submitted to a full neurological examination. The patient was alert and oriented for time and place. Memory and general knowledge were appropriate for his age. His speech was slow and quiet, and rather monotonous, almost devoid of natural voice inflexions. His face was impassive and he rarely blinked. A mild resting tremor was present in the orofacial musculature, which diminished on speaking or swallowing.

His strength was intact, and deep tendon reflexes were normal. There was cogwheel rigidity upon passive movement of the limbs. The 'pill-rolling' 4–6 Hz tremor of the right thumb and index fingers was abolished by volitional movement. The patient's gait was rather slow. If given an abrupt push, he could not quickly restore his posture, and was at risk of falling. Cutaneous sensation and proprioception were intact.

The patient was diagnosed with Parkinson's disease and was prescribed L-dihydroxyphenylalanine (L-DOPA) with carbidopa. The doctor discussed the prognosis with the patient and his wife.

This case gives rise to the following questions:

1. Why was the patient given L-DOPA with carbidopa, and are there any therapeutic alternatives?
2. What is the long-term prognosis for this patient?

Case history

Gavin Porter continued to take L-DOPA with carbidopa for 6 years. Initially, the patient complained of nausea and tiredness. The drug improved his motor symptoms, especially during the first year. However, the dose administered had to be increased gradually, and during the last year he had started suffering from totally unpredictable complete immobility, although he was taking his medication regularly. Sometimes, episodes of immobility alternate with abnormal violent movement of his limbs, which he cannot control and finds extremely embarrassing. His sleep is disturbed and he complains of nightmares. He has frequent falls, and his wife finds it very difficult to lift him. He has become very apathetic and withdrawn, and has lost interest in any activities that he used to enjoy before he became ill.

The condition of this patient after 6 years of treatment raises the following questions:

1. Was the prescription of L-DOPA with carbidopa the best choice when treatment was initiated?
2. What could be done to alleviate the additional problems that have emerged in this case?

increased resistance to movement, combined with tremor, leads to the 'cogwheel' phenomenon. Manipulating the patient's limbs feels like manipulating a lead pipe; hence the term 'lead pipe' rigidity.

Other motor and non-motor manifestations of Parkinson's disease

Abnormalities of posture and gait are associated with this disease and tend to appear at a later stage. The gait of a parkinsonian patient becomes slow and shuffling, and the posture is flexed (see Fig. 10.2). Patients have a marked tendency to fall, which is partly due to the rigidity of limb and trunk muscles, but is also a consequence of the failure of postural adjustment movements, such as holding out the arms. As the disease progresses, 'freezing' also begins to appear. Patients become 'frozen' when trying to initiate walking, when passing through narrow spaces or when turning. This immobility can be overcome using sensory cues, such as drawing lines on the floor, and asking the patient to step over them.

The handwriting is altered (Fig. 10.3), and as the disease evolves it becomes small and indecipherable (micrographia). The skin may have a greasy appearance (seborrhoea), and constipation is common. Other autonomic abnormalities, such as urinary dysfunction (in particular, urinary incontinence due to bladder detrusor hyperreflexia), increased sweating and sexual dysfunction, are also encountered in parkinsonian patients.

In the late stages of the disease, many patients present with memory impairment, confusion and disorientation, and other features of dementia. Cognitive deficits represent a serious clinical problem and may be compounded by the unwanted effects of medication. It is estimated that dementia occurs in about 30% of parkinsonian patients, especially when the disease is diagnosed after the age of 70 years. Depression is also very common, at any stage of the disease, and may be reactive or part of the disease process (Box 10.4).

The diagnosis of PD is made entirely on the basis of the symptoms, and does not involve additional laboratory investigations or imaging procedures. PD is diagnosed by: (1) finding at examination at least two out of several signs of a movement disorder (e.g. rigidity, resting tremor, bradykinesia, or problems with posture and gait); and (2) a positive response to dopamine substitution treatment.

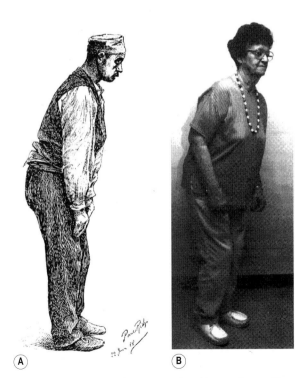

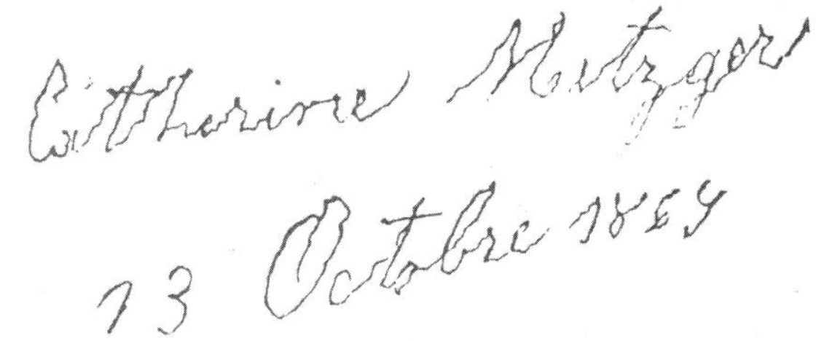

(A)   (B)

Fig. 10.2 (A) Rigid posture of a patient with Parkinson's disease. (B) Characteristic flexed posture of a patient with Parkinson's disease. (A) Drawn by Paul Richer, a former intern of Charcot's. From Richer (1888), in Koller WC, ed. Handbook of Parkinson's Disease. Marcel Dekker, 1987. (B) From Hauser RA, Zesiewicz TA. Parkinson's Disease—Questions and Answers. Merit Publishing International, Basingstoke, 1996.

Fig. 10.3 A specimen of the handwriting of a patient with paralysis agitans under the care of Professor Charcot at the Hôpital St Louis in 1869. From Charcot (1872), in Koller WC, ed. Handbook of Parkinson's Disease. Marcel Dekker, 1987.

The presentation in the patient described in Boxes 10.1 and 10.2 is typical of PD. His muscle strength is not affected, but his symptoms reflect difficulties in initiating and coordinating simple motor acts, and impaired posture and gait. The patient has no gross sensory impairment. Furthermore, no muscle weakness, paralysis or spasticity are detected, which rules out a lesion of the UMNs or LMNs. The motor abnormalities have global effects on his performance of motor acts that form part of normal daily activities, and also his posture. This suggests an abnormality of motor systems that is not strictly localized. The onset of this dysfunction in motor performance is gradual, which rules out a vascular event and is suggestive of a neurodegenerative process. There is no pattern of relapse and remission, and the state of the patient is constantly deteriorating. Thus, as the pathological process may be continuous, it is important to understand the rationale of any treatment attempted and establish whether therapeutic strategies can at least slow down the neurodegenerative process and improve the patient's quality of life.

All parkinsonian syndromes (Table 10.1) are characterized by akinesia, rigidity and tremor at rest. It is important to differentiate between idiopathic PD (i.e. no detectable cause for the disease) and secondary parkinsonism, which may be due to other causes, such as vascular lesions in the basal ganglia, carbon monoxide or manganese poisoning, repeated head trauma ('boxer's parkinsonism'), or chronic blockade of dopaminergic receptors in the basal ganglia (use of neuroleptic drugs in schizophrenic patients). Idiopathic PD is an irreversible neurodegenerative disease. In the final stages of the disease, patients become bedridden, and death is due to medical complications (Table 10.2).

Pathophysiology of Parkinson's disease

The pathological hallmark of PD is the degeneration of the nigrostriatal dopaminergic pathway. Post-mortem analysis of specimens from patients with PD shows a striking absence of dopaminergic cells in the substantia nigra (Fig. 10.4). *In vivo* imaging of dopaminergic neurones, using, for example, a labelled precursor of dopamine, or markers of the dopamine neuronal reuptake system, also confirms the loss of striatal dopaminergic terminals (see below). Unfortunately, when the diagnosis is made, it is likely that more than 70–80% of dopaminergic neurones in the substantia nigra will have been already lost.

Nigrostriatal dopaminergic neurones are tonically active and exert a modulatory influence on the striatum and the striatonigral and striatopallidal efferent pathways, through D_1 and D_2 receptors, respectively. According to the prevailing model, dopamine facilitates the activity of striatal projection neurones in the direct pathway through D_1 receptors, and inhibits the activity of striatal projection neurones in the indirect pathway via D_2 receptors. Under normal conditions, as a result of the activity in the two pathways, and the neuromodulatory effect of dopamine, there is adequate thalamocortical excitatory input (see Fig. 10.1A), and facilitation of movement.

Table 10.1 Classification of parkinsonian syndromes

Idiopathic Parkinson's disease
Secondary parkinsonian syndromes
Infectious or post-infectious
Toxic
Drug-induced
Metabolic
Post-traumatic
Vascular
Tumour

Parkinsonian syndromes as part of other neurodegenerative disorders
Multiple system atrophy
Progressive supranuclear palsy
Corticobasal ganglionic degeneration
Diffuse Lewy body disease

Table 10.2 Hoehn and Yahr staging of Parkinson's disease

Stage 1
Signs and symptoms on one side only
Symptoms mild
Symptoms inconvenient but not disabling
Usually presents with tremor of one limb
Friends have noticed changes in posture, locomotion and facial expression

Stage 2
Symptoms are bilateral
Minimal disability
Posture and gait affected

Stage 3
Significant slowing of body movements
Early impairment of equilibrium on walking or standing
Generalized dysfunction that is moderately severe

Stage 4
Severe symptoms
Can still walk to a limited extent
Rigidity and bradykinesia
No longer able to live alone
Tremor may be less than earlier stages

Stage 5
Cachectic stage
Invalidism complete
Cannot stand or walk
Requires constant nursing care

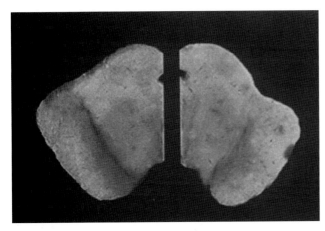

Fig. 10.4 Neurodegeneration in Parkinson's disease. Brain sections from the midbrain of a normal patient (left) and a Parkinson's disease patient (right). The Parkinson's disease hemisphere on the right shows a loss of melanized dopaminergic neurones in the substantia nigra. From Alexi et al. Progress in Neurobiology 2000; 60: 418.

Oxidative stress in Parkinson's disease

(a) $\quad DA + O_2 + H_2O \xrightarrow{MAO} 3,4\text{-DHPA} + NH_3 + H_2O_2$

(b) $\quad DA + O_2 \longrightarrow SQ^\bullet + {}^\bullet O_2^- + H^+$

$\qquad DA + {}^\bullet O_2^- + 2H^+ \longrightarrow SQ^\bullet + H_2O_2$

(c) $\quad H_2O_2 + 2GSH \longrightarrow GSSG + 2H_2O$

(d) $\quad H_2O_2 + Fe^{+2} \longrightarrow OH^\bullet + OH^- + Fe^{+3}$

Fig. 10.5 Oxidation processes in the basal ganglia. Examples of reactions involving dopamine and leading to formation of free radicals, and oxidation of protective substances such as glutathione. DA, dopamine; H_2O_2, hydrogen peroxide; 3,4-DHPA, 3,4-dihydroxyphenylacetaldehyde; OH^-, hydroxyl ion; OH•, hydroxyl radical; GSH, reduced glutathione; GSSG, oxidized glutathione; Fe^{2+}, ferrous iron; Fe^{3+}, ferric ion; •O_2^-, superoxide radical; MAO, monoamine oxidase; SQ•, quinones.

As illustrated in Figure 10.1B, the degeneration of the dopaminergic nigrostriatal cells leads to an imbalance in striatal output pathways. The loss of dopamine appears to lead to an increase in the activity of GABAergic striatal neurones in the indirect circuit, and a decrease in the activity of GABAergic striatal neurones in the direct circuit. The decreased inhibition in the direct pathway leads to increased activity of inhibitory GABAergic nigrothalamic projections, and diminished thalamocortical input, and therefore less activation of the motor cortex. The slowness of normal movement (bradykinesia) or lack of movement (akinesia) seen in parkinsonism is considered to be a consequence of this increased inhibition of thalamic neurones that project to the cortex. The increased activity in the indirect pathway leads ultimately to a similar consequence, through disinhibition of the subthalamic nucleus, which provides an excitatory glutamatergic projection to the substantia nigra. Therefore, in PD, the excitatory input to cortical areas involved in motor control is reduced. In other diseases of the basal ganglia, such as Huntington's disease, the opposite happens, leading to a hyperkinetic syndrome (see below). However, this is a simplified view of the functioning of the basal ganglia, and the limitations of this functional model become apparent as the disease evolves, and as complications of treatment emerge.

PD is characterized by the massive loss of nigrostriatal dopaminergic melanized cells, but the pathological examination also reveals other abnormalities. For example, another characteristic, although not pathognomonic, finding in idiopathic PD is the presence of Lewy bodies. These are concentric eosinophilic cytoplasmic inclusions with peripheral halos and dense cores, and are consistently immunoreactive to the proteins α-synuclein and ubiquitin. Lewy bodies are a frequent incidental finding at postmortem examination in elderly patients. In idiopathic PD, Lewy bodies and other signs of neurodegeneration can be found in the substantia nigra and also in other structures, such as the locus coeruleus, the nucleus basalis of Meynert, the pedunculopontine nucleus, the dorsal motor nucleus of the vagus, the cerebral cortex and the spinal cord. There is thus evidence that the neurodegenerative process in PD does not exclusively affect dopaminergic systems; as the disease evolves, significant changes in noradrenergic, serotonergic and cholinergic neurones can be detected.

Causes of Parkinson's disease

PD is one of the most common neurological disorders leading to major disability and ultimately death. It affects 1/1000 of the population and is rising in both incidence and prevalence, due to increased longevity and improvements in treatment. It affects both sexes equally, and occurs in all races. It is the second most common neurodegenerative disease, affecting 1% of the population above the age of 65 years.

The cause of primary PD is unknown. There is evidence for a role of both environmental and genetic factors. The effects of exposure to certain toxic agents, such as manganese oxide, and also the association of parkinsonism with viral encephalitis lethargica, clearly show that environmental precipitating causes cannot be ruled out. A minority of cases, represented by familial forms of the disease, are associated with a genetic abnormality. Thus, mutations in α-synuclein are associated with autosomal-dominant forms of PD, whereas mutations in the gene *parkin* are associated with autosomal-recessive juvenile-onset PD. However, the majority of cases of PD are not associated with a clearly defined cause. Dopaminergic cell loss in the substantia nigra occurs naturally with increasing age, but appears to be accelerated in PD. This may be due to increased oxidative stress, or to selective neurotoxins, which may preferentially target dopaminergic cells that are rich in neuromelanin, such as those in the substantia nigra. The oxidation of endogenous dopamine leads to the formation of H_2O_2 and highly reactive free radicals (Fig. 10.5). Neuromelanin,

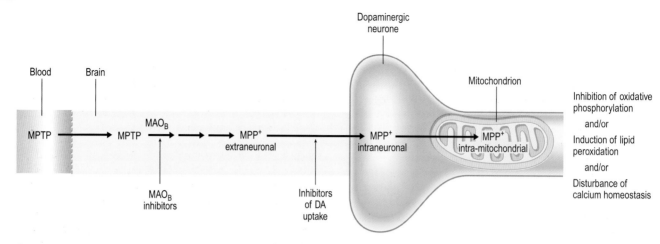

Fig. 10.6 The fate of MPTP after systemic administration, and mechanisms underlying its toxicity for dopaminergic neurones. MPTP, 1-methyl-4-phenyl-1,2,3,6-tetrahydropyridine; MPP$^+$, 1-methyl-4-phenylpyridinium ion; MAO$_B$, monoamine oxidase B; DA, dopamine.

which gives nigral dopaminergic cells their characteristic colour, is an oxidation product of dopamine. Post-mortem studies show evidence of oxidative damage and decreased activity of complex I of the mitochondrial electron transport chain in the substantia nigra in PD. Patients also have increased iron levels in the substantia nigra pars compacta and a reduced concentration of the iron binding protein transferrin, which makes iron more available for oxidation reactions. There is also evidence of increased lipid peroxidation in PD.

The reported development of severe parkinsonian symptoms in young drug addicts following accidental exposure to 1-methyl-4-phenyl-1,2,3,6-tetrahydropyridine (MPTP) lends strength to a neurotoxic cause of PD, through exposure to environmental neurotoxins. MPTP can be produced during the synthesis of the opiate pethidine. MPTP is very lipophilic, and crosses the blood–brain barrier (BBB) without difficulty. It is converted into a toxic metabolite, the 1-methyl-4-phenylpyridinium ion (MPP$^+$), through the action of the enzyme monoamine oxidase type B (MAO$_B$). MPP$^+$ is taken up by the plasma membrane dopamine transporter into nigral dopaminergic neurones, and selectively destroys them by inhibiting complex I of the respiratory chain in mitochondria (Fig. 10.6). The administration of MPTP in primates replicates all the clinical signs of PD, including tremor, rigidity, akinesia and postural instability.

Treatment of Parkinson's disease

The pharmacological treatment of PD attempts to compensate for the loss of nigral dopaminergic cells and the imbalance in input thus created in the striatum (Box 10.5). Dopamine replacement therapy has been the major treatment for PD for the last three decades.

Dopaminergic medication

L-DOPA

Dopamine does not cross the blood–brain barrier (BBB), so direct systemic supplementation with dopamine is not therapeutically useful. L-DOPA (or levodopa), a precursor in the biosynthetic pathway of dopamine (Fig. 10.8), can be used in order to increase dopamine concentrations in the deficient areas. After oral administration, L-DOPA is absorbed into the systemic circulation through the energy-dependent saturable activity of a neutral amino acid transporter in the duodenum. The same transporter also facilitates the passage of L-DOPA across the BBB. In the brain, L-DOPA is taken up into dopaminergic neurones and can be converted into dopamine in the remaining cells in the substantia nigra. Conversion of L-DOPA into dopamine is catalysed by an aromatic amino acid decarboxylase (also called DOPA decarboxylase). This conversion occurs not only in the brain but also at the periphery. The conversion at the periphery can be blocked by co-administration of a DOPA decarboxylase inhibitor such as benserazide or carbidopa. L-DOPA can also be metabolized at the periphery by catechol-*O*-methyl transferase (COMT). The administration of L-DOPA with COMT inhibitors, such as entacapone, significantly improves the central bioavailability of the precursor (Fig. 10.9) and leads to fewer variations in plasma concentration. As other amino acids compete with L-DOPA for intestinal absorption through the same transporter, dietary protein intake can change the bioavailability of L-DOPA.

Prior to the introduction of L-DOPA into clinical use, the life expectancy following diagnosis was about 10 years. L-DOPA has increased the quality of life, particularly in the early years of treatment, and has improved survival. L-DOPA remains the most efficacious anti-parkinsonian

Box 10.5 Dopaminergic systems and receptors

Dopamine is a catecholamine neurotransmitter associated with numerous physiological and pathological processes, including motor activity, emotion, cognition, addiction, endocrine regulation, and cardiovascular and renal function. Because of the variety of effects induced by dopamine, one of the major challenges is to develop dopaminergic drugs that affect selectively these processes.

In the central nervous system, dopamine-containing neurones form three main pathways (Fig. 10.7).

1. The nigrostriatal pathway: cell bodies lie in the substantia nigra, and the axons innervate the caudate nucleus and the putamen. This system is mainly involved in the integration of sensory information and the control of movement.
2. The mesolimbic/mesocortical pathway: cell bodies are situated mainly in the ventral tegmental area (which is medial to the substantia nigra), and the axons innervate the nucleus accumbens (considered by some authors to be the most ventral part of the striatum), the olfactory tubercle, the amygdala and the cortex (in particular the prefrontal and cingulate cortices). This system is associated with reward and reinforcement mechanisms (involved in addiction), emotional behaviour and cognition.
3. The tuberoinfundibular pathway: cell bodies are located in the arcuate nucleus in the hypothalamus, and the axons project to the median eminence. In this system, dopamine acts as a modulator of the hypothalamic–pituitary axis (for example, it inhibits prolactin secretion).

Dopamine exerts its effects through five receptor subtypes: D_1, D_2, D_3, D_4 and D_5. These can be grouped into two classes: the D_1-like receptors (this includes the D_1 and D_5 receptors) and the D_2-like receptors (this includes the D_2, D_3 and D_4 receptors). Additional complexity is conferred by the existence of multiple receptor isoforms within a receptor subtype. All dopamine receptors are G-protein-coupled receptors. They are associated with several signal transduction systems. The two main classes of receptor may exert opposite effects on the same signalling mechanism. For example, D_1-like receptors activate adenylate cyclase, whereas D_2-like receptors inhibit this enzyme. D_1 and D_2 receptors are the predominant dopamine receptor subtypes in the central nervous system. They are present at moderate to high densities in the projection areas of the dopaminergic pathways. Dopamine receptors can be located postsynaptically or presynaptically. In the latter case, they may act as autoreceptors, which regulate dopaminergic signalling, but also as heteroreceptors, through their location on non-dopaminergic terminals.

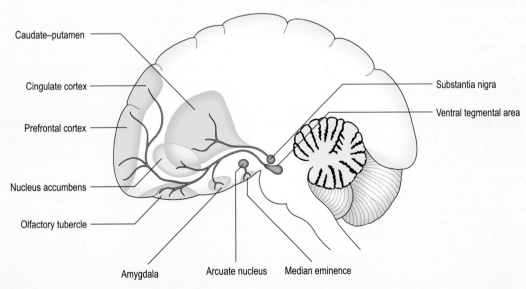

Fig. 10.7 Dopaminergic projections in the central nervous system.

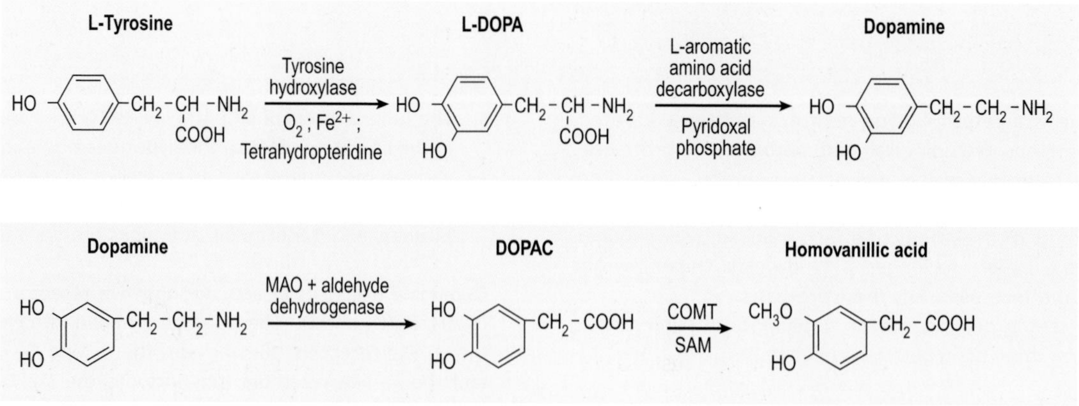

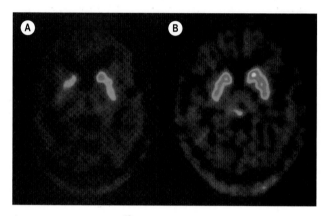

Fig. 10.8 Biosynthesis and metabolism of dopamine. L-DOPA, L-dihydroxyphenylalanine; DOPAC, dihydroxyphenylacetic acid; COMT, catechol-*O*-methyl-transferase; SAM, *S*-adenosylmethionine; MAO, monoamine oxidase.

Fig. 10.9 PET studies on [^{18}F]6-L-fluorodopa accumulation in a subject with Parkinson's disease (Hoehn and Yahr stage 3): (A) a scan after administration of L-DOPA without entacapone; (B) a scan at the same level after administration of L-DOPA with entacapone. Note that striatal uptake of fluorodopa is enhanced in the presence of entacapone. From Olanow et al. Trends in Neurosciences 2000; 23(10 Suppl): S123.

Table 10.3 Complications of L-DOPA therapy
Motor fluctuations (end-of-dose deterioration, 'on–off' phenomenon, delayed or no 'on' responses)
Dyskinesias ('on'-period dyskinesia, biphasic dyskinesias, 'off'-period dystonias)
Non-motor complications (tingling, pain, akathisia, autonomic dysfunction)
Neuropsychiatric complications (hallucinations, delirium, mood changes, hypersexuality, sleep fragmentation, nightmares)

drug, and almost all patients respond to this drug. However, the use of L-DOPA is associated with a wide range of unwanted effects and long-term additional drug-induced problems: nausea, vomiting, postural hypotension, hallucinations and paranoid delusions, and complex acute and delayed motor complications, such as dyskinesias (abnormal involuntary movements) and the 'on–off' effect (Table 10.3).

The nausea and vomiting are due to conversion of L-DOPA into dopamine at the periphery and activation of dopamine receptors in the chemoreceptor trigger zone (in the area postrema in the medulla), which is outside the BBB. This can be largely prevented by co-administration of L-DOPA with DOPA decarboxylase inhibitors (in this example, L-DOPA is given to the patient with carbidopa). Nausea can also be treated with domperidone, which is a dopamine receptor antagonist that does not cross the BBB. Hallucinations are due to the increased production of dopamine in mesolimbic dopaminergic neurones. The

motor complications of long-term therapy with L-DOPA are particularly disabling (Box 10.4). The pathogenesis of late complications is only partly understood. They occur in 75–80% of patients who have received L-DOPA for more than 4–5 years, and can occur in patients who have received it for less time than this. They do not appear immediately after initiation of L-DOPA therapy, but require chronic exposure to L-DOPA, with intermittent dosing. Dyskinesias can be subdivided into chorea-like movements (hyperkinetic, purposeless dance-like movements) and dystonias (intense and sustained muscle contractions). Peak-dose dyskinesia and wearing-off dystonias are due to fluctuations in the level of dopamine produced intracerebrally after each dose of L-DOPA. The 'on–off' effect refers to dramatic fluctuations in motor performance, which are not always related to the intake of L-DOPA. Patients experience normal mobility ('on') followed suddenly by total 'freezing' ('off'). This has been likened to switching a light on and off. A majority of patients treated with L-DOPA for several years also experience an increasingly rapid wearing-off of the clinical benefit after each dose of precursor (also called 'end-of-dose deterioration'). This may be due to the altered pharmacokinetics of L-DOPA, with exacerbations of peaks and troughs in the concentration of dopamine produced, and changes in the sensitivity of dopaminergic receptors. In patients with marked motor fluctuations, benefit may be derived from controlled-release forms of

L-DOPA/carbidopa or L-DOPA/benserazide. Their bio-availability is 70–80% that of normal L-DOPA/carbidopa or L-DOPA/benserazide combinations. In extreme cases, L-DOPA may also be administered continuously by the intravenous or intraduodenal routes. Surgical intervention may also be attempted to relieve L-DOPA-induced dyskinesia and dystonia (see below). Furthermore, several new drugs are at present under development to specifically treat L-DOPA-induced dykinesias. These include α$_2$-receptor antagonists, glutamate receptor antagonists (acting at 4-amino-3-hydroxy-5-methyl-4-isoxazole propionic acid (AMPA), N-methyl-D-aspartate (NMDA) and metabotropic glutamate receptors), 5-HT$_{1A}$ receptor antagonists and D$_4$ receptor antagonists. If proven successful, they may make the benefit of L-DOPA prescription less short-lived.

Dopaminergic agonists

Dopamine agonists, such as bromocriptine, pergolide, lisuride, pramipexole and ropinirole, can be used when adequate control of the symptoms can no longer be achieved with L-DOPA/carbidopa, or significant unwanted effects of this combination (dystonia and dyskinesia) have developed. A significant number of patients may improve on dopaminergic agonists alone, especially at the beginning of the disease. The early introduction of dopaminergic agonists might be beneficial in delaying the onset of dyskinesia and 'on–off' effects seen with L-DOPA. These agents do not have the same efficacy as L-DOPA, so ultimately L-DOPA must be prescribed. Dopamine agonists can induce nausea and vomiting, which can be treated with domperidone. They can also induce hallucinations, cardiac arrhythmias and postural hypotension. Their potential for causing dyskinesia and dystonia is much less than that of L-DOPA/carbidopa (Fig. 10.10). Agonists with longer half-lives, such as cabergoline (Table 10.4), appear to be the best, and avoid the peaks and troughs in plasma concentration seen with short-acting compounds such as L-DOPA and other agonists. A pulsatile profile of stimulation of receptors is considered to be at least partly responsible for the onset of dyskinesias after the administration of short-acting compounds. Apomorphine is an agonist that can be used subcutaneously (intermittent or continuous administration) in patients who experience major loss of efficacy of L-DOPA. Agonists in clinical use at present do not discriminate between D$_1$ and D$_2$ receptors, or have a slightly higher affinity for D$_2$ receptors. New agonists (e.g. cabergoline) also have affinity for D$_3$ receptors. Rotigotine is an agonist which can be used transdermally and thus provide continuous drug delivery and added pharmacokinetic benefit compared to agents that need to be taken orally several times a day.

Monoamine oxidase B inhibitors

MAO$_B$ is an isoform of monoamine oxidase that is involved in dopamine metabolism (see Fig. 10.10). The inhibition of MAO$_B$ by selegiline (alternative name deprenyl) can increase the levels of dopamine, and may also protect against xenobiotics that may be converted

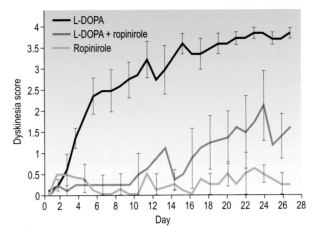

Fig. 10.10 Dyskinesia in 1-methyl-4-phenyl-1,2,3,6-tetrahydropyridine (MPTP)-treated monkeys. Frequency of dyskinesia in MPTP-treated marmosets treated with L-DOPA, ropinirole, or L-DOPA with ropinirole. Note the significantly higher dyskinesia score in L-DOPA-treated animals. After Olanow et al. Trends in Neurosciences 2000; 23(10 Suppl): S120.

Table 10.4 Half-life of dopaminergic drugs

L-DOPA/carbidopa	1–1.5 h
Bromocriptine	12–15 h
Pergolide	7–16 h
Ropinirole	6–8 h
Pramipexole	8–12 h
Cabergoline	>24 h

into neurotoxic species, in a manner similar to MPTP (see above). MAO$_B$ inhibitors are used as adjunctive therapy. Used in conjunction with L-DOPA, selegiline allows dose reduction and prolongation of the duration of action of L-DOPA. It can be used as monotherapy only at a very early stage of the disease.

Non-dopaminergic medication

Anticholinergic agents

Anticholinergic medication is used in order to redress the dopamine–acetylcholine imbalance that may develop in the parkinsonian striatum. Dopamine exerts an inhibitory effect on striatal cholinergic cells. Its loss leads to cholinergic hyperactivity. Antimuscarinic agents, such as benzhexol, benztropine, procyclidine and orphenadrine, are particularly effective in reducing tremor. They produce only minor improvement in bradykinesia. Their side effects include dry mouth, difficult micturition, constipation and confusion. Their use is problematic in the elderly.

Amantadine

Amantadine was initially developed as an antiviral compound, and its antiparkinsonian effects were discovered

Surgery in Parkinson's disease (or finding the right answers through trial and error)

Surgical intervention was relatively common in the management of Parkinson's disease before the introduction of L-DOPA. In 1930, Polack and Davis performed posterior rhizotomies (cutting of sensory nerve roots), which led to some improvement in rigidity but no improvement in tremor. Later on, Bucy excised Brodmann's cortical area 4, which led to decreased tremor but was accompanied by contralateral hemiparesis. In the 1950s, lesions to the caudate, ansa lenticularis and pallidum led to reduction in tremor and rigidity in 40–70% of patients, but with high mortality rates. In 1952, while attempting a pedunculotomy in a parkinsonian patient, Cooper damaged and then ligated the anterior choroidal artery. This led to reduction in tremor and rigidity, which was attributed to an ischaemic lesion in the medial pallidum, the ansa and the fasciculus lenticularis, and the ventrolateral nucleus of the thalamus. This focused attention on two important targets for lesioning or stimulation: the thalamus and the medial pallidum. Benabid in the mid-1990s showed that stimulation of the subthalamic nucleus was an equally interesting approach. In recent years, continuing advances in stereotaxic procedures, brain imaging and electrophysiological recording have gradually made surgery much more precise and accurate, and have considerably reduced the morbidity and mortality associated with such procedures.

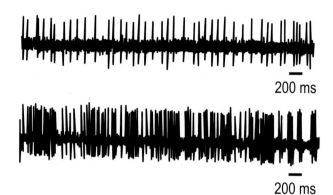

Fig. 10.11 Changes in neuronal activity after experimental nigrostriatal lesion: firing of neurones in control rats (top) and rats whose nigrostriatal projections are lesioned unilaterally with 6-hydroxydopamine (bottom). Note that the lesion changes the spiking activity from a regular pattern of discharge to bursting activity. After Hirsch et al. Trends in Neurosciences 2000; 23(10 Suppl): S83.

later, by serendipity. It appears to increase dopamine release, and it can inhibit dopamine uptake and block NMDA glutamate receptors. It is well absorbed and has a half-life of approximately 24h. Its efficacy is moderate. Its side effects include confusion, hallucinations, nightmares, ankle oedema and livedo reticularis (an erythematous rash of the lower extremities).

Other strategies

Surgical intervention

Surgical procedures were attempted for the first time in PD in the early years of the 20th century (Box 10.6). The introduction of L-DOPA therapy led to a relative loss of interest in surgical intervention. However, in recent years there has been a renewed interest in this approach, and it has been playing an increasingly important role in the management of advanced PD, especially in patients with motor complications due to treatment.

The rationale for such treatment is offered by the alterations in neuronal firing in the basal ganglia that accompany the degeneration of nigrostriatal neurones. The loss of nigral cells, combined with intermittent stimulation of dopamine receptors, may lead to abnormal firing patterns

in striatal output pathways. There may be reduced activity of neurones in the external part of the globus pallidus, in parallel with a significant increase in the activity of neurones in the substantia nigra pars reticulata, the internal globus pallidus and the subthalamic nucleus. For example, after nigral lesion, neurones in the subthalamic nucleus change their activity from a spiking pattern to a bursting pattern (Fig. 10.11). These abnormalities may underlie parkinsonian symptoms, and also the dyskinesia/dystonia induced by long-term L-DOPA replacement therapy. Stereotactic lesions can be carried out in the thalamus or the internal segment of the globus pallidus. Targeting the thalamus may prove particularly useful in patients with intractable tremor, whereas pallidotomy may alleviate rigidity and L-DOPA-induced dyskinesia/dystonia. Furthermore, the wearing-off and 'on–off' phenomena may also be significantly reduced. Chronic electrical stimulation at various sites in the basal ganglia can also be performed. For example, stimulation of the subthalamic nucleus can induce a depolarizing block of the neurones, and alleviation of rigidity and akinesia. The surgical procedure involves the implantation of an electrode with an exposed tip into the target. The electrode is connected to a wire running beneath the skin to a stimulator placed in the chest. The stimulator can be adjusted externally with a programmer. If a side effect occurs due to electrical stimulation, the stimulation can be reduced. Figure 10.12 illustrates these techniques and the clinical improvement associated with their successful use. The improvement can last for years, and may allow a very significant reduction in the doses of drugs taken by the patient. These surgical treatments are not yet used routinely in large number of patients.

Cell grafts

Considering the localized neurodegeneration in PD, neural grafting would appear to be a particularly well-suited strategy for replacement of the lost dopaminergic cells. Cell

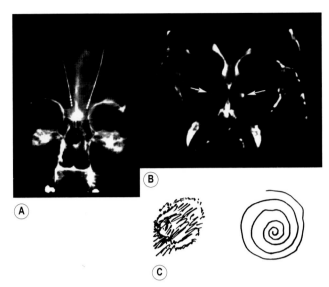

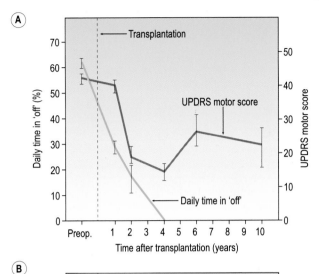

Fig. 10.12 Surgical intervention in Parkinson's disease. (A) Bilateral implantation of electrodes for stimulation in the subthalamic nucleus. (B) Bilateral pallidotomy (arrows indicate the lesions). (Both (A) and (B) courtesy of Dr S. Karanth.) (C) Improvement in handwriting in a patient who received a unilateral thalamic lesion. After Narabayashi C. In Stern G, ed. Parkinson's Disease. The Johns Hopkins University Press, 1990: 609.

Table 10.5	Cell-based therapies in Parkinson's disease
1970–72	Experimental adrenal medulla and fetal nigral cell grafts in the anterior eye chamber
1979	Experimental grafts of fetal nigral cells in animals with nigrostriatal lesions
1985	Adrenal medulla grafts in patients with Parkinson's disease
1988	Fetal nigral grafts in patients with Parkinson's disease
1997	Fetal pig nigral grafts in patients with Parkinson's disease
1998	Experimental grafts of embryonic stem cells in animals with nigrostriatal lesions

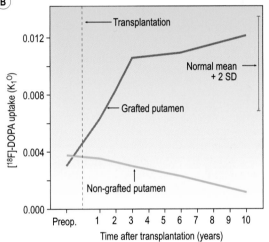

Fig. 10.13 Effect of nigral transplants in PD. (A) Percentage of the day spent in the 'off' phase and motor examination score on the Unified Parkinson's Disease Rating Scale (UPDRS), preoperatively and after intrastriatal grafting. (B) [^{18}F]DOPA uptake before and after transplantation. Note the concomitant increase in [^{18}F]DOPA uptake and the clinical improvement after grafting. After Piccini et al. Nature Neuroscience 1999; 2(12): 1138.

replacement therapies for PD have evolved over the last three decades of the 20th century, as summarized in Table 10.5. In experimental animals, autologous fetal dopaminergic cells transplanted into the striatum survive and adopt a morphology and neurochemical phenotype consistent with dopaminergic reinnervation. Initial attempts in patients involved the use of homografts of adrenal medulla, which contains catecholamine-secreting cells. However, follow-up studies showed poor survival of the grafts, modest clinical improvement accompanied by numerous side effects, and a high level of morbidity and mortality. Human embryonic nigral grafts were tried subsequently, and the accumulated observations so far show that they can lead to significant and long-lasting clinical improvement. Furthermore, positron emission tomography (PET) studies offer evidence

of regulated dopamine release from such grafts. As illustrated in Figure 10.13, in the case of a patient who unilaterally received ventral mesencephalic tissue from four human embryos in the anterior, posterior and middle putamen, clinical improvement was paralleled by improvement in dopamine storage capacity, as reflected in accumulation of DOPA. Furthermore, PET analysis with the use of [^{11}C]raclopride, an *in vivo* marker of D_2 receptors, showed that the endogenous dopamine produced by the graft can be released by agents such as methamphetamine, and thus displace the marker from the receptors, which further confirms the functionality of the graft.

Other grafting attempts have involved the use of dopaminergic xenografts from porcine donors, non-neuronal cells engineered to secrete dopamine-synthesizing enzymes (thus acting as a pump that provides the deficient amine) and, more recently, stem cells. Embryonic stem cells are derived from the blastocyst stage of the embryo, before implantation in the uterus. They are capable of multiple divisions and can differentiate into a variety of cell types, including dopaminergic neurones. After transplantation, stem cells can integrate into the host tissue and differentiate into neurones and glia. Their high plasticity offers enormous potential, but their unrestrained and uncontrolled growth could lead to tumour formation.

The experimental and clinical observations on intracerebral grafts suggest that cells used for transplantation should have the capacity to: (1) grow neurites; (2) establish connections with the appropriate neurones in the host tissue (for example, in PD the grafts are placed ectopically in the striatum); (3) differentiate successfully into dopamine-releasing cells; and (4) resist destruction by any neurotoxic latent process.

Neurotrophic factors

Neurotrophic factors are endogenous substances that control cell proliferation and differentiation in the nervous system. Trophic effects are essential during development, but also at the adult stage, in the immediate aftermath of injury and during regeneration. Many neurotrophic and growth factors are present in the substantia nigra and/or the striatum. Experimental evidence shows that several of these neurotrophic factors support the survival and differentiation of mesencephalic dopaminergic neurones. These factors include epidermal growth factor, basic fibroblast growth factor, brain-derived neurotrophic factor and glial cell line-derived neurotrophic factor. These factors have also been shown to reverse dopaminergic deficits in animal models. However, neurotrophic factors are large molecules, and will not cross the BBB after systemic administration. Direct injection of these factors into the cerebral ventricles or parenchyma is unlikely to become a routine clinical procedure in the near future. An alternative is the cerebral implantation of encapsulated cells engineered to produce and secrete neurotrophic factors. Encapsulation would protect against a host immune response and would counter the danger of abnormal growth.

General management strategy and long-term prognosis in Parkinson's disease

There is no cure at present for PD, as progression of the neurodegenerative process cannot be stopped. The evolution of the disease is highly variable between individuals. Some patients maintain reasonable function 12–15 years into the disease, while others experience rapid worsening of symptoms very early. The current treatments are only symptomatic, but have improved the patients' overall quality of life, especially in the early years of treatment, and have increased average life-expectancy. Patients usually experience improvement in symptoms when L-DOPA therapy is first introduced. The response is relatively stable throughout the day, and this is probably due to the ability of remaining nigrostriatal neurones to produce dopamine from L-DOPA, store it and release it in a relatively physiological manner. In spite of the medication, degeneration continues and disability becomes more severe. This leads to a tendency to increase the dose of dopaminergic drugs. However, the number of nigral residual cells is very small, and the levels of dopamine produced from L-DOPA supplementation will start to fluctuate widely. Patients first notice a much shorter duration of improvement after taking a dose of medication, and also develop peak-dose dyskinesias. At this point, further increasing the doses of drugs leads to more severe dyskinetic episodes, which are not necessarily accompanied by significant improvement in the dyskinesia-free intervals. The importance and complexity of successfully managing a patient who presents with a combination of akinesia and dykinesia cannot be overstated, and the strategies chosen depend on preference and experience of the specialist in charge of the case (see example in Table 10.6). In parallel with pharmacological adjustments, the surgical options are important additional options in such cases.

Some patients develop dementia and also experience major postural problems. Postural imbalance is not improved significantly by drugs, is a cause of morbidity and mortality, and increases the strain on the carers. Dopamine agonists often offer only transient improvement of motor symptoms. In the early phases of the disease, the stigma of tremor may be restrictive and a serious threat to employment. Thus, each aspect of the disease requires careful consideration and specific rehabilitative management. A view that has emerged recently is that the optimum management of young (i.e. <50–60 years) patients and elderly patients may differ. Figure 10.14 offers a possible algorithm of differential treatment to illustrate this point. In particular, the introduction of L-DOPA is delayed as much as possible in younger patients, because L-DOPA-induced dyskinesias and dystonias seem to be more marked in young patients. Therefore, for young patients, symptomatic therapy may be better initiated with a dopamine agonist. Dopamine agonists may adequately control symptoms for several years, after which L-DOPA introduction becomes inevitable. Finally, it is important to stress that the successful management of parkinsonian patients, particularly in the middle and late stages of the disease, involves a multidisciplinary approach, combining medical treatment with physiotherapy, speech therapy and occupational therapy (Table 10.7), and also providing specialist nursing care. In the case presented here, it may have been wiser to delay the introduction of L-DOPA therapy. The complications could be initially treated with a controlled-release L-DOPA preparation, with or without a dopaminergic agonist.

Huntington's disease

Huntington's disease is a neurodegenerative disease associated with a loss of striatal efferent pathways, in particular the early massive loss of striatopallidal followed by loss of striatonigral GABAergic projection neurones. Striatal interneurones are relatively spared. Huntington's disease is

Table 10.6 Treatment recommendations for motor fluctuations and dyskinesias in Parkinson's disease including akinetic crisis

1. End-of-dose deterioration (wearing-off)
Take L-DOPA well before meals (30–60 min)
Add dopamine agonist
Add selegiline
Change to, or add, L-DOPA administration and reduce size of individual doses to avoid overdosage
Take the first L-DOPA dose immediately on rising
Eat a low-protein diet during the day
Take L-DOPA as a dispersible or liquid formulation for early-morning or afternoon akinesia

2. Paroxysmal 'on–off'
See the preceding recommendations on wearing-off
Fewer, higher doses of L-DOPA, however, may be preferable in some patients
Administer apomorphine by subcutaneous intermittent injections or continuous infusion (mini-pump)

3. Peak-dose mobile dyskinesias
Discuss with the patient whether the dyskinesias are an acceptable price to pay for mobility (mild to intermediate dyskinesias often bother the carer more than the patient)
Discuss whether the patient prefers increase of time 'on' with dyskinesia or less time 'on' with less dyskinesia
Suggest intake of drug with meals (may help peak-dose dyskinesias)
Adding a long-acting dopamine agonist should help reduce 'troughs' of dopaminergic stimulation; it may also permit lower doses of L-DOPA to be used, and hence often reduce the severity of dyskinesias
Try controlled-release L-DOPA preparations (peak-dose dyskinesias can increase)
Administer subcutaneous apomorphine by injection or infusion pump
Add amantadine

4. Biphasic dyskinesia
Overlapping doses of L-DOPA and use of controlled-release preparations often result in permanent dyskinetic chaos
May be worsened by protein meals
Take higher doses less often, going through complete cycle to 'off' again before taking next dose

5. Off-period dystonia
Dispersible L-DOPA preparation or apomorphine injection, especially as first dose to get rid of early-morning dystonia
Controlled-release L-DOPA during day or at bedtime
Add agonist during day or at bedtime
Add anticholinergic
Local administration of botulinum toxin in selected cases

6. Akinetic crisis
Intensive care facilities should be available
Ancillary measures: parenteral fluids with electrolyte and caloric substitution, antithrombotic prophylaxis, physiotherapy, skin care
Restart L-DOPA at a slightly lower dose than before and increase gradually to the previous dose over 1–2 days if akinetic crisis is the result of L-DOPA withdrawal
Increase L-DOPA dose by 100–200 mg/daily until response is observed if akinetic crisis is due to underdosing
Administer single injection of apomorphine by subcutaneous continuous infusion (initially 1–2 mg/h; increase by 0.5–1 mg every 12 h with an 8–12 h break at night; maximal daily dose 170–240 mg). If domperidone cover is required, give 20 mg three times daily before staring apomorphine; in emergencies, give 50–60 mg domperidone 30–60 min before apomorphine, if necessary via nasogastric tube

After Oertel and Bandman (1999).

an autosomal-dominant disease due to a mutation in a gene present on the short arm of chromosome 4, which encodes the protein huntingtin. A DNA test can now identify the gene. Individuals at risk can be offered genetic testing, after suitable counselling. Prenatal genetic testing can also be carried out. The onset of the disease is in middle life, and progression to death takes place over 10–12 years. It occurs in 5–10/100 000 of the population. The transmission can occur through parents of either sex, and penetrance is complete.

The function of huntingtin is unknown. The protein is present in all tissues and is essential for life, as homozygous knockout mice are not viable. The mutation leads to an abnormal number of repeats of glutamine (encoded by the codon CAG) in the protein. Interestingly, several other neurological diseases are associated with the expansion of a CAG repeat in the genome. Examples are spinobulbar muscular atrophy, dentatorubropallidoluysian atrophy and different types of spinocerebellar ataxias. Huntingtin (as well as the other proteins containing polyglutamine repeats) can directly interact with transcription factors and thus modify the expression of genes. Curiously, only specific subsets of neurones are vulnerable in each of these diseases, although the relevant proteins are present throughout the brain and other organs.

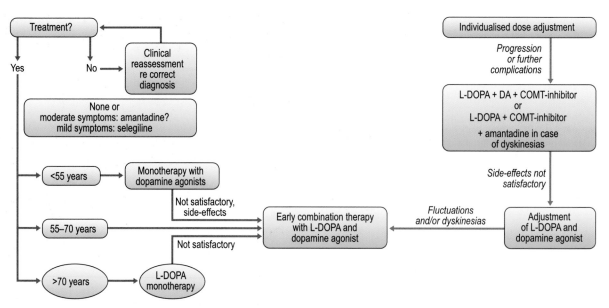

Fig. 10.14 Algorithm for treating akinetic rigid Parkinson's disease patient. COMT, catechol-*O*-methyltransferase; DA, dopamine. Adapted from Braune HJ, Moeler JC, Oertal WH. In Lewitt PA, Oertal WH eds., Parkinson's Disease: The Treatment Options. London: Martin Dunitz, 1999:251

Table 10.7 Motor control deficits and corresponding physical therapy in Parkinson's disease

Motor control deficits	*Corresponding physical therapy*
Truncal stiffness	Exercises involving trunk movements
Mis-scaling of movement amplitude	Use large-amplitude movements
Respiratory complications and impairment	Breathing exercises with relaxation techniques
Slowed gain, stepping cadence	Gait exercises, especially varying walking cadence exercises
Stride length	Rhythmic auditory stimulation
Balance instability, falling	Self-initiated and external perturbations
	Side-to-side rocking motion and facilitation of anterior/posterior motion
	Pre-gait-type activities
Problems with simultaneous and sequential movements	Repetitive practice of functional activities, simultaneous sequencing of different motor programmes, rising from seated position
Impaired prediction of movements, inability to start movements ('freezing')	Rhythmic activities with cueing signals, polysensory cueing
	Selection of proper cueing frequencies
Hastening	Biofeedback and relaxation techniques
Dyskinesia and dystonia	Slow stretching exercises
Tremor	Upper-body karate training
	External damping device for the upper extremity
Speech impairment	Delayed auditory feedback device, prosodic exercises, rhythmic stimulation
Dysphagia	Reclining neck at 60° with head support
Psychological symptoms and problems	Relaxation and cognitive restructuring, training in social skills specifically adapted to Parkinson's disease, teaching programmes for relatives

After Pohl et al. (1999).

The length of the polyglutamine tract varies between individuals. Individuals with more than 40 repeats will almost certainly develop Huntington's disease. The number of repeats is also inversely correlated with age at onset of the disease. The mutation of huntingtin leads to a 'gain of function', which may be ultimately associated with abnormal energy metabolism. Proteins with polyglutamine repeats can aggregate and form fibrils similar to the amyloid β-fibrils in Alzheimer's disease. The mutant protein can be found in the cytoplasm and is also present in large intranuclear inclusions. Striatal projection neurones receive a significant glutamate input from the cortex, so they may be at increased risk of stimulation of glutamate receptors and subsequent uncontrolled rises in cytoplasmic Ca^{2+}, leading to cell death. Therefore, it has been suggested that the loss of cells in the striatum is due to excitotoxicity. The intrastriatal administration of excitatory amino acids, such as kainic acid, ibotenic acid or quinolinic acid, leads to massive striatal neurodegeneration. Agonists at the NMDA glutamate receptor, such as quinolinic acid, injected intrastriatally in experimental models, lead to a pattern of neuropathology that is very similar to the pattern found in Huntington's disease. Mitochondrial poisons, such as 3-nitropropionic acid, which compromise energy metabolism, also lead to striatal degeneration. It cannot be ruled out that metabolic compromise leads to secondary excitotoxicity, through uncontrolled release of glutamate. However, there is still a missing link in the pathophysiology, between the effects of a protein with expanded CAG repeats and the triggering of excitotoxicity at the cellular level.

As illustrated in Figure 10.1C, the loss of striatal efferent pathways leads to disinhibition of the glutamatergic thalamocortical input, and the emergence of abnormal movements that define a very characteristic hyperkinetic syndrome. The patients affected present with chorea, i.e. an involuntary, jerking movement that affects the limbs and the axial muscle groups. Patients try to suppress the movements and incorporate them into more purposeful ones. It is important to note that chorea can be due to a variety of causes. It can be associated with a hereditary disease (e.g. Huntington's disease), but it can also be induced by drugs (e.g. antiparkinsonian drugs and oral contraceptives) or alcohol, or have an immunological or metabolic cause. Sydenham's chorea is post-infectious, and associated with rheumatic fever.

Chorea must be differentiated from hemiballismus, in which movements are more violent and jerky, and affect only one side of the body, as a result of damage to the subthalamic nucleus on the contralateral side. Writhing movements are also associated with athetosis, another dyskinesia. In this case, movements are slower, and reflect gradual transitions from one dystonic posture to another. Athetosis is typically encountered in cerebral palsy.

MRI and CT scanning show that in advanced Huntington's disease there is atrophy of the caudate and putamen, and atrophy of the cerebral cortex. In some cases, the brain weight may be reduced by one-third (Fig. 10.15).

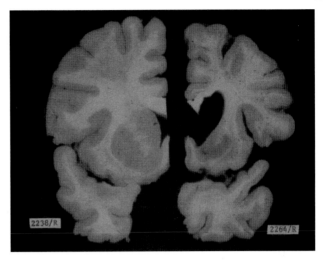

Fig. 10.15 Neurodegeneration in Huntington's disease: brain sections taken through the caudate putamen of a normal patient (left) and a Huntington's disease patient. The Huntington disease hemisphere on the right shows degeneration of the caudate nucleus adjacent to the lateral ventricle, which has enlarged in response to striatal atrophy. From Alexi et al. Progress in Neurobiology 2000; 60: 435.

The loss of striatal efferent pathways appears to lead to dopaminergic hyperactivity. Antidopaminergic medication, e.g. dopaminergic antagonists such as haloperidol or chlorpromazine, can alleviate the symptoms. Depletion of vesicular amine stores in dopaminergic terminals, by drugs such as tetrabenazine, may also help. Many patients develop depression, which responds to antidepressant medication (e.g. tricyclic antidepressants).

Huntington's disease is an irreversible neurodegenerative disease, and in the last stages of the disease cardiovascular and respiratory complications due to increased debility are a common cause of death. One of the possible strategies for treating this disease is based on the principle of inhibition of expression of the mutant allele. However, inhibition of the mutant allele must not disrupt in parallel the expression of the normal allele, which is required for development. Antigene (i.e. blockade of transcription) or antisense oligonucleotide (blockade of translation) strategies have been tried experimentally, but have so far had limited success. It remains to be seen whether an antisense-based approach can be effective in humans. The nature of the degenerative process in Huntington's disease has also led to much research on cell replacement strategies, as has happened with PD. For recovery of normal movement, complete restoration of striatal efferent circuits is required. Fetal striatal cells are commonly used for transplantation in animal models of Huntington's disease. Encouraging results have led to trials in patients, with autografts or xenografts (porcine donors). There is preliminary evidence that grafts of fetal striatal cells implanted in the striatum of patients with Huntington's disease may survive and lead to long-lasting cognitive and motor improvement. This offers new hope for the treatment of this devastating disease.

STROKE AND HEAD INJURY

Chapter objectives

After studying this chapter you should be able to:

1. Define the terms ischaemia, stroke, infarction, thrombus, atherosclerosis, embolism, intracerebral haemorrhage, subarachnoid haemorrhage, aneurysm, arteriovenous malformation and transient ischaemic attack.

2. Describe the main arterial circulation of the brain.

3. Describe the venous drainage of the brain.

4. Define autoregulation and the factors that affect brain blood flow.

5. Describe the mechanisms of cell damage that occur in cerebrovascular accident.

6. Relate the main cortical functional regions to the arterial system and recognize symptoms associated with damage to major brain arteries.

7. Recognize the main vascular structures in angiograms.

8. Define coma, concussion, raised intracranial pressure and mass effect.

9. Describe the main pathophysiological mechanisms in traumatic head injury.

10. Describe treatment strategies for stroke and head injury.

Introduction

The blood supply to the brain provides it with oxygen, nutrients and a means to excrete metabolic waste. If the blood supply is interrupted in any way, then devastating consequences can ensue. The brain has an intense metabolism, and the capacity for anaerobic metabolism is minimal; interruption of the oxygen supply for a few minutes can cause irreversible damage. The vascular system is a supporting system, and diseases of vascular origin will cause secondary alterations in other neural systems. Vascular disease is often identified by its characteristic temporal profile of sudden onset, with rapid appearance of specific combinations of neurological symptoms.

A stroke or cerebrovascular accident is characterized by a temporary, or permanent, loss of function of brain tissue caused by interruption of the vascular supply. Stroke is the third leading cause of death after heart disease and cancer. It is most often due to disease or trauma. In the UK, someone has a stroke every 5 min and approximately 150 000 people have a stroke each year with

64 000 dying from stroke. In the USA, there are 550 000 strokes per year with 160 000 deaths. The incidence and mortality rate are higher in older patients. Of patients who have had their first stroke, 24% will die within a month and 42% within a year; the mortality rate increases with subsequent strokes. Of those who survive, one-third make a good recovery and another one-third to one-half are disabled, requiring some form of care; there are about 350 000 people with stroke-related disabilities in the UK. The cost of stroke to the National Health Service in the UK is estimated to be over £2.3 billion ($25 billion in the USA), and this is expected to rise by about 30% over the next 20 years. Currently, stroke patients occupy approximately 20% of all acute hospital beds and 25% of long-term beds. Brain infarctions account for 75% of strokes, and cerebrovascular accidents such as subarachnoid or intracerebral haemorrhages account for a further 15%.

Head (or traumatic brain) injury accounts for about 1% of deaths in developed countries, one-third of all trauma deaths and up to one-half of road traffic accident-related deaths. It is, like stroke, a common cause of death and disability. In the USA, up to half a million people suffer traumatic brain injury each year. In the UK, for every 100 survivors, 60% make a good recovery, 20% have minor psychiatric/psychological problems, 15% are severely disabled and 5% remain in a persistent vegetative state. The mortality rate is 20–30 people per 100 000. There is much overlap in the neurological symptoms presented by patients with head injury and those with cerebrovascular disease.

This chapter describes the vascular supply to the brain and how it is visualized using angiography. Following stroke injury, it is important to identify the type of stroke, minimize its size and evaluate what treatment options are available to either prevent the problem from reoccurring or to maximize recovery of function after the event. Similarly, acute head injury management aims to control secondary mechanisms of injury: hypoxia, haemorrhage and raised intracranial pressure.

Box 11.1 Case history

Mr Arthur Attack is a 71-year-old who arrives at Accident and Emergency accompanied by his wife. Mrs Attack says that he had just finished his fried breakfast 2 hours ago and was doing nothing in particular when suddenly, in mid-conversation, he became unable to speak. Arthur appears perfectly aware of his surroundings but is unable to understand anything that his wife or the doctor says to him or writes down for him. Arthur has difficulty in speaking, and when he does speak, the speech is unintelligible. On examination, he is found to weigh 108 kg and is hypertensive. Neurological examination reveals increased reflexes and some weakness of his right arm and face; somatosensation on the right side of his face and arm is also absent. His doctor tells his wife that he has just had a stroke, and he is immediately prescribed a drug called Alteplase (tPA). Ten days later, there has been some improvement in his condition. All sensation has returned and he is now able to understand verbal and written commands. However, he is still unable to speak properly, and the motor symptoms remain.

This case gives rise to the following questions:

1. What are the main causes of stroke?
2. What is the blood supply to the brain?
3. How does the main arterial blood supply relate to the main functional areas of the cerebral cortex?
4. What are the mechanisms underlying cell injury in stroke and how does this influence treatment?
5. What is the prognosis for this patient?

Physiological control of cerebral blood flow

Brain cells are dependent on aerobic metabolism for their survival; if deprived of oxygen for 20 s (anoxia), the brain lapses into unconsciousness as the affected neurones cease electrical activity. This can become irreversible if it extends beyond 5 min. It takes longer for this process to occur in the brainstem and spinal cord. The brain represents approximately 2% of the body weight but uses 20% of the available oxygen and 15% of the cardiac output. Blood flow is about 750 mL/min, and this remains constant throughout the day, whether we are asleep, awake, lying down or standing up. The average blood flow is 50–55 mL/100 g of brain tissue per minute. If this falls to less than 30 mL/100 g per minute, then ischaemia (lack of bloodborne oxygen) ensues, and infarction (tissue cell death) occurs below 20 mL/100 g per minute.

Maintaining a constant blood flow depends on a constant blood perfusion pressure and vascular resistance. The cerebral perfusion pressure is defined as the mean arterial pressure minus the intracranial pressure, rather than cerebral venous pressure. This is because the brain is enclosed within the skull, and it is the pressure within this 'closed box' that is effectively acting on the outside of the arteries and thus is the one that opposes arterial pressure. The cerebral perfusion pressure does not always remain constant, and as mean arterial pressure is closely regulated within narrow ranges, changes must occur in the cerebral vascular resistance to compensate for changes in perfusion pressure. This occurs through mechanisms intrinsic to the brain: when perfusion pressure decreases, vascular pressure decreases; if perfusion pressure increases, so does the resistance. Cerebral blood flow is kept relatively constant by several processes. Metabolic mechanisms involve the action of vasodilating agents such as adenosine, K^+, H^+ and nitric oxide (NO), which regulate arteriole size. Autoregulation is a major homeostatic mechanism whose function is to keep blood flow constant over the pressure range 60–150 mmHg. It is closely related to local metabolic processes, and uses chemical and neurogenic mechanisms to control pressure, the most important being the levels of carbon dioxide and oxygen. Hypoxia or hypercarbia cause an increase in cerebral blood flow, whereas hypocarbia causes a decrease in blood flow, by constricting or relaxing the arteriole smooth muscle. These changes are brought about by alterations in the H^+ concentration in the extracellular fluid compartment surrounding the blood vessels. Another source of autoregulation is the level of intraluminal pressure within the arterioles. Any increase in pressure produces a direct, myogenic response that is sufficient to maintain a steady state of perfusion. These processes are not controlled by the sympathetic nervous system, as drugs that affect blood pressure do not, in general, have any effect on cerebral blood flow.

Too much oxygen can also have deleterious effects on brain cells. Increased levels of extracellular oxygen can lead to the formation of free radical ions, which can damage brain cells by the process of excitotoxicity (see later). Free radicals also destabilize neurotransmitters by changing the tissue pH, and causing them to spontaneously oxidize, which can further exacerbate the toxicity.

Not all areas of the brain are equally active at the same time. Oxygen is shunted around to areas (and cells) that need it most for a particular task at a particular time because they are more metabolically active. For example, there is relatively more blood flow to the motor cortex when someone is performing a motor task. This suggests that blood is shunted around to whichever area needs it. A consequence of this is that areas that are not actively processing information have a decreased blood flow. This observation has led to the development of brain scan techniques that measure regional cerebral blood flow to functionally active areas following injection of a radioactive isotope of the inert gas xenon (^{133}Xe) into an artery. This was the first method used to provide detailed insight into how various brain areas functioned in normal and pathological conditions, because of the direct relationship between blood flow and cellular metabolic activity.

Blood supply to the brain

Blood is supplied to the brain via the anterior and posterior circulations. The anterior circulation supplies supratentorial structures (the cortex and diencephalon), whereas the posterior circulation supplies the structures in the posterior fossa (cerebellum and brainstem). Both circulations initially arise from the aortic arch, but the posterior circulation enters the skull cavity through the foramen magnum, while the anterior circulation enters through the foramen lacerum (Fig. 11.1).

The anterior circulation carries 80% of the blood supply to the brain. It is derived from the internal carotid arteries (ICAs), which branch off from the common carotid arteries and enter the brain cavity through the carotid canal (in the skull vault) to emerge on its interior surface via the foramen lacerum (which is only visible in a dried skull, as in life it is filled with cartilage). The arteries make a series of stepwise turns, passing through the cavernous sinus, before emerging, on each side, next to the optic chiasm, where they divide into their major branches, the middle cerebral artery (MCA) and anterior cerebral artery (ACA). The two anterior cerebral arteries are connected by the anterior communicating artery.

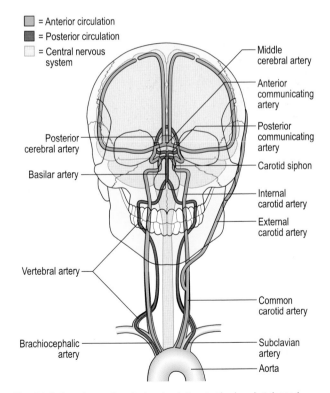

= Anterior circulation
= Posterior circulation
= Central nervous system

Middle cerebral artery
Anterior communicating artery
Posterior communicating artery
Carotid siphon
Internal carotid artery
External carotid artery
Common carotid artery
Subclavian artery
Aorta

Posterior cerebral artery
Basilar artery
Vertebral artery
Brachiocephalic artery

Fig. 11.1 Anterior and posterior circulation to the head. Adapted from McNeill EM. Neuroanatomy Primer, Colour to Learn, Lippincott, Williams and Wilkins, 1997.

The posterior circulation comprises the vertebral, basilar and posterior cerebral arteries (PCAs), and they convey the remaining 20% of the arterial supply to the posterior fossa brain structures and inferior surface of the posterior aspects of the cortex.

The anterior and posterior circulations are connected together at the base of the midbrain around the optic chiasm by a network of arteries called the circle of Willis, first described by Thomas Willis, doctor to King James II, in 1664. The arteries that form the circle of Willis are a single anterior communicating artery, a pair of ACAs, ICAs, PCAs, and a pair of posterior communicating arteries (Fig. 11.2). There is a substantial amount of anatomical variation between individuals in the arrangement of this circle, due to developmental changes. During embryonic development, the ICA supplies the ACA, MCA and PCA, but as the brain develops, the PCA develops from the basilar artery, as the posterior communicating artery atrophies. However, in approximately 20% of people, the embryonic pattern remains and the PCA branches off the anterior circulation. Common variations in the circle of Willis include absence of one or both posterior communicating arteries, origination of the PCAs from an enlarged posterior communicating artery, or multiple small anterior communicating arteries. These anastomoses allow for a certain amount of shunting of blood from the anterior to posterior circulation or from one side to the other in the event of arterial occlusion, but generally the anastomoses are not effective against total occlusion of one of the major supply arteries.

Main terminal branches of the anterior system

The ICA gives rise to several small branches at its proximal portion before dividing into its two main terminal branches, the MCA and ACA. The hypophysial artery forms a plexus around the pituitary stalk. The ophthalmic artery is the most proximal branch of the ICA. It supplies the orbit, the eye muscles and the retina, and eventually connects to the external carotid (facial and superficial temporal) arteries through anastomoses with arteries of the forehead and nose (ethmoidal, nasal, supraorbital and supratrochlear). Occlusion of the ophthalmic artery is an important diagnostic sign in transient ischaemic attacks (Box 11.2). Another artery that is important in providing anastomoses between different arterial systems is the posterior communicating artery, which links the carotid and vertebral systems. Clinically, this is one of the most frequent sites for aneurysm formation, at the junction where it leaves the ICA (see later).

The MCA is the largest and most important branch of the ICA, and receives 80% of the carotid blood flow (Fig. 11.3). Its proximal part gives off three deep branches. The lateral and medial striate arteries supply the striatum and the internal capsule regions of the brain. Occlusion of these deep arteries is the chief cause of classic stroke,

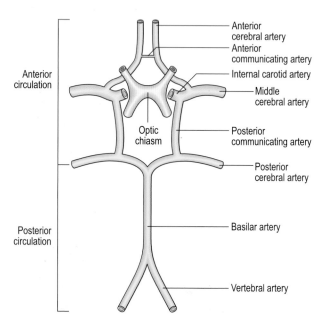

Fig. 11.2 Schematic view of the circle of Willis.

Anterior circulation

Posterior circulation

Anterior cerebral artery
Anterior communicating artery
Internal carotid artery
Middle cerebral artery
Optic chiasm
Posterior communicating artery
Posterior cerebral artery
Basilar artery
Vertebral artery

and the most common location is the putamen and internal capsule. The anterior choroidal artery supplies parts of the limbic system, the hippocampus and amygdala, in the medial temporal lobe, the posterior part of the internal capsule, the optic radiation and the choroid plexus of the inferior horn of the lateral ventricle, which is important in the formation of cerebrospinal fluid (CSF). Occlusion of this artery may cause hemiparesis, hemianaesthesia, hemianopsia and loss of short-term memory.

The more distal part of the MCA travels laterally through the lateral fissure and then separates into superior and inferior branches that supply most of the lateral side of the brain (frontal, parietal, temporal and occipital regions). This ramification is known as the middle cerebral candelabra (from angiographic studies). The branches are named with respect to the cortical region that they supply (see Fig. 11.3).

The ACA supplies the medial side of the frontal and parietal lobes as far back as the parieto-occipital sulcus, and overlaps onto the orbital and lateral surfaces of the brain. It winds around the genu of corpus callosum before dividing into two main terminal branches. The callosomarginal artery supplies the cingulate and frontal gyri and the paracentral lobule (Fig. 11.4). The pericallosal artery supplies the corpus callosum. On the lateral surface of the brain, its branches anastomose with terminal branches of the MCA. The ACA gives off one proximal branch, the recurrent artery of Heubner, which supplies the ventral part of the basal ganglia and the anterior limb of the internal capsule. It anastomoses with the lateral striate arteries of the MCA. Occlusion of this artery is rare but can cause 'clumsy hand' syndrome, with contralateral weakness of the arm and face.

Main terminal branches of the posterior system

The vertebral arteries are derived from the subclavian and brachiocephalic arteries and pass through the transverse foraminae of the C1–C6 vertebrae before entering the skull cavity via the foramen magnum to travel along the ventral surface of the brainstem. The main branches

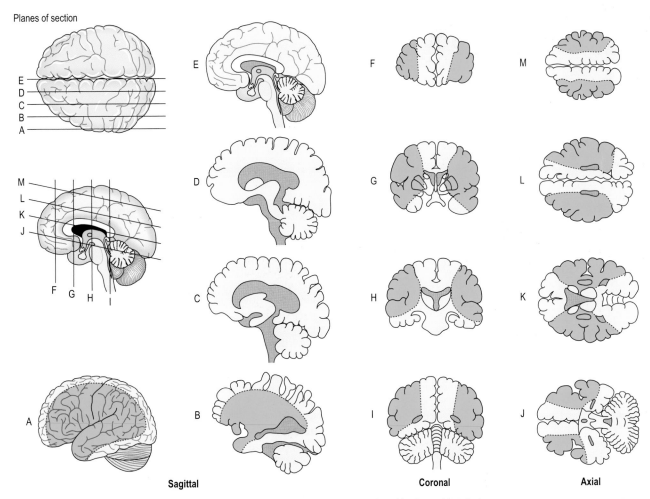

Planes of section

Sagittal   Coronal   Axial

Fig. 11.3 Distribution of the middle cerebral artery in the sagittal (A–E), coronal (F–I) and horizontal (J–M) planes.

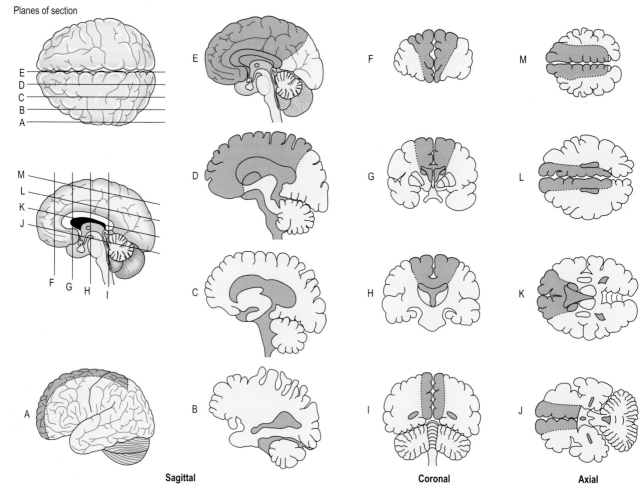

Planes of section

Sagittal　　　　Coronal　　　　Axial

Fig. 11.4 Distribution of the anterior cerebral artery in the sagittal (A–E), coronal (F–I) and horizontal (J–M) planes.

are the anterior and posterior spinal arteries, which supply the spinal cord (see Chapter 4), and the posterior inferior cerebellar artery, which supplies the medulla and cerebellum. The two vertebral arteries join to form the basilar artery at the pontomedullary junction. The basilar artery runs in the basilar sulcus on the ventral surface of the pons and ends at the midbrain, where it divides to form the PCA, which travels along the ventral surface of the midbrain, passing around cranial nerve III, to anastomose with the posterior communicating artery. The details of the blood supply to the brainstem are described in Chapter 6. The deep cortical branches of the PCA supply the thalamus and posterior limb of the internal capsule (via the thalamogeniculate and posterior choroidal arteries). Other branches supply the inferior and medial surfaces of the temporal lobe (limbic region) and the occipital lobe. The main terminal branches are the calcarine and parieto-occipital arteries. Terminal branches of the PCA extend onto the lateral surface of the brain to anastomose with terminal branches of the MCA (Fig. 11.5).

Venous system

The cerebral drainage is through valveless superficial and deep veins (Fig. 11.6). The superficial veins are located in the subarachnoid space above each hemisphere; they collect blood from the neocortex and subcortical white matter, and empty into the cranial venous sinuses. The upper part of the hemisphere drains via the superior cerebral vein into the superior sagittal sinus, the middle part (via the inferior cerebral veins) into the cavernous sinus, and the lower part into the transverse sinus. The deep cerebral veins that drain blood from the caudate nucleus and thalamus (thalamostriate and choroidal veins) join to form the internal cerebral vein on each side, and these unite to form the great cerebral vein of Galen. The anterior and deep cerebral veins unite to form the basal vein, which also empties into the great cerebral vein. This pierces the tentorium cerebelli to join with the inferior sagittal sinus, which drains the falx cerebri, and then joins with the straight sinus that connects to the transverse sinus.

Planes of section

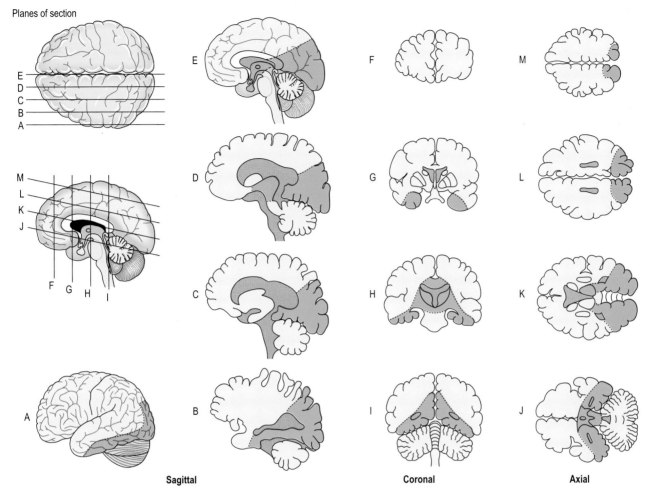

Sagittal   **Coronal**   **Axial**

Fig. 11.5 Distribution of the posterior cerebral artery in the sagittal (A–E), coronal (F–I) and horizontal (J–M) planes.

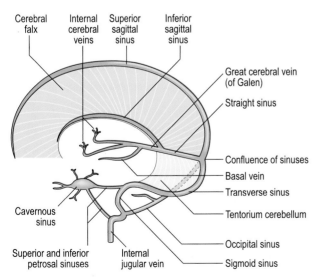

Fig. 11.6 Schematic plane of the cerebral venous circulation.

The cavernous sinus drains into the transverse sinuses via the petrosal sinuses. The two transverse, the straight and the superior sagittal sinuses meet at the confluence of sinuses. Blood drains away 'downhill' through the transverse sinuses to the sigmoid sinus and into the internal jugular vein (at the jugular foramen). The internal jugular vein receives venous drainage from the face, scalp and neck before draining into the subclavian vein and returning to the heart via the brachiocephalic vein and superior vena cava.

Functional anatomy of the cerebral vasculature

Any brain dysfunction of vascular origin will result in certain clinical signs and symptoms. Thus, it is essential to have a clear understanding of how the blood supply relates to the functional areas of the brain. This is shown

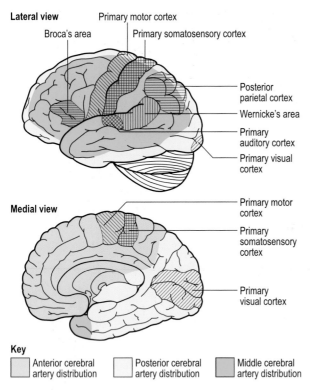

Lateral view

Broca's area

Primary motor cortex

Primary somatosensory cortex

Posterior parietal cortex

Wernicke's area

Primary auditory cortex

Primary visual cortex

Medial view

Primary motor cortex

Primary somatosensory cortex

Primary visual cortex

Key

☐ Anterior cerebral artery distribution

☐ Posterior cerebral artery distribution

☐ Middle cerebral artery distribution

Fig. 11.7 Distribution of the main cerebral arteries with respect to major functional cortical areas.

Table 11.1 Functional areas associated with the main cerebral arteries

Cerebral artery	Cortical area
Anterior cerebral	Paracentral lobule: primary motor cortex and primary somatosensory cortex regions (hip to feet) Supplementary motor area (movement) Prefrontal and orbitofrontal cortex (cognition and emotion) Corpus callosum Septal nucleus (pleasure)
Middle cerebral	Frontal lobe: primary motor cortex (hip to head), premotor area, frontal eye field Parietal cortex: primary somatosensory cortex (hip to head), primary taste cortex Temporal lobe: primary auditory cortex (hearing), primary olfactory cortex (smell) Basal ganglia (movement initiation) Optic radiation (vision) Uncus (emotion) Dominant hemisphere: language centres—Wernicke's area (receptive speech) and Broca's area (expressive speech) Non-dominant hemisphere: contralateral awareness of self and surroundings
Posterior cerebral	Visual cortex (primary and association) Hippocampus (long-term memory) Thalamus Hypothalamus (autonomic function)

in Figure 11.7 and Table 11.1. It is essential to be able to distinguish whether a vascular lesion is located within the anterior or the posterior arterial systems.

Angiography

It is not possible to directly examine the cerebral blood vessels in patients (unless it is at post-mortem!). Instead, angiography is used (Fig. 11.8). This method can detect three different types of abnormality: structural abnormality due to stenosis or occlusion, alteration in blood vessel position (due to displacement by a mass lesion), and alterations in flow patterns such as occur in arteriovenous malformations or during stenosis or partial vessel occlusion (Figs. 11.9, 11.14 and 11.15).

Stroke

Stroke can be associated with a variety of causes. The risk factors for stroke and their likely effects are detailed in Table 11.2.

There are two main types of stroke: ischaemic and haemorrhagic (Fig. 11.10). Each has a different cause and both can result in infarction, or death, of brain tissue. Ischaemic stroke occurs when a blood clot blocks an artery, disrupting the bloodborne supply of oxygen to the brain, and it results in non-mass lesions. It can result from stenosis or thrombosis of the arteries, or from the presence of thromboemboli in arteries. Atherosclerosis is the most important cause of ischaemic stroke (Box 11.3).

Stenosis is narrowing of an artery due to build-up of plaque material so that blood flow is restricted. If 50% of the normal blood pressure is not maintained, then brain damage will occur. Very often, an ischaemic stroke is the result of a build-up of cholesterol and other debris in the arteries over many years. Thrombosis refers to the total blockage of a main brain artery by a blood clot (thrombus), plaque or embolus. A thromboembolism is a piece of plaque that has broken off from a thrombus elsewhere in the body, e.g. the heart, and travels through the arterial system until it lodges in a brain artery, cutting off the supply beyond this point. If this occurs in the small blood vessels deep within the brain, the type of stroke is termed a lacunar stroke. The infarcts produced by this type of stroke are small (0.5–10 mm). Lacunar infarcts can also occur in the brainstem.

Classification of stroke

Stroke can be classified as stroke in evolution, where progression of neurological defects occurs over 24–48 h, suggesting an ongoing infarct, or completed stroke, where

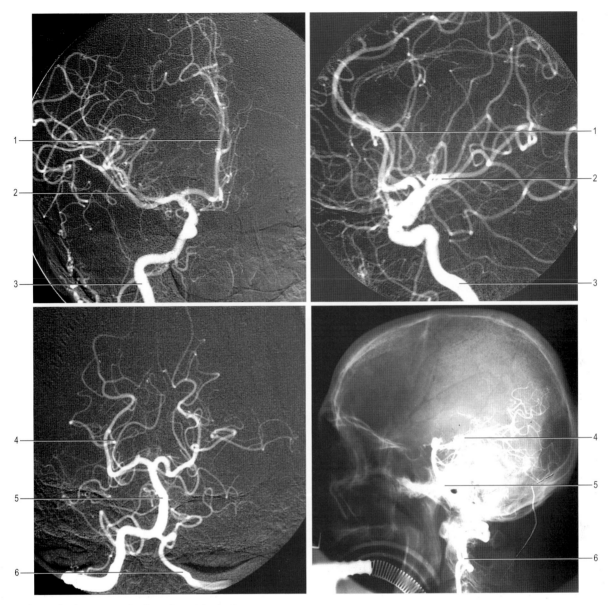

1. Anterior cerebral artery.
2. Middle cerebral artery.
3. Internal carotid artery.
4. Posterior cerebral artery.
5. Basilar artery.
6. Vertebral arteries.

Fig. 11.8 Normal angiogram of anterior (top pair) and posterior (bottom pair) circulations viewed in coronal (left) and sagittal (right) planes.

infarction is complete and the patient's neurological deficits do not increase further. The latter is the most common type seen. The term stroke is apt because of its distinct temporal profile; for most sufferers, the symptoms come on literally 'at a stroke'. The key symptoms include a sudden numbness, weakness or paralysis on one side of the body. Signs of this may be a drooping arm, leg or eyelid, or a dribbling mouth, sudden slurred speech, difficulty in finding words or understanding speech, sudden blurring, disturbance or loss of vision, especially in one eye, dizziness, confusion, unsteadiness and/or a severe headache.

The effects of a stroke vary enormously, depending on which part of the brain is damaged and the extent of that damage, which in turn depends on which vessel is affected. Classification is based on artery territory, and there are four main syndromes that correspond to different vascular territories:

1. total anterior circulation stroke that results from occlusion of the MCA with or without the ACA

2. partial anterior circulation stroke that results from occlusion of branches of the MCA or isolated ACA occlusion

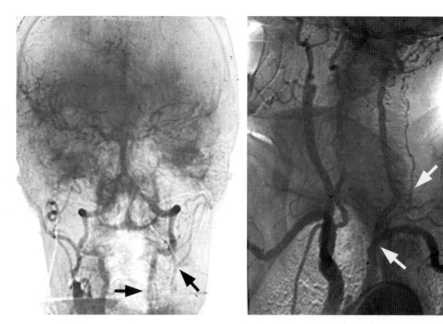

Fig. 11.9 Angiogram showing occlusion of the left common carotid artery (black arrows) and left vertebral artery (white arrows) caused by atheroma.

3. posterior circulation stroke affecting the brainstem, cerebellum or occipital lobe

4. lacunar stroke produced by occlusion of the deep brain (thalamostriate) arteries.

The symptoms associated with each type of stroke are detailed in Table 11.3.

The second main type of stroke is haemorrhagic stroke, when a blood vessel in or around the brain bursts, causing a bleed or haemorrhage within the skull cavity. Long-standing, untreated hypertension is the most common cause of this type of stroke. Intracranial arteries differ from those found elsewhere in the body, in that they are thin-walled and susceptible to blockage or rupture. Thus, untreated hypertension increases the strain on the artery walls, increasing the risk of bursting and bleeding. Onset is sudden, without warning, usually while the patient is awake. Headache is often present but is not a diagnostic feature. Loss of consciousness is also common.

There are several types of haemorrhagic stroke (see Fig. 11.10):

1. A haemorrhagic stroke may be due to an intracerebral haemorrhage, in which a blood vessel bursts within the brain itself. The blood may form a haematoma (a pool of congealed blood) within the brain parenchyma (tissue), resulting in a focal mass effect (Fig. 11.13), or in existing spaces such as the subdural or subarachnoid spaces (non-mass effects). Parenchymal haemorrhages occur most frequently in the basal ganglia (50%), thalamus (10%), hindbrain (pons or cerebellum, 20%) or lobular white matter (20%). White matter strokes are often severe and cause extensive neurological deficits by interrupting the passage of axon tracts such as the internal capsule.

2. A subarachnoid haemorrhage occurs when a blood vessel on the surface of the brain bleeds into the subarachnoid space, the area between the brain and the meninges. The most common cause is head injury (see later).

3. An aneurysm is due to a weakness of the thin-walled intima layer of arteries that causes a localized dilatation of the artery lumen. Blood collects in these 'berry-like' swellings, called Berry aneurysms. They often occur in the circle of Willis (Fig. 11.14). Eventually, as the pressure builds, the aneurysm bursts and bleeds into the subarachnoid space, causing an increase in intracranial pressure, which can be fatal if not treated. Also, the filling of the aneurysm balloon can lead to raised intracranial pressure by a mass effect that may cause brain damage. Normally, aneurysms go undetected and they are akin to ticking time-bombs. They may be fortuitously detected in angiograms that are being performed for other reasons. If detected, they may be clipped during a neurosurgical operation (see Fig. 11.14). The classic presentation of a burst aneurysm is a sudden, severe headache, neck stiffness and vomiting, and loss of consciousness. Often, there are focal neurological signs.

4. Arteriovenous malformations are congenital abnormalities that result from defective developmental communications between arteries and veins without the intervening capillaries. They appear in angiograms as a Medusa-like tangle of

Table 11.2 Risk factors for stroke

Risk	Consequence
Untreated hypertension	Damages arterial walls
Atrial fibrillation	Increased risk of formation of clots in the heart that may dislodge and travel to the brain (irregular heartbeat)
Smoking	Increases blood pressure and has adverse effects on arterial walls
Diabetes	Increased risk of high blood pressure and atherosclerosis
Diet	Diets high in saturated fat lead to arterial stenosis, high salt levels and raised blood pressure
Heavy drinking	Over time, excessive drinking raises blood pressure; alcohol binges can rapidly increase blood pressure, causing blood vessels to burst
Age	Strokes are more common in people older than 55 years of age, probably because atherosclerosis takes a long time to develop and arteries become less elastic with increasing age
Gender	Men are at greater risk than women, especially if aged less than 65 years
Family history	Having a close relative with a history of stroke increases the risk, as factors such as diabetes and high blood pressure have a genetic component
Contraceptive pills	Make blood more likely to clot and/or raise blood pressure
Genetic	Complex interaction between genes and environmental cues. Candidate genes include angiotensin-converting enzyme, endothelial nitric oxide synthase, apolipoprotein E and β-fibrinogen
Haematological disorders	Thrombocytosis (platelet disorder that may predispose to cerebral ischaemia). Polycythemia (increases number of blood cells, leading to blood thickening). Haemophilia (blood thinning prevents it from coagulating). Sickle cell disease (causes thrombosis in young black people). Hyperuricaemia (gout; increased uric acid in the blood that may precipitate in blood and block the blood vessel)
Drug abuse	Amphetamine or cocaine abuse leads to a rapid rise in blood pressure (minutes to hours); most haemorrhages are in the subcortical white matter
Vascular inflammatory disorders	Giant cell arteritis. Systemic lupus erythematosus (inflammatory changes stimulate platelet adhesion on damaged surfaces)
Ethnic background	Asians, Africans and Afro-Caribbeans have a higher risk; this is linked to other risk factors such as high blood pressure (Africans) and diabetes (Asians)
Previous transient ischaemic attack (TIA)	20% of patients with TIA will go on to have a full-blown stroke

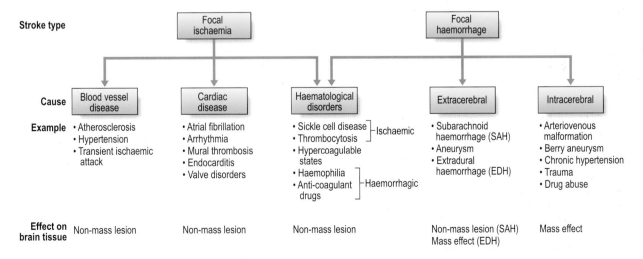

Fig. 11.10 Causes of ischaemic and haemorrhagic stroke.

Box
11.3   Atherosclerosis

Atherosclerosis is the most important cause of ischaemic stroke. It is a generalized vascular disease of unknown aetiology that tends to primarily affect large-calibre blood vessels such as the carotid arteries (at their bifurcation points) and the circle of Willis at the junction of the internal carotid artery and middle cerebral artery and vertebral and basilar arteries (Fig. 11.11).

The basic pathological lesion is the atherosclerotic plaque. Damage to the intima layer of the arterial cell wall produces focal desquamation, exposing the underlying connective tissue to circulating platelets. These aggregate and stick to the arterial wall. Aggregation causes platelets to secrete substances that, in conjunction with certain lipids, react to form a fibrous plaque that projects into the arterial lumen. With further arterial damage, this process is repeated and the plaque enlarges, causing stenosis of the vessel (Fig. 11.12).

Because the plaque slows blood flow, a secondary consequence of this process is a thrombus that may form on the plaque. A thrombus is formed by platelets and fibrin sticking together via interactions with clotting factors that convert soluble fibrinogen to insoluble fibrin. Thrombus formation is particularly likely in veins where blood flow rate is slower and blood pressure is lower; in addition, the presence of valves provides pockets of stagnant flow. Anything that causes hypercoagulation of the blood, such as inherited protein C or S deficiency or increased amounts of clotting factor VII or fibrinogen (as occurs in pregnancy or after surgery), increases the risk of thrombosis. If an embolus then breaks off a thrombus, it can become lodged in a distal vessel. The combination of changes in the vascular wall, reduced blood flow and increased blood coaguability are known as Virchow's triad.

Drugs such as aspirin or drugs that selectively inhibit the enzyme thromboxane synthase (which converts prostaglandin H_2 to thromboxane A_2, a potent platelet aggregator and vasoconstrictor) or stimulate the production of endothelial prostacyclins (which dilate blood vessels) are useful in preventing thromboembolism complications in atherosclerotic stroke.

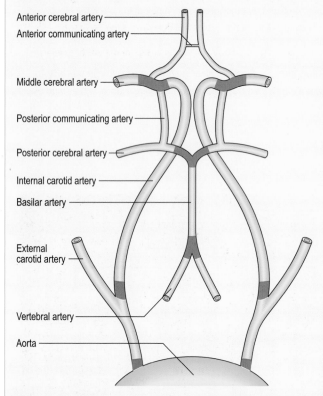

Anterior cerebral artery

Anterior communicating artery

Middle cerebral artery

Posterior communicating artery

Posterior cerebral artery

Internal carotid artery

Basilar artery

External carotid artery

Vertebral artery

Aorta

Fig. 11.11 Locations of severe atherosclerotic blockage of the anterior and posterior circulations.

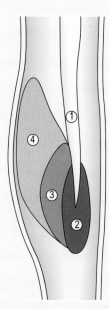

1. Tear in intima wall.
2. Formation of atheromatous plaque by circulating platelets.
3. Emboli settle on the plaque to form a mural thrombus.
4. Blood dams up behind the occlusive thrombus to form a stagnant thrombus.

Fig. 11.12 Formation of an atherosclerotic plaque.

Table 11.3 Neurological signs associated with stroke in the anterior or posterior arterial circulations

Stroke type	Symptoms
Total anterior circulation (high mortality long-term morbidity rates)	Contralateral flaccid hemiplegia (MCA + ACA) Contralateral hemisensory loss (MCA + ACA) Homonymous hemianopsia (MCA—anterior choroidal) Global aphasia (dominant hemisphere, MCA) Sensory neglect (non-dominant hemisphere, MCA) Dysarthria and dsysphagia (MCA) Incontinence (ACA) Gait apraxia (ACA) Perception difficulties such as prosopagnosia (recognizing familiar objects or knowing how to use them). There may also be problems with abstract concepts such as telling the time Although vision may not be affected directly, it may be difficult for the brain to interpret what the eyes see Cerebral dementia involving cognitive problems such as thinking, learning, concentrating, remembering, decision-making, reasoning and planning (frontal lobes)
Partial anterior circulation	Different combinations of the above deficits, depending on which area is affected. Some of the more common ones are: MCA inferior branches—receptive aphasia, constructional apraxia, expressive aphasia, neglect, perception difficulties; ACA branches—split-brain syndrome (pericallosal artery), dyspraxia
Posterior circulation	Cortical: contralateral homonymous hemianopsia; cortical blindness (visual agnosia); alexia (inability to read); amnesia; disturbances of higher mental function Brainstem: dissociated hemiparesis (ipsilateral face, contralateral body); dissociated hemisensory loss (ipsilateral face, contralateral body); diplopia; dysphagia; dysarthria; vertigo; ataxia
Lacunar	Pure motor hemiparesis (face, arm and leg weakness on one side; no other symptoms except dysarthria; lesion in internal capsule) Pure hemisensory stroke (loss of superficial sensation and paraesthesia of one side of the body; thalamic lesion) Ataxic hemiparesis (distal leg weakness, arm–leg incoordination; Babinski sign and inability to walk unaided; lesion in internal capsule, cerebellum or pons) Dysarthria and clumsy hand syndrome (moderate to severe dysarthria and clumsiness of hand movement and facial weakness on one side; lesion in internal capsule or pons)

MCA, middle cerebral artery; ACA, anterior cerebral artery.

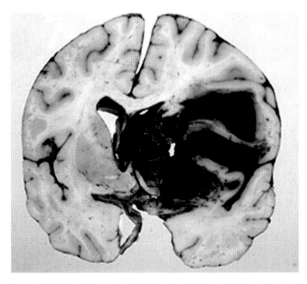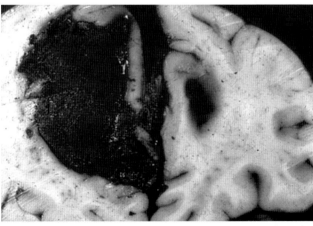

Fig. 11.13 Examples of fatal intracerebral haemorrhage. Left: infarct of the lenticulostriate arteries of the middle cerebral artery. Right: anterior cerebral artery. Both cause death through the consequences of the mass effect (see text for details).

distorted and contorted blood vessels (Fig. 11.15) that may be atrophied, and therefore prone to rupture, or hypertrophic. Often, rapid shunting of blood occurs, producing ischaemia in neighbouring parts of the brain that may result in tissue infarction or seizure activity.

5. Intraventricular haemorrhage is the most common neurological complication in about 40% of premature babies (<1.5 kg body weight). The hypoxic pressure exerted on the baby's head during delivery can cause haemorrhage. The prognosis for large haemorrhages is poor, but for smaller ones it is good. Children may be left with variable degrees of neurological deficit.

Massive haemorrhages may rupture brain tissue and leak into the ventricles, resulting in blood in the CSF. A fatal outcome occurs when brain herniation occurs due to the mass effect of the oedema and haematoma. Clinical presentation depends on the site of haemorrhage. The most common site for hypertensive haemorrhage is in the basal ganglia. The clinical features of hypertensive intracerebral haemorrhage in various brain regions are detailed in Table 11.4.

In the case history presented in Box.11.1, it is likely that Arthur is suffering from atherosclerosis. He has several risk factors that predispose him towards ischaemic stroke: his age, high blood pressure and the fact that he is overweight. His hypertension accelerates the atherosclerotic process and increases the risk of blood vessel damage. Additionally, in older people, the blood vessels have less elasticity, predisposing them to stenosis. The doctor is able to make the diagnosis based on the history (sudden onset) and neurological examination (in this case, it is a partial anterior circulation stroke). Whether the stroke is ischaemic or haemorrhagic cannot be reliably distinguished

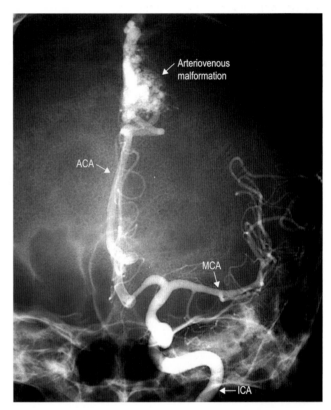

Fig. 11.15 Angiogram showing an arteriovenous malformation located in the anterior cerebral artery (ACA). MCA, middle cerebral artery; ICA, internal carotid artery.

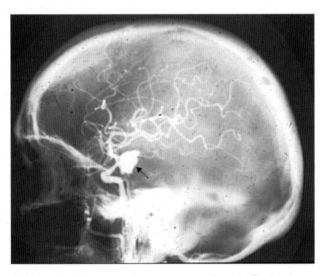

Fig. 11.14 Angiogram revealing an aneurysm (arrow) affecting the posterior cerebral artery.

Table 11.4 Clinical features of hypertensive haemorrhage

Location	Coma	Pupil reaction (to light)	Sensorimotor disturbance	Hemianopsia
Basal ganglia (putamen)	Common	Normal	Hemiparesis	Common
Thalamus	Common	Small, sluggish	Hemisensory loss	Transient
Subcortical white matter	Rare	Normal	Hemiparesis and/or hemisensory loss	Common
Cerebellum	Delayed (12–24 h)	Small, reactive	Gait ataxia	No
Pons (often fatal)	Immediate	Pinpoint, non-reactive	Quadriplegia	No

clinically but, as Arthur did not lose consciousness, it is more likely to be ischaemic. However, there are several tests and investigations that can be performed to confirm the diagnosis. These are detailed in Box 11.4.

Mechanisms of cell injury in ischaemic stroke

The brain has a very high rate of oxidative metabolism. Anaerobic metabolism in the brain is negligible, and as a consequence the brain is extremely vulnerable to hypoxic damage. Cell death occurs in stroke because of anoxia and the resultant loss of ability of the cell to maintain the integrity of the cell membrane through the activity of the energy-dependent ATPase pumps. The pathophysiological consequences of stroke involve a complex sequence of events that evolve over time and space (Fig. 11.16) and set up several vicious circles that ultimately lead to brain

---

Box 11.4 Recognizing and diagnosing stroke

The major signs of stroke can be recognized using the **FAST** system:

F for facial weakness (assessed by asking the person to smile or observation of a drooping face or eyelid)
A for arm weakness; assessed by asking the person raise both arms
S for speech; is the person's speech clear and can they understand what you say?

If the person has failed any of these tests then it is

T time to call the emergency services.

At hospital, a number of investigations can help identify the type of stroke that has occurred and the best treatment options. The precise tests will differ from person to person, but common tests performed in every stroke patient include:

- Blood pressure measurement.
- Blood tests to check blood glucose, blood clotting, cholesterol levels, thyroid function, erythrocyte sedimentation rate, plasma viscosity and the presence of haematological disease.
- Chest X-ray to check for cardiac or respiratory problems.
- An electrocardiogram to measure the rhythm and activity of the heart, or an echocardiogram.
- Brain scans or angiograms to determine the type and location of the stroke and to look for signs of damage. These are the most definitive diagnostic procedures currently available.
- Doppler ultrasound scans of the carotid arteries to check blood flow to the brain.
- Cerebrospinal fluid examination for diagnosing subarachnoid haemorrhage.

---

cell death. The main mechanisms involved include excitotoxicity, inflammation and programmed cell death, and the molecular pathways for these have been extensively studied (Fig. 11.17). The mechanisms involved are different in different areas of the stroke region: at the site of infarct, the core region, hypoxia is most severe and brain tissue rapidly dies. Surrounding the core is an area called the ischaemic penumbra, where there is residual blood flow and where brain cells undergo potentially reversible electrophysiological and metabolic failure. These cells have not yet entered signal cascades that lead to cell death. The size of the penumbra is variable. The importance of this penumbra is that here the cell damage may be reversible, and those drug treatments that block the release and action of excitotoxins may reduce or limit the amount of functional deficit.

When the brain becomes hypoxic, ATP levels start to fall and the ATP-dependent Na^+ pumps in the neuronal and glial cell membranes become dysfunctional. The Na^+ that enters the cells, either during action potentials or because of the ongoing leaks in the membrane, cannot be pumped out, causing membrane depolarization. This creates an inward osmotic force, as the influx of Na^+ (and Cl^-) is much greater than the efflux of K^+, and the cells swell due to the passive influx of water, causing oedema. Cells eventually burst as the cell membrane fails; this is necrotic cell death. The brain is encased in a rigid box, the skull, so if the neurones start to swell, this will increase the intracranial pressure, leading to compression of the ventricles and the cerebral blood vessels. Compression of the blood vessels, especially the veins, reduces the blood flow and hence further decreases the oxygen supply. A vicious circle is set up that leads to a rapid decline in cerebral perfusion. Brain oedema is one of the earliest events in stroke (or head injury), and its magnitude is one of the major factors that determine whether the patient will survive beyond the first few hours.

The reuptake process that removes glutamate from the synaptic cleft and stabilizes glutamatergic transmission is also energy-intensive, and thus requires ATP. As soon as oxygen levels fall and ATP levels decline, the reuptake process slows down. Consequently, glutamate begins to

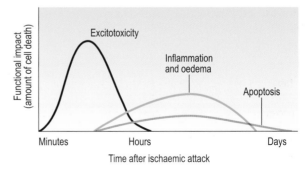

Fig. 11.16 Time course of pathophysiological changes occurring in ischaemic stroke. In the earliest stages, excitotoxic mechanisms damage both neurones and glial cells and contribute to the genesis of inflammation and cell death. Adapted from Dirnagl U. et al. Trends in Neuroscience,1999; 22: 391-7.

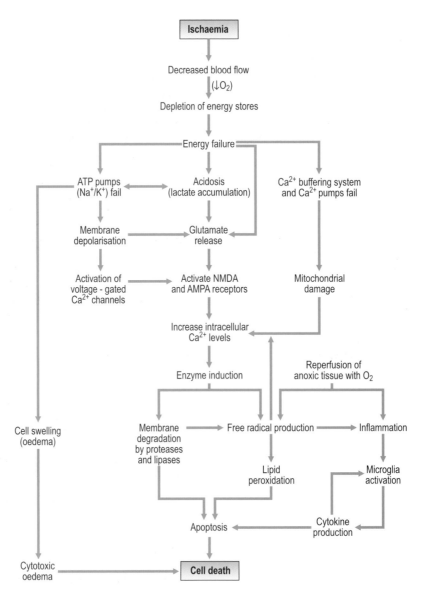

Fig. 11.17 Mechanisms contributing to neurotoxicity in ischaemia. Disruption of normal blood flow results in activation of multiple and complex signal cascades that ultimately result in cell death. The key event is excitotoxicity, leading to increased intracellular Ca^{2+} levels, which result in the generation and activation of free radicals that damage the cells and cause further inflammatory responses. Paradoxically, reperfusion of ischaemic tissue with oxygen can also lead to neuronal damage—reperfusion injury—by causing free radical formation. NMDA, N-methyl-D-aspartate; AMPA, 4-amino-3-hydroxy-5-methyl-4-isoxazole propionic acid. Adapted from De Kayser J. et al. Trends in Neuroscience, 1999; 22: 535-9.

accumulate in the synaptic cleft and, with the associated rise in extracellular K^+, further depolarization of cells may occur. This leads to more hyperexcitability and more glutamate release, and yet another vicious circle.

Activation of the N-methyl-D-aspartate (NMDA) glutamate receptor leads to Ca^{2+} influx into neurones. This receptor is normally tightly regulated by a number of factors, so that Ca^{2+} entry into neurones is closely controlled. Excessive extracellular glutamate levels lead to prolonged neuronal depolarization via 4-amino-3-hydroxy-5-methyl-4-isoxazole propionic acid (AMPA) receptors, which in itself is not harmful. However, the depolarization of the postsynaptic cell also activates the NMDA receptor

(which is held inactive at normal resting potentials by an Mg^{2+} block of the receptor), which in turn leads to further Ca^{2+} entry. This is where critical processes are triggered, due to Ca^{2+} overload as the Ca^{2+} buffering systems of neurones, the mitochondria and endoplasmic reticulum, fail. The rise in internal Ca^{2+} level activates many second messenger systems, which all demand energy in the form of ATP or other substrates. However, because of hypoxia, this energy is not available. Disruption of neuronal Ca^{2+}-induced processes leads to the formation of free radicals, such as the superoxide anion (O_2^-), via the activation of NO production (Box 11.5). These free radicals are very reactive and initiate cell damage by reacting with many cell components

Box 11.5 The enigmatic role of nitric oxide in stroke

Nitric oxide (NO) is produced from arginine via the enzyme nitric oxide synthase (NOS). NO is a powerful vasodilator of blood vessels. The well-known therapeutic actions of nitrates or nitrites given to angina sufferers are due to their vasodilator action on coronary arteries. NO has been found to be a vasodilator of cerebral blood vessels, and NOS is found in the endothelial cells lining cerebral blood vessels. Blockade of NO synthesis reduces cerebral blood flow and attenuates the response of cerebral vessels to hypercapnia. However, there are problems with the hypothesis that NO is the intrinsic cerebral vasodilator control substance. If this were the case, NO levels would be expected to increase during cerebral hypoxia, as this is known to be a powerful stimulant of cerebral vasodilatation. However, blockade of NO synthesis does not block hypoxia-induced vasodilatation in the brain. In fact, rather than NO production being part of a protective mechanism against hypoxia, there is considerable evidence that the opposite may be true: release of NO in some cases appears to be a fundamental step in the excitotoxic response. Following cerebral hypoxia, NO reacts with the superoxide anion to form peroxynitrite, which destroys cell membranes. NO also decreases the activity of superoxide dismutase (which inactivates the superoxide anion).

If NO is part of a mechanism that supports oxygen delivery in neurones, why is it also involved in the excitotoxic mechanisms of cell death? There are three different isoforms of NOS, neuronal, endothelial and inducible (found in macrophages), and they have different functions. Endothelial

NOS normally functions as a vasodilator. Increases in endothelial NOS levels that occur in stroke may contribute to reperfusion-induced cell death through production of NO, which can interact with free radical ions.

Neuronal NOS is found in a small proportion of neurones and is upregulated in cells after stroke. Glutamate activates neuronal NOS via Ca^{2+} influx. Here, NOS can act as a death mediator. Interestingly, NOS-expressing neurones appear to be unusually resistant to hypoxic damage, and so the NO released by these cells during extreme hypoxia may cause the death of others. Could the excess NO released during hypoxia act as a selective 'culling' process, so that when life-threatening levels of hypoxia occur, some neurones are actively sacrificed before others? Not all cells in any one brain area may have the same importance to the organism. Cells that have a history of high levels of activity might have high levels of intracellular reducing agents such as vitamin C or glutathione, which would initially protect them from the consequences of NO attack. In contrast, cells that had been relatively inactive before the hypoxia would have less biochemical protection and might be the first to die. In such a way, the brain could attempt a 'damage limitation exercise', to protect the cells that have been most active in the past from the effects of a hypoxic crisis.

NOS inhibitors show neuroprotective effects in animal models of ischaemia, and thus offer a therapeutic option for stroke treatment. However, none of the few clinical trials that have assessed these inhibitors so far has shown a beneficial outcome.

(e.g. lipid peroxidation reaction). This eventually damages the cell so badly that it undergoes necrosis (see Fig. 11.17). Thus, glutamate toxicity is a prominent cause of necrotic cell death.

The brain has a number of natural defence molecules to protect against free radical damage. These molecules are reducing agents. They prevent other molecules being oxidized, and react with free radicals or oxidizing agents to form inert products. Three of the most important protectors are vitamin C (ascorbic acid), vitamin E (α-tocopherol) and glutathione. Vitamin C is a powerful water-soluble reducing agent that is present in high levels in the central nervous system, in both neurones and glial cells, and is also found in CSF. Vitamin C is released into the CSF by neuronal depolarization, and also by increases in neuronal activity. Its CSF levels rise sharply following ischaemic hypoxia, and this may be a protective measure to 'mop up' free radicals produced by hypoxic metabolism. Vitamin E is a lipid-soluble reducing agent that eliminates free radicals in cell membranes and other lipid-rich structures, and acts synergistically with vitamin C. Glutathione is a peptide that can react with a number of oxidizing agents and free radicals

via the enzyme glutathione peroxidase, to render them harmless.

Increased intracellular Ca^{2+} levels can trigger the formation of the cytokines tumour necrosis factor-α, interleukin-1β and platelet-activating factor. It also leads to increased activity of the enzyme cyclo-oxygenase 2 (COX-2), which contributes to post-ischaemic inflammation. The cytokines activate microglia, which then release more cytokines, glutamate and other neurotoxins, and attract immune cells that express inducible nitric oxide synthase (iNOS). High intracellular Ca^{2+} levels also damage mitochondria and induce apoptosis (cell suicide) via activation of caspases, particularly within the penumbra region. This mechanism operates on a slower time scale, occurring over a period of hours to days after the initial focal ischaemic event (see Fig. 11.16). Apoptotic cells do not swell and burst; they shrivel and implode.

Rehabilitation of stroke patients

At least one-third of stroke patients who survive the initial event are left with considerable disability. Recovery from disabling stroke can take at least 3–12 months. The length of time varies widely from person to person. Some of this is due to spontaneous resolution of acute problems such as oedema, compensatory brain plasticity and the effects of drugs that rescue cells in the penumbra. It is now recognized that patients recovering in specialist stroke units, as opposed to general wards, make a better recovery. This is because of the availability of specialist multidisciplinary teams that aim to optimize each patient's recovery and maximize the plasticity of the intact brain.

The purpose of rehabilitation is to help people re-learn skills that they have lost (reablement), learn new skills, and find ways to manage any permanent disabilities that they may have been left with.

Medical rehabilitation involves a problem-solving process focused upon disability and handicap by:

1. Assessment, which aims to discover the level of disability, prognostic factors and the patient's goals.

2. Goal planning, which covers the areas of accommodation, personal support and social role of the patient. This is an essential part of the rehabilitation process, and should be discussed by the patient, family and carers.

3. Intervention, which tries to reduce the risk of subsequent attacks by addressing potentially treatable risk factors (see Table 11.2).

4. Evaluation by neurological examination.

A rehabilitation programme includes methods designed to help with posture, balance and movement, together with specialist help for specific difficulties such as speech and language. Many different professionals may be involved in this, but the patient's motivation and efforts are equally important. Key experts include: doctors and nurses (specialist stroke nurses or community nurses) to oversee medical management; physiotherapists to help with problems of posture and movement; occupational therapists to help with everyday activities at home, leisure and work; speech and language therapists to help with communication problems; and clinical psychologists to help with problems affecting mental processes and emotions. As well as reablement, the patient needs resettlement, which may involve adaptation or alteration of their environment (housing and social lifestyles), and involve other professionals such as social workers and dieticians.

Prognosis for recovery

It is imperative that patients receive medical treatment as soon as possible after vascular injury. Time is of the essence, as the faster the treatment initiation, the better the probability of saving more brain tissue and reducing functional deficits. The initial aim is to stabilize the condition, control blood pressure and prevent the acute complications of stroke, such as aspiration pneumonia or immobility; these account for 35% of acute deaths. The doctor may prescribe drugs designed to prevent a further stroke and to treat any underlying conditions, such as high blood pressure or high cholesterol levels (see below).

The brain is capable of great plasticity. In the weeks and months following a stroke, many partially damaged cells recover and start to work again. Meanwhile, other unaffected parts of the brain take over tasks that were previously performed by the brain cells that were destroyed. This is part of the aim of rehabilitation. The length of time it takes to recover varies widely from person to person. It is common to have an initial spurt of recovery in the first few weeks after the stroke. As a rule, most of the recovery takes place during the first year to 18 months, but many people continue to improve over a much longer period.

It is now recognized that patients who suffer small haemorrhagic strokes often make a better recovery than those with ischaemic stroke. Haematomas more often irritate brain tissue rather than physically damage it. The brain absorbs some of the blood from these haemorrhages, and as it does so the affected area heals and begins to function again, making it possible for normal function to be completely regained after small haemorrhagic strokes.

Stroke treatment and neuroprotection

There are two main strategies: prevention and neuroprotection. Drugs that treat accessory conditions, such as angiotensin-converting enzyme (ACE) inhibitors, and diuretics that lower blood pressure, reduce the risk of stroke. Statins (HMG-CoA reductase inhibitors) are a family of drugs that reduce cholesterol levels by blocking its synthesis. They do have a very rare and important side effect, in that they cause myopathy, resulting in muscle pain and weakness. Statins reduce the risk of stroke by 20–30%. For people who have already suffered a stroke, secondary prevention measures are required. They are strongly advised to change their lifestyle in order to reduce the relevant risk factors (see Table 11.2).

Other preventive measures include administration of agents that prevent platelet aggregation and blood coagulation. Aspirin inhibits the enzyme COX, and chronic treatment with aspirin (50–300 mg/day) reduces the relative risk of stroke by 25% in those who have had a TIA or stroke. Heparin is the drug of choice for acute anticoagulation therapy, while warfarin is used for long-term therapy and is given to patients with atrial fibrillation. Both are used after a TIA and may be used for stroke in evolution. Other clot-busting anticoagulants include streptokinase, argatroban and tissue plasminogen activator (tPA). Streptokinase was the original clot-busting agent, but is now not used, due to the high mortality associated with intracerebral haemorrhage. Argatroban (factor VIIa inhibitor) is an anticoagulant that may work by dissolving the primary clot and improving the microcirculation.

tPA (alteplase) is the only recognized drug that improves outcome with stroke. It must be given within 8 h of stroke onset, and is useful for treatment of stroke in evolution. However, due to its limited therapeutic time frame, it is only used in a minority of stroke patients.

Neuroprotective drugs are aimed at preventing or reducing secondary cell death in the penumbra region. Although much is now known about the molecular pathways of apoptosis, excitotoxicity and oxidative stress, clinically effective treatments remain elusive. Several drugs that have been shown in animal models of stroke to be neuroprotective have so far failed to achieve their preclinical promise in all phase III clinical trials (Table 11.5).

The question often asked is why? Is it the drug, the trial design or the model? The answer is probably all three. Animal models of ischaemia generally fall into one of two categories: reversible or permanent. In stroke patients, both types occur, so that animal models never

really mimic the clinical situation. Preclinical models use standardized methods to evoke reproducible ischaemic lesions in previously healthy young animals, whereas the typical stroke patient is usually elderly with numerous risk factors and complicating diseases, such as hypertension or heart disease. Therefore, animal models need to reflect the human condition more accurately. Additionally, in clinical trials, young and old patients are grouped together, as are the types of stroke that they present with. Thus, it is not surprising that no benefit is demonstrated when a drug designed to target a specific pathophysiological problem is given to such a heterogeneous population of patients. A single drug treatment is not applicable to all stroke types; the appropriate drug should be given for the pathophysiological disturbance that it was designed to treat.

Doses of drugs that are neuroprotective in animal models often have adverse effects in humans. Good examples of these are the anti-excitotoxic drugs, such as

Table 11.5 Results of clinical phase III trials in stroke with neuroprotective drugs

Target	Drug	Time frame	Treatment duration	Outcome
Ca^{2+} channels	Nimodipine (channel blocker) Flumazenil	48 h	(Up to) 3 weeks	No neurological or functional improvement (3 weeks to 12 months later). Negative haemodynamic effects
Na^+ channels	Fos-phenytoin (channel blocker)	4 h	3 days	No neurological or functional improvement at 3 months
Glutamate receptors (NMDA)	Selfotel (receptor antagonist)	6 h 8 h	Bolus 2 weeks	Unfavourable risk/benefit ratio
	Aptigave Eliprodil			No neurological or functional improvement at 3 months
$GABA_A$ receptors	Clomethiazole ($GABA_A$ agonist)	12 h	24 h	No neurological or functional improvement at 3–12 months
Free radicals	Lubeluzole* (decreases NOS activity)	6 h 6 h	5 days 3 days	No reduction in mortality No functional improvement at 3 months
	Tirilazad†	48 h	2 weeks	
	Ebselen‡			
Cell membrane	Citicholine	24 h	6 weeks	No neurological or functional improvement at 3 months
	Piracetam (increases cAMP levels)	12 h 6 h	12 weeks 5 days	No neurological or functional improvement at 1 month
	Enlimomab (antibody to endothelial adhesion molecule)			Unfavourable risk/benefit ratio

NMDA, N-methyl-D-aspartate; GABA, γ-aminobutyric acid; NOS, nitric oxide synthase.
Modified from de Keyser J et al. Trends in Neuroscience 1999; 22: 535–540.
*Also inhibits glutamate release, and Na^+ and Ca^{2+} channels.
†Also has glutathione peroxidase activity.
‡Also inhibits lipid peroxidation.

the NMDA receptor antagonists. These induce psycho-mimetic effects such as delirium, hallucinations, paranoia, catatonia and sedation, which preclude their use. In some instances, the dose is reduced to suboptimal levels because of overemphasis on safety aspects, even though the side effects may be properly controlled. Additionally, it is not known how long neuroprotective therapies should be continued for. Fear of side effects reduces the dose level and the duration of treatment to levels that are insufficient to have an effect because the plasma concentrations are too low.

Finally, analysis of outcome in animal and human studies is different. In animal models, infarct size is quantified so that the effect of a drug can be evaluated, usually over a short time span. In humans, neurological and functional scores—National Institutes of Health stroke scale (NIHSS, Table 11.6) and Barthel index—are commonly used at 3 or 6 months after stroke. These may be less amenable to statistical analysis, and may be less sensitive than anatomical markers of infarct size. The latter could be assessed with the use of sophisticated imaging methods such as positron emission tomography (PET), and diffusion-weighted and perfusion MRI, to measure the penumbra and infarct size before and after treatment. Recent evidence suggests the NIHSS score strongly predicts outcome; patients who score 6 or less at 3 months have a good outcome whilst those that score 16 or more are likely to die or have severe disability.

The Barthel Index consists of 10 activities that specifically measure a person's daily living and mobility. These include feeding, bathing, moving from wheelchair to bed and return, grooming, transferring to and from a toilet, walking on level surface, going up and down stairs, dressing, continence of bowels and bladder. They are weighted according to whether they have received help while doing the task using scores of 0 (unable), 5, 10, or 15 (independent). Middle scores imply that over 50% of the effort comes from the patient. The scores for each activity are summed to create a total score of up to 100. This is used as a record of what the patient can do independently, without help, but using aids if necessary. The assessment is used to monitor improvement in activities of daily living over time. The higher the score, the more 'independent' the person. In the UK, often the 5, 10 and 15 scores are substituted by 1, 2 and 3. This gives a potential maximum of 20 rather than 100.

All clinical trials conducted so far have used drugs to target one specific pathway of the ischaemic cascade. Most preclinical observations indicate that combinations of clot-lysing drugs and neuroprotective drugs have synergistic effects. They reduce reperfusion injury and inhibit apoptosis cascades, and decrease the dosages for each, thereby reducing their adverse effects. For example, combination of intravenous tPA with clomethiazole (GABA$_A$ agonist) or lubeluzole (NOS inhibitor) have been used in recent clinical trials. Thus, drug combinations that promote cell survival, extend the therapeutic time window and target multiple pathways may prove to be the way forward in treating stroke.

Another quite different approach to helping stroke patients is the use of hypothermia. Prolonged submersion in icy water is known to protect the brain, and promotes a favourable neurological outcome, especially in children. In contrast, raising body temperatures, even by 1°C, worsens the outcome two-fold. Dropping the core body temperature by 2–3°C is sufficient to reduce neuronal death

Table 11.6 The NIH stroke scale (each examination is assessed independently from previous examinations)

Category	Score
1. Level of consciousness	
General response	0 = alert, 1 = drowsy, 2 = stupor, 3 = coma
Response to two questions	0 = both correct, 1 = one correct, 2 = none correct
Response to two commands	0 = both correct, 1 = one correct, 2 = none correct
2. Gaze	0 = normal, 1 = partial gaze palsy, 2 = forced eye deviation
3. Visual fields	0 = normal, 1 = bilateral quadrantonopia, 2 = homonymous hemianopsia, 3 = cortical blindness
4. Facial movement	0 = normal, 1 = minor paresis, 2 = partial paresis, 3 = complete palsy
5. Motor function: arms, legs	0 = no drift, 1 = minor drift, 2 = some effort against gravity, 3 = no effort against gravity, 4 = no movement
6. Limb ataxia	0 = absent, 1 = unilateral presence in arm or leg, 2 = unilateral presence in arm and leg or bilateral, 9 = untestable (no motor function or coma)
7. Sensory	0 = normal, 1 = mild loss, 2 = severe loss (unilateral)
8. Language (aphasia)	0 = none, 1 = expressive or receptive aphasia (mild–moderate), 2 = global aphasia (severe), 3 = mute
9. Dysarthria	0 = normal articulation, 1 = mild–moderate, 2 = unintelligible, 9 = untestable
10. Neglect	0 = none, 1 = partial (can recognize stimuli on right or left but not both), 2 = complete (bilateral neglect)

from asphyxia, particularly in neonates. Several questions remain unresolved, such as the duration of hypothermia and onset time after stroke. Long-term (12–24 h) hypothermia seems to have a favourable outcome if initiated soon after stroke. The mechanisms involved remain unclear, but the simple explanation is that lower temperatures slow metabolic demand. In addition to this mechanism, recent research indicates that hypothermia decreases intracellular acidosis, iNOS-induced NO generation, apoptosis, microglial activation, excitotoxicity, free radical generation and cerebral oedema. Thus, hypothermia seems to target many of the neuronal death pathways. Several clinical trials are underway to assess hypothermia in ischaemic stroke in combination with thrombolytic agents.

Head injury

Very severe head injuries involve forces incompatible with life, and death is immediate. With most severe head injuries, however, there is a variable period of survival, and the usual cause of death is raised intracranial pressure (Box 11.6), as a result of either brain swelling or a haemorrhage accumulating inside the skull, which distorts the brain and produces damage in vital structures

(Box 11.6). Post-traumatic disability depends on the location and amount of brain damage; the most usual neuropathological causes of long-term disability after a head injury are damage to axons and hypoxic–ischaemic damage, sustained at the time of injury.

There are two important mechanisms involved in head injury: impact to the head, and movement of the brain; these result in slightly different patterns of injury. In the human situation, of course, there is almost always impact, with variable amounts of brain movement. Because excessive movement alone can damage the brain, it is important to remember that it is not necessary for the head to hit anything for a severe head injury to occur.

The severity of head injury can be assessed in several ways: by the level of consciousness (Box 11.7), by pupil reactions to light, and by neurological and radiological investigations. The Glasgow Coma Scale (GCS) is an important indicator of head injury severity. The clinical assessment of the degree of coma is done by using the Glasgow Coma Scale (Table 11.7). This method is easily reproducible, and is very useful for monitoring changes in the conscious level. The Glasgow Coma Score is calculated from the patient's eye-opening, verbal and best motor responses. Scores in each category range from 1 (no response) to a maximum of between 4 and 6 (for a normal response), and are summed to give a score ranging

---

Box 11.6 Brain swelling and raised intracranial pressure

Cerebral swelling after head injury may be caused by either cerebral oedema or vascular haemorrhage. There are three types of cerebral oedema:

1. Vasogenic. This is due to accumulation of water outside cells, as a result of disruption of the blood–brain barrier. After trauma, damaged plasma constituents move into the extracellular space, causing the extracellular compartment to increase in volume, so leading to brain swelling.
2. Cytotoxic. As the brain swells due to vasogenic oedema, the tissue becomes ischaemic, cell membranes become damaged, and Na^+/K^+ pumps fail to maintain the membrane ionic gradient. Intracellular Na^+ accumulation leads to cell swelling, resulting in cytotoxic oedema.
3. Interstitial. This is a consequence of an increase in the volume of the extracellular fluid in the absence of disruption to the blood–brain barrier, e.g. due to insufficient antidiuretic hormone secretion.

In the context of head trauma, vasogenic and cytotoxic oedema are important.

The cranial vault contains the brain and the meninges, the cerebrospinal fluid and the vascular supply, within a

fixed volume. Any increase in volume of one of these must occur at the expense of the others, if the pressure is to remain unchanged. Any uncompensated increase in volume of any of the constituents causes raised intracranial pressure. While raised intracranial pressure is always seen with space-occupying lesions, pressure may rise in the absence of a mass lesion. Brain swelling and hydrocephalus are the two most common generalized causes of raised intracranial pressure.

The brain is only perfused because systemic arterial pressure is higher than intracranial pressure. As intracranial pressure rises, the blood flow to the brain will decrease, unless the arterial pressure rises in compensation. This compensatory rise does occur when intracranial pressure starts to rise, but cerebral perfusion rapidly falls off as intracranial pressure rises still higher. Tissue ischaemia then leads to cytotoxic oedema, and so more swelling.

Rising intracranial pressure causes a number of nonspecific symptoms, including headache (from stretching and distortion of dura and blood vessels), vomiting (from pressure on the floor of the fourth ventricle), papilloedema (from pressure on the optic nerve sheath), and falling consciousness levels (from pressure on the diencephalon and upper brainstem).

Box 11.7 Basic mechanisms of consciousness and coma

There are two separate components to consciousness: being awake or alert, and being aware. In order to be fully conscious, a person needs to have both an intact ascending reticular activating system in the brainstem, and a functioning cerebral cortex.

Coma is a state of unrousable unresponsiveness, caused by damage to either the diencephalon/midbrain or the hemispheres. After head injury, it may be due to:

- generalized brain swelling causing pressure on the reticular formation
- temporal lobe herniation through the tentorial notch that compresses or distorts the midbrain
- traumatic damage to axons (which effectively leads to deafferentation of the cortex)
- severe hypoxic damage to neurones in the cortex (e.g. from cardiac arrest or impaired cerebral perfusion).

Concussion, on the other hand, is a reversible state of unconsciousness of brief duration, without structural pathological alteration. Its pathophysiological mechanism is unknown but may represent some form of brain shock.

Table 11.7 The Glasgow Coma Scale

Category	Score
Eye-opening response	
Spontaneous	4
On command	3
In response to pain	2
None	1
Verbal response	
Speaks freely, coherently and purposefully	5
Speaks in a confused, disoriented fashion	4
Uses inappropriate words	3
Makes incomprehensible sounds	2
No response	1
Best motor response	
Obeys commands freely	6
Makes purposeful movements in response to noxious stimuli	5
Withdraws from noxious stimuli	4
Shows flexion after noxious stimuli (decorticate posturing)	3
Shows extension after noxious stimuli (decerebrate posturing)	2
No response	1

between 3 and 15. Patients with a score of <8 are in coma, and have a severe head injury. A score of 9–12 indicates a moderate head injury, and a score >12 indicates a mild head injury. The GSC has prognostic value, as the scores both immediately after the injury and 24 h later correlate with the degree of long-term impairment.

The damage seen in head injury can be classified in a number of ways. Clinically, the most useful is as focal or diffuse injury (Table 11.8). Focal injury indicates pathology that can be seen on a CT or MRI scan, and which may be neurosurgically treatable. Diffuse brain injury refers to microscopic damage that cannot be demonstrated with any of the current imaging techniques, but which clinicians diagnose because they have an unconscious patient whose scan shows very little obvious damage.

Focal pathology in relation to vascular injury

Skull fractures

See Fig. 11.18.

A skull fracture is of relevance because it is an indication of the force of the impact on the head. A depressed fracture, in which an area of skull is driven inwards, needs to be repaired by a neurosurgeon. Depressed fractures may tear arteries or the meninges, leading to haemorrhage. Infection is a possible secondary consequence of skull fractures in which the scalp is torn. Skull base fractures are difficult to see on X-ray images. They

Table 11.8 Patterns of damage during head injury

Damage	Example
Focal damage	
Scalp	Contusions (bruises) Lacerations
Skull	Fracture
Meninges	Extradural and subdural haemorrhages
Brain	Contusions and lacerations Intracerebral (parenchymal) haemorrhage Axonal damage
Diffuse damage	
Brain	Diffuse axonal injury Hypoxic–ischaemic damage Diffuse brain swelling

are associated with physical signs such as CSF bleeding through the nose, as there is communication with the nasal sinuses, Battle's sign (Fig. 11.18B) or bleeding into the middle ear.

Blows around the eyes may fracture the orbit. The medial and inferior walls are paper-thin, and indirect injuries that displace the orbital walls produce 'blow-out

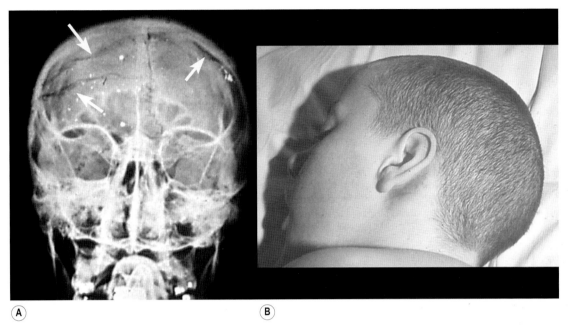

Fig. 11.18 (A) Radiograph showing skull fractures (arrows). (B) Skull base fracture in a baby showing Battle's sign (bruising behind the ear), indicating petrous bone skull fracture.

fractures', which may involve damage to the air sinuses. Orbital fractures often produce intraorbital bleeding, producing pressure on the eyeball and 'black eyes', as the blood accumulates in the soft tissues around the eye. Orbital fractures may damage the cavernous sinus and thus the blood/nerve supply to the eye. The abducens nerve and ICA run in its substance, and the oculomotor, trochlear ophthalmic and maxillary nerves run in its lateral wall. Infection can spread to the cavernous sinus via the ophthalmic vein as a result of such fractures.

Meninges

Bleeding in the spaces around the brain is a common feature of closed head injury. In trauma, bleeding may be extradural, subdural or subarachnoid. Extradural and subdural haemorrhages usually need to be evacuated neurosurgically, and if left untreated are important causes of death, because they act as mass lesions (Box 11.8).

Extradural haemorrhage

Extradural haemorrhage (EDH) occurs in approximately 10% of severe head injuries, and in up to 15% of fatal head injuries. It is important to understand the anatomy and natural history of EDHs, because if an EDH is not diagnosed and treated, it will kill the patient. EDH is an impact phenomenon. It occurs when a blood vessel running between the skull and the dura is torn, in association with a skull fracture. The blood vessel damaged is either an artery or one of the large venous sinuses (the veins are thin-walled, with little muscle or elastic tissue and no valves). In many cases, it is the middle meningeal

artery that is torn. This artery lies beneath the pterion, where the skull is thinnest, and is relatively easily fractured by a blow to the side of the head. Although the blood flow from the bleed may be rapid, EDHs accumulate slowly, usually over a period of hours, because the dura strongly adheres to the inner aspect of the calvarium, and the enlarging clot slowly strips the dura from the bone. The patient may appear to be lucid immediately after the injury, and only becomes unconscious as the haemorrhage enlarges, and begins to press on the brain (Fig. 11.20). Because there is so little reserve volume inside the skull, haematomas of more than 75 mL are usually fatal; death is caused by a combination of mass effect and raised intracranial pressure.

On CT or MRI images, EDHs appear convex (See Fig. 11.23) as their spread is limited by the bone sutures because the dura mater is tightly adhered to the sutures and so they expand inward toward the brain rather than along the skull margin.

Subdural haemorrhage

Acute subdural haemorrhage (SDH) is completely different from EDH. It is principally caused by movement of the brain, and not by impact. The movement responsible is acceleration, with or without deceleration. When the head is accelerated, the inertia of the brain causes its movement to lag behind that of the skull. This leads to traction on bridging veins running between brain and dura mater, which get torn. Blood from the ruptured vessels spreads slowly and freely through the subdural space (an artificial region within the dura created by the separation of the *arachnoid mater* from the *dura mater*

Box 11.8 The effects of a mass lesion inside the skull

The cranial cavity is subdivided by the relatively rigid tentorium and falx cerebri into three compartments, with limited capacity to accommodate accumulations of blood or swelling due to oedema without an increase in pressure. Differences in pressure between two adjacent intracranial compartments or between an intracranial compartment and the spinal canal cause the brain to be displaced into the lower-pressure compartment (i.e. internal herniation). Raised intracranial pressure can also lead to external herniation of brain tissue through a skull fracture or craniotomy.

There are three sites where herniation tends to occur (Fig. 11.19):

1. subfalcine—herniation of the cingulate gyrus under the falx cerebri
2. tentorial—herniation of the uncus of the temporal lobe through the tentorial notch
3. tonsillar—herniation of the cerebellar tonsils through the foramen magnum and onto the respiratory and cardiac centres of the medulla.

Apart from distorting and causing pressure on the brain, internal herniation compresses blood vessels, leading to secondary ischaemic damage. Cranial nerves are often also compressed, causing focal neurological signs.

With herniation there is downward displacement of diencephalic structures and descent of the brainstem, resulting in buckling of the brainstem, with traction on the external portions of the arterial supply and compression of their internal parts. This creates foci of haemorrhagic necrosis in the midbrain and pons. It is this brainstem damage, along with the rise in intracranial pressure, that leads to death.

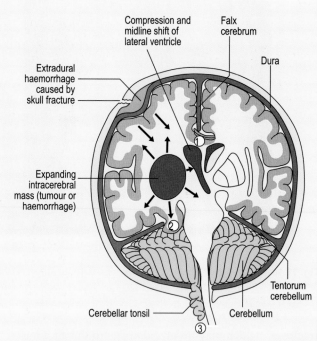

1. Subfalcine herniation. 3. Tonsillar herniation.
2. Uncal herniation.

Fig. 11.19 Schematic showing the neuroanatomical basis for brain herniation syndromes. An increase in the volume of the contents in the skull, such as a brain tumour or intracranial bleed, can cause brain tissue to be displaced at one of the three sites shown.

---

and not between the dura mater and arachnoid mater, as its name suggests). SDH can envelop the entire hemisphere (Fig. 11.21, upper image) and may spread into the subarachnoid space below. The bleeding tends to stop spontaneously. Sometimes, the symptoms (headache, drowsiness and confusion) may take days to months to become apparent. Because of the forces involved in producing an SDH, there is very often damage to axons in the underlying brain as well. This is in contrast to an EDH, where the underlying brain tissue is not usually severely damaged. If the blood is not removed, it will compress the brain tissue, leading to infarction.

SDHs are more frequent than EDHs, and are common findings in child abuse cases such as shaken baby syndrome. Acute subdural bleeds have a mortality rate of 60–80% if left untreated. They are also common in chronic alcoholics and the elderly where cortical atrophy is common, increasing the tension on the bridging veins increasing the likelihood of damage with shearing forces. On CT

and MRI images, an SDH often appears crescent shaped with the concave side facing away from the skull and they may also track along the dural folds (See Fig. 11.23).

Subarachnoid haemorrhage

Subarachnoid bleeding in trauma is almost always insignificant, and is seen on the surface of the hemispheres in relation to fracture sites or contusions. It most often results from penetrating brain injury. Occasionally, if a vessel at the base of the brain is damaged, a large amount of blood collects in the subarachnoid space over the base of the brain. On CT or MRI images, fresh blood can be seen invaginating between the cerebral gyri, making the sulci appear white (See Fig. 11.23). Spontaneous subarachnoid haemorrhage is quite different from traumatic subarachnoid haemorrhage, which results from rupture of an aneurysm on a vessel of the circle of Willis (e.g. a Berry aneurysm) (Fig. 11.21, lower image). The latter

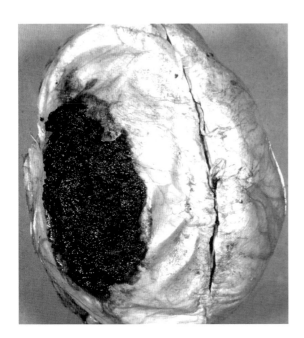

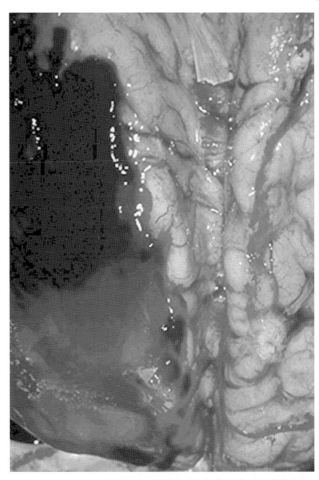

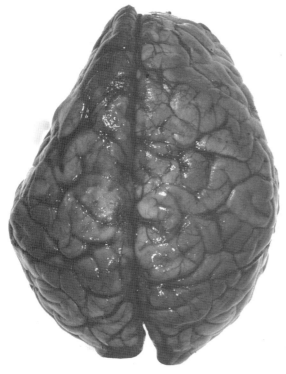

Fig. 11.20 Extradural haematoma (EDH). Top: an example of an EDH caused by rupture of the middle meningeal artery. Bottom: effects of an EDH on the underlying brain tissue, showing severe compression of the left frontal lobe.

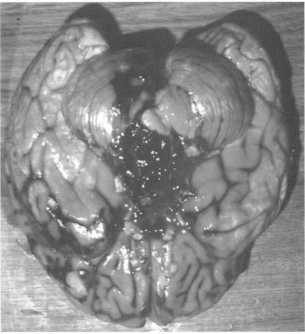

Fig. 11.21 Two examples of subdural haemorrhage (SDH), where blood distributes and collects over the surface of the front of the brain (upper figure) or collects at the base of the brain (lower figure).

type of subarachnoid haemorrhage is a form of haemorrhagic stroke.

Brain contusions and lacerations

Contusions are caused by impact, and can be thought of as brain 'bruises'. They occur on the crests of gyri, particularly where the brain moves over the roughened floor of the skull (Figs 11.22 and 11.23), namely the inferior surface of the frontal lobes, the lateral and inferior surfaces of the temporal lobes, region adjacent to the lateral fissures or at the orbital poles.

At their mildest, contusions are very small superficial areas of haemorrhagic necrosis, confined to the cortex. Larger contusions involve the underlying white matter, and may be associated with considerable oedema and a degree of mass effect. Contusions occur at the site of impact ('coup'), and at sites opposite the point of impact ('contre-coup'), depending on the type of blow. The prefrontal cortex and the temporal lobe poles are the parts of the brain most often injured in acceleration–deceleration trauma. They are rarely life-threatening on their own, however, and with increasing time of survival, the necrotic brain tissue is resorbed. It is not uncommon to see the remnants of contusional injury as an incidental finding at post-mortem. The term 'laceration' is used when the arachnoid mater and brain are damaged, usually at the site of a fracture, or by a penetrating injury or a large intracerebral haematoma.

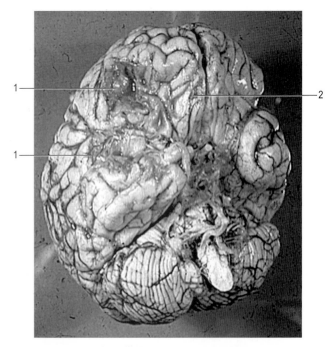

1. Lesion.   2. 'Hollow tooth'.

Fig. 11.22 Traumatic lacerations of right orbital cortex and coup and contre-coup lesions of temporal lobes. The right olfactory bulb is also damaged, as are the crests of the gyri, producing a split hollow tooth appearance.

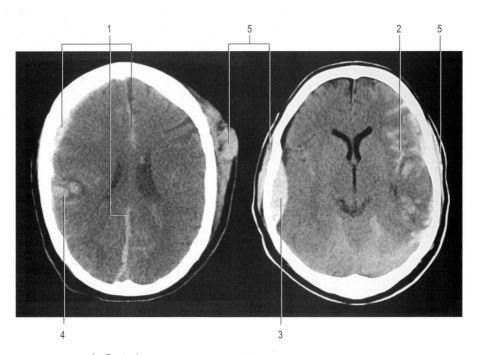

1. Subdural bleed.   4. Contusion.
2. Subarachnoid bleed.   5. Soft tissue injury (extra-cranial).
3. Extradural bleed.

Fig. 11.23 MRI images showing different types of pathology present in head injury. Left image courtesy of Mr. A. Elsmore; right image courtesy of Dr Andrew Downie.

Intracerebral (parenchymal) haemorrhage

Bleeding within the brain tissue is usually the result of penetrating head wounds, such as that caused by high-velocity impacts, e.g. bullets. Low-velocity focal impact may result in bone fragment penetration from a skull fracture. When parenchymal haemorrhage is the result of a closed head injury, it commonly affects the frontal and temporal lobes.

Diffuse pathology

Diffuse axonal injury (DAI) is the term given to widespread damage to axons, caused by acceleration of the head, with or without deceleration, that stretches the axons to the point of rupture. It differs from acceleration–deceleration injuries during trauma, which primarily result from the brain rubbing against the bony protuberances of the skull vault. Like SDH, this is primarily a non-impact phenomenon. Brain damage may also occur as a consequence of acceleration–deceleration injury in the absence of impact, as in 'shaken baby' syndrome, where young babies are violently shaken by adults. The anterior temporal lobes and prefrontal cortex region are most affected by acceleration–deceleration injury. A patient with DAI is usually unconscious from the time of injury, remains in prolonged coma, and is severely disabled or vegetative until death.

Hypoxic–ischaemic damage is also very common in head injury. The injured brain is extremely sensitive to hypoxia, and the primary aim of emergency head injury treatment is to maintain oxygenation and cerebral perfusion. Head injuries frequently occur in settings in which there are multiple injuries: injuries to the ribs may interfere with breathing, and therefore oxygenation of the blood, while major bleeding will cause shock and hypotension.

Diffuse brain swelling is often seen in head injury, particularly in children, probably partly as a result of failure of cerebral autoregulation (see earlier). Any significant swelling will, of course, cause intracranial pressure to rise, and so reduce cerebral perfusion. Diffuse brain injury can impair mental functions such as long-term memory and problem-solving, and result in neglect and prosopagnosia (inability to recognize faces) and an inability to synthesize and analyse information.

Axons are as vulnerable as other intracranial structures to traumatic damage, and it is now generally believed that a degree of axonal damage occurs in most head injuries. Experimental work suggests that mild reversible axonal injury is the cause of concussion symptoms, and that scattered irreversible axonal damage may be responsible for a number of the behavioural and cognitive sequelae of mild head injuries, such as the 'punch-drunk syndrome' seen in boxers. With more severe injuries, the amount and distribution of axonal damage often determine the outcome.

With all forms of traumatic axonal injury, whether very mild or very severe, it is clear that the damage does not become irreversible until several hours, possibly days, after injury, providing a 'therapeutic window' during which it may be possible to prevent, or at least minimize, the damage caused.

Treatment of head injury

The aim of treatment is similar to that of stroke treatment, i.e. to prevent secondary brain damage. It focuses on maintaining adequate oxygenation and reducing intracranial pressure. For EDH, surgical aspiration of the clot is a life-saving technique; a ventricular shunt can be done to reduce hydrocephalus, or drugs such as mannitol (an osmotic diuretic) or dexamethasone (an anti-inflammatory drug) can be used to reduce oedema. Hyperventilation and its consequent hypocapnia also reduce intracranial pressure, as does hypothermia and hyperbaric oxygen, or drugs such as phenothiazines.

Even mild head injuries (e.g. concussion) can impair mental processes such as perception, attention and memory. Even though in some cases there may not be anatomical damage, most traumatic head injury patients suffer from long-term complications and disabilities that are physical (pain and headache, epilepsy, hearing, visual or sensory impairment, motor weakness or disequilibrium) and/or mental (memory loss, inability to concentrate, personality and emotional changes, language difficulties and depression).

The pharmacological management of head injury is still limited, although encouraging results have been obtained in recent years with drugs such as dexamphetamine, methylphenidate, bromocriptine, amantadine, L-DOPA/carbidopa, tacrine and rivastigmine, which increase attention and heighten arousal levels. The neuroprotective mechanism of action of such a wide range of compounds, from dopamine agonists such as bromocriptine to acetylcholinesterase inhibitors such as tacrine, which appear to exert some beneficial effects, is still unclear. Protection may be directly related to their pharmacodynamics, or may result from some other yet undiscovered property. In the case of head trauma, in a similar manner to stroke, the use of combined medications may have many advantages that are still incompletely explored.

Rehabilitation methods are similar to those used in stroke, but often with a special emphasis on cognitive therapy. In general, head injury patients tend to have a better prognosis than stroke patients, partly because head injury patients are in better vascular health and are often younger.

Comments on the case history

Once Arthur's stroke had been diagnosed, immediate treatment was begun. This should result in a favourable prognosis. Pharmacological treatment was aimed at reducing infarct size and rescuing brain cells in the penumbra region, which would otherwise die from ischaemia. Prompt administration of Alteplase (tPA), a clot-lysing agent, dissolved the thrombus and restored the cerebral circulation to this region. This resulted in resolution of the sensory loss and the language disabilities, suggesting that blood flow was restored to the parietal and temporal lobes. The core region appears to reside in the frontal lobe, and this accounts for the residual motor deficits, including language articulation. It is unlikely that further improvement will occur, and rehabilitation programmes will be needed, to allow Arthur to cope with his disabilities. A change of lifestyle is also required to reduce the risk of subsequent strokes.

INFECTION IN THE CENTRAL NERVOUS SYSTEM

Chapter objectives

After studying this chapter you should be able to:

1. Describe the structure and function of the meninges and the blood–brain barrier.

2. Classify the major causative agents of brain infections.

3. Be able to recognize the major features of bacterial and viral meningitis.

4. Describe the treatment of meningitis and be aware of the specific problems in immunocompromised patients.

Introduction

Normally, the central nervous system (CNS) is protected from infection by the blood–brain barrier (BBB). However, this can be breached, and the CNS can be infected by a wide variety of organisms. Box 12.1 illustrates the significant neurological consequences of infections.

Types of infection of the central nervous system

There are many different organisms that can infect the CNS. The causative agents of infections are summarized in Table 12.1. Infections of the CNS fall into three groups,

Box 12.1 Case history

On returning home after attending nursery school, 4-year-old David complains of a headache. Shortly afterwards, he says that he feels sick and is tired. He goes to lie down in his bedroom and asks that the curtains be drawn, even though it is only 2 p.m. After he has actually been sick, his mother notices a rash on his feet while she is changing his clothes. Remembering a leaflet about meningitis she saw in the doctor's surgery, the mother immediately calls an ambulance and David is taken to the local hospital. On examination by the doctor, he is shown to have a fever and neck stiffness, with a positive Kernig's sign. Examining the rash more closely, the doctor notices that it does not go pale when pressed. David is immediately given an intravenous injection of benzylpenicillin and chloramphenicol. The doctor takes blood samples and a throat swab. By this time, David has a deteriorating level of consciousness and he is transferred immediately to the intensive care department. Subsequent culture of the throat sample identifies the presence of *Neisseria meningitidis*. David is very ill for a few days but, because of his mother's prompt action, his illness is not as dangerous as it might have been. The other members of David's family are given antibiotics, as are the other children at the nursery school. Following his successful treatment, David is tested to find out if he has any lingering problems.

This case gives rise to the following questions:

1. What types of infection can occur in the central nervous system?
2. What are the meninges and what is their function?
3. What is the blood–brain barrier and what are its functions?
4. What is meningitis and what are its causes?
5. How is meningitis diagnosed and treated, and what is the likely prognosis?

depending on which part of the CNS tissue is affected and the extent of the infection.

The most well-known type of generalized brain infection is meningitis, an inflammation of the meninges surrounding the brain. This type of infection is the subject of a large amount of public information, concerning both the need for early identification of the condition and rapid treatment (which in many cases is essential), and raising awareness of the vaccines that are available. The most severe forms of meningitis are caused by bacteria, and if these are suspected to be the causative agents, then antibiotics should be given immediately.

When the brain tissue (parenchyma) itself becomes infected, this is called encephalitis and is most often caused by viruses. In many cases, the disease is mild and self-limiting, but there are some types of encephalitis that cause significant mortality.

A number of viruses can cause specific localized infections. One of the most well-known is polio virus, which infects the lower motor neurones of the spinal cord and brainstem, causing paralysis, which may be permanent. Fortunately, this occurs rarely in the UK, because of an extensive vaccination programme, but it still occurs in many less developed countries. Herpes zoster virus, the causative agent of chickenpox, can infect the dorsal root ganglion cells. It remains dormant but can be reactivated later in life to cause shingles. Another virus that infects specific nerve ganglia is herpes simplex virus (HSV). The type 1 virus infects the trigeminal nerve ganglion, and can also be reactivated periodically to produce cold sores. The type 2 virus infects the dorsal root ganglion in the sacral region, and its reactivation causes genital herpes.

Table 12.1 Examples of central nervous system infections and their causative agents

Bacteria	*Neisseria meningitidis**, *Streptococcus pneumoniae**, *Haemophilus influenzae*, *Escherichia coli*, *Mycobacterium tuberculosis* (these all cause meningitis), *Mycobacterium leprae* (leprosy), *Treponema pallidum* (syphilis), *Borrelia burgdorferi* (Lyme disease)
Viruses	Herpes simplex (encephalitis), herpes zoster (shingles), poliovirus, rabies, human immunodeficiency virus (HIV), mumps
Protozoa	*Plasmodium falciparum* (malaria), toxoplasmosis, trypanosomiasis (sleeping sickness)
Metazoa	Encysted tapeworm larvae (hyatid disease, cysticercosis)
Fungi	*Cryptococcus neoformans*, *Histoplasma capsulatum*, *Coccidioides immitis*
Prions	Creutzfeldt–Jacob disease (CJD) and new variant CJD

*These two organisms account for about 70% of cases of meningitis in the UK.

When the infection of the brain is due to a localized bacterial infection, a cerebral abscess is produced. The accumulation of pus causes a typical expanding mass in the brain, with many of the signs and symptoms seen in the presence of brain tumours and other space-filling lesions. These can be very severe because of the rapidity of growth of the abscess.

A disease that was first described in the 1920s but has recently received much attention is Creutzfeldt–Jakob disease (CJD), a degenerative disease of the elderly causing characteristic spongiform changes to the brain. The disease, which is related to bovine spongiform encephalitis (BSE) in cattle, and scrapie in sheep, is thought to be due to the presence in the brain and lymphatic tissue of abnormal forms of a protein called a prion. CJD can be transmitted following neurosurgery, as the infective agent is not destroyed by normal sterilization procedures. It has also been transmitted by growth hormone treatment of children of small stature. Interest in this rare disease has been stimulated by the appearance since 1994 of a new form of the disease, which, unlike classic CJD, occurs in young people. The presence of an epidemic of BSE in British cattle, allied with the suggestion that this new variant CJD (nvCJD) is due to the consumption of beef from these infected animals, has not only stimulated much research on this subject, but has also led to the widespread slaughter of beef herds, and changes in animal feed and slaughter practices in the UK. However, the widely feared epidemic of nvCJD has not yet occurred and as of November 2009, the UK National CJD Surveillance Unit had confirmed 166 cases of nvCJD and the number of suspected cases per year seems to be falling.

The meninges

The meninges are a series of membranes that surround the brain and spinal cord. They are separated by cerebrospinal fluid (CSF), which acts as a cushion, supporting the weight of the brain and protecting it from damage that might be caused by movement. Suspending the brain in fluid reduces the effective brain weight, and prevents it from being squeezed by its own mass. The meninges are made up of three distinct layers, called the dura mater, the arachnoid mater and the pia mater, each of which has a specific role (Fig. 12.1).

Dura mater

The outermost layer is the dura mater (dura = hard or tough). This thick, leathery membrane forms the outer protective layer surrounding the brain. It is formed from two layers: the periosteal layer, which lies close to the periosteum (the inner surface of the skull), and the meningeal layer, which lies closer to the brain. In most areas of the brain, these two layers are fused, but in some regions they enclose blood-filled cavities called dural sinuses, which collect venous blood and eventually drain into the internal jugular vein.

The meningeal layer extends inwards in several places to form septa that partition the brain into separate areas and limit the movement of the brain within the skull (Fig. 12.2). The falx cerebri (falx = sickle) is a sickle-shaped sheet that extends into the longitudinal fissure, separating the two cerebral hemispheres. At the front of the brain it is attached to the crista galli, a projection of the ethmoid bone, and its free edge curves over the corpus callosum to the rear of the skull, above the cerebellum. Here it attaches to another dural septum, the tentorium cerebelli (tentorium = tent). This extends horizontally into the transverse fissure, which extends between the rear of the cerebral cortices and the cerebellum, arching over the posterior cranial fossa. Like the falx cerebri, it does not form a complete sheet; its free edge forms a U-shape, enclosing the midbrain and attaching at the front to the clinoid processes of the sphenoid bone. The cranial region below this is the infratentorial

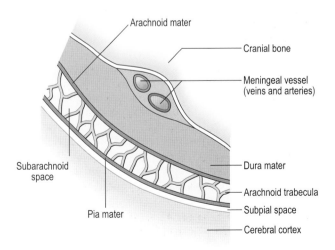

Fig. 12.1 Anatomy of the meninges. The thick dura mater, the arachnoid mater and the pia mater enclose the brain and contain the cerebrospinal fluid.

Box 12.2 Papilloedema and fundoscopy

The meninges also enclose the optic nerve all the way to the retina. This means that raised intracranial pressure will be transmitted through the subarachnoid space surrounding the optic nerve and the blood vessels of the retina, the central artery and the central vein. Increased pressure will compress the central vein, leading to enlargement of the retinal veins and oedema of the optic papilla, which can be seen when the rear of the retina, the fundus, is examined with an ophthalmoscope (see Box 7.2).

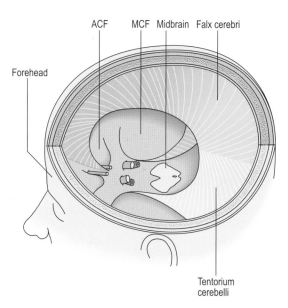

Fig. 12.2 Drawing of the meninges showing the falx cerebri and tentorium cerebelli with the vault of the cranium removed. MCF, middle cranial fossa; ACF, anterior cranial fossa.

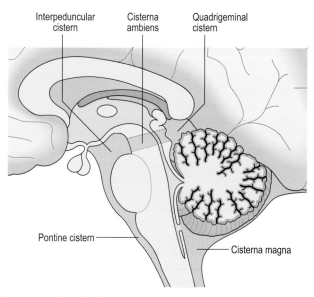

Fig. 12.3 Subarachnoid cisternae. Enlargements of the subarachnoid space form cisternae that contain cerebrospinal fluid.

compartment, and the region above is the supratentorial compartment. A third sheet, the falx cerebelli, runs along the midline of the cerebellum, along the vermis. The dura mater of the spinal cord has only a single meningeal layer, which extends from the rim of the foramen magnum to the level of the second sacral vertebra (S2).

The sensory innervation of the dura mater is provided by the trigeminal and upper cervical spinal nerves. If the dura is inflamed, then these nerves are stimulated, giving specific patterns of pain that depend on which areas of the dura are involved (see below).

Arachnoid mater

Lying immediately under the dura mater, separated only by the narrow subdural space, is the arachnoid mater (arachnoid = spider-like). This thin membrane, which completely encloses the wide subarachnoid space, is composed of fibrous material and cells connected by tight junctions that seal the space. Extending from the arachnoid mater across the subarachnoid space to the pia mater are numerous thin extensions, called trabeculae, whose web-like appearance gives the arachnoid mater its name. The arachnoid space is filled with CSF. Within the fluid are also many major arteries, which then project down into the brain tissue. In specific areas, particularly around the brainstem, because the arachnoid mater does not dip into the contours of the brain, the subarachnoid space enlarges to form cisterns (Fig. 12.3). The largest of these is the cisterna magna, which lies between the cerebellum and the medulla. Folds of the arachnoid mater project through the dura mater into the superior dural sinuses. These are called arachnoid villi or arachnoid granulations. These are involved in the reabsorption of CSF into venous blood (see below).

Pia mater

The third layer of the meninges is the pia mater (pia = gentle). This very fine layer of connective tissue follows the contours of the brain, dipping down into the sulci. It is highly vascularized, with small blood vessels, and is permeable to CSF. Where small arteries enter the brain, the pia mater is carried down for short distances into the perivascular space.

Cerebrospinal fluid production and circulation

The CSF that bathes the brain has an ionic content broadly similar to that of blood plasma, with some slight differences (Table 12.2). Under normal conditions, it contains very little protein, no red cells and very few leukocytes. It contains glucose, at about 60% of the level found in plasma. It has a total volume of about 140 mL and is clear in appearance.

CSF is produced at a rate of about 500 mL/day. Most of this (60%) is secreted by the choroid plexuses, found in the lateral, third and fourth ventricles. The remaining 40% is produced by capillary filtration and metabolic water. The choroid plexuses consist of loops of capillaries covered by a layer of specialized epithelial cells. These capillaries, unlike most brain capillaries, are fairly permeable, allowing fluid to filter in from the blood. However, the epithelial cells are linked by tight junctions that prevent the free flow of this filtrate. The choroid epithelial cells selectively transport ions and glucose into the ventricles, with water following osmotically (Fig. 12.4). The CSF then flows through the ventricles into the subarachnoid space, via the lateral and

Table 12.2 Comparison of blood plasma and cerebrospinal fluid (CSF) composition

	CSF	Plasma
Protein (mg/dL)	35	7000
Glucose (mg/dL)	60	90
Na^+ (mmol/L)	138	138
K^+ (mmol/L)	2.8	4.5
Ca^{2+} (mmol/L)	2.1	4.8
Mg^{2+} (mmol/L)	2.3	1.7
Cl^- (mmol/L)	119	102
pH	7.33	7.41

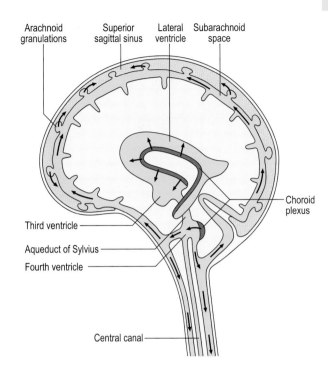

Fig. 12.5 Production and flow of cerebrospinal fluid (CSF). CSF is secreted into the lateral, third and fourth ventricles, and flows into the subarachnoid space. Arrows indicate flow of CSF.

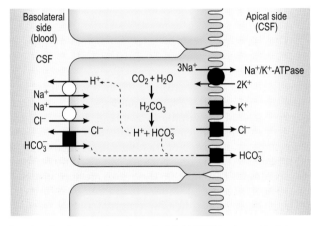

Fig. 12.4 Production of cerebrospinal fluid (CSF) by the epithelial cells of the choroid plexus. Filled circle, primary active transport; open circles, secondary active transport; filled rectangles, facilitated diffusion.

Box 12.3 Hydrocephalus

Hydrocephalus (or water on the brain) is the abnormal accumulation of cerebrospinal fluid (CSF). This can occur if the flow of CSF through the ventricles and over the brain is impaired, if there is a reduction in the reabsorption of CSF, and rarely, if there is excess CSF production. The commonest cause of hydrocephalus is the obstruction of the CSF flow from the fourth ventricle into the subarachnoid space, with a consequent enlargement of the ventricles. In babies, whose cranial sutures have not yet fused, this causes enlargement of the head with thinning of the cerebral hemispheres. In adults, because the skull is rigid, the increased pressure compresses blood vessels and damages brain tissue.

median apertures of the fourth ventricle. The ventricles are lined with ependymal cells. These are simple epithelial cells with numerous microvilli and one or two cilia on their apical surface. Their basolateral surface is in contact with astrocytic processes. After leaving the ventricles, the CSF flows through the cisternae at the base of the brain, and then travels across the cerebral and cerebellar hemispheres (Fig. 12.5). It is aided by the movement of the microvilli and cilia of the ependymal cells that line the ventricles, and by its reabsorption into the venous sinuses. This reabsorption involves the movement of all of the CSF into the venous blood, and has been suggested to be produced by the movement of large vacuoles across the arachnoid epithelium. Some of the fluid drains into cervical lymph nodes via the sheaths of the cranial nerves and into the spinal veins through arachnoid projections. In some cases, CSF can accumulate (Box 12.3).

Very little CSF flows through the central canal of the spinal cord, which is not patent in most adults, but some CSF flows within the subarachnoid space through the foramen magnum, towards the lumbar region, reaching the end of the spinal meninges in about 12 h. As the meninges of the spinal cord extend to the second sacral vertebra (S2) but the spinal cord extends only as far as the first or second lumbar level (L1, L2), the space below L2 forms a large lumbar cistern containing CSF that can be sampled by lumbar puncture (see Box 4.2). There is little danger of damaging the freely floating spinal nerves, as they will drift away from the point of the needle. However, lumbar puncture should not be performed under circumstances of increased intracranial pressure, as this can cause herniation of the brain.

The blood–brain barrier

The BBB is formed from endothelial cells, which make up the continuous capillaries of the brain. These are surrounded by a layer of basement membrane, which itself is covered by a layer consisting of the endfeet of glial astrocytes (Fig. 12.6). These do not touch the endothelial cells but are important in producing factors that induce specific characteristics in the endothelial cells. These characteristics include high transendothelial resistance, which is due to the length and complexity of the tight junctions between the endothelial cells. There are also very few pores, either small or large, that cross the endothelium, and transcytosis is limited.

The brain endothelium is more restrictive, by a factor of 50–100, than other continuous capillaries. It is this 'tight' barrier that prevents bloodborne compounds from entering the brain, unless specifically transported. Other BBB characteristics include the presence of specific populations of transporters that move molecules in and out of the brain. Sugars and amino acids are transported in, while P-glycoprotein acts to transport lipophilic molecules out. The action of this efflux pump, while protecting the brain from many xenobiotics, has the effect of reducing the movement of many therapeutic drugs across the BBB. This has important consequences for the treatment of brain-specific illness, as the drugs have to gain access to the brain by travelling through the BBB in some way.

Substances injected into the CSF can travel freely into the brain. The ependymal cells that line the ventricles are not connected by tight junctions. However, in the choroid plexus, although the endothelial cells are 'leaky', a blood–CSF barrier is produced by tight junctions between the choroid epithelial cells.

Meningitis

Meningitis is an inflammation of the pia and arachnoid mater, and is indicated by an increase in the number of white cells in the CSF. Meningitis is most commonly caused by a wide variety of infective agents; however, there are also non-infective causes, such as contrast medium, drugs and tumour cells. It is normally confined to the subarachnoid space, rather than the subdural space. Infective agents can access the CSF directly via the sinuses or the nasopharynx, through fractures of the skull or, most commonly, from the bloodstream.

Meningitis occurs as a result either of organisms crossing the BBB during systemic infection, or of a breakdown of the barrier due to a skull fracture or neurosurgery. A contiguous infection of the middle ear or paranasal sinuses can also lead to infection of the meninges. However, the most common route is through the blood, across the BBB. How the barrier is breached is not known. It may be that toxins produced by bacteria in the blood stimulate an increase in the permeability of either the BBB or the blood–CSF barrier. A further possibility is that organisms cross into the brain in areas such as the area postrema, where there is no BBB.

Bacterial meningitis

There are about 2000–2500 formally notified cases per year of bacterial meningitis in England and Wales, and over half of these are caused by infection with *Neisseria meningitidis* or are cases of meningococcal meningitis. It should be noted that other bacteria can also be associated with meningitis (Table 12.3). Most cases are sporadic; only about 1% of cases are secondary to other known cases.

There are several different serogroups of *N. meningitidis*, which are associated with different risk groups. Most meningitis occurs in children under the age of 4 years, with the greatest age-specific risk being at 6–12 months. This is mainly due to serogroup B, but also to serogroup C. There is a second peak of meningitis in late adolescence, largely due to serogroup C. Serogroup A infection occurs mainly in non-industrialized countries, and is associated with epidemics.

In the UK a conjugate vaccine against *N. meningitidis* serogroup C strains is now given to young children, while university students are being given a polysaccharide-only

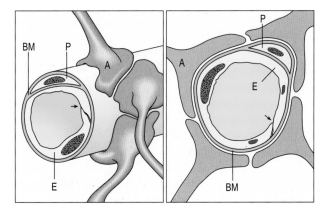

Fig. 12.6 Cells forming the blood–brain barrier. E, endothelial cell; A, astrocyte; BM, basement membrane; P, pericyte. The arrow indicates the inter-endothelial tight junctions.

Table 12.3 Possible causes of bacterial meningitis
Neisseria meningitides (meningococcus)[*]
Streptococcus pneumoniae (pneumococcus)[*]
Staphylococcus aureus
Haemophilus influenzae (type b)[†]
Escherichia coli
Mycobacterium tuberculosis
Lysteria monocytogenes
[*]*Major causes of meningitis.* [†]*Almost eliminated due to vaccination.*

vaccine, because they show a reasonable response to T-cell-independent antigens. This has almost completely abolished deaths due to serogroup C. However, there is at present no vaccine against serogroup B.

Meningococci are ubiquitous Gram-negative diplococci. Many people carry meningococci in the nasopharynx, but most strains are non-pathogenic. However, up to 1% of the population may carry pathogenic strains. The main risk seems to be the recent acquisition of a new strain, but it is unknown why a small minority develop meningitis and most people do not.

A particular symptom of meningococcal meningitis is a haemorrhagic rash. This is due to leakage of blood from capillaries into the skin. This can produce petechiae, which are small skin haemorrhages that vary in size from pinpoints to a few millimetres. The rash does not blanch on pressure and can be seen clearly when a glass is pressed on the skin. However, this sign may be sparse and does not occur in all cases, being most common in the more severe forms of the disease. Septicaemia is a dangerous complication of meningitis (Box 12.4).

Even in the absence of septicaemia, meningitis is still a medical emergency, with the main pathology being cerebral oedema. In the subarachnoid space there are relatively few phagocytic cells and low levels of complement. This enables invading bacteria to multiply rapidly. Lipopolysaccharide components of the bacterial cell walls stimulate the production of inflammatory cytokines, such as interleukin-1 and tumour necrosis factor, which increase the permeability of the BBB and attract neutrophils. Protein leaks across the endothelium, and water follows due to the increase in interstitial colloid osmotic pressure, producing cerebral oedema. This raises the intracranial pressure, and

the associated risk of herniation. A poor prognostic feature is depression of consciousness.

There are two other main bacterial causes of meningitis. These are *Haemophilus influenzae* type b, and *Streptococcus pneumoniae*. *Haemophilus influenzae* infection usually occurs in young children (<5 years), but since the introduction of the Hib vaccine in 1992, this has all but disappeared in the UK. *Streptococcus pneumoniae* infection is usually associated with young infants, the elderly with respiratory infections, or otitis media (inflammation of the middle ear lining). In neonates, the most common causative agents are *Escherichia coli* and group B *Streptococcus*.

A further cause of bacterial meningitis, which is more common in developing countries, is infection with *Mycobacterium tuberculosis*, which causes tuberculous meningitis. This form of meningitis is slow in onset and may occur years after the primary infection; it may be preceded by non-specific symptoms.

Other bacteria, such as *Staphylococcus aureus* and *Listeria monocytogenes*, have been associated with meningitis, particularly in immunocompromised patients (see Table 12.4).

Aseptic and viral meningitis

The term aseptic meningitis is used to describe cases in which there are clinical signs of meningitis, but bacteria cannot be cultured from the CSF. This can have a wide range of causes, including viral and other non-bacterial infections, such as with fungi and protozoa (Table 12.4). Meningitis can also have non-infective, inflammatory causes such as sarcoidosis.

Many different viruses can cause meningitis, but this is usually less severe than bacterial meningitis and is self-limiting, lasting for 4–10 days. There may be continuing headaches for several weeks, but there are rarely any serious sequelae.

Box 12.4 Septicaemia and meningococcal meningitis

When the infection due to *N. meningitidis* spreads in the blood, a severe form of septicaemia can occur. There is a large drop in blood pressure, due to reduced peripheral resistance. This occurs because of the action of the bacterial endotoxin, which, via increases in nitric oxide synthesis, causes relaxation of vascular smooth muscle. There is increased secretion of a cytokine, interleukin-1, which increases capillary permeability. The flow through capillary beds becomes very slow, and eventually clotting factors can accumulate and produce inappropriate clotting in the tissues. This is called disseminated intravascular coagulation. As well as reducing blood flow still further and preventing the supply of oxygen and removal of acid products of metabolism from the tissues, this depletes the available clotting factors, allowing blood to haemorrhage from the leaky blood vessels. The severe reduction in blood flow leads to metabolic acidosis, and eventually to skin and limb necrosis.

Table 12.4 Some non-bacterial causes of meningitis

Type of organism	Examples
Viruses	Enteroviruses (echovirus, Coxsackie virus types A and B)
	Mumps
	Poliovirus
	Epstein–Barr virus
	Herpes viruses (herpes simplex and herpes zoster)
	Human immunodeficiency virus
Fungi	*Cryptococcus neoformans*
	Candida spp.
Spirochaetes	Leptospirosis, Lyme disease, syphilis

Diagnosis and treatment of meningitis

Meningitis is usually diagnosed on the basis of a combination of clinical features and laboratory diagnostic tests. However, the progression of bacterial meningitis is so rapid that when meningitis is suspected, treatment should be started before laboratory results are available. Benzylpenicillin should be given immediately, either intravenously or intramuscularly, by the first doctor to suspect meningitis. This broad-spectrum antibiotic is given because it is effective against meningococcal and pneumococcal infection. It can be combined with chloramphenicol, which is active against *Haemophilus* spp.

Meningitis usually presents with headache, often of rapid onset, fever, neck stiffness, photophobia and vomiting. In some types of meningitis there is also a rash. There may be altered consciousness, seizures and focal signs.

The headache may be due to inflammation of the supratentorial dura, which is innervated by the trigeminal nerve. The neck stiffness and reflex neck retraction are due to reflex contraction of the posterior nuchal muscles. These muscles are supplied by the cervical nerves that innervate the infratentorial dura.

Patients may show a positive Kernig's sign: after flexion of the leg at the hip, extension of the knee produces lower back pain, indicating irritation of the meninges.

Cerebrospinal fluid sampling and changes in cerebrospinal fluid composition

Meningitis can be diagnosed after sampling the CSF through a lumbar puncture (see Fig. 12.6). However, if there are any signs of focal intracranial disease or raised intracranial pressure, and if subsequent neuroimaging reveals any evidence of impaired CSF circulation, then lumbar puncture should not be carried out, as there is a risk of brain herniation. It is also contraindicated in severely ill children, as it may lead to deterioration. Throat swabs can indicate the presence of meningococcal infection.

Normal CSF is clear and contains very few cells. Inflammation of the meninges will increase the number of immune cells present. In bacterial meningitis, these will be predominantly neutrophils, while in other types of meningitis they are mainly lymphocytes (Table 12.5). The presence of bacteria will make the CSF turbid or even clearly pus-containing, and, reflecting the breakdown of the BBB, there will be higher than normal levels

of protein. Because of the utilization of CSF glucose by metabolizing bacteria, the levels will be abnormally low in bacterial meningitis. CSF pressure is raised, and CSF flow may be impaired due to adhesions of the meninges and the presence of pus.

Culture of CSF (and blood) can reveal the type of bacterial infection present. This is important not only in order to determine the optimal antibiotic combination to use in further treatment, but also to obtain data about the antibiotic sensitivity of the bacteria. While *N. meningitidis* remains sensitive to penicillin, a significant number of *H. influenzae* strains and some *S. pneumoniae* strains show antibiotic resistance (Box 12.5).

Bacteria in cases of meningitis can be identified by examining cultures. Morphology and Gram staining will differentiate between the three main bacterial causes, and the Ziehl–Nielsen stain identifies acid-fast bacilli, such as *Mycobacterium*. However, these are only seen in about 20% of cases of tubercular meningitis. Indian ink can be used to stain fungi.

Box 12.5 Antibiotic resistance

Both the penicillins and cephalosporins are β-lactams, and act by inhibiting one of the final stages of the synthesis of peptidoglycan, which forms the cell wall of Gram-positive bacteria. However, some bacterial strains have developed resistance to some of these antibiotics. One of the main mechanisms of this resistance is the production by bacteria of β-lactamases, which destroy the antibiotics by cleaving the β-lactam ring. This has led to the development of β-lactam antibiotics that are β-lactamase resistant, such as flucloxacillin. Chloramphenicol acts in a different way from the β-lactams, by inhibiting bacterial protein synthesis. Resistance to chloramphenicol is due to the production by the bacteria of acetyltransferase enzymes, which inactivate the antibiotic by acetylation.

Meticillin-resistant *Staphylococcus aureus* (MRSA) is a particular problem, as only vancomycin and teicoplanin are effective in most cases, and there are even reports of resistance to these drugs. New groups of antibiotics such as the streptogramins and the oxazolidinones are still effective against MRSA.

Table 12.5 Comparison of cerebrospinal fluid in different types of meningitis

Type	Cell count	Cell types	Protein	Glucose
Bacterial	>200/μL	Polymorphs	>1.5 g/L	<40% of that in blood
Viral	50–200/μL	Lymphocytes	<1.0 g/L	Normal
Normal	<5/μL	Lymphocytes	<0.45 g/L	>60% of that in blood

One of the problems with culturing CSF (and blood) is that it can take some time, and in the case of tuberculosis may take many weeks. Newer tests may enable the causative agents to be identified more quickly. Antigen detection of specific polysaccharides present on the bacterial cells walls in the CSF or urine can be used to detect some bacteria. The bacterial DNA of *N. meningitidis* can now be identified with the technique of DNA amplification by the polymerase chain reaction (PCR).

Treatment of meningitis

It is very important that antibiotic treatment is initiated immediately on suspicion of bacterial meningitis. The treatments of choice for meningococcal and pneumococcal infection are benzylpenicillin and cefotaxime, respectively; cefotaxime and chloramphenicol can be used to treat *H. influenzae*. If the causative agent has not yet been identified, then a combination of these drugs should be used. The antibiotic treatment should be continued for 7 days after the fever has ceased (14 days for pneumococcal infections).

Other treatment should be aimed at reducing the fever, and pain relief for headaches. Anticonvulsants (diazepam) should be used for patients with seizures. In cases of septicaemia, fluid balance must be strictly monitored and, if possible, controlled. Septicaemia can lead very rapidly to severe shock, disseminated intravascular coagulation and multi-organ failure.

The β-lactam antibiotics disrupt the bacterial cell walls, releasing more of the lipopolysaccharides that cause the inflammatory response. In this way, the treatment can exacerbate the pathology. In cases of infection with *H. influenzae* and *S. pneumoniae*, there is some evidence that pretreatment with steroids can reduce the subsequent cerebral oedema and reduce the potential after-effects, such as deafness. However, this has not been shown for *N. meningitidis*, and the need for rapid antibiotic therapy would make any delay dangerous.

Tuberculous meningitis is treated for the first 2 months with a combination of isoniazid (with pyridoxine to prevent side effects due to pyridoxine deficiency), rifampicin and pyrazinamide. Treatment with isoniazid and rifampicin must then be continued, along with regular monitoring, for at least another 10 months.

Bacterial meningitis can progress extremely rapidly, and any delay in treatment can increase the morbidity and mortality. The most serious form of meningococcal meningitis involves septicaemia, and this accounts for most of the 20% mortality associated with this type of meningitis. If septicaemia is not present, then the mortality rate drops to 3%, which is lower than those for *H. influenzae* (4–5%) and *S. pneumoniae* (10%).

Long-term sequelae of meningitis include hydrocephalus, cranial nerve palsies, visual and motor deficits and epilepsy. In children, there may be behavioural disturbances, learning difficulties, hearing loss and epilepsy.

Meningitis and meningococcal septicaemia are statutory notifiable diseases in England and Wales and should be reported to the local Consultant in Communicable Disease Control (CCDC). Any contacts and family members of a patient with meningococcal meningitis are at increased risk (800-fold), and should be given rifampicin or ciprofloxacin in order to eradicate bacteria in the throat.

Encephalitis

Viral encephalitis can be produced by several viruses (Table 12.6); the infections can be sporadic, epidemic or transmitted by animals. Many of these sporadic infections cause a mild illness, with headache and drowsiness, which is self-limiting, but in more severe cases patients have altered behaviour, seizures, confusion or coma. Brain swelling is common, with its associated risk of brain damage.

In the UK, the most dangerous form of viral encephalitis is that caused by HSV. While HSV can be identified in CSF with the use of viral antigen immunoassays and amplification of viral DNA with PCR techniques, this is usually too slow to be of clinical use. For this reason, patients with acute encephalitis should be treated with acyclovir immediately, especially if there is evidence of brain swelling on computed tomography (CT) scans (Box 12.6). There are no other specific treatments for encephalitis, except ganciclovir, which is active against cytomegalovirus. Patients may need treatment for seizures and cerebral oedema.

Encephalitis may occasionally be caused by other organisms, such as *Mycoplasma*, *Rickettsia* (typhus) and *Histoplasma*.

Cerebral abscesses

A range of bacteria, fungi and protozoa (e.g. *Streptococcus*, *Staphylococcus*, *Bacteroides* and *Proteus*) can cause focal areas of infection, i.e. abscesses, in the brain and spinal cord. The infection usually reaches the brain from infectious sites elsewhere in the body, so identification and treatment of

Table 12.6 Causes of viral encephalitis
Sporadic
Herpes simplex (HSV)
Herpes zoster
Cytomegalovirus
Epstein–Barr virus
Adenovirus
Human immunodeficiency virus
Epidemic
Arboviruses
Eastern equine encephalitis virus
Japanese B arbovirus

Acyclovir and antiviral therapy

While there are many effective antibacterial agents that target specific bacterial processes, there are far fewer steps that can be selectively blocked by drugs that will inhibit viruses without harming the host, because viruses survive by utilizing many of the normal metabolic processes of the host cell. Acyclovir exploits the need of the virus to produce new viral DNA, which it does using a viral DNA polymerase that is different from the mammalian enzyme. Acyclovir is a guanine derivative that is converted to the monophosphate by thymidine kinase. This occurs most rapidly in the virus-infected cells, as the viral kinase is much more effective than the host enzyme. The host cell kinases then convert the monophosphate to acyclovir triphosphate. This is then incorporated into the growing DNA chain, where it acts as a chain terminator.

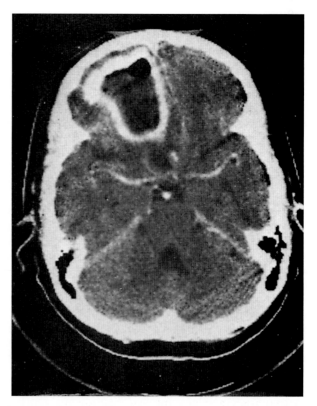

Fig. 12.7 Enhanced axial computed tomography scan showing a right frontal abscess. From Forbes CD, Jackson WF. Colour Atlas and Text of Clinical Medicine, 3rd edn. Mosby International Ltd, 2002.

the source of the infection should form part of the overall treatment.

The patient usually has a combination of progressive headache, focal neurological signs, seizures and fever. The investigation of choice is a CT or MRI scan. Lumbar puncture should not be carried out, because of the risk of herniation. A few weeks after infection, the abscess becomes encapsulated and can be seen clearly (Fig. 12.7). The central area of the abscess will have a low-density appearance, there will be prominent ring enhancement of the lesion, which appears bright, and there will be an oedematous surrounding area of low density. Because of the mass effect of the abscess, there may also be a shift in the midline and compression of the ventricles.

Treatment involves surgical decompression and drainage of the abscess, antibiotics (broad spectrum until the causative agent has been identified) and treatment for cerebral oedema.

Brain infections in the immunocompromised patient

An increasing number of patients have compromised immune systems. This may result from treatment with cytotoxic drugs or immunosuppressant steroids, or long-term severe general illness. In these patients there is an increased risk of infection with bacteria and fungi . However, the largest group of immunocompromised patients are those with immune deficiency due to infection with human immunodeficiency virus (HIV).

Infection with HIV can cause neurological disease at any stage, but most problems occur when patients have progressed to AIDS, with significant impairment of their immune systems. Like other immunocompromised patients, they are prone to a wide range of infections, both with organisms that are normally pathogenic but cause more severe infections in these patients, and with organisms that are not normally pathogenic (i.e. opportunistic infections).

HIV can infect and replicate in the microglial cells of the brain, which can act as a reservoir of infection. The active replication of HIV in the brain leads to increased permeability of the BBB, allowing easier access to infecting organisms, and in consequence, 80% of HIV-positive patients develop some neurological disease. Any future treatment to eradicate HIV must also be able to eradicate the virus present in the brain, because the movement of macrophages across the BBB could result in re-infection.

A condition specific to HIV infection is called HIV-associated dementia. This is a slowly developing dementia that is thought to be due to a direct effect of HIV infection of the brain. It is dealt with in more detail in Chapter 14.

EPILEPSY

13

Chapter objectives

After studying this chapter you should be able to:

1. Define epilepsy and describe the main types.

2. Discuss the use of electroencephalography in the investigation of neuronal function and the diagnosis of epilepsy.

3. Give an outline of mechanisms that underlie seizures.

4. Describe the treatment for epilepsy.

5. Discuss the implications of epilepsy for the quality of life of patients.

Introduction

In adults, once the brain has reached maturation, control over sensorimotor and autonomic functions is expected, as well as complete awareness of one's behaviour and reactions under various social circumstances. One of the commonest neurological diseases, epilepsy, often deprives an adult of this control and leads to a dramatic loss of contact with reality, through loss of consciousness. An illustration of this is given in the case history in Box 13.1. As will be discussed in this chapter, epilepsy is a major medical problem that poses a challenge therapeutically, can significantly disrupt the course of a normal life and its quality, and may bring social stigma to the sufferer.

General description of epilepsy

A seizure is an uncontrolled sustained discharge of a large group of neurones in the brain. Epilepsy is the name given to a heterogeneous group of conditions in which there is a tendency for seizures to reoccur; that is, there have been at least two before diagnosis. The types

of seizure that occur in epilepsy are very varied, ranging from the generalized seizure with loss of consciousness, muscle spasms and coma (commonly known as grand mal), to the much less overwhelming petit mal (absence seizure), the only sign of which is that the person stops what they are doing and appears to be staring into the distance. Seizures are generally self-limiting phenomena. However, in some cases, generalized seizures are not self-limiting, and the patient will have recurrent seizures for 10–20 min, without regaining consciousness between them. This is known as status epilepticus and is a serious, life-threatening medical emergency.

In a broad sense, there are two categories of epilepsy: partial epilepsy, in which the seizures begin focally in the brain, and generalized epilepsy, which involves both hemispheres of the brain from the outset. However, the clinical situation is much more complex, as reflected in the present classification of the epilepsies. There is a detailed classification system, devised by the International League Against Epilepsy (ILAE), for seizure types. A simplified form of this classification is shown in Table 13.1.

The different types of seizure are associated with different patterns of muscular activity. Myoclonic seizures involve either localized or widespread, rapid, irregular jerking of muscles, while in tonic seizures there is a sudden rigidity of muscles, either extended or flexed. Clonic seizures involve the rhythmic jerking of many muscles, and in tonic–clonic seizures there is clonic jerking after initial tonic rigidity.

Epidemiology of epilepsy

Epilepsy is a common neurological disorder. The prevalence in the world is 0.5–1%, and the lifetime incidence is 1–3%. Symptomatic epilepsy can be caused by problems such as brain tumours or meningitis, and metabolic

Box 13.1 Case history

Gaby is a 22-year-old student who is studying to become a teacher. She has no previous serious medical history. One day, as she relaxes with her fellow students after an examination, she feels strange, with butterflies in her stomach and a sensation of fear and anxiety. She then collapses rigidly onto the floor. She has strong convulsions for about 2 min, during which she knocks against a chair. Her body then relaxes, and for the next 3 min she cannot be roused. When she wakes up she is confused and tired, and also bruised from hitting the chair. She is taken to hospital by her colleagues, where the doctor tells her she has had a seizure. There is no family history of seizures. She undergoes a series of tests, including an electroencephalogram (EEG) and a brain scan. A few weeks later she has a second seizure at home, and following a consultation with the hospital specialist, she starts taking sodium valproate. She is advised to change her type of contraceptive pill. She is very concerned about the implications of having this disease for her career choice as a teacher.

This case gives rise to the following questions:

1. What is epilepsy?
2. What does an EEG measure and how is it used in the diagnosis of epilepsy?
3. What are the mechanisms of excitation and inhibition in the brain and how are seizures produced?
4. What types of epilepsy are there?
5. How is epilepsy treated?
6. What restrictions are there for patients with epilepsy?

Table 13.1 International classification of epileptic seizures (simplified)

Partial (focal) seizures	Simple partial seizures (consciousness not impaired)
	Complex partial seizures (consciousness lost)
	Partial seizures evolving to secondary generalized seizures
Generalized seizures	Absence seizures
	Myoclonic seizures
	Clonic seizures
	Tonic seizures
	Tonic–clonic seizures
	Atonic seizures
Unclassified seizures	

abnormalities such as hypoglycaemia and uraemia (Table 13.2). However, most cases of epilepsy have no immediately obvious cause and are termed idiopathic (i.e. without an apparent cause in a patient without neurological deficits) or cryptogenic (a cause is suspected but not proven). There are several predisposing factors for the development of epilepsy, but in many cases there is no history to suggest a cause. Some types of seizure can be induced by flashing lights, such as flickering fluorescent lights, computer or television screens, and strobe lighting.

Types of epileptic syndrome

The aetiologies and types of seizure disorder are age-dependent. Some of the common childhood epileptic syndromes are shown in Table 13.3. In children, generalized seizures occur more than partial seizures. Epilepsy in children is predominantly idiopathic. In contrast, in adults there is an increasing incidence of acquired epilepsy, which is secondary to head injury, tumours, stroke or infections. In adults, partial seizures are the predominant seizure type.

The classification of seizures and epilepsy is extremely complex, and a simpler approach, which leads to a 'decision-tree' system, may be more useful to the general medical practitioner. This works on the idea that seizures can be classified better by their frequency, what provokes them and any identifiable underlying cause.

Patients with epilepsy have a high frequency of depression and a higher risk of suicide than the general population. In addition, three distinct patterns of psychosis are associated with epilepsy. They occur either during (ictal), after (postictal) or between (interictal) seizures. Interictal psychosis may be produced by an unwanted effect of the antiepileptic therapy, and postictal psychosis may require antipsychotic treatment.

Diagnostic investigations of epilepsy

A patient with suspected epilepsy must be given a complete neurological examination. This could reveal deficits that reflect specific structural changes.

When diagnosing epilepsy, it is first important to make sure that there is no confusion with conditions that produce similar clinical signs, such as syncope, transient ischaemic attacks (TIAs), hypoglycaemia, migraine or pseudoseizures (psychogenic seizures). Once the diagnosis of epilepsy is confirmed, it is important to obtain additional information and determine possible causes. In an adult with no previous history of epilepsy, it is important to carry out a brain scan in order to exclude the possibility of a tumour or other mass-filling lesion as the cause of the seizures. Establishing whether there is a family history of epilepsy is also important (Box 13.2).

Electroencephalography and magnetoencephalography

Electroencephalography and magnetoencephalography are based on the generation of electrical and magnetic fields as a consequence of the electrical activity of neurones. An EEG is a non-invasive method of measuring the surface electrical activity of the brain. When neurones in the brain are active, the electrical currents that flow across

---

Table 13.2 Some of the causes and predisposing factors of epilepsy

Metabolic disturbances (especially electrolyte imbalances and uraemia)

Hypoxia

Chronic alcohol abuse (either during heavy drinking or during withdrawal)

Some neuroactive drugs (either in overdose or at normal levels in susceptible patients)

Drug withdrawal states (especially phenobarbitone and benzodiazepines)

Strokes (haemorrhagic or infarction)

Aneurysms

Perinatal trauma and anoxia

Central nervous system infection (meningitis, encephalitis, cerebral abscess)

Traumatic brain injury

Family history

Intrauterine infections (e.g. rubella)

Developmental abnormalities

Craniotomy

Degenerative brain disorders

Brain tumour

Table 13.3 Some of the common childhood epileptic syndromes

Syndrome	Age of onset	Features
Childhood absence epilepsy (CAE)	3–12 years	Many absences Convulsions rare
Juvenile absence epilepsy	7–17 years	Fewer absences than with CAE Convulsions common
Juvenile myoclonic epilepsy (Janz syndrome)	10–20 years	Myoclonic jerks on waking Generalized tonic–clonic seizures Occasional absences
Infantile spasms (West's syndrome)	3–7 months	Flexor spasms, tonic and atonic seizures, progressive mental handicap

There is a strong correlation between epilepsy and family history, with about 30% of patients having a close relative with epilepsy. Results obtained in the past decade show that several types of idiopathic epilepsy are associated with gene mutations. For most epileptic syndromes, the mode of inheritance is complex. For example, common forms of idiopathic epilepsy, such as juvenile myoclonic epilepsy or juvenile and childhood absence epilepsy, do not follow a simple Mendelian mode of inheritance. Identification of the genes mutated in idiopathic epilepsies shows these forms of epilepsy to be channelopathies; that is, they are due to mutations in voltage- or ligand-gated ion channels (e.g. nicotinic receptors, Na^+, K^+ and Ca^{2+} channels, and $GABA_A$ receptors). These mutations ultimately lead to altered neuronal excitability. However, the details of the mechanisms that underlie the development of epilepsy in each case are still incompletely understood.

Box
13.3   Cerebral cortical neurones and the generation of electrical signals

The cerebral cortex is organized into six distinct layers, with layer 1 lying just beneath the pia mater and layer 6 just above the white matter. Within these layers, there is a relatively similar arrangement of the different cell types throughout the brain, although the thickness of the layers varies in the different functional regions of the cortex. The cells with the largest cell bodies in the cortex are the pyramidal cells, which are found in layers 2, 3 and 5, orientated with their apex with its long dendrite running upwards towards the brain surface. From their base, long axons descend through deeper layers and leave the cortex. Areas rich in pyramidal cells are mainly output layers. The cortex also contains non-pyramidal cells, which are usually smaller and have no specific orientation of their dendrites. Their axons terminate locally, in the same layer or immediate vicinity. Non-pyramidal cells are involved primarily in receiving inputs from thalamic and other afferents and in the local processing of information. As pyramidal cells are orientated with their dendrites at right angles to the cortical surface, when they are active the potentials generated in the extracellular fluid give the largest signal at the brain surface.

the neuronal cell membranes also set up extracellular currents that flow through the extracellular space. Recordings of these currents can be made at sites distant from where the currents are generated. In the case of an EEG, these currents can be measured by electrodes placed on the scalp. The changes in electrical potential measured by the EEG are the summated ionic currents produced by the large numbers of neurones found under the electrodes, in the cortex (see Box 13.3). The electrodes are positioned according to a standard pattern, and the potential difference is measured between pairs of electrodes (Fig. 13.1).

While the largest signal generated by neurones is the action potential, it is a very short-lasting event, and unless action potentials occur simultaneously, they cannot summate to produce a large enough extracellular electrical potential to be measured by the surface electrodes. Therefore, most of the electrical activity measured in an EEG comes from the summation of postsynaptic potentials. Although these are smaller than action potentials, they are much slower in their development and can therefore summate. The direction of the waves recorded by the EEG electrodes will depend both on whether the postsynaptic potential is excitatory or inhibitory and on the depth of the activity within the cortex. Within the cortex, much of the activity is usually contained within individual local areas, with outputs to distant areas, allowing for extensive parallel and serial processing of sensory and motor information. However, when the activity of several groups of neurones is synchronized, a seizure can occur.

Normal EEG patterns

A clinician uses an EEG to obtain information about the activity in the brain. It is a sensitive indicator of behaviour

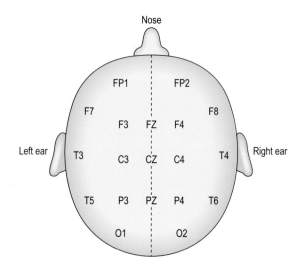

Fig. 13.1 Standard placement of EEG leads. The letters and numbers correspond to specific anatomical positions. For example, F = frontal.

and shows characteristic patterns when a person is alert, drowsy or asleep. The amplitude of the EEG waves depends on the synchronicity in activity of the underlying neurones. A frequency that is too high or too low is indicative of impaired cortical function. In addition, the presence of unusual waveforms, such as sharp spikes, spike-and-wave potentials or unusually slow waves, indicates a brain lesion or seizure disorder.

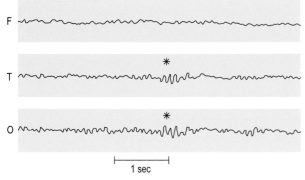

F

T

    *

O

    *

|— 1 sec —|

Fig. 13.2 Normal electroencephalogram patterns from the frontal, temporal and occipital lobes recorded at rest. The frontal lobes (F) show low-amplitude, high-frequency beta activity, while higher-amplitude, lower-frequency alpha activity (*) is seen in the temporal (T) and occipital (O) lobes.

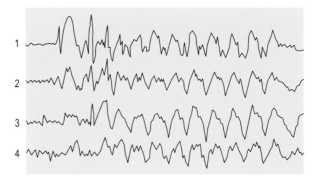

Fig. 13.3 An electroencephalogram showing activity typical of generalized epilepsy, with large spikes and waves that are synchronized in all four leads.

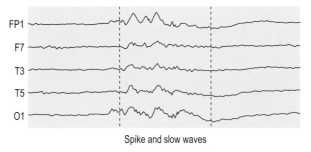

FP1

F7

T3

T5

O1

Spike and slow waves

Fig. 13.4 Spike and slow-wave interictal activity in a patient with generalized epilepsy.

Although the EEG pattern of every individual is unique, there are several common patterns that can be related to specific brain states (Fig. 13.2). In general, an EEG pattern that is of low amplitude and high frequency, with no obvious pattern, indicates an alert or awake state. These are beta waves, and have a frequency of 14–25 Hz. This type of activity is called desynchronous, and occurs because the brain neurones are all working independently, so that many of the different frequencies of activity cancel each other out. However, when a person is relaxed, especially with their eyes closed, as in sleep or quiet contemplation, the amplitude increases but the frequency is low. This rhythm of activity is the alpha rhythm, and occurs because neurones are now firing synchronously. These slow synchronous waves are of low amplitude and have a frequency of 8–13 Hz. They are largest in the parieto-occipital region, but if a relaxed person is disturbed or opens their eyes, or becomes anxious, the alpha rhythms abruptly stop. Theta and delta waves are not normally seen in awake adults. Irregular theta waves (4–7 Hz) are common in children and are seen in adults in early and rapid eye movement (REM) sleep. Low-frequency (4 Hz or less), high-amplitude delta waves are only seen in deep sleep or during anaesthesia or coma. Other characteristic EEG patterns can occur, such as the sudden high-amplitude bursts called sleep spindles, which happen during stage 2 sleep. If the brain dies, the EEG pattern becomes a flat line.

Electroencephalogram patterns in epilepsy

The EEG is an essential component in the diagnosis of epilepsy. It provides important information about background activity and epileptiform discharges, and is required for the diagnosis of specific syndromes. This guides selection of antiepileptic medication and prognosis. There are dramatic and characteristic changes in the EEG patterns of patients with epilepsy during seizures (Fig. 13.3), but unless the recording is prolonged, the patient may not

have a seizure during the EEG procedure. The pattern of activity during a fit is called the ictal phase.

However, 50–70% of patients will show characteristic epileptiform activity between seizures; this is the interictal activity. In some cases, it is also possible to induce abnormal activity by forced hyperventilation (3 min) or flashing lights (stroboscopic photic stimulation). Interictal changes may take the form of spikes and waves (Fig. 13.4), which are thought to reflect the underlying depolarization of the cortical neurones. Up to 15% of patients with epilepsy show no abnormal interictal activity, while a significant number (0.5–2%) of randomly selected individuals without epilepsy show similar interictal electroencephalogram patterns. This rises to 5–10% in first-degree relatives of patients with confirmed epilepsy.

During a seizure, the EEG shows large-amplitude spikes and waves. They may be generalized, occurring in all electrodes, or they may only occur in a subset of the recordings. For example, in absence seizures, the EEG shows a rhythmic 3–4 Hz spike and wave potential from most scalp electrodes, whereas in grand mal fits, the EEG shows higher-frequency, irregular, large-amplitude waves from most recording sites. In some cases, the EEG may show the focal discharges spreading across the brain to give a generalized pattern. The region of origin of partial epilepsy can be determined by the pattern of the EEG abnormalities. This is necessary in the surgical treatment of epilepsy.

An interesting future development based on EEG recording is the potential prediction of seizures. There is accumulating evidence that seizures develop minutes to hours before their clinical expression. In the future, it may be possible to define the exact characteristics of the EEG changes that precede a seizure, and devise a therapeutic strategy to prevent the onset of the clinical seizure. There is some evidence that seizures can be predicted from clear changes in the EEG at least 20 min before they occur, with some more subtle changes occurring up to 90 min before seizure onset. An implantable device could warn of the impending seizure, and intervene with focal stimulation or focal application of drugs, so that the seizure is aborted.

Other diagnostic techniques

Structural changes in the brain can be studied with the use of techniques such as magnetic resonance imaging (MRI) and computed tomography (CT). Magnetic resonance spectroscopy (MRS) can detect changes in the biochemistry of the brain. Positron emission tomography (PET) can be used to study brain activity, and single photon emission computed tomography (SPECT) is used to locate seizure foci. Especially when they are used in combination, they can be of help in devising the best therapeutic strategy.

MRI can reveal previously undetected structural abnormalities. MRI scanning is useful for investigating aetiology, and for selecting patients for surgical treatment. The technique can reveal several types of cerebral abnormality, such as hippocampal sclerosis, small lesions (invisible on CT scans) and cortical dysgenesis.

The analysis of nervous tissue proton MRS spectra shows three major peaks: A N-acetylaspartate (NAA), creatine and phosphocreatine, and choline-containing compounds. A reduction in the NAA peak is generally viewed as reflecting neuronal loss or dysfunction. A reduction in the NAA peak and a concomitant increase in the other two major peaks may indicate gliosis and neuronal loss. MRS spectra can also provide information on tissue inositol, lactate, γ-aminobutyric acid (GABA) and glutamate concentrations. MRS can help in the detection of hippocampal sclerosis and cortical foci.

Different types of seizure

The different types of partial and generalized seizures have very diverse presentations.

Partial seizures

Simple partial seizures

Simple partial seizures occur when the seizure activity is limited to a focal area. There is no loss of consciousness.

The origin of focal seizures leads to symptoms that depend on the area involved. For example, convulsive limb movements on one side of the body indicate an epileptic focus in the motor cortex on the contralateral side. The patient may experience weakness in the affected muscles after the seizure. Other focal symptoms include tingling, hallucinations (visual, olfactory or gustatory) and swallowing or chewing movements. The latter are indicative of temporal lobe epilepsy, which is the commonest form of focal epilepsy. Because of the temporal lobe involvement in memory, it is not surprising that the focal symptoms can include a feeling of *déjà vu* (i.e. 'having been there before'), a feeling of a rush of memories, or memory loss. The patient may appear detached and slow, and may have repetitive movements, such as lip-smacking and chewing movements, and make noises. Sometimes this behaviour is more complex and may be aggressive. Focal epilepsies are often associated with focal structural disease, which can include developmental abnormalities in the young, and trauma or tumours in older patients.

Complex partial seizures

These focal epilepsies are associated with impaired consciousness. They are often more severe forms of temporal lobe epilepsies and may last for between 30s and 1–2 min. Although the patient may be unable to communicate or respond to commands, consciousness may not be completely impaired. During the seizure, patients may be able to continue simple motor behaviour.

Partial seizures with secondary generalization

Focal epilepsy may sometimes spread over the cerebral cortex, first on the side of the initial focus and then to the opposite hemisphere. This can be seen in the EEG by a gradual increase in the ictal activity, starting with the focal area and gradually including all the traces. A particular example of this type of seizure is known as Jacksonian epilepsy, in which the focal signs start either in the face or at the extremities of a limb. Movements then rapidly spread across the face or ascend the limb, leading to a generalized seizure (see below). Because the focal seizure may spread very rapidly and the patient may not remember the focal start of the seizure, the only indication that this is not a primary generalized seizure (apart from an EEG, which may be hard to obtain) is the evidence of focal movements (as reported by an observer) and unilateral postictal motor weakness (Todd's paralysis), which may be seen if the focus of the seizure is in the motor cortex.

Generalized seizures

Generalized seizures involve both hemispheres of the brain, and abnormalities can be seen simultaneously in all the EEG traces. Seizures of this type are thought to originate from midline structures such as the thalamus, which diffusely innervate the entire cortex, thus triggering a generalized seizure.

Absence seizures

This type of seizure, also known as petit mal, usually starts in childhood and may occur many times each day, lasting for only 5–15 s. The condition is reminiscent of 'daydreaming', with the patient staring vacantly, sometimes with eye-blinking and eye-rolling. The EEG shows a characteristic bilateral 3-Hz waveform, seen in all traces with synchronized spike–wave patterns. This type of epilepsy is often diagnosed following poor school performance by an inattentive child. It has been suggested that this type of seizure results from abnormalities in T-type Ca^{2+} channels.

Tonic–clonic seizures

This is the type of seizure suffered by Gaby (see Box 13.1). These seizures, also called grand mal, are the most typical type seen in adults. Prior to an attack, some patients may experience vague symptoms, called an 'aura'. This may be a smell or a taste, or just 'feeling strange'. It may last for a few seconds, which may be enough for the patient to be able to lie down, thus preventing injury due to falling during the seizure. However, many patients have no warning. The typical seizure of this type has three phases. The first is the tonic phase, which lasts for about 10–40 s. The patient becomes very rigid, as all the muscles in the body undergo tonic, sustained contraction. The patient falls rigidly, and as the respiratory and laryngeal muscles are also contracted, may let out a cry or grunt as air is forced out of the chest through the taut vocal cords. During this time, there is no respiration, so the patient becomes cyanotic. This is followed by the clonic phase, during which the muscles go into strong, random contractions. This limb-jerking may be accompanied by urinary and faecal incontinence, and there may be tongue-biting and frothing at the mouth. Breathing is jerky and inefficient and there is tachycardia. This phase usually lasts for 2–3 min, although it can last for longer. The third phase is a coma, in which the patient's breathing becomes regular and their colour returns to normal. The length of this period is related to the duration of the previous tonic–clonic phases. When patients wake, they may be confused and have a headache.

During a seizure of this type, the levels of neuronal activity are very high, but because of the reduction (or lack) of respiration, the blood oxygenation is poor. During this time, there is an accumulation of lactic acid in the brain, and it is this hypoxia and acidosis which is probably the cause of the coma. Blood tests show a raised pH and a low pO_2. There are increases in creatine phosphokinase and serum prolactin levels.

Repeated seizures can lead to neuronal degeneration, which is thought to be due to the excessive release of glutamate during the seizure. This can cause cell death through the mechanism known as excitotoxicity, a mechanism that is also implicated in cell death due to stroke (see Chapter 11).

Febrile convulsions

This type of seizure, which may be generalized or focal, occurs commonly in young children under the age of 5 years, and is triggered by fever. Comparison of the EEGs of children and adults shows that the electrical activity of the adult brain is more stable than that of children, and this instability seems to be increased by fever. These seizures cause anxiety in parents, worried about the future development of epilepsy. However, these seizures usually occur only once, and in the small proportion of cases in which the child does develop epilepsy later, there are other associated risk factors (see Table 13.3).

Status epilepticus

Usually, epileptic seizures are self-limiting, but sometimes the seizures continue without the patient regaining consciousness. Status epilepticus is defined as recurrent seizures for 30 min or more. When these are generalized seizures without the patient regaining consciousness (convulsive status epilepticus), this condition is a serious emergency, with a mortality of 10–15%, and is one of the reasons why the mortality of patients with epilepsy is three times that of age-matched controls. Deaths during convulsive status epilepticus are due to the hypoxia and acidosis that occur during a seizure. If there is no time for recovery between seizures, this condition worsens and can lead to cerebral oedema, brain damage and cardiorespiratory failure.

Neurobiology of epilepsy

The cellular basis of epilepsy is still unresolved, but at a very basic level, it is believed that epilepsy may be due to intrinsic neuronal hyperexcitability (e.g. due to dysfunctional voltage-gated ion channels), exaggerated activity at excitatory synapses, or insufficient activity of inhibitory circuits. As mentioned elsewhere in this book, the major neurotransmitters mediating fast neurotransmission in the brain are the amino acids glutamate and GABA. These neurotransmitters play a large part in controlling the excitation–inhibition balance in the central nervous system (CNS).

Glutamate transmission

Glutamate receptors can be divided into two main types: ionotropic and metabotropic (see Chapter 15). The fast, ionotropic receptors are divided into N-methyl-D-aspartate (NMDA) and non-NMDA receptors. NMDA receptors are permeable to both Na^+ and Ca^{2+}, and are blocked at normal resting potentials by Mg^{2+}. This blockade is removed by depolarization, so NMDA receptors can only be activated in a neurone that is already partially depolarized. NMDA receptors are involved in a process called long-term potentiation (LTP see Chapter 14). During LTP, the simultaneous activity of multiple inputs to a neurone will activate NMDA receptors which consequently strengthens the connection between the active neurones which is why the indiscriminate blockade of NMDA receptors may have very unfavourable effects on cognition.

The non-NMDA receptors are AMPA named after a preferred agonist, 4-amino-3-hydroxy-5-methyl-4-isoxazoleproprionic acid and kainate receptors. They can be activated at normal resting potentials, and their activation leads to depolarization. When activity levels are high, the neurone will be sufficiently depolarized for both NMDA and non-NMDA receptors to be activated. This will allow Ca^{2+} to enter the cell, where it acts as a second messenger. Glutamate receptor agonists, such as kainic acid and ibotenic acid, can induce various types of seizure in animals. Furthermore, structural changes in glutamate receptors have been found in surgical specimens from epileptic patients. The pyramidal cells of the cortex are glutamatergic, and there is some evidence that glutamatergic dysfunction may be associated with certain types of epilepsy. However, NMDA receptor antagonists have limited antiepileptic activity and induce unacceptable adverse effects; therefore, they cannot be used clinically.

GABA transmission

There are two main types of GABA receptor: $GABA_A$ receptors, which are ionotropic receptors, and $GABA_B$ receptors, which are G-protein-linked receptors. When activated, $GABA_A$ receptors, which are multimeric proteins composed of several subunits, open an integral Cl^- channel. This tends to clamp the neuronal potential closer to the resting potential. $GABA_A$ receptors are postsynaptic, whereas $GABA_B$ receptors are found both post- and presynaptically. There are many different types of inhibitory non-pyramidal cell in the cortex. Many of these cells do not have dendritic spines and are termed non-spiny neurones. Some of these inhibitory cells have synapses on the pyramidal cells that are close to the cell body, while excitatory inputs tend to arrive on the pyramidal cell dendrites. This means that activity in inhibitory synapses that use GABA will have a powerful influence on the firing patterns of the excitatory pyramidal cells. Inhibitory postsynaptic potentials are the mechanism by which neurones are prevented from firing. Some theories of the genesis of epilepsy postulate that a reduction in GABAergic activity allows the uncontrolled discharge of large numbers of neurones. Lower than normal numbers of GABAergic neurones have been found in tissue from patients with epilepsy refractory to treatment. Furthermore, increasing GABAergic activity is the mechanism of action for several of the drugs used to treat epilepsy.

Mechanisms underlying seizures and epileptogenesis

Experiments carried out in animal models of epilepsy have investigated the events underlying interictal and ictal electrical activity. There are several different ways of producing epileptiform activity in animals. Some of these involve drugs that either inhibit GABA or increase glutamate activities. $GABA_A$ antagonists such as bicuculline or picrotoxin, and glutamate agonists, can all produce seizure activity. Another model is called 'kindling', in which repeated high-frequency stimulation of parts of the limbic system can produce long-term changes in excitability, so that seizures can be produced by quite low levels of stimulation for months after the initial stimulation period. Some models analyse changes in brain tissue slices where the layered structure of the brain and local electrical circuits can be maintained. Intracellular and extracellular recordings from these preparations reveal some common underlying patterns.

Neurones in a region with epileptogenic activity fire bursts of action potentials. This is thought to be underlined by a slow depolarizing shift, called a 'paroxysmal depolarization shift'. This induces action potentials from a group of neurones, and these are superimposed on the shift (Fig. 13.5). This is followed by a period of hyperpolarization, during which the activation of both voltage- and Ca^{2+}-sensitive K^+ channels stops the spiking activity.

When the interval between interictal spikes shortens, the period of hyperpolarization is reduced. As a result of the increased neuronal firing, there is an increase in extracellular K^+ levels, which depolarizes neurones and puts them closer to the firing threshold. However, the mechanism by which local inhibition is reduced sufficiently to allow the synchronous discharge of large numbers of neurones is not known.

In one type of epilepsy, mesial temporal sclerosis (MTS), where seizures originate in the hippocampus, possibly due to neuronal damage in infancy, there are losses of neurones in specific areas called CA1 and CA3. In response to the cell loss, there is sprouting of the axons of excitatory glutamatergic granule cells (also known as mossy fibres) (Fig. 13.6). These form connections with other granule cells of the dentate gyrus, which are not inhibited by the normal inhibitory connections. This leads to a set of excitatory loops that have a high propensity to produce seizures.

Another theory of epileptogenesis involves the Chandelier cells of the cortex. These are widespread, inhibitory interneurones that release GABA onto pyramidal cells, particularly on the initial segment of the axon (Fig. 13.7).

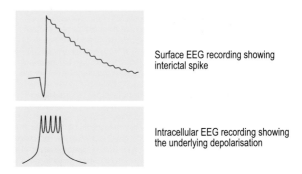

Surface EEG recording showing interictal spike

Intracellular EEG recording showing the underlying depolarisation

Fig. 13.5 An interictal spike produced by slow depolarization underlies the burst firing of cortical neurones. EEG, electroencephalography.

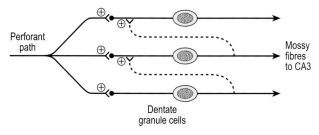

Fig. 13.6 Structural changes in hippocampal sclerosis. Sprouting of mossy fibres can lead to the formation of excitatory loops that lack normal inhibition.

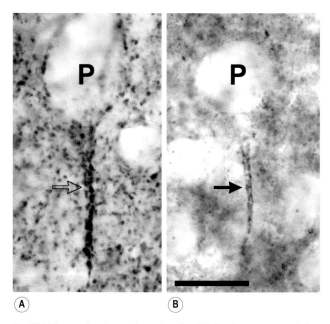

Fig. 13.7 Pre- and postsynaptic markers for GABAergic neurotransmission. Chandelier cells labelled with GAT-1 (A) synapse onto pyramidal neurones (P) labelled with an antibody against the GABA$_A$ receptor (B). From Volk, Lewis. Physiology and Behaviour 2002; 77: 501–505.

These cells express high levels of the GABA transporter GAT-1, which can be used as a marker for their presence. In some forms of epilepsy there is a loss of Chandelier cells, as shown by a loss of GAT-1. It is suggested that loss of just a few of these cells would have a significant effect on the excitability of the pyramidal cell. The theory also suggests that, because of the normal individual variation in the number of GABAergic neurones, loss of Chandelier cells would be sufficient to produce epilepsy in an individual with lower than average numbers of inhibitory neurones.

Ion channel changes in epilepsy

Neuronal membrane excitability is controlled by complex mechanisms, which depend on the coordinated activity of multiple ion channels. The rising phase of the action potential is caused by a current that flows through fast-inactivating Na$^+$ channels. This current is also associated with a slow-inactivating component. The blockade of this component can lead to a switch in the firing of neurones from regular spiking to burst firing. Certain types of genetically determined epilepsies, such as the familial generalized epilepsies with febrile seizures, are associated with changes in the molecular structure of Na$^+$ channels. Such mutations decrease the rate of inactivation of Na$^+$ channels (Fig. 13.8).

K$^+$ channels also have a role in excitability; in particular, they are critically involved in the repolarization of the membrane. The blockade of the K$^+$ M current (which is inhibited by the activation of muscarinic acetylcholine receptors) leads to a shift towards greater depolarization of the membrane. The K$^+$ channel subunits KCN2 and KCN3 contribute to this current, and mutations in these genes are associated with the phenotype of benign neonatal familial convulsions.

Finally, Ca^{2+} currents are also an important element of control of neuronal excitability, and converging evidence suggests that dysfunctional Ca^{2+} channels may be associated with epileptogenesis. Absence epilepsies have been associated with overexpression of a low-threshold Ca^{2+} current in reticular thalamic neurones.

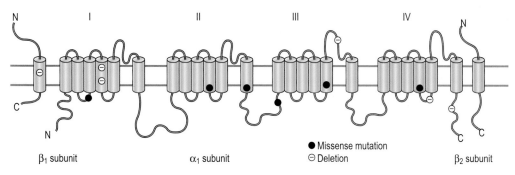

Fig. 13.8 Mutations in Na$^+$ channel subunits associated with idiopathic epilepsy.

Pharmacological treatment of epilepsy

There is a wide range of drugs available for the treatment of epilepsy (Table 13.4). In the past decade, many new drugs have been introduced, as well as improved formulations of first-generation anticonvulsant drugs. Because patients already have epilepsy when they are diagnosed, all these drugs are, strictly speaking, anticonvulsants; that is, they prevent the established seizure activity. In cases where epilepsy is likely to develop, e.g. following head trauma or perinatal hypoxia, drugs that could prevent the future development of seizures, true antiepileptics, would be useful, but no such compounds have yet been developed for clinical use. Active attempts are being made in animal models of epilepsy to understand the mechanisms that underlie epileptogenesis. However, evidence suggests that even when drugs are introduced early and they at least partly control the seizures, they do not affect the progression of epilepsy.

It is important to note that primary generalized seizures are usually more easily controlled than focal epilepsies. Many patients can, after a period of remission, stop their treatment, but there may be a recurrence of seizures which may have consequences for employment and activities such as driving (see below).

Mode of action of anticonvulsant drugs

Ion channel inhibitors

Several different drugs inhibit voltage-sensitive channels, thus reducing neuronal excitability.

Phenytoin blocks voltage-sensitive Na^+ channels preferentially in their inactive state. This occurs just after the channel has been open, which means that the blockade is use-dependent. This therefore tends to block activity in those pathways showing high-frequency repetitive discharges. Phenytoin blocks the spread of seizures but has little effect against the epileptic focus. The pharmacokinetics of this drug are complex and can change over the therapeutic range. It is saturation (or zero order) kinetics.

Table 13.4 Anticonvulsant drugs

Established drugs	New drugs
Phenytoin	Lamotrigine
Sodium valproate	Vigabatrin
Carbamazepine	Topiramate
Phenobarbitone	Tiagabine
Acetazolamide	Gabapentin
Clobazam	Levetiracetam
Ethosuximide	
Clonazepam	
Primidone	

Small increases in the dose can lead to significant increases in plasma concentration, so monitoring of the plasma concentration is required. Phenytoin is an inducer of hepatic microsomal enzymes. It has a number of side effects, including gum hypertrophy, acne and hirsutism, and it is teratogenic. It is used in all forms of epilepsy, with the exception of absence seizures, which it can aggravate.

Carbamazepine has a mode of action on Na^+ channels similar to that of phenytoin. It can induce rash, hepatotoxicity and blood dyscrasia. It is also an enzyme inducer and has teratogenic effects. It can be used for simple and complex partial seizures and tonic–clonic generalized seizures.

Ethosuximide, which is effective in preventing absence seizures, acts by blocking the T-type Ca^{2+} channels found in the thalamic neurones, which are thought to generate this type of seizure activity.

Valproate has a complex pharmacology, but one of its mechanisms of action is the inhibition of Na^+ channels. The drug can also block L-type Ca^{2+} channels. Furthermore, it may increase GABAergic transmission, by stimulating GABA synthesis and inhibiting its metabolism. It is effective in patients with all types of seizure, is easy to use and is generally well tolerated, although it can induce unwanted effects such as tremor and weight gain.

Some of the new antiepileptic drugs also affect the function of ion channels. Lamotrigine induces use-dependent blockade of Na^+ channels, and also reduces Ca^{2+} currents. Gabapentin is also associated with a reduction in voltage-dependent Ca^{2+} currents. Topiramate has a complex pharmacology, but part of its mechanism of action is also the blockade of Na^+ channels. Levetiracetam has no effect on voltage-dependent Na^+ or L-, P-, Q- or T-type Ca^{2+} channels, but selectively inhibits N-type Ca^{2+} channels with no effects of other channels. Zonisamide blocks both Na^+ and Ca^{2+} channels.

GABA receptor ligands

Benzodiazepines such as clonazepam and clobazam, and barbiturates such as phenobarbitone, act by binding to the $GABA_A$ receptor. $GABA_A$ receptors are pentameric proteins, made up of five subunits surrounding a Cl^- channel. The majority of $GABA_A$ receptors in the brain contain α-, β- and γ-subunits, each of which can be transcribed from a family of genes (for more detail see Chapter 16). On the $GABA_A$ receptor complex there are binding sites for GABA, and also modulatory binding sites for a number of other compounds. There are sites for both benzodiazepines and barbiturates, and these compounds act as positive allosteric modulators at the $GABA_A$ receptor; that is, they amplify the response to GABA. Benzodiazepines increase the frequency of opening of the Cl^- channel, whereas barbiturates increase the duration of opening of the channel. At high concentrations, barbiturates can have intrinsic effects, independent of the presence of GABA. They commonly induce sedation, and their therapeutic window is much narrower than that of benzodiazepines. Clobazam is used as adjunctive therapy, whereas clonazepam is used for generalized seizures and also absence seizures (if ethosuximide fails), and can also be used for status epilepticus. Both compounds suppress the spread of seizures but have little effect at the epileptic focus. In contrast, phenobarbitone can suppress activity at the epileptic focus. Primidone is metabolized in the body to phenobarbitone.

Agents that increase the levels of GABA

The metabolism of GABA is a cycle, involving glutamate and glutamine, occurring between neurones and glial cells (Fig. 13.9). After its release into the synaptic cleft, GABA is transported into surrounding neurones and glial cells by high-affinity transporters, such as GAT-1. It is then broken down by GABA transaminase (GABA-T) to produce glutamate. Glutamate is metabolized to glutamine, which is then transported back into the neurone or glia. GABA is synthesized in neurones from glutamate, by the action of glutamic acid decarboxylase (GAD). This shunt enables the carbon skeleton of GABA to be returned to the neurone via glutamine, which has no neurotransmitter action.

Two anticonvulsant drugs act on elements of this cycle to increase GABA concentrations. Tiagabine blocks the reuptake of GABA by the GABA transporter GAT-1, while vigabatrin is a selective irreversible inhibitor of GABA-T. Sodium valproate can also inhibit GABA-T. Both vigabatrin and tiagabine can be used as adjunctive therapy in partial seizures.

Other drugs

As illustrated above, the pharmacology of epilepsy is complex, and some of the compounds in present use may have efficacy because of the multiple targets they affect. For example, the same drug can inhibit voltage-gated ion

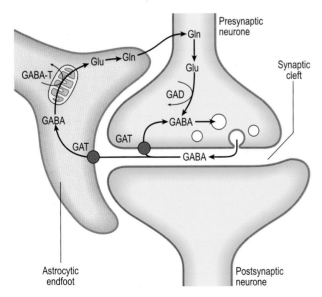

Fig. 13.9 Cycle of γ-aminobutyric acid (GABA) synthesis and degradation. GABA released from neurones is transported into surrounding neurones and glial cells by a high-affinity transporter (GAT-1). Glu, glutamate; Gln, glutamine.

channels, act at the benzodiazepine site of the GABA$_A$ receptor, and suppress the release of monoamines! Which component of such a spectrum is the most important is not always clear, and it may be that synergism is an important concept in the design of new drugs. However, many of these new second-generation antiepileptic drugs have so far failed to show significantly more efficacy than the established first-generation drugs. This may be because new drugs are tested preclinically on the same animal models as the old drugs, and such models may be inadequate and fail to reveal new targets with entirely new mechanisms of action. Furthermore, in some cases, although the rationale for the new target is sound, the drugs may induce unacceptable side effects.

General comments on anticonvulsant medication

The unwanted effects induced by anticonvulsant drugs are numerous, and some of the drugs used to treat epilepsy interact with other drugs. Some do this by inducing metabolizing liver enzymes, thus increasing the metabolism of other medications, including warfarin and the contraceptive pill, as well as other antiepileptics. Sodium valproate, used in the case history given in Box 13.1, inhibits the liver metabolism of some drugs, increasing their half-life.

Many of the drugs used to treat epilepsy are teratogenic and this may determine the treatment given to women patients who wish to become pregnant. A lower dose of a safer drug plus, in some cases, folate supplements and early screening for fetal abnormalities, are of benefit.

Anticonvulsant drug concentrations can be measured in blood, and this is particularly useful in optimizing the dose of drugs such as phenytoin, which have a relatively narrow therapeutic window. Knowledge of drug levels may also be useful in assessing compliance, particularly in cases where a patient is brought into hospital unconscious.

To conclude, different drugs are recommended for use in patients with generalized or focal epilepsies (Table 13.5), and some drugs are preferred in different age groups.

Characteristics of the ideal drug and strategy for the treatment of epilepsy

The choice of a drug usually depends upon the patient's seizure type (see Table 13.5). The pharmacokinetic characteristics, including absorption, elimination and potential for drug interactions (e.g. through potentiation or inhibition of common metabolic pathways), are of critical importance for patients who take medication for other conditions, and for patients with impaired renal or hepatic function. The ideal drug would have a rapid absorption rate, low plasma protein binding, and rapid CNS penetration. It would be eliminated predominantly by the kidneys. The new anticonvulsant drugs do not prompt the same concerns about interactions, because

Table 13.5 Efficacy of antiepileptic drugs against common seizure types

| Drug | Seizure type | | | | |
	Partial	Secondary generalized	Tonic–clonic	Absence	Myoclonic
Phenytoin	+	+	+	−	−
Carbamazepine	+	+	+	−	−
Valproate	+	+	+	+	+
Lamotrigine	+	+	+	+	+
Gabapentin	+	+	?+	?	−
Topiramate	+	+	+	?	+
Clobazam	+	+	+	?+	+
Phenobarbitone	+	+	+	0	?+
Tiagabine	+	+	?+	−	?

0, ineffective; ? + , probably effective; +, proven efficacy; ?, unknown; −, worsens seizures.

they have much better pharmacokinetic profiles than the older drugs (such as phenytoin or carbamazepine) and therefore require less monitoring for potential interactions. The potential interaction of anticonvulsant therapy with the contraceptive medication used by a young woman with epilepsy is illustrated in the case history given in Box 13.1. The new antiepileptic drugs—vigabatrin, gabapentin, lamotrigine and tiagabine—do not affect the metabolism of the contraceptive pill. However, caution is still warranted concerning the effects of the new drugs on the fetus: there is insufficient information to determine whether the new antiepileptic drugs are teratogenic or not.

The goal of antiepileptic therapy is to keep the patient free of seizures, with no adverse effects on brain function. However, many of the drugs used to treat epilepsy have considerable side effects, both on the CNS and on other organs. In order to ensure patient compliance over what will probably be an extended period of time (sometimes a lifetime), it is important to test different drugs until a satisfactory drug regimen is established. Usually, a patient will be given a single drug (monotherapy) and the dosage varied until either seizure activity is stopped or there are adverse effects. Other drugs should be tried on a monotherapy basis before additional drugs are included, because of lack of efficacy of the monotherapy. It is not usual to give more than three drugs simultaneously. About 60% of patients are controlled with a single drug. In other patients, better results are obtained by adding a second and even a third drug. If a patient still suffers seizures after the addition of multiple drugs this is referred to as refractory epilepsy. Unfortunately, up to 40% of individuals suffer from this intractable, pharmacoresistant epilepsy (Box 13.4).

Box 13.4 Pharmacoresistance in epilepsy

The phenomenon of pharmacoresistance in epilepsy is significant. Fewer than 5% of patients who are refractory to first-generation anticonvulsant drugs are free of seizures with the new drugs. Intractability of seizures is associated with various factors, such as onset of seizures in the first year of life, structural brain lesions (e.g. hippocampal sclerosis), brain tumours and neurodevelopmental abnormalities. Pharmacoresistance is frequent in patients with partial seizures. It has been suggested that pharmacoresistance is due to genetic factors, disease-related factors or drug-related factors. Thus, genetic polymorphism may underlie lack of response to a drug. On the other hand, the resistance may be due to the ongoing reorganization of neuronal networks triggered by the seizures. Last, but not least, drug uptake into the brain may be drastically reduced by the overexpression of multidrug transporters in the blood–brain barrier, whose activity leads to significant drug efflux. If this is the case, then inhibitors of these transporters, or drugs that are not substrates of these transporters, may be the answer to the problem of resistance.

Other treatments for epilepsy

Surgery

In patients with focal epilepsy that cannot be adequately controlled by drugs, surgical removal of the epileptic focus may be possible if it is in an area of the brain that can be removed without leaving a major neurological deficit. The area to be removed can be pinpointed using MRI and EEG recordings. The aim of the surgery is to obtain either complete freedom from seizures, or an amelioration of the seizure frequency. The types of epilepsy most amenable to this type of treatment are epilepsy due to MTS or tumours. Other rare surgical interventions include separating the two hemispheres of the brain by sectioning of the corpus callosum (callosotomy) in order to prevent seizures becoming generalized to both hemispheres.

Nerve stimulation

Vagus nerve stimulation is currently the most widely used adjunctive therapy in pharmacoresistant partial epilepsy. Since its introduction in the late 1990s, it has been used on several thousand patients worldwide. The left vagus nerve is stimulated with electrodes that are connected to a pulse generator in the left part of the chest. Intermittent stimulation of the nerve has been shown to reduce seizure frequency by 50% in up to 43% of patients with pharmacologically refractory partial-onset seizures. However, in some patients there is a delay of several months before a beneficial effect can be seen. Transcranial magnetic stimulation or stimulation through scalp depth electrodes has also been attempted with some success. A possible mode of action is disruption of the neural patterns required to initiate seizure activity.

Dietary

The ketogenic diet is one of the oldest available treatments for epilepsy, and one of the most successful treatments for medically intractable epilepsy in children. The principle is based on the physiology of starvation. The brain usually uses glucose as its energy source, but in starvation can metabolize ketones. In the ketogenic diet, carbohydrate intake is very limited and most of the calorie intake is in the form of fat. The metabolism of fat leads to production of ketone bodies (ketogenesis). While on the diet, children also receive vitamins and minerals, in particular calcium supplementation. This diet was proposed initially more than 80 years ago, and it was based on observations that date back to the Middle Ages, on the effect of fasting on epilepsy. Prospective and retrospective studies have confirmed the efficacy, tolerability and safety of this diet, but randomized controlled studies are still required, and its mechanism of action remains unknown.

Treatment of status epilepticus

Treatment is in three parts. First, the patient must be given immediate resuscitation (Airway, Breathing and Circulation). Then, drugs are given to control the seizures, and finally identification and possible treatment of the underlying cause of the status are required. Drugs given initially are usually diazepam (or other benzodiazepines such as lorazepam). If these are ineffective at suppressing seizure activity, the barbiturate phenobarbitone or the anticonvulsant phenytoin are used in large intravenous doses. If seizures continue for more than 30 min, then general anaesthesia using thiopentone should be applied, with ventilation and intensive care treatment.

Some patients will have a previous diagnosis of epilepsy. Their condition may be caused by a failure to take their medication, which can be determined by measuring drug blood levels. If this is the case, their normal medication should be reapplied; otherwise, treatment should be as for new cases. In patients with no previous history of epilepsy, status epilepticus may be caused by several factors, such as trauma, alcohol abuse, drug overdose, tumours or stroke.

Social consequences of epilepsy

There is a significant social stigma associated with a diagnosis of epilepsy. Social stigma is the term given when a person's social, physical or mental condition influences other people's views of them or their behaviour towards them. Members of the general public may be uneasy with someone with epilepsy. This may possibly be overcome by informing them exactly what the seizures entail, but because of fears of rejection, many epileptics try to hide their condition.

A diagnosis of epilepsy may have severe consequences for a person's present or future employment prospects. Some jobs are completely inaccessible to people with epilepsy, such as the police and fire services or the armed forces. They cannot fly aircraft or drive trains.

There are strict regulations governing whether a person with epilepsy can hold a UK driving licence. They cannot hold an ordinary licence unless they have been free from any seizure for at least 1 year or have only had seizures while asleep for more than 3 years. Further restrictions apply as regards heavy goods vehicles and passenger service vehicles. This directly limits the type of occupation available to someone with epilepsy, and depending on where they live and their need for a car as a means of transport, it may limit their choice among jobs not requiring a driving licence.

There are occupations that may be difficult for someone with poorly controlled epilepsy, such as teaching young children, or working at height. There may be reluctance among employers to employ someone with epilepsy, because of fears that their customers or other employees might be upset by someone having a seizure, or that they may be held responsible if the epileptic person injures themselves during a seizure.

A person with epilepsy may be advised about the dangers of certain leisure activities. Water sports and climbing should not be done unsupervised, and riding a bicycle, particularly on the public highway, may be dangerous. Some simple measures, such as not locking the bathroom door, may be advisable. Patients with photosensitive epilepsy may be advised to sit further away from the television than normal and avoid computer games with flashing lights. Stroboscopic disco lights usually operate at too low a frequency to induce seizures, but highly sensitive individuals may be affected by striped objects and Venetian window blinds.

DEMENTIA

14

Chapter objectives

After studying this chapter you should be able to:

1. Define and classify dementia and its causes.

2. Describe the mechanisms underlying learning and memory and explain how they underlie neuronal plasticity.

3. Describe Alzheimer's disease and its pathophysiology.

4. Describe the treatment of Alzheimer's disease.

Introduction

Dementia is a generic term that describes a progressive and irreversible loss of higher mental function, particularly memory. Cognitive decline is associated with other significant alterations in mood and behaviour that lead to complete disintegration of the personality. This disease can become a terrifying experience for both patients and carers, although in many cases the patients may not be as aware of their condition as their carers. It occurs mainly in the elderly, and patients become progressively more and more dependent. Changes may be slow and insidious, and may be ignored initially, so dementia may be at an advanced stage at the time of diagnosis. Alzheimer's disease (AD) is the commonest form of dementia in the elderly (especially in Europe and the USA) but there are also other causes of dementia, especially cerebrovascular. Dementia may also occur in younger patients, e.g. secondary to other conditions, as in patients infected with the human immunodeficiency virus (HIV). Dementia currently affects over 750 000 people in the UK and more than 4 million people in the USA.

Causes and diagnosis of dementia

Dementia leads to a gradual loss of cognitive function, without impairment of consciousness. It is related to, but distinct from, the mental retardation due to brain damage in early life. In the latter case, development of impairment is both slow and limited. Pseudo-dementia is a form of impaired thinking that occurs in some patients with severe depression. It can be distinguished from acute confusion by several criteria (Table 14.1). In acute confusional states, the patient responds to some stimuli in a purposeful manner but is often disoriented, sleepy, inattentive or agitated (delirium). There are often autonomic disturbances (fever, tachycardia and sweating) and motor abnormalities (tremor and myoclonus).

As dementia is a generic term, it covers diseases and syndromes that may have a variety of causes (Table 14.2). The degenerative/inherited types of dementia are largely non-reversible. However, many of the other causes are either reversible or can at least be partially reversed or halted with treatment.

Irrespective of dementia being of a primary or secondary nature, a key element in the diagnosis is the psychological testing of the patient. The testing of the higher mental functions of a patient involves their speech abilities and requires appropriate attention, although some aspects can be tested without speech. Patients also need to be able to hear or read instructions.

Cognitive function can be examined initially using standard tests such as the Mini Mental State Examination (Table 14.3). This test is a simple method of scoring mental performance. However, this test cannot detect small degrees of impairment, and results depend on the patient's initial cognitive abilities. The maximum score is 30, and a score below 24 indicates dementia.

Certain types of dementia are also associated with very specific behavioural and personality changes (e.g. moral disinhibition in frontotemporal dementia).

Dementia can be associated with atrophy of the brain, enlarged ventricles and widening of the sulci, which can be

Box 14.1 Case history

Gary P., a 78-year-old man, is seen by his general practitioner after his wife expresses concern about his condition. He has gradually become very forgetful over the last 1–2 years. His wife says that he recently got lost when out shopping, even though they had lived in the same place for years, and that at a recent family gathering he had not been able to remember the names of some of the younger family members. He has always managed the household bills, but recently his wife has taken over, as he complains that 'things are getting too complicated'. He complains that he cannot find things around the house because his wife keeps moving them, which she denies.

He has had no significant medical problems in the past, and his physical examination is normal. He looks fit and he takes no medication. He speaks fluently but makes frequent errors, either using incorrect words or substituting made-up words instead. He can name three objects but cannot recall them later. When asked the name of the current Prime Minister, he says 'I've never met him.'

Gary's wife is very anxious and asks the doctor whether her husband is developing Alzheimer's disease, as his own mother died 'senile' 20 years ago. She wants to know about any treatment that could help him and slow down his mental decline.

This case gives rise to the following questions:

1. How do you test for mental disease?
2. Does this man suffer from dementia?
3. How are memories formed and maintained?
4. What is Alzheimer's disease and what are its causes?
5. What is the treatment for dementia and can its progression be stopped?

Table 14.1 Differences between acute confusion and dementia

Criteria	Acute confusion	Dementia
Level of consciousness	Impaired	Normal
Course	Acute/fluctuating	Chronic/progressive
Autonomic dysfunction	Present	Absent
Prognosis	Usually reversible	Generally irreversible

detected using computed tomography (CT) and magnetic resonance imaging (MRI) scans (Fig. 14.1). Other dementia subtype-specific pathological changes can also be detected (e.g. spongiform changes in Creuzfeldt–Jakob disease (CJD)). However, such changes may occur late in the evolution of the disease (see discussion below). Blood tests can identify reversible causes of dementia, such as hypothyroidism and vitamin deficiencies. They can also identify HIV status. Liver function tests can identify Wilson's disease, and analysis of cerebrospinal fluid can be used to diagnose neurosyphilis and meningitis. CT and MRI scans can also identify tumours, haematomas and hydrocephalus.

Neurobiology of learning and memory

Loss of memory is a most striking feature of AD, and of other dementias. Learning is the acquisition of new facts and behaviours through experience, and memory is the storage and recall of those facts and behaviours. In order to learn, the brain must be able to change in response to experience; that is, it must show plasticity.

Learning can be divided into two types:

1. Declarative learning is acquiring new facts about the world. This leads to the formation of two types of memory—episodic memory (remembering events such as last year's holiday), and semantic memory (remembering facts such as Ulan Batur is the capital of Mongolia).

2. Procedural (motor) learning is learning complex actions such as how to ride a bicycle (or walk!).

Table 14.2 Some causes of dementia

Degenerative/inherited	Alzheimer's disease
	Pick's disease (frontotemporal dementia)
	Lewy body dementia
	Huntington's disease
	Wilson's disease
	Parkinson's disease
	Multiple sclerosis
Vascular	Vascular dementia
	Cerebral vasculitis
Space-occupying lesions	Chronic hydrocephalus
	Normal pressure hydrocephalus
	Tumour
	Chronic subdural haematoma
Infection	HIV-associated dementia
	Creutzfeldt–Jakob disease
	Abscess
	Syphilis (now rare)
	Post-meningitis
	Post-encephalitis
Traumatic	Post head trauma
	Punch-drunk syndrome (dementia pugilistica)
Toxic	Cerebral anoxia (due to cardiac arrest, respiratory failure or carbon monoxide poisoning)
	Alcohol and drugs (e.g. barbiturates)
	Occupational exposure to toxins
	Heavy metal poisoning
Metabolic or nutritional causes	Hypothyroidism
	Hypocalcaemia
	Vitamin B_{12}/folic acid/niacin deficiency
	Thiamine deficiency (often in alcoholics) leading to Korsakoff's syndrome and Wernicke's encephalopathy

Table 14.3 Mini Mental State Examination

Test	Maximum score
Orientation	
What is the year, month, day, date, season?	5 (1 mark per item)
Where are you (country, county, town, hospital, ward)?	5 (1 mark per item)
Retention	
Name three objects and then repeat these named objects	3 (1 mark for each object)
Calculation and attention	
Count up in 7s five times or spell 'world' backwards	5 (1 mark for each correct addition or correct letter)
Recall	
Recall the three objects named earlier	3 (1 mark per object)
Language	
Name a pencil and a watch	2 (1 mark for each object named)
Repeat 'No ifs, ands, or buts'	1
Give a three stage command	3 (1 mark for each stage)
Read and obey the written command 'Close your eyes'	1
Write a sensible sentence, with a subject and a verb	1
Copy two intersecting pentagons	1

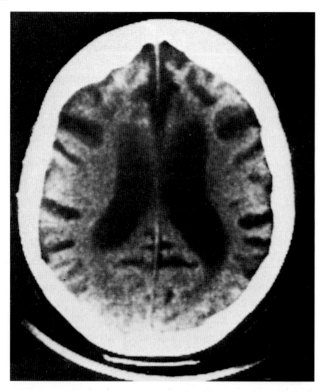

Fig. 14.1 Computed tomography scan of the brain, showing enlarged ventricles and widened sulci. This patient has Alzheimer's disease but a similar picture could be seen in other disorders. From Forbes CD, Jackson WF. Colour Atlas and Text of Clinical Medicine, 3rd edn. Mosby, 2002.

Damage to specific areas of the brain shows that episodic memories are stored in specific areas of the frontal cortex, whereas semantic memories are distributed across a number of areas, each dealing with a characteristic of the memory, such as the appearance or sound. Semantic knowledge uses categories such as fruit or animals. This is shown by very particular lesions, which lead, for example, to patients being unable to name all types of fruit.

Declarative learning is relatively easy to acquire; many memories only need a single exposure. They require conscious recall and may be forgotten. In contrast, procedural learning is slow, in that for many skills, repeated practice is required. Its recall is unconscious and it is not easily lost.

Short-term and long-term memory

Short-term memory, such as remembering a new telephone number, is easily disrupted until it has been stored in long-term memory, a process called consolidation. After consolidation, it can remain permanently, although the ability to retrieve it from long-term store depends on factors such as how often it is retrieved. Only a small number of short-term memories are consolidated, and this depends on the level of arousal and attention, which will depend on the personal significance of the information.

Short- and long-term memory are separate processes, and items do not have to pass through short-term memory in order to reach long-term memory. This is shown in the few patients whose short-term memory is damaged but who can still consolidate memories into long-term memory.

Amnesia

Memory loss occurs in two ways. Loss of recent memory, including the inability to form new memories, is anterograde amnesia, and suggests that there is a defect in the memory storage process. A failure in recall leads to the inability to retrieve previously stored memories, producing retrograde amnesia. This type of amnesia may be progressive, with more recent memories being lost first. The patient is left with memories that reach further and further back into the past.

Models of learning and memory

Learning and memory have been studied in several model systems. Simple invertebrates, such as the marine mollusc *Aplysia californica*, have been used to elucidate possible changes in ion channel activity and intracellular signalling underlying simple learning patterns. The fruit fly, *Drosophila melanogaster*, has been used to probe genetic aspects of learning. However, in mammals, it is the study of changing patterns of synaptic activity in the hippocampus and the cerebellum that forms the basis for current theories regarding memory.

Involvement of the hippocampus in memory formation

Much evidence, particularly from clinical cases, shows that the hippocampus is central in the consolidation of newly acquired memories, particularly declarative memory. Patients with either accidental lesions of the hippocampus, with surgical removal of the hippocampus (for intractable temporal lobe epilepsy) or who have suffered transient hypoxia, sufficient to destroy neurones in the hippocampus, suffer from severe anterograde amnesia. They retain short-term memory and can recall previously stored long-term memories, but are unable to consolidate new memories.

Central to theories of memory formation is the idea that there are long-term changes in synaptic connectivity, either by acquisition of new connections or by strengthening of existing synapses. This is known as Hebb's rule, after Donald Hebb, who wrote an influential book on the subject. It states that if two neurones are excited simultaneously, then active synapses between them will be strengthened. This means that Hebbian synapses can act as coincidence detectors, measuring the correlation between pre- and postsynaptic firing. This property would seem to be a requirement for any sort of associative learning, in which the stimulus and the response are closely paired.

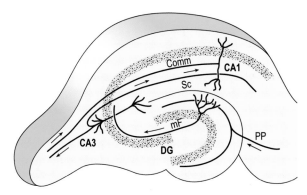

Fig. 14.2 Circuitry of the hippocampus. PP, perforant path; mF, mossy fibres; Sc, Schaffer collaterals; Comm, commissural fibres; DG, dentate gyrus. Stippled areas represent granule cell bodies in the dentate gyrus and pyramidal cells in CA3 and CA1.

Long-term potentiation in the hippocampus

The hippocampus, which is part of the limbic system and lies in the medial temporal lobe, has a laminar structure and relatively simple circuitry. This means that thin tissue slices, which can be maintained *in vitro*, can be used to study changes in connectivity. It is possible to stimulate inputs to the neurones in the slices and record the responses of other neurones in the circuits.

Information processed by the sensory neocortex provides inputs to the hippocampus via the entorhinal cortex (Brodmann's area 28). This projects through the perforant path to the granule cells of the dentate gyrus (Fig. 14.2). The granule cell axons, called mossy fibres, synapse on large pyramidal cells in the CA3 hippocampal region. CA stands for cornu ammonis, or ram's horn, referring to the shape of this area. There are two outputs from these CA3 neurones.

First, fibres leave the hippocampus via the fornix and travel to the hypothalamus, which then connects with the thalamus. Outputs from the anterior nucleus of the thalamus project to the cingulate cortex and the entorhinal cortex. This is known as the Papez circuit, and it functionally links the hippocampus to the cortical regions.

Second, the CA3 axonal projections to the CA1 cells, called Schaffer collaterals, synapse on large numbers of neurones in the CA1 region. Some CA3 fibres cross in the ventral commissure of the hippocampus and innervate the contralateral septal nucleus, forming a highly interconnected network. The CA1 outputs convey the results of hippocampal processing, via the subiculum, back to the entorhinal cortex and the sensory neocortex. The hippocampus also receives diffuse innervation, via the fornix, from a number of other brain regions, particularly, in relation to AD, a cholinergic input from the septal nucleus.

Stimulation of Schaffer collaterals results in an excitatory postsynaptic potential (EPSP) in the CA1 neurones. The phenomenon of long-term potentiation (LTP) is the long-lasting increase in synaptic strength, as measured by the size of the EPSP, that is observed after high-frequency stimulation of the Schaffer collaterals (typically 100 stimuli

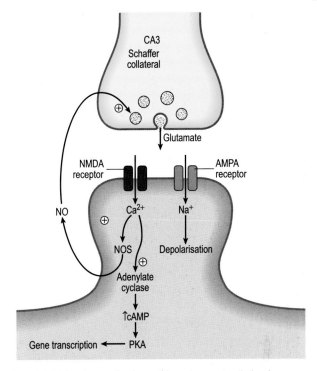

Fig. 14.3 Molecular mechanisms of long-term potentiation in the hippocampus. NMDA, N-methyl-D-aspartate; AMPA, 4-amino-3-hydroxy-5-methyl-4-isoxazole propionic acid; NOS, nitric oxide synthase; PKA, proteininase kinase A.

at 100 Hz). This potentiation is input-specific, in that LTP is not induced at all synapses but only at those with the high-frequency input. It is also state-dependent; if the CA1 neurones are already depolarized when stimulated, the degree of stimulation necessary to produce LTP is less, but only if the activity is closely linked in time. In this way, LTP has many of the properties required of a Hebbian synapse. LTP has also been shown to occur in the neocortex, the amygdala and other structures.

Molecular mechanisms of long-term potentiation

The mechanisms underlying the increased responsiveness of the postsynaptic neurones involve two populations of glutamate receptors on the CA1 cells: the 4-amino-3-hydroxy-5-methyl-4-isoxazole propionic acid (AMPA) and N-methyl-D-aspartate (NMDA) receptor types (Fig. 14.3). AMPA receptors can open in response to released glutamate and allow influx of Na^+, which depolarizes the neurone, producing an EPSP. However, there are also NMDA receptors, which at normal resting membrane potentials are blocked by Mg^{2+}. This blockade is released by depolarization, so during high-frequency input, or if the neurone has already been depolarized, NMDA receptors can be activated as well as AMPA receptors. Activation of NMDA receptors allows the influx of both Na^+ and Ca^{2+}, and it is the Ca^{2+} influx that is critical for the development of LTP. In the absence of extracellular Ca^{2+}, or if the intracellular Ca^{2+} is buffered, LTP does not occur.

There seem to be two types of LTP maintenance. If the high-frequency input only occurs once, LTP lasts for about 3h and decays. This transient, early LTP is not dependent on protein synthesis, as it cannot be prevented by protein synthesis inhibitors. However, if the high-frequency input is repeated a few times, then a form of late LTP occurs that lasts for at least 24h and is dependent on protein synthesis. Late LTP requires Ca^{2+} to activate, via the second messenger cyclic AMP (cAMP), a cascade of enzymes (such as protein kinase A), which culminates in the activation of genes and changes in gene activity. In this way, LTP can change the long-term structure of synapses.

However, the final steps have not been resolved. There are two potential explanations, which are not mutually exclusive, and each of which has some support:

- Postsynaptically, in early LTP, there are increases in the numbers and sensitivity of AMPA receptors. In late LTP, new synapses are formed.

- Presynaptically, in early LTP, there is an increase in the release of glutamate. This requires the presence of a chemical messenger, a retrograde transmitter, which travels across the synaptic cleft. It has been suggested that nitric oxide (NO) or even carbon monoxide (CO) are possible candidates. In late LTP, an increased number of release sites increases the amount of glutamate release.

Long-term depression in the cerebellum

If LTP were the only mechanism acting to encode memories, then there would be very limited fine-tuning of signal strengths in the central nervous system (CNS), as all active synapses would eventually end up being strong. As a necessary balance to learning-enhanced activity, there is also activity-dependent long-term depression (LTD). This can be observed in the hippocampus, where low-frequency, long-period stimulation (1 Hz, 10–15 min) depresses the EPSP for several hours. LTD and LTP are mutually exclusive, suggesting that they act via similar mechanisms.

A completely different form of LTD is observed in the cerebellum, where it is thought to be involved in procedural (motor) learning. Purkinje cells in the cerebellum receive inputs from climbing fibres and parallel fibres. Parallel fibre firing results in activation of both AMPA receptors and metabotropic glutamate receptors (mGluRs) on the Purkinje cells. These mGluRs are linked to phospholipase C and the production of the second messengers inositol 1,4,5-tris-phosphate and diacylglycerol, and subsequent rises in intracellular Ca^{2+}. Climbing fibres activate AMPA receptors, the depolarization of which results in the opening of voltage-dependent Ca^{2+} channels and a large rise in intracellular Ca^{2+}. The final outcome of the simultaneous activation of both the climbing and parallel fibres is a cascade involving cyclic GMP and a number

of protein kinases, and possibly NO. This eventually decreases the responsiveness of the AMPA receptors and reduces Purkinje cell firing.

Learning in the amygdala

Aversive learning, in which a noxious stimulus (unconditional stimulus) is associated with a neutral stimulus (conditional stimulus) until the neutral stimulus can evoke the same response (conditional response) as the normal response (unconditional response) to the noxious stimulus, involves neurones in the amygdala. Neurones in the amygdala fire in patterns that correlate with the development of the conditioned response. Lesions of the amygdala prevent this occurring and prevent expression of the acquired responses. The amygdala activates pathways that are involved in the response of the sympathetic nervous system to stress: the 'fright, flight or fight' response.

Alzheimer's disease

AD manifests as a progressive loss of memory, particularly recent memories, and of other cognitive functions. In the last stages of the disease, patients require round-the-clock care, which puts a tremendous strain on carers. Hallucinations and confusion are common, and aggression, depression and parkinsonism also occur in some but not all patients. Death occurs inevitably after 3–15 years. More than 12 million people are affected worldwide by AD. Age is the major risk factor for developing AD, so a healthcare crisis is very likely in countries with ageing populations if no treatment is found to protect against the disease, or at least delay or stop its progression.

AD is predominantly a disease of the elderly. The prevalence of late-onset AD is about 5% in 70-year-olds and over 20% in people aged over 80 years. However, it can be found in younger people, in some cases from the age of 30 years onwards. Early-onset AD represents less than 5% of cases of AD.

Risk factors for developing AD include a genetic predisposition (i.e. increased risk if there are already cases of AD in the family). Environmental factors are also important. For example, there is a significant association between serious acute head injuries and the risk of later developing AD. Similarly, there is a link between the repeated, subchronic damage suffered by boxers due to repeated punching, and the development of dementia pugilistica (punch-drunk syndrome), which is a form of AD (see Table 14.2).

When making a diagnosis of AD, it is important to exclude other possible causes of dementia, some of which may be treatable (see Table 14.2).

The early diagnosis of AD is an area of much interest. It is likely that it would be easier to slow down the pathogenic process if the treatment were started at a very early stage of the disease. Such a stage may be represented by mild cognitive impairment (Box 14.2).

Mild cognitive impairment—a
prodrome to Alzheimer's disease?

Mild cognitive impairment (MCI) is an age-related syndrome that may be the precursor to Alzheimer's disease (AD). MCI is characterized by significant memory impairment in the absence of dementia. Patients with MCI have memory deficits that are at least one and a half standard deviations below the mean of the population. It is important to look for verbal memory impairment, since this is one of the primary deficits in patients who progress to AD. Impaired delayed recall is also a good predictor of progression to AD. MCI as a clinical entity is likely to be very heterogeneous: some patients with MCI may have very early AD, whereas others may never progress to AD. However, in many cases, MCI is a transitional stage between normal ageing and AD, the annual conversion rate reaching 15%. It is important to identify which MCI patients will progress to AD. At present, there is no reliable clinical method to determine which patients will progress to AD and which patients will not. In future, the choice of appropriate AD biomarkers (see Box 14.5) will help to identify such patients. MCI patients represent the most promising population of patients for whom prophylactic treatment could be initiated in order to delay the onset of AD.

Genetics of Alzheimer's disease

Although AD is very probably caused by a number of different factors, most likely acting in concert, the final result is a common neuropathology. The majority of AD cases are sporadic and of late onset (>60 years), but some cases are of early onset (<60 years) and occur repeatedly in families. Not much is known about the genetics of late-onset AD, but the analysis of familial early-onset cases has already provided some clues about the genes linked with AD. It is also important to note that if a family has members affected by the early-onset form of the disease, it is not exempt from development of late-onset forms of AD.

Amyloid precursor protein

AD can occur with a very early onset (30–40 years), particularly in people with Down's syndrome. Almost all individuals with Down's syndrome who live beyond the age of 30 years show some symptoms of AD, and neuritic plaques can be detected in the brain much earlier. Down's syndrome is caused by the presence of an extra chromosome 21 (hence the name trisomy 21), and this suggests that there may be a link between chromosome 21 and AD. The amyloid peptide, which is involved in the neuropathology of AD (see below), is formed from the amyloid precursor protein (APP). It has subsequently been discovered that the gene for APP is located on chromosome 21,

so in Down's syndrome it is possible that an excess of APP leads to AD. Mutations in the APP gene have been shown to be associated with several rare, early-onset, familial forms of AD.

Presenilins and early-onset Alzheimer's disease

Linkages have been found between genes located on chromosomes 14 and 1 and early-onset familial AD. The two genes involved, namely those encoding the proteins presenilin-1 (PS-1) and presenilin-2 (PS-2), have now been located and sequenced and have been found to code for homologous proteins. The PS-1 gene is associated with about 2% of all AD cases (and 30–40% of all early-onset cases), while the PS-2 gene is linked to the disease developing in families of Volga German descent (approximately 1% of early-onset cases). The PS-1 gene is fully penetrant, whereas the PS-2 gene shows incomplete penetrance, as individuals can live to an old age and not show symptoms of the disease. PS-1 and PS-2 are proteins involved in the γ-secretase enzyme complex (see below).

The *APOE* gene and late-onset Alzheimer's disease

Although there is no linkage between a single genetic mutation and late-onset AD, there is a clear association between susceptibility to AD and a particular allelic variant of the gene that encodes apolipoprotein E (apoE), at the *APOE* gene locus on chromosome 19. ApoE is involved in the storage, transport and metabolism of cholesterol. The *APOE* locus has three alleles; ε2, ε3 and ε4. Susceptibility to AD depends on the combination of alleles inherited from both parents, not on any mutation in the genes themselves. The risk of developing AD increases and the mean age of onset decreases with each copy of the ε4 allele inherited. Conversely, inheritance of the ε2 allele decreases the risk and increases the mean age of onset, which indicates a protective role for this allele (Table 14.4). The presence of ε4 does not cause AD, but does increase the likelihood of the disease developing at an earlier age.

As well as being applicable to late-onset, sporadic AD, this correlation also has validity in early-onset familial cases. Estimates vary, but it has been suggested that between 60% and 90% of total AD cases could be associated with the *APOE* genotype. Although exact allelic frequencies vary between racial and ethnic groups, the most common allele in the US population as a whole is ε3 (~74%), followed by ε4 (~16%) and ε2 (~10%). This means that the rarest combination is ε2/ε2, which is present in less than 1% of the population, and the most deleterious combination, ε4/ε4, is present in about 2.5%. When *APOE* genotypes were compared in two US groups of 176 AD patients and 91 non-AD controls, 17% of AD patients had the ε4/ε4 genotype, compared with 2% of the controls. The ε3/ε4 genotype was also more prevalent in the AD patients: 43% compared to 21% of the controls. Similar results were shown in a study of Japanese AD patients, although the

Table 14.4 *APOE* genotypes alter the mean age of onset of Alzheimer's disease (AD)

APOE genotype	Mean age of onset of AD (years)
2/2	? (rare genotype)
2/3	>90
2/4	80–90
3/3	80–90
3/4	70–80
4/4	<70

frequency of ε4 alleles is lower (~9%) in Japan. This leads to a predicted lower number of ε4/ε4 and ε3/ε4 individuals in the population, and correlates with a lower prevalence of AD in Japan, with a higher mean age of onset.

Neuropathology of Alzheimer's disease

AD is associated with a complex pattern of neuronal degeneration. There is atrophy of the brain, with loss of neurones and loss of synapses, in both cortical and subcortical regions. Neuronal loss is significant in the hippocampus, in the frontal, parietal and anterior temporal lobes, in the amygdala and in the olfactory system. Brain weight can be reduced by 30–40% and MRI scans show dramatically enlarged ventricles and widened sulci (see Fig. 14.1). There is wide interindividual variation in the degree of cell loss, but in many patients there is a large reduction in the marker for cholinergic neurones, choline acetyltransferase (CAT), which is caused by the loss of neurones in the basal forebrain cholinergic nuclei.

There are also significant losses in other neurotransmitter systems, such as the noradrenergic (e.g. losses in the locus coeruleus), serotonergic and glutamatergic systems. In particular, there are losses in the glutamatergic pathways projecting to and from the hippocampus. This leads to functional isolation of the hippocampus and probably underlies the inability to form long-term memories that is common in AD.

Although the exact pattern of neuronal loss may vary from patient to patient, the appearance of the brain at the cellular level shows two characteristic features in AD: the neuritic plaques and the neurofibrillary tangles (Fig. 14.4). In fact, the only certain way of confirming a provisional diagnosis of AD at present is by the post-mortem examination of the brain for these features. The patient in the case history given in Box 14.1 is likely to be suffering from AD at an early stage, although this could only be confirmed after death.

Neuritic plaques

Neuritic plaques are extracellular structures that consist predominantly of insoluble deposits of β-amyloid

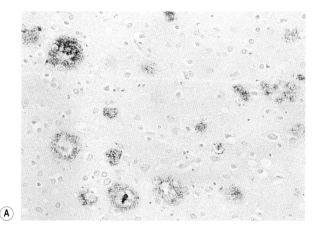

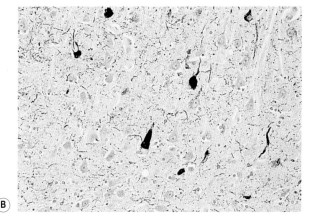

Fig. 14.4 (A) Neuritic plaques, stained for Aβ protein. (B) Neurofibrillary tangles, stained for tau protein (T). From Stevens A, Lowe J. Pathology, 2nd edn, 2000.

peptide (Aβ); hence the alternative name, amyloid plaques. However, there are also many other proteins associated with plaques, including apoE, components of the complement cascade and cytokines. The plaque core is surrounded by dystrophic neurites and reactive astroglia and microglia. While neuritic plaques are particularly prevalent in areas of the AD brain showing substantial neuronal loss, neuritic plaques are also seen, albeit usually at a lower frequency, in normal elderly people without AD. Thus, the number of plaques does not seem to be invariably related to AD, as there are normal elderly people with large numbers of plaques, and some AD patients who have few, if any, plaques.

Neurofibrillary tangles

Neurofibrillary tangles (NFTs) are dense aggregates of long, unbranched filaments that are found in the cytoplasm of neurones, in particular cortical pyramidal cells. Electron microscopy shows that they consist of two 10-nm filaments that are twisted in a helix, with a period of about 160 nm, to form paired helical filaments (PHFs). These filaments are composed of the microtubule-associated protein tau, in an abnormally phosphorylated form that

Biomarkers in Alzheimer's disease

It is becoming increasingly important to define potential disease biomarkers in Alzheimer's disease (AD). Once identified, these would consolidate the diagnosis, and also allow us to follow the evolution of the disease and the success of treatment regimens.

It has been suggested that there are two possible biomarkers in the cerebrospinal fluid (CSF) of AD patients: (1) the 42 amino acid form of Aβ amyloid peptide (i.e. $A\beta_{1-42}$); and (2) the phosphorylated tau protein.

The concentration of $A\beta_{1-42}$ is decreased in the CSF of AD patients. There is a significant correlation between the decrease in $A\beta_{1-42}$ concentration and the increased number of amyloid plaques in areas such as the neocortex and hippocampus.

The level of soluble tau protein in the frontal cortex is highly predictive of the degree of cognitive impairment, and some studies have shown that levels of total soluble tau in CSF are raised in AD patients. However, there is at least a 20% overlap between CSF levels in normal and in AD patients, so the test is not specific enough. However, the level of the phosphorylated form of tau protein is also significantly increased in the CSF of AD patients. This may reflect the hyperphosphorylated state of the protein in the brain parenchyma, and appears to be a test with more specificity for AD.

Neuroimaging can also be used as a biomarker. Computed tomography (CT) and magnetic resonance imaging (MRI) can add to the specificity of diagnosis of certain subtypes of dementia. At the same time, these techniques can also show the significant overlap between dementias: AD can be associated with white matter lesions revealed by MRI, whereas vascular dementia can be associated with temporal lobe atrophy revealed by CT and MRI. Functional MRI is a more recent technique that provides information on blood flow and cerebral metabolism. It provides better identification rates than MRI, and used in conjunction with psychological testing can enable the location of function in the brain, the monitoring of deficiencies, and observation of the effects of treatment.

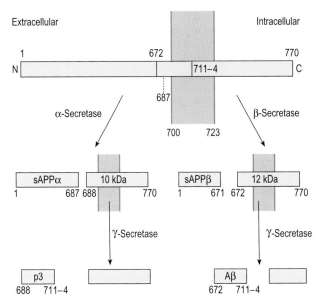

Fig. 14.5 Structure of amyloid precursor protein (APP) and its processing by α-, β- and γ-secretase enzymes. Aβ represents the amyloid peptides.

The amyloid hypothesis

The main component of neuritic plaques, Aβ, is a peptide containing between 39 and 42 amino acids. Aβ is cleaved by proteases from the amyloid precursor protein (APP), which is an integral membrane protein with a single transmembrane segment, a C-terminal cytoplasmic domain and an N-terminal extracellular domain. APP is processed by at least three proteases, named α-, β- and γ-secretases (Fig. 14.5).

α-Secretase cleaves membrane-associated APP at a site (residue 687) just outside the membrane. The N-terminal fragment is secreted (sAPPα), leaving an 83 amino acid C-terminal fragment, which is cleaved by γ-secretase to produce a smaller peptide, called p3. APP can also be cleaved by β-secretase at residue 671. This results in a smaller fragment, sAPPβ. The remaining 99 amino acid fragment is then further cleaved by γ-secretase in the region 711–714, to produce the Aβ peptide (672–711 to 714). Although Aβ occurs in a range of lengths, some forms, particularly the longer ones, are more able to form plaques. As the α- and β-secretases cleave the same precursor in different positions, cleavage of APP by the α pathway cannot produce Aβ, and the p3 peptide does not appear to form plaques. Thus, processing of APP down the α-secretase pathway does not appear to be involved in AD. However, processing of APP by alternative pathways seems to be involved, and it has been suggested that increased processing via the β-secretase pathway leads to excess production of Aβ, and plaque formation.

Under normal conditions, the Aβ peptide that is secreted is soluble, and seems to have no adverse effects on cells. However, in AD, the peptide forms aggregates of insoluble β-pleated sheets of fibrillar Aβ protein (hence the name β-amyloid). The conformational change from soluble

self-assembles to form the PHFs. Although NFTs are also seen in other neurodegenerative diseases, the number of NFTs correlates well with the severity of the dementia. Remnants of dead cells that contained NFTs can also be seen as extracellular 'ghost' tangles. In AD, neurones in the entorhinal cortex are often very enriched in tangles.

Studies on the main components of plaques and tangles have led to suggestions concerning possible biomarkers in AD (Box 14.3), and have also given rise to two theories of the aetiology of AD. These are:

1. The 'β-amyloid hypothesis', which centres around the abnormal deposition of Aβ in plaques.

2. The 'tau and tangle hypothesis', in which the key event is the formation of PHFs and tangles.

to fibrillar forms seems to be a spontaneous event and no trigger is known. The fibrillization is increased with higher concentrations of Aβ and with the longer forms of Aβ, particularly Aβ$_{1-42}$, so any production of larger amounts of Aβ than normal, or production of the larger, less soluble forms of Aβ, will tend to increase plaque formation. Once the Aβ plaque has started to form, other molecules can interact with the nascent plaque to eventually produce the mature plaque, with associated areas of cell death.

Although the manner in which the formation of plaques could cause cell death is unproven, it has been shown that aggregates of Aβ can disrupt Ca^{2+} homeostasis in neurones. Even a relatively small reduction in the ability of cells to regulate intracellular Ca^{2+} could leave them vulnerable to damage by excitotoxicity, ischaemia and free radicals.

The tau and tangle hypothesis

While the amyloid hypothesis is seen by some to be central to the pathophysiological process in AD, there is a competing hypothesis, which proposes that it is the formation of fibrillary tangles and the subsequent disruption of axonal transport that is the key pathological event and the reason for cell death. This idea is supported by the good correlation between the severity of dementia and the frequency of tangles.

Although tangles have been shown to contain many different proteins, the core of the tangle is made up of tau protein. Physiologically, the tau protein binds to microtubules and may form cross-bridges between microtubules that stabilize the microtubules, promoting tubulin polymerization and microtubule bundling, which are essential for axon elongation and maintenance. Tau is a phosphoprotein, and the ability of tau to bind to microtubules is reduced by phosphorylation.

The tau protein isolated from PHFs is hyperphosphorylated (tau-HP) when compared to normal tau, and this greatly reduces its ability to bind to microtubules. Phosphorylation seems to inhibit both tau–tau and tau–tubulin binding. Tau–tau (and tau–tubulin) binding occurs at a site that is masked by phosphorylation of tau. It has been suggested, on the basis of in vitro experiments, that it is only normal tau that can self-aggregate, by undergoing a critical conformational change that allows self-association, and that it is an autocatalytic event in which the presence of altered tau can promote the alteration of other tau molecules. This has been compared to the action of prion proteins, in which the normal α-helical form is thought to be converted to the pathogenic β-sheet form of the protein by the presence of the β-form, which induces the switch (see below).

These considerations do not explain why PHFs do not accumulate in normal brain if there are no abnormal modifications necessary to produce tau aggregation. Also, they do not explain the presence of tau-HP in PHFs. Other factors may be needed to fully explain the paradox.

The role of apoE

ApoE protein is involved in the recycling of cholesterol during membrane repair and remodelling and ApoE binds to both lipoproteins and to the low-density lipoprotein (LDL) receptor. The affinity of binding to the different types of lipoprotein and to the LDL receptor varies with the different apoE isoforms (ε1–4), but the significance of these different interactions is not clear. It has been suggested that the ε4 isoform is less effective than ε2 and ε3 at repairing membrane damage. Neurones may be particularly susceptible to reductions in the effectiveness of apoE, as the other apolipoproteins—apoB and apoA1—are not found in the brain.

ApoE has also been shown to bind to both Aβ and tau proteins both in vivo and in vitro. After a long period of incubation (days), apoE and Aβ form fibrils, but these are not the same as the types of fibril seen with Aβ alone or in in vivo plaques. ApoE binding to plaques is extracellular, but apoE has also been shown to enter the neuronal cytoplasm, a necessary property if it is to interact with tau proteins in vivo.

Other factors involved in the causation of Alzheimer's disease

As reviewed above, the pathophysiology of AD involves several different processes. Historically, the 'amyloid hypothesis' and the 'tau and tangle hypothesis' postulated two distinct phenomena as roots of the pathology. However, recent evidence suggests that these two aspects may be interconnected. One example of this possible link is the enzyme glycogen kinase-3 (GSK-3), which phosphorylates tau. It has been shown that inhibition of this protein results in reduced production of Aβ peptides.

Furthermore, although much research effort has been focused on the role of Aβ, tau and apoE in the pathogenesis of AD, there are also other factors that are considered to play a critical role in the development of AD. Two such examples are given below.

Alzheimer's disease has a neuroinflammatory component

Microglia are activated and proliferate locally at the sites of AD lesions. Microglia then produce cytokines and free radicals, which could produce a chronic inflammatory response. In both head injury and ischaemia, activation of microglia and increases in APP expression appear very rapidly. Aβ is known to activate microglia. Whether activated microglia secrete Aβ or not is a contentious issue. The complement receptor, C1q, binds to Aβ, triggering the complement cascade. In this way, the inflammatory process may be both initiated and potentiated by Aβ. There is possibly a critical role of proinflammatory cytokines in AD. Interestingly, the chronic use of non-steroidal anti-inflammatory drugs (NSAIDs) has been associated with a decreased risk of developing AD (see below).

Abnormal glycation of proteins and Alzheimer's disease

With increasing age, there is an accumulation of abnormally glycated proteins, called advanced glycosylation end-products (AGEs), and an increase in the production of free radicals, consistent with a permanent state of oxidative stress. Owing to the reduced rate of protein turnover with age, this leads to an increased accumulation of damaged proteins and lipids. Several features have suggested that these mechanisms are exacerbated in AD, leading to abnormal modifications of proteins, including Aβ and tau, which can stimulate their aggregation. It has been shown that AGE-modified Aβ can act as a template for further deposition of soluble Aβ. Tau protein from AD but not from normal brains is also AGE-modified and undergoes oxidation-induced cross-linking. However, why some aged individuals develop AD and others do not is not known, although if apoE4 is significantly less able to repair damaged neurones, this could lead to greater oxidative stress and the development of AD. In injury-related AD, it is possible that an increase in oxidative stress due to high levels of cell damage, both acute and chronic, could act as a triggering factor for the development of AD.

Treatment of Alzheimer's disease

An integrated view of the aetiopathology of AD is that this disease may begin early in life, and that it is underlined by genetic factors and various environmental stressors. However, regardless of the major primary cause, a cascade of irreversible events is triggered that compromises neurotransmission and leads to cell death and major synaptic loss.

The existing treatments for AD address the disruption of neurotransmission, as discussed in detail below. However, emerging therapies are attempting to address the primary cause of the disease, and thus not only reverse the symptoms, but also modify the disease process (Table 14.5).

Cholinesterase inhibitors

In AD there is a significant loss of forebrain cholinergic projection neurones. These represent an important part of the cholinergic neurone population in the CNS (Box 14.4). The role of acetylcholine (ACh) in cognition is well established in experimental models. For example, cholinergic receptor antagonists such as the muscarinic antagonist scopolamine impair learning and memory. Therefore, the cognitive deficit seen in AD is at least partly due to the deficit in ACh. A deficit in cholinergic transmission is also supported by a significant decrease in CAT activity in the cortex and hippocampus of patients with AD. It has been shown that there is a correlation between the loss of cortical cholinergic synapses and cognitive decline, and also the loss of cholinergic receptors.

Table 14.5 Selected therapeutic strategies in Alzheimer's disease (AD)

Target	Therapeutic agent
Cholinergic	Cholinesterase inhibitors
Glutamatergic	Memantine
Antioxidants	Vitamin E
	Selegiline
Anti-inflammatory	Non-steroidal anti-inflammatory drugs (NSAIDs)
Reduction of risk factors	Statins
	Vitamins B_6 and B_{12}
	Folic acid
Anti-amyloid	Secretase inhibitors
	Immunization
Tau hyperphosphorylation	Kinase inhibitors

Inhibiting the cholinesterase activity that inactivates ACh would lead to potentiation of the failing cholinergic signal. There are two types of cholinesterase: acetylcholinesterase (AChE) and butyrylcholinesterase (BuChE). The two types are related structurally, but their distribution in the body, their substrate specificity and their functional roles differ. AChE is present in the brain, and its main function is to hydrolyse the released acetylcholine. BuChE is present in the brain but also in the skin, gastrointestinal tract, liver and plasma, and has a broader substrate specificity than AChE. Tacrine was the first cholinesterase inhibitor to be approved for treatment of AD, at the beginning of the 1990s. This drug inhibits both AChE and BChE and improves the Mini Mental State Examination score. However, it is associated with a high incidence of gastrointestinal side effects, such as diarrhoea, nausea and vomiting. It also induces hepatotoxicity in some patients. Its pharmacokinetics are very poor; tacrine must be administered four times a day because of its short half-life.

Donepezil is a non-competitive, non-selective, reversible inhibitor of AChE, whose long half-life makes possible once-daily dosing. In clinical trials it has been shown that the administration of donepezil to patients with moderate to severe AD leads to improved cognition and daily functioning, compared to patients who receive placebo. However, when treatment is stopped, there is an immediate and accelerated deterioration in all measures, and by the time the drug washout is completed, the scores of patients receiving the drug and those receiving placebo become the same. Therefore, it is unlikely that cholinesterase inhibitors modify, even in a minor way, the disease process.

Rivastigmine is another example of a cholinesterase inhibitor. It is a pseudo-irreversible inhibitor of AChE and

The cholinergic system in the forebrain

Acetylcholine (ACh) is a neurotransmitter present in several large clusters of projection neurones in the central nervous system (CNS) (Fig. 14.6), as well as in numerous inter neurones. The human cholinergic systems in the basal forebrain include neurones in the septal and diagonal complex and in the basal nucleus (nucleus basalis) of Meynert.

Several subgroups can be distinguished:

- Group Ch1 of the medial septum comprises 10% of the cells in this area.
- The diagonal band of Broca comprises groups Ch2 and Ch3.

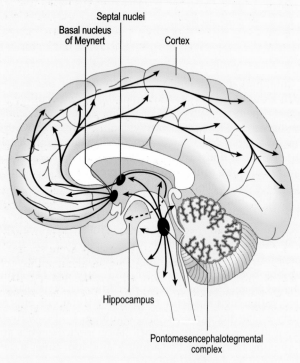

Fig. 14.6 The cholinergic system in the forebrain.

- The largest group of cholinergic cells in the basal forebrain (around 90%), Ch4, is represented by the basal nucleus of Meynert. The number of cholinergic cells in Ch4 is approximately 210 000 per hemisphere.

Groups Ch1 and Ch2 provide cholinergic input to the hippocampus, the Ch3 cells provide innervation to olfactory areas, and the Ch4 cells innervate the cortex and amygdala. All cholinergic cells in the basal forebrain express the high- and low-affinity receptors for the neurotrophin nerve growth factor (NGF). This suggests that this neurotrophin is critical for their survival. However, attempts to use NGF therapeutically in Alzheimer's disease (AD) have not had much success so far.

ACh is synthesized from acetyl-CoA and choline. Choline is present in the extracellular fluid and is taken up into the terminal through an active uptake system. Dietary supplements of choline have been tried, to boost the falling levels of ACh in the brain in AD, but this strategy has had very limited success.

ACh can bind and activate both nicotinic and muscarinic receptors. The former are ligand-gated ion channels, whereas the latter are metabotropic receptors. Positron emission tomography (PET) studies suggest that nicotinic receptor deficits are an early phenomenon in AD. Interestingly, it has been shown that Aβ peptides can block the interaction of nicotinic agonists with their receptors, suggesting a direct link between the amyloid pathology and neurotransmission.

The muscarinic receptors, M1 to M5, have a widespread distribution in the body. M1 and M2, and to a lesser extent M5, are present in the CNS. M1 receptors mediate excitatory effects, whereas M2 receptors have mainly inhibitory effects, and a predominantly presynaptic location. Using non-selective muscarinic ligands, PET studies have shown that age and AD lead to decreased muscarinic receptor binding in the cortex. It has been reported that M1 agonists may decrease the levels of Aβ amyloid. Thus, a therapeutic strategy based on muscarinic agonists may not only improve cognition but might also have a disease-modifying effect, by interfering with plaque formation.

is not metabolized by liver microsomes. It is claimed to have fewer unwanted effects than tacrine and donepezil.

Galantamine is a cholinesterase inhibitor and also a positive allosteric modulator of nicotinic receptors. The latter property may offer an advantage compared to the other inhibitors, as the drug may enhance the signal mediated by nicotinic receptors. It appears to have fewer and milder side effects than the other inhibitors, and there is less tolerance to its effects.

Overall, the tolerability of cholinesterase inhibitors is reasonable. Most inhibitors have unwanted gastrointestinal effects that are more prominent in the first year of

treatment. The inhibitors induce a global improvement in cognitive performance, although the response is variable between patients. It is still unclear how beneficial these compounds are in the severe forms of the disease. Starting therapy early increases the likelihood of a better outcome and may significantly delay admission to nursing homes. There is not enough evidence to prove the superiority of one agent over another.

Based on the same rationale, of decreased cholinergic signalling in AD, muscarinic receptor agonists and nicotinic receptor agonists or allosteric modulators (such as galantamine) are also being actively researched, and they may offer distinct advantages, such as reduced toxicity compared with the cholinesterase inhibitors named above.

Glutamatergic agents

Glutamate is a key excitatory transmitter both in cortico-subcortical projections and in corticocortical fibres. It is likely that the physiopathology of AD involves an excitotoxic component, which may be due to dysregulated glutamatergic transmission. Furthermore, the toxicity of glutamate is enhanced by amyloid peptides. In addition, the activation of glutamatergic transmission through NMDA receptors enhances the production of phosphorylated tau.

Memantine is an uncompetitive NMDA receptor antagonist that has relatively strong voltage-dependency and rapid unblocking kinetics. The interaction of memantine with the NMDA receptor channel is reminiscent of the action of Mg^{2+}, which blocks the channel under resting conditions. Because of its voltage dependency and fast kinetics, it has been suggested that memantine does not interfere with normal glutamatergic transmission, but blocks increased transmission under chronic conditions. It has been shown that memantine significantly slows down the rate of cognitive and functional decline, and that it has a positive synergistic effect with cholinesterase inhibitors such as donepezil, without adding to the burden of unwanted effects.

Antioxidants

Like other neurodegenerative diseases, AD has been associated with increased levels of oxidative stress and free radical-induced damage. Both the monoamine oxidase type B (MAO_B) inhibitor selegiline and vitamin E have been shown to have mild beneficial effects in AD. Similarly, the herbal extract of *Ginkgo biloba* may provide some neuroprotection. This extract is approved in some countries for use in dementia, but its effectiveness remains controversial.

Non-steroidal anti-inflammatory drugs

Epidemiological evidence shows that the use of NSAIDs such as ibuprofen reduces the risk of AD developing. However, clinical trials designed to confirm and further investigate such observations have failed overall to show significant neuroprotection with NSAIDs. However, it is not contested that AD physiopathology involves an inflammatory component, so a better understanding of this component may help in the elucidation of the exact role of anti-inflammatory drugs in the management or prophylactic treatment of AD.

Reduction of risk factors

There is a possible link between cholesterol and AD, and several epidemiological studies have shown that the use of statins, which decrease the production of cholesterol, leads to a decreased risk of developing AD. Cholesterol reduction leads to a reduction in the activity of β-secretase and possibly γ-secretase, and an increase in α-secretase. Large-scale prospective studies are required to confirm these observations, as well as to clarify the role of cholesterol in the middle or late stage of the disease.

Similarly, a link has been suggested between increased circulating homocysteine levels and AD. Present trials are investigating the possible neuroprotective role of a combination of vitamin B_6, vitamin B_{12} and folic acid, in order to decrease homocysteine levels.

Anti-amyloid strategies

Inhibition of secretases

The amyloid cascade starts with production of amyloid peptides, in particular the $A\beta_{1-42}$ form, through proteolysis of APP by secretases. Inhibition of β- or γ-secretase could lead to decreased production of amyloid peptides, and a reduced risk of aggregation and subsequent formation of plaques.

Vaccines against amyloid peptides

Much hope was generated when it was shown that transgenic mice made to overproduce amyloid peptides showed a reduced plaque burden when vaccinated with $A\beta_{1-42}$. This beneficial effect could also be obtained by direct administration of anti-amyloid antibodies. This effect may have two mechanisms: (1) antibodies bind to the plaque and activate the surrounding microglia to phagocytose the plaques; and (2) antibodies act as a peripheral 'sink', and pull out the peptides from the brain into the circulation, where the peptides are cleared. However, trials in patients with AD using an Aβ vaccination strategy were stopped, due to development of brain inflammation in a number of patients. More studies are required to make this approach safe in patients, but it holds promise. The principle may be applicable not only in AD, but also in other types of dementia, such as prion diseases (Box 14.5).

Tau hyperphosphorylation

Inhibition of the activity of kinases that hyperphosphorylate tau can be achieved with various compounds, including drugs such as lithium and sodium valproate, whose strong inhibitory effect on kinases such as GSK-3β was rather unexpected. Lithium can reduce amyloid peptide levels in a mouse transgenic model, so this approach has considerable potential.

Other types of dementia

Vascular dementia

After AD, vascular dementia is the second most common type of dementia in the elderly. It is caused by reoccurring

Immunization against neurodegeneration—a hope for the future?

Use of vaccination has been associated in the history of medicine with the treatment of infectious disease. Therefore, its possible relevance for neurodegenerative disease was ignored for a long time. Another reason for this was that the central nervous system (CNS) was considered to be a place where primary immune responses do not occur. Any involvement of the CNS in immune reactions was, rather, considered to be harmful.

In 1999, Schenk and collaborators showed that immunization with Aβ peptide can reduce amyloid load, and this turned the attention of the public and of the scientists to vaccination as a treatment approach in neurodegeneration. This report was followed by the observation that even the administration of antibodies could reduce the amyloid component. It was shown that antibodies 'coated' brain amyloid plaques and could trigger a classic immune response, culminating with the removal of the labelled plaques by activated microglia. Immunization could reverse the cognitive impairment, and this was confirmed in two different transgenic mouse models.

These studies noted that the cognitive improvement was likely to be due to a reduction in a pool of non-deposited Aβ, perhaps in an oligomeric form, as the reduction was seen in diffuse deposits but not in fibrillar deposits. Subsequent work also led to the suggestion that the beneficial effect of immunization is not necessarily associated with penetration of the antibody into the CNS. What was seen after passive immunization was a massive increase in the plasma Aβ concentration. Hence, the antibody could act as a 'sink' that promotes efflux of amyloid from the CNS, thereby clearing the brain parenchyma indirectly.

A third possibility is that the antibodies prevent the formation of oligomers and protofibrils, thus ultimately protecting against formation of large insoluble plaques. Whatever the mechanisms involved in the effects of vaccination, when the experimental studies were transferred to the clinic, several patients developed brain inflammation, which led to the cessation of the clinical trial. This reaction was likely to be due to a stimulation of T-cell-mediated immunity. It is hoped that slight modifications of the immunization strategy may avoid the activation of T-cells and its potentially fatal consequences.

It is hoped that with a better understanding of the mechanisms involved in antibody-mediated clearance of abnormal proteins, this strategy could be extended to other types of neurodegenerative disease, such as Huntington's disease.

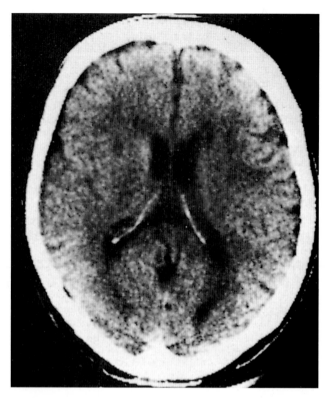

Fig. 14.7 Computed tomography scan in multi-infarct dementia. The ventricles are normal in size, but there are patchy radiolucencies throughout the white matter. These indicate the presence of demyelinated patches, which result from multiple small infarcts in the brain. From Forbes CD, Jackson WF. Colour Atlas and Text of Clinical Medicine, 3rd edn. Mosby, 2002. Reproduced by permission of Mosby International Ltd.

accompanied by brief periods of impaired consciousness and visual or sensory loss. Patients often show signs of vascular disease, such as coronary heart disease and peripheral vascular disease. The progression of the disease can be halted if further strokes can be prevented, so treatment is limited to the reduction of cardiovascular risk factors. The increase in life-expectancy is associated with an increased risk of stroke, so an increase in this type of neuropathology is likely in the future.

HIV-associated dementia

Infection with HIV often causes cognitive and motor dysfunction, and prior to the introduction of effective retroviral therapies, large numbers of infected adults (one-third) and even more children (one-half) developed HIV-1-associated dementia (HAD). Worldwide, HAD is the commonest form of dementia in those under the age of 40 years. HIV enters the CNS through infected monocytes. Many of the drugs used to treat HIV infection do not penetrate well into the brain, and so CNS infection of macrophages and microglia creates a reservoir that is not affected by peripheral treatments. Patients with advanced HAD show cerebral atrophy, with losses of up to 30% of

thromboemboli from either extracranial sources or, more commonly, small vessels in the brain. Unlike with AD, onset is rapid and progression of the disease is stepwise with focal neurological defects, which is consistent with multiple, small infarcts (Fig. 14.7). These infarcts may be neocortical neurones. Neurones may be either damaged directly by HIV proteins or killed by compounds released from infected cells. Neurones themselves are not infected with HIV, but it is thought that infected macrophages and microglia release neurotoxic compounds, such as glutamate, which can trigger excitotoxicity (see Chapter 11), and inflammatory cytokines. The appearance of many apoptotic neurones and the fact that large neurones seem to be more susceptible than small ones support the theory that free radical production, metabolic compromise and oxidative stress play a role in neuronal death.

Creutzfeldt–Jakob disease

Creutzfeldt–Jakob disease (CJD) is a rare disease characterized by rapidly progressing dementia, myoclonus and ataxia. These patients have a characteristic pattern in their electroencephalogram and there is widespread neuronal loss. The appearance of vacuoles within the brain gives the other name for this disease, subacute spongiform encephalopathy (Fig. 14.8). The transmissible agent responsible for the disease is a prion protein (see Chapter 12). Prions can multiply in the host latently for years. They are devoid of nucleic acids, and the prion protein (PrP) is encoded by a gene that is present and expressed to the same extent in the cells of normal and affected individuals. The functions of the normal variant of PrP (named PrP^c) are unknown. Prions are composed of an abnormal, protease-resistant form of PrP, designated PrP^{Sc}, which differs from PrP^c by its β-sheet structure (as opposed to α-helices, which characterize the structure of PrP^c). The increased presence of β-sheets leads to formation of fibrils, which ultimately deposit in the brain. It is unknown how PrP^c converts into PrP^{Sc} (possibly a spontaneous conversion) and how the fibrillary deposits are responsible for generalized neurodegeneration. There is at present no treatment for this disease.

Dementia with Lewy bodies

Lewy bodies are intraneuronal proteinaceous structures with radiating filaments. The protein detected in the Lewy bodies is α-synuclein, which is present in the bodies in an aggregated form (see Chapter 10). Lewy bodies can also be detected in the brains of patients with Parkinson's disease (PD), where they are found in nigrostriatal neurones. However, in dementia with Lewy bodies, they are more widely distributed. Patients with this type of dementia have visual hallucinations, fluctuations in cognitive function and some evidence of parkinsonism, but paradoxically a worsening of their condition is caused by even small amounts of anti-parkinsonian drugs. Pure AD, by definition, has no Lewy bodies, but modern sensitive techniques show that Lewy bodies can also be found in AD. The presence of synuclein in the Lewy bodies has led to the suggestion that dementia with Lewy bodies and PD are both synucleinopathies.

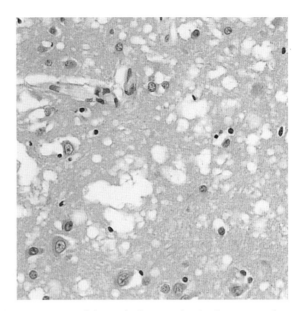

Fig. 14.8 Section of the cerebral cortex, showing large areas of vacuolation, characteristic of spongiform encephalopathy. From Stevens A, Lowe J. Pathology, 2nd edn. Mosby, 2000.

Thus, new treatment based on this common pathogenesis may be equally effective in the two diseases.

General considerations in the management of Alzheimer's disease and other types of dementia

The pharmacological and non-pharmacological management of dementia poses numerous challenges. Patients and their carers are affected not only by the cognitive loss, but also by all the other symptoms that may be comorbid with dementia, such as psychosis, aggression or depression, and the generalized change of personality. Such neuropsychiatric disorders occur in up to 90% of dementia patients, and are one of the main causes of admission to institutions.

Depression in dementia is widely studied, because of the difficulties of differential diagnosis between a depressive syndrome and the early stage (or prodromal stage) of dementia. Often, depression is reactive at the beginning (as a consequence of the psychological impact of the diagnosis), but later on may increase in severity and be due to changes in the corticolimbic circuitry. Preference is given to treatment with antidepressant drugs such as the selective serotonin reuptake inhibitors, as these are generally better tolerated than other antidepressant drugs, and they have no anticholinergic effects that may accelerate cognitive decline.

Psychosis is treated with antipsychotic drugs. New antipsychotics, such as risperidone and quetiapine, are preferable because of the reduced anticholinergic component, and also because they are better tolerated overall.

It is also important to make sure that pain and infection, or any other cause of distress, are kept under control, and that the patient is placed in a supportive environment.

Care strategies must also take into account what has long been neglected: care-giving to a patient with dementia can itself lead to pathology in the carers. Therefore, preventive healthcare strategies must also be developed for carers, and respite care must be made more available. The move from care at home to institutional care must be better planned, and should not only be a reaction to a crisis or the consequence of carer burnout.

SCHIZOPHRENIA

Chapter objectives

After studying this chapter you should be able to:

1. Describe the main symptoms of schizophrenia and the natural evolution of the disease.

2. Give an outline of corticolimbic circuits.

3. Describe the treatment for schizophrenia.

4. Discuss the main principles of long-term management of chronic psychoses.

5. Give examples of schizophrenia-like syndromes in childhood.

Introduction

One of the most complex aspects of brain function concerns the processes of cognitive control, of development of appropriate patterns of behaviour within a social context, and of congruent emotional reactions. In patients who present with psychoses, behaviour is profoundly altered, and the symptoms that emerge are diverse, bizarre and disturbing, often leading to a gradual and irreversible alienation. Psychoses challenge our understanding of higher brain functions, and their pathophysiology is much more complex than that associated with sensory or motor dysfunction. Schizophrenia is a major psychosis, and it is illustrated in the case history in Box 15.1. In order to understand the pathology of psychoses, it is important to identify the cerebral circuits and neurotransmitters that play key roles in consciousness, cognition, emotions and moral reasoning.

Schizophrenia: the clinical diagnosis

The patient described in Box 15.1 was previously diagnosed with schizophrenia, and your analysis of this case will start with a brief mental state examination, in order to reassess the following: (1) appearance and behaviour; (2) speech; (3) affect; (4) thoughts; (5) perceptions; (6) cognitive state; and (7) insight.

The examination (Box 15.2) confirms the abnormal behaviour and distorted mental perceptions, which are indicative of major psychosis in the absence of an organic cause. Furthermore, the mood of the patient is depressed, and there is a clear risk of suicide.

The symptoms encountered in schizophrenic patients can be divided into several categories:

- abnormal ideas
- abnormal perceptions
- motor, volitional and behavioural disorders
- formal thought disorder
- emotional disorders.

Abnormal ideas

The main abnormal idea in schizophrenia is delusion, i.e. a belief that is erroneous and out of keeping with the individual's background, and is held by the patient with intense conviction. Patients may present with various types of delusion: delusions of persecution (e.g. external

---

Box 15.1 Case history

Jane was a 22-year-old physics undergraduate. She also used to work in the evenings as a proofreader. Two years ago, in her final year at university, she visited her doctor accompanied by her parents, who were very concerned about changes in her behaviour and communication at home. She had become withdrawn and rather obsessed with religion. Finally, she confessed to her parents that she had a mission to save the country from a nuclear disaster and said that her 'internal voices' would guide her. Jane was diagnosed with schizophrenia, and was prescribed a neuroleptic. However, although the medication helped a little and 'the voices' became less persistent, she complained that she felt rather dizzy and tired for most of the time, and that she put on weight. The drugs made her feel so strange that at times she did not take them. She could not continue her studies, and she started drinking immoderately. She claimed that she felt 'mentally numb'.

You see Jane as a specialist, after a recent suicide attempt. Following this, an antidepressant drug was added to her antipsychotic medication. Her family continue to wonder what may have caused this disease and want to know if their daughter will ever recover. They are distraught and ask if you can prescribe a better treatment.

This case gives rise to the following questions:

1. What is the explanation for the symptoms presented by this patient?
2. What are the neurobiological mechanisms underlying this type of mental dysfunction?
3. What has triggered this major disruption of normal behaviour?

Box 15.2 Case history (continued)

The patient's appearance is striking: she is dishevelled and her clothes are untidy and unsuitable for the season. This suggests little interest in personal grooming, which is confirmed by the inappropriate choice of clothes. She is quiet during the interview and needs prompting to answer questions. Her face lacks expression. She tells you that the voices are still visiting her, but are much kinder now. They come mostly during the night, and she thinks they know that she cannot sleep, especially since she started taking the new drug added to her old medication. The cognitive assessment reveals that Jane has a significant attention deficit. Towards the end of the interview, she says abruptly that she hates her life.

The questions that need to be addressed are:

1. Is this patient receiving the most appropriate treatment?
2. Is this patient still at risk of taking her own life?
3. What is the long-term prognosis?
4. Is there a role for the family in the successful management of this patient?

forces are trying to harm the patient or damage his or her reputation), grandiose delusions (e.g. patients may believe that they have a divine purpose, or that they have supernatural powers), hypochondriacal delusions (e.g. a belief that the body is rotten and diseased) and delusional mood (e.g. everything seems strange or full of a hidden intricate meaning).

Abnormal perceptions

The cardinal symptom in this class is the hallucination, which is a perception without an object. Hallucinations may occur in any sensory modality: auditory, visual, somatic, olfactory and gustatory. Auditory hallucinations (hearing voices) are by far the most prominent and are considered to be the commonest symptom of schizophrenia. They can be the first sign of schizophrenia, or may appear at a later stage of the disease. The source of the voices can be difficult to locate: voices can surround the patient or come from a particular point in space, or may originate within the patient's head or body. They can be menacing, encouraging, mocking, or simply neutral and observing (Box 15.3). The importance of auditory hallucinations in schizophrenia has led certain specialists to consider them as typical 'first-rank symptoms', i.e. of particular relevance for the diagnosis of schizophrenia.

Box 15.3 Dialogue with 'voices'

These are notes made by a patient of what he heard. Statements in parentheses are questions inwardly directed by the patient to his voices.

(Why are you speaking in me?)
'You must eat blood … Because we are poor blockheads … We'll bring you later to an asylum … We inhale you.'
(Why do you torment me?)
'We think the best of you … Because we are frightfully fond of you … We weep laughing tears. Because we ourselves are tormented. … Every human being must laugh at you … You are in many things an absolute child, an absolute fool.'
(What is your real object?)
'We wish to kill you. You have offended divine providence. Our object is morally irrelevant. Our object is your cleansing. We love and hate you…'
(Are you human beings or spirits?)
'We are human beings … We weep about you. … You have been very prudent. Now then, little spirits! Little folk, brownies!'
(Are you near?)
'No, far away … No, in the middle of your head.'

From Kraepelin (1913).

Motor, volitional and behavioural disorders

Bleuler (1911) provided the first description of 'peculiar forms of motility, stupor, mutism, stereotypy, mannerism, negativism, spontaneous automatism and impulsivity'. Stereotypies are purposeless acts that are carried out repetitively, such as rocking or rubbing hands. Patients may also present with strange mannerisms (for example, when they eat they put the hand round the back of the head to bring the food to the mouth) or bizarre postures. Facial expressions may be altered by grimacing. In states of catatonia, the patient sits or lies expressionless, motionless and mute, sometimes in very uncomfortable and contorted postures. In contrast, in states of catalepsy (waxy flexibility), the patient's limbs can be manipulated by the observer, and the patient may maintain the final position for a long time.

Patients may present with bouts of extreme hyperactivity, which may be associated with destructiveness: they may destroy furniture and crockery, or take off their clothes and run around naked. The impulsive behaviour may lead to very violent acts, such as murder, for which the patient cannot give any explanation.

Formal thought disorder

This refers to disturbances in thinking that lead to unintelligible speech. Speech may suffer from derailment and loosening of associations (a tendency to be deflected from the main point of the discussion and a failure to follow a train of thought through to its conclusion) and may also abound in neologisms (new words invented by patients). There is poverty of content of speech, and although speech may be abundant, it fails to convey any information (Box 15.4).

Emotional disorders

One of the most typical examples of emotional dysfunction in schizophrenia is affective flattening. Patients lose natural reactions to usual social cues. Facial expression is reduced, and there is an apparent indifference to emotive topics. Patients may come across as cold and detached, and unable to establish a rapport. Schizophrenics may also display inappropriate affect (e.g. smiling or laughing when discussing death or attending a funeral) and shallowness of emotions.

Positive and negative symptoms

It is important to note that the five main categories of symptoms discussed above may occur either in isolation or in combination, and evolve during the disease. In addition, certain combinations of symptoms appear with great regularity, and this has led to a classification of schizophrenia into subtypes. Finally, the symptoms of schizophrenia can also be divided into two classes: positive (or type 1) and negative (or type 2). Thus, positive

Examples of formal thought disorder

Incoherence

Interviewer: Have you been nervous or tense lately?
Patient: No, I got a head of lettuce.
Interviewer: You got a head of lettuce? I don't understand. Tell me about lettuce.
Patient: Well, lettuce is a transformation of a dead cougar that suffered a relapse on the lion's toe. And he swallowed the lion and something happened. The … see, the … Gloria and Tommy, they're two heads and they're not whales.

Poverty of content of speech

Interviewer: Are you feeling unwell?
Patient: It's hard to live on your own in this society. I get fears of violence and death—feeling that I'm all negative inside—you know—I always have a clash with authority. They have too much power to incarcerate me and you. The alternative is death: I would have done myself in.

Neologisms

- snortie—to talk through walls
- trominoes—tiny people who live in one's body
- split-kippered—to be simultaneously alive in Lancashire and dead in Yorkshire.

From McKenna (1994).

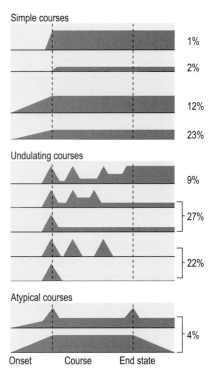

Fig. 15.1 Examples of disease courses of schizophrenia. The diagram illustrates various possible courses of schizophrenia, and the relative percentage of patients affected within a subtype. From Bleuler (1978). In McKenna PJ ed. Schizophrenia and Related Syndromes. Oxford: Oxford University Press, 1994: 55.

symptoms are those characterized by the existence of an abnormal phenomenon, and include delusions, hallucinations, thought disorder, bizarre behaviour and catatonia.

Negative symptoms are characterized by the absence or diminution of normal function and reactions. Examples of negative symptoms are: apathy, affective blunting, incongruity of emotions, lack of insight, social withdrawal, impaired judgement, poor initiative, motivation and drive, lack of interest in personal hygiene, difficulty in planning and impaired problem-solving.

Apart from being another mode of classification of symptoms, this positive–negative distinction has clinical implications. Positive symptoms are associated in particular with acute episodes, whereas negative symptoms underlie the severe disability associated with chronic schizophrenia. There is evidence that positive and negative symptoms respond differently to treatment, and that the relative balance between the two has prognostic implications.

Classification and epidemiology of schizophrenia

Schizophrenia is a very broad diagnosis, and includes a multitude of clinical presentations. This clinical heterogeneity

suggests differences in the underlying mechanisms. Clinical subtypes can be defined by identifying symptoms that co-occur. The current classification of schizophrenia according to the Diagnostic and Statistical Manual of Mental Disorders, 4th Edition (DSM-IV), includes five subtypes:

- paranoid (dominated by delusions and hallucinations)
- disorganized (hebephrenic) (characterized by emotional blunting and meaningless behaviour)
- catatonic (characterized by motor stereotypies, stupor and abnormalities of posture)
- undifferentiated (mixed characteristics)
- residual (predominant negative symptoms).

The presence of positive and/or negative symptoms is crucial for the diagnosis of schizophrenia. Diagnosis also requires evidence of gradual and sustained deterioration in work, interpersonal relationships, communication and self-care. DSM-IV requires a duration of symptoms of at least 6 months. If these criteria are satisfied and there is no evidence of an organic cause, the diagnosis of schizophrenia is very likely. The natural evolution of the disease is complex and variable (Fig. 15.1). There are cases in which several acute episodes are followed by what appears to be full recovery. The intensity of the episodes may vary. Other cases are characterized by gradual deterioration and resistance to treatment. Finally, other cases stabilize

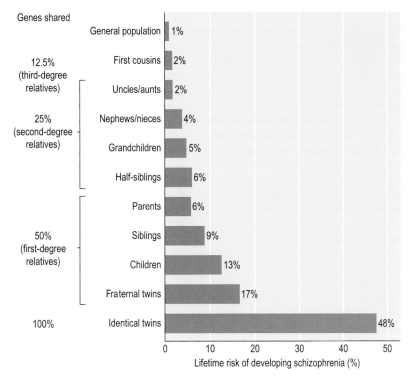

Genes shared

Fig. 15.2 Correlation between genetic relatedness and lifetime risk of developing schizophrenia. From Barondes SH. *Molecules and Mental Illness*. New York: Scientific American Library, 1993: 150.

at a moderate level of disability. Schizophrenia has a constant prevalence throughout the world (about 1%), with apparently no significant influence of culture, ethnic background or socio-economic group. There is a slightly increased prevalence in urban areas. No overall difference exists between the sexes. However, the average age of onset appears to be earlier in men (between 15 and 25 years) than in women (between 20 and 30 years). Men also have a poorer response to treatment than women, and a worse long-term outcome.

Aetiology of schizophrenia

Genetic aspects

Family, twin and adoption studies suggest that schizophrenia has a significant genetic component. Relatives of schizophrenic patients have a higher risk for developing the illness. The risk is positively correlated with the degree of genetic relatedness (Fig. 15.2). However, schizophrenia does not follow a classic genetic Mendelian model. Monozygotic twins have a concordance rate of 50% for schizophrenia, but this falls to 15–18% in dizygotic twins. Schizophrenia is not associated with a single major locus, but with multiple genetic loci of modest effect, which are epistatic (i.e. interactive), thus leading to a high cumulative risk. Nevertheless, 89% of patients have parents who are not schizophrenic, 81% of patients have no affected first-degree relatives, and 63% of patients have no family history of the disease.

Environmental factors

Environmental factors may be involved in the aetiology of schizophrenia. There is a higher risk of schizophrenia for people born in winter months (i.e. a 5% increase in risk associated with birth between December and May), and also after viral epidemics, which may affect development *in utero*. Events that occur during gestation may have an effect on the normal development of the brain, and infections that will affect the mother and indirectly the fetus have a peak incidence in winter and early spring. Obstetric complications (e.g. oxygen deprivation at birth) may also be relevant, in particular in association with a genetic risk.

Family theories

The theory that factors of a psychological nature in childhood (e.g. a style of parenting that is characterized by highly expressed emotion) are critical for the development of schizophrenia has received much less support in recent years than it did in the 1950s. In particular, the idea of a 'schizophrenogenic mother', characterized by aggressive behaviour and emotional detachment, has not been supported by carefully controlled studies. What has become apparent, though, is that more parents of schizophrenic patients are psychiatrically disturbed than parents of normal children, and they may be involved more often in situations of conflict. What is also probable is that certain life events are associated with acute schizophrenic episodes, but the association is complex, and not necessarily a direct one.

The patient in the case history presents with auditory hallucinations (hearing 'voices') and delusions of influence, social withdrawal and decreased personal grooming. The general low mood and the previous suicide attempt, as well as the loss of interest in personal appearance, reflect the co-existence of significant depression. The depressive symptoms may be part of the illness, or may be a secondary psychological reaction.

Neurobiology of schizophrenia

Structural, functional and neuropathological studies

The profound behavioural alterations seen in schizophrenia may lead us to believe that very significant pathognomonic changes in brain structure accompany this disease and that such changes are specific. However, early post-mortem studies failed to show any significant abnormalities in schizophrenic brains. The exploration of more subtle structural changes became possible with imaging techniques. The last 15–20 years of CT and MRI analysis suggest that one of the frequent abnormalities is lateral ventricular enlargement (Fig. 15.3). This change seems to be present mainly in male schizophrenics. Furthermore, the difference between schizophrenics and control patients may be quite small: it may not be greater than the difference between an average normal man and an average normal woman. Temporal lobe and prefrontal cortex abnormalities have also been reported, as well as possible alterations in the thalamus and the basal ganglia.

Functional analysis of the brain has also led to rather limited conclusions. Although electroencephalogram abnormalities are reported to be present in up to 80% of schizophrenic patients, the changes are relatively nonspecific, and may be encountered, although at a lower frequency, in normal individuals. Studies analysing cerebral blood flow and metabolism have led to the suggestion of 'hypofrontality' in schizophrenia. For example, cerebral blood flow can be monitored while schizophrenic patients and controls are performing the Wisconsin Card Sorting Test (Box 15.5).

The schizophrenic patients' performance is worse than that of controls on this test. This impairment is accompanied by smaller increases in blood flow to the prefrontal cortex during the task. Such differences are not found when a control psychological task is used. Therefore, schizophrenia may be associated with dysfunction in prefrontal cortical circuits. This conclusion is also supported by studies that have reported a reduction in cortical thickness in the dorsal prefrontal cortex of schizophrenic patients. This reduction appears to be associated not with a decrease in neurone numbers, but with a

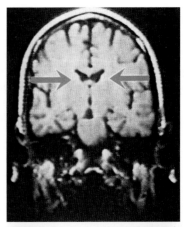

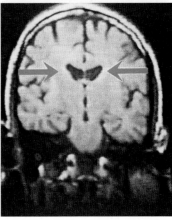

Fig. 15.3 Magnetic resonance imaging (MRI) analysis of schizophrenic brain. The images show the MRI scans of the brains of a pair of identical twins, only one of who suffers from schizophrenia (bottom). Note that the twin with schizophrenia has much larger ventricles. After Barondes SH. Molecules and Mental Illness. New York: Scientific American Library, 1993: 153.

Box 15.5 Cognition and executive function: the Wisconsin Card Sorting Test

In this test, the subjects are expected to sort cards, according to rules that are regularly changed (see Chapter 3). The rule can be: sorting by colour, sorting by shape, or sorting by number. Patients with frontal lobe lesions can learn the initial rule, but have major difficulties when they are required to switch to a new rule. They persevere and apply the old rules, and although they are aware of this incorrect perseverence, they cannot correct it. Therefore, it appears that lesions in the frontal lobes lead to difficulties in the planning, initiation and execution of complex sequences of behaviour. In particular, they significantly affect the ability to assess critically the results of behavioural sequences and to amend them appropriately.

decrease in the number of distal dendrites and dendritic spines, and axon terminals. Altered packing of neurones can lead to significant differences in laminar cell density in the schizophrenic brain. Such changes may profoundly alter the dynamics of cortical circuits (Box 15.6). Recent studies using high-resolution MRI have shown a gradual loss of grey matter, affecting the parietal, temporal and frontal cortices, during the evolution of schizophrenia in some patients.

Psychophysiological changes

One of the reproducible findings in schizophrenia is that of event-related potential (ERP) abnormalities. ERPs reflect different stages of information processing in the brain. ERP abnormalities reflect a deficit in the processing of sensory information, which is associated in particular with medial temporal lobe dysfunction. Eye-tracking (i.e. ability to follow a moving target with the eyes) changes are also reported in about 50% of schizophrenic patients. The changes are likely to reflect dysfunction in the connections between the frontal eye fields (i.e. regions of the frontal lobe that show increased activity during execution of eye movements) and the temporal and parietal cortices. Eye-tracking deficits are particularly robust phenotypic markers of familial risk for schizophrenia.

Schizophrenia and corticolimbic circuits

The results of structural and functional imaging studies suggest critical involvement of cortical and limbic structures in schizophrenia. The term 'limbic' was coined by the French neurologist Broca in 1878, and referred initially to the medial surface of the brain, in particular structures that form a ring around the ventricles and the brainstem. According to this definition, the limbic system includes the cingulate gyrus and the cortex on the medial surface of the temporal lobe, in particular the hippocampus (Fig. 15.4). Broca's anatomical concept of a 'limbic lobe' was subsequently expanded and given a functional dimension by the American neurologist James Papez. He suggested that limbic structures are interconnected, and that the cingulate cortex plays a major role in emotional behaviour.

The view put forward by Papez was essentially correct, inasmuch as the limbic system and its connections are important in the control of emotions. However, the limbic system must be seen in the context of the other cortical areas, with which it has abundant direct or indirect connections. In recent years, particular attention has been given to the study of the connections between limbic structures and the prefrontal cortex. This cortical area is the part of the frontal lobe that is situated in front of Brodmann area 6 (premotor and supplementary motor areas) and Brodmann area 8 (the frontal eye field). The prefrontal cortex receives information from the cingulate gyrus, and also from the parietal, occipital and temporal lobes. Fibres connect it reciprocally with the mediodorsal nucleus of the thalamus. The thalamus is connected with the globus pallidus and with the amygdala. Therefore,

Box 15.6 Cortical organization

The cerebral cortex contains billions of neurones, and in mammals (particularly primates and humans) it quantitatively dominates the rest of the nervous system. The activity of cortical neurones is involved in higher mental functions, such as the determination of personality, memory, cognition and emotions. All regions of the neocortex have the same basic six-layer structure, with cells of similar morphological characteristics defining distinct layers. A majority of neurones in the cortex are pyramidal cells, distinguished by an axon that arises from their base, and an apical dendrite that can cross several layers situated above the layer in which the neuronal cell body lies. Layer 1 contains fibres and very few cells. Layer 2 and layer 4 contain cells with small bodies, densely packed. Layer 3 contains medium-sized pyramidal cells, and layer 5 contains large pyramidal cells. Layer 6 contains cells that have heterogeneous shapes. From a functional point of view, layer 2 and layer 4 predominantly receive input, whereas pyramidal cells in layers 3 and 5 are the source of cortical output, either directed at other cortical areas (layer 3) or directed subcortically (layer 5). Layer 6 is also largely efferent.

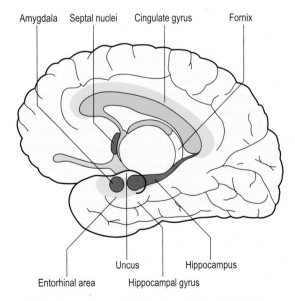

Fig. 15.4 Limbic structures. The diagram represents the right hemisphere (medial aspect). Areas represented in light or dark yellow represent limbic structures. From Brodal P. The Central Nervous System – Structure and Function. Oxford: Oxford University Press, 1998: 556.

the prefrontal cortex integrates information about all sensory modalities and about the motivational state of the individual. Much has been learned about the roles of the prefrontal cortex from cases of lesions (Box 15.7). Changes observed in limbic structures and in the prefrontal cortex in the brain of schizophrenic patients suggest that at least some of the circuits connecting these brain areas become dysfunctional in schizophrenia.

The neurodevelopmental hypothesis of schizophrenia

Despite the onset of the disease in adulthood, it has been hypothesized that abnormalities in the brain of schizophrenic patients occur early during development. This may explain the association between increased risk of schizophrenia and prenatal problems. Brain cytoarchitectural abnormalities reported in some patients have led to suggestions that the development and maturation of cortical circuits are disrupted in schizophrenic patients. Neuronal dysfunction may result from abnormal synapse formation and/or stabilization. The lesion, which may

---

Box 15.7 The prefrontal cortex and its role in cognitive function and emotional expression

The first insight into the importance of the prefrontal cortex was offered by the case of Phineas Gage, in 1848. This 25-year-old foreman had a tamping iron pushed through his skull, through the accidental blasting of explosives used on the construction site where he was working. The metre-long iron rod entered his head below the left eye, and after passing through the left frontal lobe, exited through the top of the head. The hole through the skull was more than 9 cm in diameter, and significant damage was caused to both hemispheres, in particular the frontal lobes. After extraction of the rod, the patient overcame the infection that developed, and made a full recovery. However, his personality was profoundly altered. The doctor who had taken care of him described how Gage became impatient, impulsive, unpredictable and undecided, and described him 'indulging at times in the grossest profanity—which was not previously his custom'. His personality was changed so profoundly that his friends considered that 'he was no longer Gage'. His emotional behaviour and moral reasoning seemed to be affected much more than his intelligence.

Studies of lesions of the prefrontal cortex in primates, as well as clinical observations of damage to the prefrontal cortex in patients, have confirmed the initial observations made on Phineas Gage. Lesions of the prefrontal cortex lead to changes in mood and personality. The ability to alter behaviour is reduced, and attention can be easily distracted.

---

have occurred very early in development, becomes apparent when the maturation of cerebral connections is completed, early in adulthood.

Antonio Damasio and his collaborators have described the consequences of damage to the prefrontal cortex in young adult patients who had sustained brain damage prior to the age of 16 months. The patients presented with impaired decision-making, behavioural disinhibition and insensitivity to punishment, disrupted social communication and abnormal emotion. The patients had defective social and moral reasoning, which suggests that the acquisition of complex social conventions and moral rules (a 'sense of right and wrong') had been impaired. However, the patients were normal in terms of intellect, memory, language and academic achievement. This supports the contention that early dysfunction in the prefrontal cortex may result in severe and irreversible behavioural alterations, despite otherwise normal cognitive abilities.

Neurotransmitters in schizophrenia

The complex alterations that affect the behaviour and mood of schizophrenic patients have led to a quest to define the critical transmitter involved in this disease. For almost five decades, dopamine has been considered to be the key neurotransmitter in schizophrenia. The hypothesis that dopaminergic systems are involved in the pathophysiology of this disease was based primarily on pharmacological evidence. Chlorpromazine, a dopamine receptor antagonist, was the first drug that provided significant improvement in schizophrenic patients. Direct and indirect dopaminergic agonists, such as amphetamine, can induce psychotic symptoms in normal individuals, and can exacerbate psychosis in schizophrenic patients. All the drugs used at present to treat schizophrenia are dopamine receptor antagonists. Furthermore, studies in drug-free or drug-naive schizophrenic patients suggest a mild elevation in dopamine receptors. However, the initial emphasis on generalized dopaminergic hyperactivity has been replaced by the concept of imbalance between central dopaminergic systems (for more information on dopaminergic projections, see Chapter 10). In particular, it is believed that there is simultaneous hyperactivity in the mesolimbic dopaminergic system and hypoactivity in the mesocortical dopaminergic projections.

Furthermore, in the last decade, evidence has accumulated that other neurotransmitters may be involved in the pathophysiology of schizophrenia and that of psychotic states in general. Lysergic acid diethylamide (LSD), a drug that acts on several 5-hydroxytryptamine (5-HT) receptor types, and that has been widely used recreationally, especially during the hippy wave of the 1960s, is a potent psychotomimetic. Its use is associated with significant sensory alterations. Hallucinations are common, and thought processes may become completely disconnected. 'Bad trips' on LSD can also be accompanied by paranoid ideas, and murder or suicide attempts. Some of the effects of LSD can significantly outlast the exposure to the drug. Overall, these observations suggest the existence of a serotonergic link in psychosis.

Phencyclidine (also known as PCP) is a drug that was developed in the 1950s. It became rapidly obvious that its use led to unexpected complications. PCP is an antagonist at the N-methyl-D-aspartate (NMDA) glutamate receptor type (Box 15.8), and its use is associated with the development of a psychotic state. After exposure to PCP, many patients experience paranoia, hallucinations and agitation, and also social withdrawal and reduced emotional expression. These properties are shared by ketamine, a drug still used in general anaesthesia and also in pain management. PCP and ketamine can precipitate psychotic episodes (e.g. in schizophrenic patients in remission). PCP is no longer used clinically, but it is still widely abused (snorted or smoked), especially in the USA. Chronic PCP users can develop violent criminal behaviour. The effects of PCP suggest that deficits in glutamatergic transmission may be associated with schizophrenia. Such deficits may significantly affect thalamocortical projections, which are glutamatergic. Post-mortem analysis of brains of schizophrenic patients shows loss of neurones in the mediodorsal thalamus. The analysis of changes in cortical layers shows a loss of thalamic axon terminals in layer 3, and a loss of dopaminergic innervation in layer 6 of the prefrontal cortex. These observations suggest a dual cortical deficit, in dopaminergic and glutamatergic input, which is likely to affect the activity of pyramidal neurones. Finally, alterations in glutamatergic signalling may also lead to impairment of GABAergic cortical transmission. Significant alterations in a subpopulation of cortical GABAergic cells have been reported in schizophrenic patients.

Therefore, what is gradually emerging is a new approach to the pathophysiology of psychoses, and a more integrated view of the cortical transmission deficit in schizophrenia, involving several transmitters, such as dopamine, 5-HT, glutamate and γ-aminobutyric acid (GABA)—to name just those of whose importance we are currently aware.

Box 15.8 Glutamate and its receptors

Glutamate is the main excitatory amino acid in the brain. In the cortex, it either originates in cortical afferents or is present in corticocortical fibres. After release from nerve terminals, glutamate can bind to two categories of receptor: ionotropic and metabotropic.

Ionotropic receptors

These are ligand-gated ion channels, and they are divided into three main types, named after their prototype ligand: (1) the NMDA type (after N-methyl-D-aspartate); (2) the AMPA type (after amino-3-hydroxy-5-methyl-4-isoxazole propionate); and (3) the kainate type (after kainic acid). The AMPA receptor is associated mainly with Na^+ and K^+ conductance, whereas the NMDA receptor is also significantly associated with Ca^{2+} permeability. Another interesting characteristic of the NMDA receptor is its blockade by Mg^{2+} under resting membrane potential conditions. Thus, it is only when the neuronal membrane is depolarized that the channel allows passage of ions after binding of glutamate. The NMDA receptor type also requires glycine as a co-agonist for stimulation of the receptor. This complex receptor also has various other modulatory sites. Phencyclidine and ketamine are NMDA channel blockers. Glutamate receptors are involved in learning and memory (Chapter 14).

Metabotropic receptors

Metabotropic receptors for glutamate (mGluRs) are receptors coupled to G-proteins. On the basis of sequence homology, transduction mechanisms and pharmacological profile, they can be divided into three families: the mGluR I family (coupled to activation of phospholipase C activity), and the mGluR II and mGluR III receptors (coupled to inhibition of adenylate cyclase).

Treatment of schizophrenia

Despite the unclear aetiology and neuropathology of schizophrenia, the existing treatment improves the condition of a significant number of patients. The treatment of the disease is still dominated by 'the dopamine theory of schizophrenia' (as discussed above). The antipsychotic drugs (also known as 'neuroleptics' or 'major tranquillizers') consist of a wide range of dopaminergic antagonists, which belong to various chemical classes (Table 15.1). These drugs can also be divided into 'typical' neuroleptics, which are the oldest compounds, and 'atypical' neuroleptics, which have been developed more recently. The oldest class of antipsychotic drug is the phenothiazine class, with its prototype drug, chlorpromazine (Box 15.9).

All neuroleptics act as dopamine receptor blockers, with significant affinity for the D_2 type, and not the D_1 type of receptor. One of the most elegant studies in support of the importance of the blockade of dopamine receptors was published by Johnstone and her collaborators in 1978. This study compared the efficacy of the α- and β-isomers of the neuroleptic drug flupenthixol in acute

Table 15.1 Classification and examples of antipsychotic drugs

Typical antipsychotics

Phenothiazines: chlorpromazine, thioridazine, fluphenazine, trifluoperazine

Butyrophenones: haloperidol, benperidol

Thioxanthenes: flupenthixol, clopenthixol, thiothixene

Atypical antipsychotics

Substituted benzamides: sulpiride, amisulpride

Clozapine, olanzapine, risperidone, seroquel

Chlorpromazine: a milestone in the history of psychiatry

Before the advent of modern medical treatments, psychosis, also known as 'madness', was the main reason for the existence of asylums. These institutions were full of patients with varied types of psychosis, which often made them dangerous to themselves and to society. Many moving accounts exist of the life of the 'insane' in such institutions. A young psychiatrist, newly appointed to Fulbourn Mental Hospital in Cambridgeshire, wrote these notes in 1953: 'I was taken in by someone who had a key to lock the door and lock it behind you. The crashing of the keys in the lock was an essential part of asylum life then just as it is today in jail... Some wards were full of tousled, apathetic people just sitting in a row because for twenty years the nurses had been saying, "sit down, shut up". Others were noisy. The disturbed women's ward was a phantasmagoric place. The women were in "strong clothes", shapeless garments made of reinforced cotton that couldn't be torn. Many of them were "in locked boots" which couldn't be taken off and thrown.'

Prior to the 1950s, medicine had nothing to offer apart from heavy sedation and custodial care. The enthusiasm of the medical profession for various rather crude treatments waxed and waned: induction of insulin coma, prolonged narcosis with barbiturate drugs, or massive severing of fibres in the frontal lobe through lobotomy. Everything changed when the drug chlorpromazine was introduced. Preliminary experimental observations showed that chlorpromazine had a significant sedative effect. As described by Henry Laborit, the French doctor involved in its development, the drug produced 'not any loss in consciousness, not any change in the patient's mentality, but a slight tendency to sleep, and above all "disinterest" for all that goes on around him'. When the drug was tried in the clinic, aggressive psychotic patients were controlled for the first time without recourse to force. The French psychiatrists Delay and Deniker, who were involved in the first studies, coined the term 'neuroleptic'. By the mid-1950s, it became clear that chlorpromazine was going to change radically the management of schizophrenia.

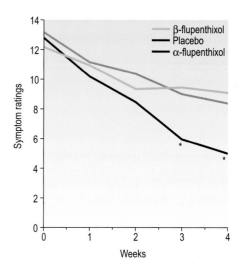

Fig. 15.5 Clinical improvement in acute schizophrenic patients treated with the two isomers of flupenthixol or with placebo. From Johnstone et al. In McKenna PJ, ed. Schizophrenia and Related Syndromes. Oxford: Oxford University Press, 1994: 144.

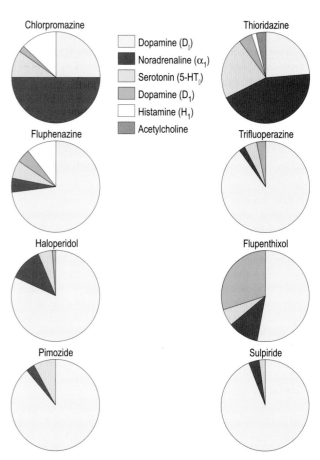

Fig. 15.6 Pharmacodynamic profiles of neuroleptics. The pie charts represent the relative receptor blocking activities of neuroleptic drugs. From McKenna PJ, ed. Schizophrenia and Related Syndromes. Oxford: Oxford University Press, 1994: 138.

schizophrenia. Only α-flupenthixol has dopamine receptor antagonist properties, and the study showed that only this isomer had antipsychotic efficacy (Fig. 15.5).

The general blockade of dopamine receptors by neuroleptics leads inevitably to extrapyramidal motor symptoms, due to disruption of nigrostriatal dopaminergic transmission, and to endocrine dysfunction (hyperprolactinaemia), due to blockade of dopaminergic transmission in the tubero-infundibular pathway. Apart from the blockade of dopamine receptors, antipsychotic drugs also act as antagonists at other receptors, such as the cholinergic muscarinic, H_1 histamine, α_2-adrenergic and 5-HT_2 receptors (Fig. 15.6). This pharmacological lack of

Table 15.2 Unwanted effects of neuroleptic drugs

Psychomotor performance

The effects on cognition and psychomotor performance are complex and depend on the subject and the task assessed. Phenothiazines in particular tend to induce drowsiness and fatigue. The sedation is related to the antihistaminergic action and the α_1-adrenergic receptor blockade

Extrapyramidal effects

Parkinsonian symptoms are the most common: tremor, rigidity, bradykinesia

Akathisia (continuous motor restlessness) can be misinterpreted as incomplete control of psychotic symptoms

Acute dyskinesia and dystonia: tonic contractions of muscles in the face, tongue and neck, and also of the truncal musles, which may lead to abnormal postures

Seizures

Many neuroleptics can lower the seizure threshold and should be used with caution in untreated epileptic patients

Endocrine effects

The disrupted dopamine control over pituitary function leads to increased prolactin release, and swelling of the breasts (gynaecomastia) and lactation (galactorrhoea)

Cutaneous effects

Chronic exposure to neuroleptics may lead to pigmentation and also photosensitivity

Hepatotoxicity

Chlopromazine in particular may induce obstructive jaundice

Haematological effects

Agranulocytosis occurs rarely with typical neuroleptics, but its incidence is much higher with clozapine. It is the most serious haematological abnormality induced by antipsychotics. It presents with fever, fatigue and prostration, and ulceration of the mouth, throat, nose, rectum or vagina. The mortality rate can reach about 30%

Cardiovascular effects

Neuroleptics can induce significant postural hypotension, with tachycardia. This is largely due to α-adrenergic receptor blockade

Metabolic effects

Weight gain induced by neuroleptics may be related to a stimulation of appetite and/or a reduction in basal metabolic rate. Excessive weight is associated with additional health risks such as hypertension and diabetes mellitus

Anticholinergic effects

These effects are due to blockade of muscarinic receptors. They include decreased salivary flow, blurred vision and impaired accommodation, constipation and urinary hesitancy or retention

Sexual dysfunction

Antipsychotics can significantly affect sexual function. They can lead to loss of sexual drive, erectile and ejaculatory dysfunction, priapism and menstrual irregularities

selectivity of action was well reflected from the beginning in the commercial name of chlorpromazine: 'Largactil'! The inevitable consequence of this lack of selectivity is the occurrence of unwanted effects, which decrease compliance.

Table 15.2 gives an overview of the main unwanted effects of neuroleptics, which affect a range of systems and physiological processes. The intensity of these unwanted effects can be very significant. For example, obesity may occur in about one-third of patients who receive fluphenazine or flupenthixol. This prevalence is four times higher than that in the general population. The host of anticholinergic effects induced by neuroleptics (constipation, difficulty in urinating, dry mouth and blurred vision) is of particular concern in elderly patients. Furthermore, the postural hypotension induced by neuroleptics, and also the interference with temperature control (hypothermia or hyperthermia), are particularly troublesome in the elderly. The choice of neuroleptic is even today often determined by its unwanted effects and their acceptability. For example, the sedation induced by chlorpromazine may be very useful in an agitated schizophrenic, whereas its antimuscarinic effects may make it quite unacceptable in an elderly patient with micturition problems. Haloperidol is less hypotensive than chlorpromazine, but has significant extrapyramidal motor effects.

Neuroleptic malignant syndrome is an idiosyncratic response to antipsychotic medication, and consists of hyperthermia (sometimes with profuse sweating), tachycardia, muscular rigidity, and fluctuating levels of consciousness. It is a rare but potentially lethal complication of antipsychotic drugs. The mortality rate can reach 20–30%. Dantrolene and dopaminergic agonists such as bromocriptine, and cooling and rehydration, have been used to treat this syndrome, which may last for several days. No particular class of antipsychotic is more or less likely to induce this syndrome. Patients may be at greater risk at the beginning of treatment or after a dose increase. Atypical neuroleptics such as clozapine may be used to manage patients who have already had an episode of neuroleptic malignant syndrome.

Some complications of neuroleptic treatment emerge after a certain duration of exposure to antipsychotic drugs. One such example is tardive dyskinesia. This includes orofacial and trunk and limb dyskinesias. The orofacial movements include protrusion of the tongue, lip-smacking, pursing and sucking movements, puffing of the cheeks and chewing. The involuntary limb movements are purposeless and jerky. The condition is both socially and physically disabling. Spontaneous fluctuations in the severity of movements may occur from day to day or even within hours or minutes. Most often, tardive dyskinesia does not disappear upon reduction of the dose or withdrawal of the neuroleptic. However, the dyskinesia may slightly improve, or stabilize over a number of years. Newer drugs, the 'atypical neuroleptics', such as clozapine, olanzapine, risperidone and seroquel, have fewer unwanted effects. In particular, the incidence of extrapyramidal effects is much lower than with the 'typical' neuroleptics, and they have higher efficacy than the old neuroleptics in treating negative symptoms. Clozapine shows efficacy in treatment-resistant patients. Unfortunately, it is associated with an increased risk of leukopenia and agranulocytosis (1–2%). Its use requires regular blood cell counts. A common characteristic of newer neuroleptics, such as risperidone, is their high affinity for $5-HT_2$ receptors. Therefore, the new antipsychotics would be better described as dopamine and 5-HT receptor antagonists. The lower potential for induction of extrapyramidal symptoms could be due to complex interactions between 5-HT and dopaminergic systems in the brain. It is not unlikely that, in the case history, Jane was initially prescribed an old type of neuroleptic, so the choice of a better, atypical compound may improve her compliance.

Some neuroleptics (e.g. haloperidol and flupenthixol) can be given as a depot slow-release preparation, which is useful when compliance with treatment is unpredictable. This approach makes chronic schizophrenia more manageable in the community, provided that adequate structures and support are available. The drugs are administered as fatty acid esters (e.g. haloperidol decanoate, fluphenazine decanoate and pipotiazine palmitate) by deep intramuscular injection at intervals of 1–4 weeks. It is less easy to control the dose administered,

especially when a reduction of the dose is required. It may take several weeks to decrease plasma concentration or to control the severity of unwanted effects.

Apart from medical treatment, schizophrenic patients may benefit from cognitive therapy and occupational therapy. Cognitive improvement, through social skill development and cognitive behavioural treatments, holds much promise, but more research is required to maximize the potential of these approaches, which are complementary to medical treatment. It is also important to note that families and carers of schizophrenic patients require long-term support, because of the distressing and unpredictable nature of this chronic disease.

Comments on the management of schizophrenia and the long-term prognosis

Schizophrenia is a serious mental illness that still poses a therapeutic challenge in a significant number of patients. It must be remembered that schizophrenia is not a homogeneous disease. There are numerous phenotypes, and each poses its own problems during long-term management. In many patients schizophrenia presents a chronic course, which is particularly disabling, especially because of the social isolation associated with negative symptoms. The evolution of schizophrenia is sometimes complicated by the use of addictive substances. Jane's use (and abuse?) of alcohol illustrates this tendency. The prognosis for each patient depends on the balance between positive and negative symptoms, their response to treatment, and also the lack of complicating factors, such as the development of drug addiction, or other circumstances involving high stress. In some patients, the response to treatment (especially the positive symptoms) is good, and they may return to an almost normal level of functioning—at least between episodes of relapse. The risk of suicide will not disappear during the course of the disease, and may be exacerbated by the presence of depression. Of patients with schizophrenia, 10–15% commit suicide. The long-term outcome in schizophrenia is variable. Schizophrenia consists in many cases of a sequence of exacerbations followed by improvements. About one-third of patients have one or a limited number of acute episodes, with full or partial remission between episodes. Another one-third of patients develop a chronic condition that is stable and is controlled to a variable extent by antipsychotic medication. Patients who relapse after cessation of treatment require constant, long-term medication on a type and dose of neuroleptic that they tolerate reasonably well (in terms of unwanted effects). The value of maintenance neuroleptic treatment in schizophrenia is supported by numerous studies. Research suggests that neuroleptics may have effects that are far more complex than the blockade of neurotransmitter receptors. Their chronic use may alter the expression of genes critically involved in the generation and maintenance of synapses. Therefore, if a deficit in synapse stabilization, partly developmental, is at the core of the pathophysiology of schizophrenia, antipsychotic drugs may address the primary cause of the disease. Future studies will be required to consolidate these observations. Finally, the remaining one-third of patients have a progressive debilitating psychosis, with increasing impairment and no return to baseline. It is important to bear in mind that it is this core of chronic schizophrenic patients who have only very moderate improvement even if treated with new neuroleptics.

Other psychoses and schizophrenia-like syndromes

Psychotic states can be induced by exposure to a variety of psychoactive compounds, some of which have been mentioned already. The differential diagnosis of schizophrenia must also take into account psychoses that may occur in the context of temporal lobe epilepsy, multiple sclerosis, alcoholism, or delirium and dementia in elderly people.

Childhood psychoses and schizophrenia-like syndromes are a complex family of disorders. Examples of such disorders are autism and Asperger's syndrome.

Autism was defined as a syndrome and introduced to the medical world by the child psychiatrist Leo Kanner in 1943. He described a distinctive syndrome in children, characterized by a solitary nature and an inability to relate to people and to situations. Other features included the performance of repetitive activities, mutism or abnormal language. The abnormalities of speech in autistic children include echolalia (repeating, like a parrot, words or sentences without any understanding) and avoidance or confusion of personal pronouns (e.g. 'he' for 'she', or 'you' for 'we'). It has been suggested that the fundamental failure in autism is the lack of development of a 'theory of the mind': autistic children have no concept of what other people think or feel, and this leads to a lack of empathy, and no or very little attachment to other people. Humans, animals and objects seem to be treated alike, more like 'tools', to satisfy the child's needs. Such children sometimes display unusual features of memory or skill. The prevalence of autism is about 2/1000 children. The typical patterns of autistic behaviour usually emerge after up to 18–20 months of apparently normal development. The aetiology of autism is unknown and there is evidence for genetic factors. It is likely that autism is a disorder with a major neurodevelopmental component: a disruption in brain formation *in utero* emerges in childhood, when the brain is growing rapidly and its connectivity evolves towards maturation. Although autism and schizophrenia are clearly different disorders, there are strong resemblances in terms of the existence of motor, speech and behavioural abnormalities. Neuropathological abnormalities have been described in various brain structures: the hippocampus, the mamillary nuclei, the amygdala and the anterior cingulate cortex. Cerebellar abnormalities (such as loss of Purkinje cells) are a constant feature. Some of the pathology appears to be age-dependent. Autism is also associated with epilepsy. Various types of epilepsy (e.g. absences, generalized tonic–clonic seizures and complex partial seizures) affect 35–45% of autistic children and adults. No definitive neurochemical abnormality has yet been defined as pathognomonic for autism, but there is converging evidence in support of dopaminergic dysfunction.

Various drug treatments have been tried in autism, without a solid scientific rationale: antipsychotic drugs, dopaminergic agonists, opiate antagonists, β-adrenergic blockers, lithium and antidepressant drugs. The benefits reported appear to be limited, and poorly reproducible between studies. Dietary interventions (e.g. supplementation with vitamin B_6 or magnesium) have been attempted, and have provided some improvement. Therapy focuses on behavioural intervention and on the development of structured education programmes. Only a very small proportion of children with autism develop into normal adults. The majority of autistic children will show psychiatric impairments throughout life. In other cases, there is some improvement, and it is possible for the patient to lead an almost independent adult life.

Asperger's syndrome has broadly similar features to autism, but is milder and does not become apparent until after 3 years of age. It is much more common in boys than in girls. Speech is impoverished and features stereotyped repetitions of phrases. Unlike with autism, intelligence may be normal. Patients affected by the syndrome may display exceptional abilities in very narrowly defined fields. However, there is failure to develop peer relationships, and very poor social reciprocity. Outcome is variable between patients. A proportion of patients with Asperger's syndrome may develop mild schizophrenia. They may display obsessive behaviour and forms of bizarre violence.

There is still some confusion about whether autism and Asperger's syndrome should be viewed as part of a continuum or as two distinct conditions. Irrespective of the best classification, it is likely that these represent two related conditions characterized by major disruption of social contact and affective reactions.

DEPRESSION AND ANXIETY

16

Chapter objectives

After studying this chapter you should be able to:

1. Define mood and anxiety disorders.
2. Give an account of the neurobiological correlates of depression and anxiety.
3. Describe the pharmacological treatment of depression and anxiety.
4. Discuss the non-pharmacological therapeutic approaches to the treatment of depression and anxiety.
5. Describe the treatment of insomnia.

Introduction

Neurological dysfunction caused by acute trauma or neuronal degeneration is reflected in specific impairment, where no confusion exists between the diseased state and the normal state. In contrast, depression and anxiety represent, in a broad sense, states experienced by almost all individuals at some point in their life. The current diagnostic criteria are somewhat arbitrary, and the efficacy of drugs is limited. It may still be believed erroneously by some that depression and anxiety are not major medical problems, but rather transient states that resolve, sooner or later, with full remission. However, as the case history in Box 16.1 indicates, this is not so, and the disease burden they represent for the patient, the family and society is significantly underestimated.

Classification of mood disorders

'If sorrow persists, then it is melancholia.'

(Hippocrates, 460–370 BC)

Descriptions of depressed states date back to Sumerian and Egyptian documents. Later, Hippocrates, Galen and other medical authors of antiquity continued to describe depression, its possible causes and treatments. The term 'melancholia' was used until the late 19th century, when Kraepelin introduced the term 'manic depression', to differentiate this severely disturbed mental state from schizophrenia.

Depression is a general term that defines a family of diseases. Table 16.1 gives the present classification of mood disorders according to the American Psychiatric Association Diagnostic and Statistical Manual of Mental Disorders IV (DSM-IV). Most of this chapter will be dedicated to the discussion of major depression disorder and bipolar disorder. The classification of depressive states is complex and still controversial. There are several reasons for this. No common causes are known that could be used for an aetiologically-based classification. Furthermore, there are no clear biological markers or objective diagnostic tests that would allow for a reliable biologically based classification.

Clinical features of mood disorders

Depression is characterized by a series of changes that gradually cause significant impairment of the activity of the individual concerned. Table 16.2 shows typical core symptoms of depression. These are psychological and somatic.

Psychological symptoms include feelings of misery, guilt, hopelessness and general pessimism. Some patients may become irritable or aggressive. Enjoyment of various activities is lost (i.e. development of anhedonia, which means 'loss of pleasure') and energy is low. Interest,

Box 16.1 Case history

William L. is a scientist who shares his time between work at the university and writing about science. Over several weeks, around his 45th birthday, he feels increasing fatigue and has trouble in sleeping. He has started going to bed early, because he feels tired all the time and because he tends to be awake at dawn, unable to go to sleep again. His wife notices that he no longer enjoys his hobbies. He is often irritable and impatient with his children. Things take a turn for the worse when William cancels a series of lectures and meetings, because he feels that he can no longer cope with his work. His insomnia is getting worse and he is losing weight. He consults his doctor, who diagnoses depression, and prescribes venlafaxine. William is sceptical about treatment and is reluctant to take the medication. He explains to his doctor that he knows that antidepressant drugs can make you feel unwell. He remembers from his childhood that his mother had been suffering from periods of depression, and had to take drugs. She had never fully recovered, up to her accidental death a few years ago. William asks his doctor whether other approaches could be used instead of drugs. He is worried about 'getting addicted' to drugs and not being able to have a normal life without them. William's doctor explains that cognitive behavioural therapy is another option, and that it may be possible later to consider using this therapy.

William starts taking the medication, and although he sees no major change in the first 2 weeks, after 3 months of treatment he feels well and fully resumes his activities. His mood is much improved, and while on a holiday he decides to stop taking the medication. Unfortunately, less than 2 years after this first episode, William feels unwell again, and he needs to stop work and start a new course of venlafaxine. The drug is less efficacious this time, and the doctor is very concerned about the feelings of guilt that William now experiences, and his heightened level of anxiety. He arranges with William to start regular sessions with a therapist, in parallel with the medication.

This case gives rise to the following questions:

1. What triggers the depressive symptoms?
2. What is the cause of depression?
3. How can drugs help and what other alternatives are there?
4. Why do patients relapse?
5. What is the long-term management of depression?

concentration and ability to function efficiently and make decisions are significantly impaired. Some patients show very severe mental and physical slow-down (retarded depression). Other patients present with a paradoxical reaction, characterized by increased activity and restlessness (agitated depression). Delusion and hallucinations

Table 16.1 DSM-IV classification of mood disorders

Major depression

Bipolar disorder

Dysthymic disorder

Depressive disorder not otherwise specified

Table 16.2 DSM-IV syndrome profile of major depression

Psychomotor retardation or psychomotor agitation

Fatigue or loss of energy

Diminished ability to concentrate

Diminished interest in social activity

Depressed mood

Feelings of guilt and worthlessness

Suicidal ideation

Insomnia

Weight loss and decreased appetite

Lack of interest and anhedonia

may develop in some patients (depression with psychotic features). These have the same negative and destructive tone as the other symptoms.

Somatic symptoms are very common, and often dominate the presentation of the case when patients consult the doctor. Sleep is almost always disturbed, with early-morning waking or difficulty in falling asleep. Most patients lose weight, but in some patients the opposite is seen: they eat more and gain weight. Patients may also suffer from nausea, constipation and headaches. Often, patients find it easier to talk about the somatic symptoms and feel rather embarrassed about revealing their psychological problems.

Depression can be rated according to a variety of scales. Examples of such scales are the Hamilton Depression Scale, the Beck Depression Inventory and the Zung Self-Rating Depression Scale. For example, in the Hamilton Depression Scale, there are 21 questions that cover the various symptoms and their intensity. The total score reflects the severity of depression (Box 16.2).

Bipolar disorder (also called manic-depressive disorder) consists of alternating episodes of depression and mania. The frequency of the episodes and their severity may increase as the disease evolves. The manic attack is characterized by symptoms that are the opposite of those seen in depression. Patients are overactive, disinhibited, unfocused and extravagant. They can become completely irresponsible and display unlimited confidence in themselves. They may engage in unrealistic business ventures, reckless driving, incredible buying sprees, and numerous

sexual liaisons. They appear to need little food or sleep. Thought and speech are intense, with a dominating flight of ideas. Thought content can be grandiose, and delusions and hallucinations with a paranoid content may develop. In extreme cases, hospital admission is required (under the provisions of the UK Mental Health Act 1983), because of the patient's loss of insight into their illness.

Dysthymic disorder is a recent diagnostic category. Symptoms of depression are generally milder than in major depression, but with a more protracted course (at least 2 years of constant low mood).

Epidemiology of depression and natural evolution of the disease

Major depressive disorder is probably the most common psychiatric disorder. It is the leading cause of disability among those aged 5 years and older, and the second leading source of disease burden, as recently defined by the World Health Organization. The prevalence and incidence are in a similar range worldwide. For example, recent estimates of the lifetime prevalence rate in the USA are 21% for women and 13% for men. Another 1.3–1.8% of the population is affected by bipolar disorder. Depression affects children, adolescents, adults and the elderly. For many patients, major depression is a lifelong disorder that consists of episodes of relapse separated by remission intervals. The mean age of onset of depression has decreased gradually from the 40–50-year age range to the 25–35-year age range. Stress is considered to be one of the main risk factors for the development of depression. Evidence suggests that negative psychosocial factors (e.g. bereavement, loss of a job or loss of social status) may trigger the first depression episode. However, this is more likely to happen in susceptible individuals (i.e. on a predisposing genetic background). Depression is associated with a 10–15% mortality rate, due to suicide. It is also a major independent risk factor for the development of coronary heart disease and stroke. Depression can also occur in association with other medical conditions, e.g. Parkinson's disease, head trauma, cancer, diabetes, or endocrine dysfunctions such as hypercortisolaemia or hypothyroidism.

Genetics of mood disorders

Twin and adoption studies support a genetic link in depression, and it is well established that first-degree relatives (parents, siblings and children) of individuals with major depressive disorder are at high risk of developing the disease. Approximately 40–50% of the risk of developing depression is genetic. Twin studies show that genetic factors may have a far greater aetiological role in bipolar depression than in non-bipolar major depression.

Box 16.2 The Hamilton Rating Scale for Depression (to be administered by a health care professional)

Patient's name
_____

Date of assessment
_____

To rate the severity of depression in patients who are already diagnosed as depressed, administer this questionnaire. The higher the score, the more severe the depression.

For each item, write the correct number on the line next to the item (Only one response per item)

_____ 1. **DEPRESSED MOOD** (sadness, hopeless, helpless, worthless)
0 = Absent
1 = These feeling states indicated only on questioning
2 = These feeling states spontaneously reported verbally
3 = Communicates feeling states non-verbally—i.e. through facial expression, posture, voice and tendency to weep
4 = Patient reports VIRTUALLY ONLY these feeling states in his spontaneous verbal and non-verbal communication

_____ 2. **FEELINGS OF GUILT**
0 = Absent
1 = Self-reproach, feels he has let people down
2 = Ideas of guilt or rumination over past errors or sinful deeds
3 = Present illness is a punishment. Delusions of guilt
4 = Hears accusatory or denunciatory voices and/or experiences threatening visual hallucinations

_____ 3. **SUICIDE**
0 = Absent
1 = Feels life is not worth living
2 = Wishes he were dead or any thoughts of possible death to self
3 = Suicidal ideas or gesture
4 = Attempts at suicide (any serious attempt rates 4)

_____ 4. **INSOMNIA EARLY**
0 = No difficulty falling asleep
1 = Complains of occasional difficulty falling asleep—i.e., more than ½ hour
2 = Complains of nightly difficulty falling asleep

_____ 5. **INSOMNIA MIDDLE**
0 = No difficulty
1 = Patient complains of being restless and disturbed during the night
2 = Waking during the night—any getting out of bed rates 2 (except for purposes of voiding)

_____ 6. **INSOMNIA LATE**
0 = No difficulty
1 = Waking in early hours of the morning but goes back to sleep
2 = Unable to fall asleep again if he gets out of bed

_____ 7. **WORK AND ACTIVITIES**
0 = No difficulty
1 = Thoughts and feelings of incapacity, fatigue or weakness related to activities; work or hobbies
2 = Loss of interest in activity; hobbies or work—either directly reported by patient, or indirect in listlessness, indecision and vacillation (feels he has to push self to work or activities)
3 = Decrease in actual time spent in activities or decrease in productivity
4 = Stopped working because of present illness

8.   **RETARDATION: PSYCHOMOTOR** (Slowness of thought and speech; impaired ability to concentrate; decreased motor activity)

_____   **0** = Normal speech and thought
1 = Slight retardation at interview
2 = Obvious retardation at interview
3 = Interview difficult
4 = Complete stupor

9.   **AGITATION**

_____   **0** = None
1 = Fidgetiness
2 = Playing with hands, hair, etc.
3 = Moving about, can't sit still
4 = Hand wringing, nail biting, hair-pulling, biting of lips

10.   **ANXIETY (PSYCHOLOGICAL)**

_____   **0** = No difficulty
1 = Subjective tension and irritability
2 = Worrying about minor matters
3 = Apprehensive attitude apparent in face or speech
4 = Fears expressed without questioning

11.   **ANXIETY SOMATIC:** Physiological concomitants of anxiety (i.e., effects of autonomic overactivity, 'butterflies', indigestion, stomach cramps, belching, diarrhoea, palpitations, hyperventilation, paraesthesia, sweating, flushing, tremor, headache, urinary frequency). Avoid asking about possible medication side effects (i.e., dry mouth, constipation)

_____   **0** = Absent
1 = Mild
2 = Moderate
3 = Severe
4 = Incapacitating

12.   **SOMATIC SYMPTOMS (GASTROINTESTINAL)**

_____   **0** = None
1 = Loss of appetite but eating without encouragement from others. Food intake about normal
2 = Difficulty eating without urging from others. Marked reduction of appetite and food intake

13.   **SOMATIC SYMPTOMS GENERAL**

_____   **0** = None
1 = Heaviness in limbs, back or head. Backaches, headache, muscle aches. Loss of energy and fatigability
2 = Any clear-cut symptom rates 2

14.   **GENITAL SYMPTOMS** (Symptoms such as: loss of libido; impaired sexual performance; menstrual disturbances)

_____   **0** = Absent
1 = Mild
2 = Severe

15.   **HYPOCHONDRIASIS**

_____   **0** = Not present
1 = Self-absorption (bodily)
2 = Preoccupation with health
3 = Frequent complaints, requests for help, etc.
4 = Hypochondriacal delusions

(Continued)

Box
16.2 The Hamilton Rating Scale for Depression (to be administered by a health care professional) (Continued)

16. **LOSS OF WEIGHT**

_____ A. When rating by history:

0 = No weight loss

1 = Probably weight loss associated with present illness

2 = Definite (according to patient) weight loss

3 = Not assessed

17. **INSIGHT**

_____ 0 = Acknowledges being depressed and ill

1 = Acknowledges illness but attributes cause to bad food, climate, overwork, virus, need for rest, etc.

2 = Denies being ill at all

18. **DIURNAL VARIATION**

_____ A. Note whether symptoms are worse in morning or evening. If NO diurnal variation, mark none

0 = No variation

1 = Worse in A.M.

2 = Worse in P.M.

B. When present, mark the severity of the variation. Mark 'None' if NO variation

0 = None

1 = Mild

2 = Severe

19. **DEPERSONALIZATION AND DEREALIZATION** (Such as: Feelings of unreality; Nihilistic ideas)

_____ 0 = Absent

1 = Mild

2 = Moderate

3 = Severe

4 = Incapacitating

20. **PARANOID SYMPTOMS**

_____ 0 = None

1 = Suspicious

2 = Ideas of reference

3 = Delusions of reference and persecution

21. **OBSESSIONAL AND COMPULSIVE SYMPTOMS**

_____ 0 = Absent

1 = Mild

2 = Severe

Total Score_____

The lifetime risk of developing the illness in relatives of patients with major depression is:

- first-degree relatives 10–20%
- dizygotic twin 15–30%.
- monozygotic twin 50–70%.

There is also evidence for a shared genetic susceptibility between major depression and bipolar disorder.

In major depression, linkage studies have suggested an association with the 5-hydroxytryptamine (5-HT) transporter, 5-HT receptor genes and dopamine receptor genes, and genes associated with GABAergic transmission.

Neurobiology of depression

Structures involved

The anatomical and physiological basis of depression is still incompletely understood. However, imaging and post-mortem analyses are providing information about the structures and circuits involved. Positron emission tomography (PET) studies of cerebral blood flow and glucose metabolism show abnormal activity in structures involved in emotional behaviour. They support the involvement of limbic, cortical and subcortical structures such as the cingulate cortex, the hippocampus, the thalamus, the amygdala and the hypothalamus. In particular, studies in unmedicated patients with depression show decreases in glucose metabolism in the dorsoanterolateral and dorsomedial prefrontal cortex and in the anterior cingulate cortex ventral to the genu corpus callosum (Fig. 16.1). In contrast, metabolism is increased in the left and right orbital/ventrolateral prefrontal cortex, the posterior cingulate cortex, the anterior insula and the left amygdala. Antidepressant treatment reverses some of these changes, e.g. the increased metabolism in the amygdala. This structure is involved in autonomic, emotional and neuroendocrine responses to stress, and there is a positive correlation between its activation and the severity of depression ratings. Furthermore, the degree of activation of the amygdala correlates with the levels of circulating cortisol under stress conditions.

Post-mortem studies also show reductions in the density and size of neurones and glia in the prefrontal cortex. These structural changes may underlie the reduction in metabolism, and may explain why antidepressants fail to alter metabolic changes in these areas. Interestingly, these structure changes occur in areas where there was previously increased glucose metabolism. The latter is closely correlated with activation of glutamatergic transmission. Therefore, it is conceivable that chronic hyperactive glutamatergic transmission leads to alterations—in particular atrophy—of the neuropil. The amygdala and the prefrontal cortex are linked by excitatory amino acid projections, and it has been shown that surgical lesions that interrupt these projections can relieve depressive symptoms that are resistant to pharmacological treatment.

Neurochemistry

Since the introduction of the first antidepressant drugs, the theory that has dominated the field has been 'the monoamine theory of depression'. This postulates that in the brain of depressed individuals, there is hypoactivity of monoaminergic systems. The emphasis has been on the noradrenergic and serotonergic ascending systems, which extensively innervate the forebrain (Fig. 16.2). The monoamine deficiency theory is now increasingly considered to be a rather simplistic model of the pathophysiology of depression. Patients with major depression do not consistently demonstrate alterations in monoamine function, although reductions in the activity of the 5-HT and noradrenaline systems can be seen in some patients. A role of monoamines in the pathophysiology of depression cannot be contested, as all drugs that are effective in the clinic act on monoaminergic systems.

The cholinergic system may also be involved in depression (cholinomimetics have depressogenic and antimanic effects, and in depression there is enhanced sensitivity to cholinergic stimulation). Reduced cerebrospinal fluid (CSF) and plasma γ-aminobutyric acid (GABA) levels have also been reported in depression, and there is evidence that antidepressant treatment may enhance GABA signalling. Finally, the existence of a glutamatergic link is also strongly supported by various observations: antidepressants reduce the expression of N-methyl-D-aspartate (NMDA) receptor subunits, and ketamine (an NMDA receptor blocker) has antidepressant effects. Furthermore, it is known that stress increases glutamate release, whereas antidepressant drugs may decrease the release and/or increase the reuptake of the excitatory amino acid.

Many depressed patients also present with neuroendocrine changes, in particular a series of abnormalities in the hypothalamus–pituitary–adrenal (HPA) axis (Table 16.3). Notable among these are the increased level of plasma cortisol and the absence of response to a dexamethasone challenge. In the dexamethasone suppression test, depressed patients cannot suppress cortisol secretion when the synthetic glucocorticoid dexamethasone is administered. The secretion of cortisol is under the control of the hypothalamus and the hormone corticotrophin-releasing factor (CRF). Hypersecretion of CRF has been reported in some depressed patients. CRF binds to two receptor subtypes: CRF_1 and CRF_2. CRF_1 antagonists have shown antidepressant potential. The excess release of cortisol is being considered as a risk factor for the development of hippocampal atrophy (which has been described after intense stress). Thus, there is a possible link between stress as a triggering factor in depression, the HPA abnormalities in patients with depression, and the structural changes reported in depression.

Treatment of depression

Pharmacological management

The treatment of depression is based on the use of drugs belonging to several classes, as shown in Table 16.4. Drugs can be classified according to their structure (e.g. tricyclic antidepressants (TCAs)) or their mechanism of action (e.g. monoamine reuptake inhibition versus monoamine oxidase inhibition). Most drugs currently prescribed act on monoaminergic transmission. For all antidepressant medications, the onset of clinical efficacy is at least 2–3 weeks after initiation of treatment. This indicates that it is not the immediate changes that follow the acute administration of these compounds that are responsible for their therapeutic effect, but the delayed secondary effects. For example, with many antidepressant drugs, chronic treatment leads to downregulation of β- and $α_2$-adrenoceptors, and $5-HT_2$ receptors.

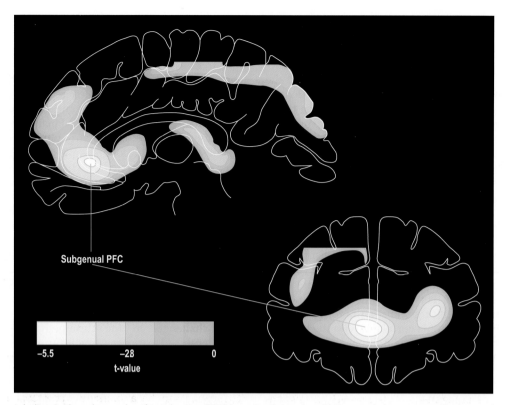

Fig. 16.1 Hypometabolism in the subgenual prefrontal cortex (PFC) in major depression. Positron emission tomography image showing an area of decreased glucose metabolism and cerebral blood flow in the subgenual prefrontal cortex in unmedicated depressed patients. From Drevets et al. Nature. 1997; 386: 824-7.

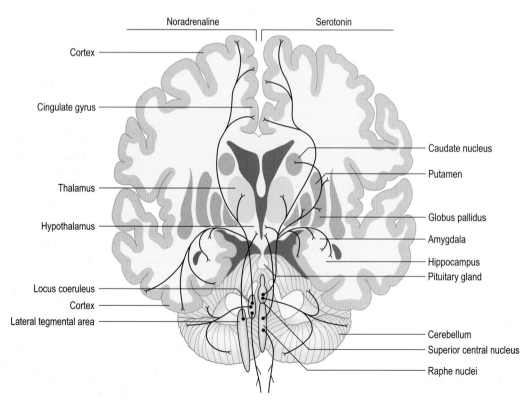

Fig. 16.2 The ascending noradrenergic and serotonergic pathways. Adapted from Snyder (1986).

Table 16.3 Abnormalities of the hypothalamus–pituitary–adrenal axis in depression

Increased plasma cortisol

Increased urinary free cortisol

Abnormal cortisol circadian rhythm

Increased CRF in the cerebrospinal fluid

Decreased response of ACTH after CRF stimulation

Decreased glucocorticoid receptor sensitivity

Increased circulating ACTH

Increased adrenal gland size

CRF, corticotrophin-releasing factor; ACTH, adrenocorticotrophin.

Table 16.4 Classes of antidepressant drug

Tricyclic and tetracyclic antidepressants

Amitriptyline, clomipramine, desipramine, doxepine, imipramine, nortriptyline, protryptiline

Monoamine oxidase inhibitors (irreversible)

Phenelzine, tranylcypromine, isocarboxazide

Monoamine oxidase A inhibitors (reversible)

Moclobemide

Atypical antidepressants

Mirtazapine, bupropion, trazodone, tianeptine

Selective serotonin reuptake inhibitors

Citalopram, fluoxetine, fluvoxamine, paroxetine, sertraline

Serotonin and noradrenaline reuptake inhibitors

Venlafaxine, duloxetine

Noradrenaline reuptake inhibitors

Reboxetine

TCAs were the first-line medication for several decades, before the development of selective serotonin reuptake inhibitors (SSRIs). Drugs in the TCA class, such as amitriptyline and imipramine, inhibit the noradrenaline and 5-HT uptake systems with variable affinities (Box 16.3). However, at clinically relevant concentrations, they also have significant affinity for various receptors (e.g. α_1-adrenergic, H_1 histaminergic and muscarinic), where they act as antagonists. This property is responsible for their numerous side effects. For example, they induce anticholinergic muscarinic effects, such as dry mouth, constipation, blurred vision and difficult micturition. They induce postural hypotension and sedation (consequences of adrenergic and histaminergic blockade). At high doses they have cardiac toxicity, and overdoses are lethal. They induce strong potentiation of the effects of alcohol; combining drinking with antidepressant drugs may lead to severe respiratory depression.

Monoamine oxidase inhibitors (MAOIs) are irreversible inhibitors of monoamine oxidases. The monoamine oxidases (MAO_A and MAO_B) are the enzymes primarily responsible for the breakdown of monoamines such as dopamine, noradrenaline and serotonin. The MAO_A and MAO_B genes are next to each other on the human X chromosome. Monoamine oxidases are located in the presynaptic terminal and are associated with the mitochondria. The inhibition of these enzymes increases the cytoplasmic concentration of amines. MAOIs do not differentiate between the two enzyme types. They were the first drugs to be introduced clinically for the treatment of depression, but they were replaced by TCAs, which had higher efficacy. There is a risk of dangerous interaction of MAOIs with tyramine-containing food (e.g. red wine, mature cheese and broad beans). Tyramine is an amine substrate of MAO_A and MAO_B, and is normally metabolized by these enzymes in the gut and the liver. Tyramine can displace noradrenaline from its storage vesicles and ultimately increase its level in the synaptic cleft. Inhibition of the monoamine oxidases leads to high levels of tyramine, and an increase in the release of noradrenaline.

The result can be a massive hypertensive crisis, with possible intracranial haemorrhage. This chain of effects is described as the 'cheese effect' (because tyramine is found in mature cheese). Indirectly acting sympathomimetic amines such as ephedrine and amphetamine can also cause hypertension in patients who are taking MAOIs. Apart from these specific unwanted complications of treatment, MAOIs can also induce postural hypotension, weight gain, antimuscarinic effects and hepatotoxicity. They also interact dangerously with the opiate analgesic pethidine: the syndrome is characterized by hypotension, restlessness and coma.

MAOIs of the reversible type are represented by the new drug moclobemide. This compound has an efficacy comparable to that of other MAOIs, but there is a significantly decreased risk of a 'cheese effect', due to the reversible nature of enzyme inhibition.

MAOIs are more effective drugs than TCAs or SSRIs in atypical depression, i.e. depression characterized by weight gain and hypersomnia, or in patients who do not respond to other antidepressants.

SSRIs, such as citalopram, fluoxetine, paroxetine and sertraline, have largely replaced other antidepressants in the treatment of most types of depression. These compounds have a higher selectivity for the 5-HT reuptake system than the TCAs (Table 16.5). The most selective is citalopram. SSRIs have a much more acceptable profile of side effects and are safer than TCAs in overdose. The unwanted effects of SSRIs include nausea, headache, insomnia and sexual dysfunction. It is important to note that although SSRI antidepressants offer significant advantages over TCAs in tolerability and safety,

Box
16.3 Monoamine transporters

A monoaminergic neurone releases amine by exocytosis, triggered by depolarization of the nerve terminal. Release is followed by diffusion of the transmitter away from the synaptic cleft, activation of pre- and postsynaptic receptors, and reuptake of the released amine into the presynaptic nerve terminal. The process of reuptake of monoamines is carried out by specialized plasma membrane transporters. The transporters for noradrenaline, 5-hydroxytryptamine (5-HT) and dopamine are termed DAT, NET and SERT, respectively, and they control the half-life of monoamines in the extracellular space (see Fig. 16.3). Psychoactive substances (e.g. cocaine and amphetamine) or therapeutic drugs (e.g. antidepressants) modify the activity of monoamine transporters. Transporters use the energy from the Na$^+$ transmembrane gradient to transport the transmitter inside the terminal. NET limits the availability of noradrenaline for diffusion. It can transport molecules that are structurally similar to noradrenaline, such as dopamine, cocaine and amphetamine. DAT is located around the active zone of the synapse and is considered to play a major role in the regulation of extracellular levels of dopamine. DAT is also a target for cocaine and amphetamine. It has been shown that the motor stimulant effects of these drugs are absent in DAT knockout mice (i.e. animals that do not express the transporter). The 5-HT transporter is part of the same transporter family, and it is the target for selective serotonin reuptake inhibitors (SSRIs). At clinically relevant doses of SSRIs, there is 70–80% occupancy of the 5-HT transporter.

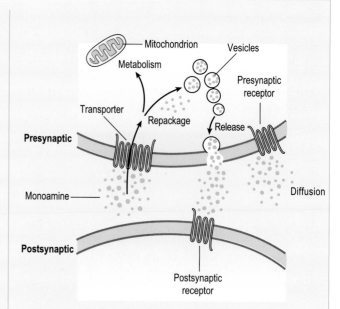

Fig. 16.3 Schematic representation of plasma membrane monoamine transporters. NET, DAT and SERT are localized in the presynaptic plasma membrane. Uptake of the neurotransmitter from the extracellular space takes place via a process that is coupled to ion transport and that can also occur in the reverse direction. The neurotransmitter can then be repackaged in vesicles for subsequent release and/or can be inactivated, e.g. by the monoamine oxidase enzymes.

Table 16.5 Selectivity of antidepressants as inhibitors of monoamine reuptake

Drug	Selectivity ratio 5-HT : NA
TCAs	
Desipramine	0.003
Nortriptyline	0.015
Imipramine	0.31
Amitriptyline	0.36
Clomipramine	5.2
SSRIs	
Fluoxetine	23
Paroxetine	33
Fluvoxamine	71
Sertraline	73
Citalopram	4000

After Heal and Cheetham (1999). 5-HT, 5-hydroxytryptamine; NA, noradrenaline; TCA, tricyclic antidepressant; SSRI, selective serotonin reuptake inhibitor.

they are not more efficacious in severe, life-threatening depression.

Atypical antidepressants include drugs such as trazodone (5-HT reuptake inhibitor and 5-HT$_2$ receptor antagonist), mirtazapine (an α_2, 5-HT$_2$ and 5-HT$_3$ antagonist), bupropion (inhibitor of dopamine and noradrenaline reuptake) and tianeptine (5-HT reuptake enhancer). These compounds have complex mechanisms of action. Overall, they have fewer side effects than TCAs and are less toxic in overdose.

Serotonin and noradrenaline reuptake inhibitors (SNRIs), such as venlafaxine and duloxetine, appear to have some advantages over SSRIs. This may be due to the synergism of blockade of 5-HT and noradrenaline uptake. In contrast with TCAs, these drugs do not have significant activity at other targets, which may explain their much milder profile of unwanted effects. Venlafaxine has also been shown to have a faster onset of action (<2 weeks) than TCAs, MAOIs or SSRIs.

Noradrenaline reuptake inhibitors, such as reboxetine, have been shown to have therapeutic efficacy in major depression similar to that of imipramine, desipramine and fluoxetine. Adverse effects include dry mouth, sweating, constipation, insomnia and blurred vision.

Non-pharmacological management

Electroconvulsive therapy

The first electroconvulsive treatment dates back to 1938 and was carried out by Cerletti and Bini. This had been preceded by the historical observations of Meduna in 1934 (Box 16.4). Although there was a high risk of significant medical morbidity, the results clearly indicated from the beginning that electroconvulsive therapy (ECT) was efficacious in severely mentally ill patients. Unfortunately, evidence of its success led to a rather indiscriminate use in its early phase. The use of general anaesthesia and muscle relaxants has made ECT much safer.

ECT is reserved for second-line treatment of patients who fail to respond to antidepressant drugs. It is particularly useful in very disturbed patients, who are at high risk for suicide. ECT is administered two or three times a week, over several weeks. Electrodes can be placed unilaterally or bilaterally, on each side of the head. If cognitive side effects following treatment become significant, electrodes can be placed only unilaterally, and the frequency of treatments reduced. Several factors can affect the seizure threshold, either by increasing it (age, anticonvulsants or dehydration) or decreasing it (caffeine or hyperventilation).

Headache and nausea are common side effects of ECT, but the major problems with ECT are its effects on learning and memory, which may be considered unacceptable by some patients. Patients lose the memory of events that preceded the treatment (retrograde amnesia). However, the loss is transient, and the patient usually recovers after a few weeks. Patients who respond to treatment have a better quality of life than before, and consider that the lost memories are an acceptable price to pay. Other patients feel very affected by the loss of memory and feel alienated, in both their private life and their work.

ECT can be used only for a short time. However, continuation and maintenance can be used to prevent relapse of depression after a successful first course of ECT. The information available so far suggests that long-term use (>1 year) of ECT is efficacious and relatively well tolerated, and reduces hospital use for a population of chronically depressed patients refractory to various types of medication.

According to a recent report, about 11000 patients receive ECT annually in the UK. ECT is used not only in major depression, but also in other psychiatric disorders: mania, schizophreniform psychoses, neuroleptic malignant syndrome and catatonic states. Patients treated with ECT or with a combination of drugs and ECT show a better response than patients treated only with drugs. The mechanism of action underlying the efficacy of ECT in a wide spectrum of disorders is still unclear. It has been shown that seizures upregulate the expression of neurotrophic factors, such as nerve growth factor and brain-derived neurotrophic factor. They also increase hippocampal neurogenesis (i.e. production of new neurones)

It is possible that the first attempt by Meduna to use ECT therapeutically was encouraged by the benefits reported by Wagner-Jauregg, who used induction of fever to treat the dementia associated with neurosyphilis. The underlying idea was that of treating a disease with another disease. Interestingly, Meduna tried the idea of inducing the seizure therapeutically in a patient with schizophrenia. What follows is the account of that first attempt (recounted by Fink in 2001).

'At 10.30 on the morning of January 24, 1934, the Hungarian neuropsychiatrist Ladislas Meduna approached the bed of Zoltan, a 30-year-old Budapest labourer who appeared lifeless. Zoltan had hardly spoken or cared for himself for more than 4 years; his mental condition of catatonic schizophrenia was considered hopeless. No remedy was available and none looked for, as the doctors believed the illness to be an immutable genetic fault, laid down at the moment of conception. Meduna injected an oily extract of camphor into the patient's right buttock. Soon the patient's heart raced, sweat rose on his brow, and he became increasingly fearful, and after 45 minutes, his eyes suddenly closed, his jaw clenched, breathing stopped and he lost consciousness. With a deep and noisy sigh, his arms and legs extended, he convulsed, and his bed thumped rhythmically, as the attendants caught him as he was about to roll on the floor. His skin became ashen and he wet the bed. As suddenly as the spasm started, it ended. His eyes opened and a pink colour slowly returned to his cheeks. Zoltan continued to stare and was as speechless as before. He had survived an induced grand-mal epileptic fit. Meduna injected camphor at 3–4 day intervals, and 2 days after the 5th seizure, Zoltan awakened, looked about, got out of bed, asked where he was, and requested breakfast. He did not believe that he had been in hospital for 4 years, and knew nothing of the intervening history. Later that day, he again relapsed into stupor. After each of the next seizures Zoltan remained alert and interested for longer and longer periods, until after the 8th injection he left the hospital to return to his home and work. His mental condition was relieved and five years later he was well and working.'

and hippocampal synaptic plasticity. The technique is continuously optimized (e.g. novel electrode placements, optimization of electrical stimulus parameters, and treatment frequency). New methods for inducing more localized seizures are also under development, such as transcranial magnetic stimulation. The use of magnetic fields provides more control over the site and extent of stimulation than ECT. This enhanced control is a means of focusing the treatment on target cortical structures that may be critical for the antidepressant response, and reducing spread to the medial temporal regions implicated in the cognitive unwanted effects of ECT.

Other stimulation therapies

Other stimulation methods used in depression include vagus nerve stimulation and deep brain stimulation. Both of these techniques are also used in other pathologies, i.e. epilepsy and Parkinson's disease, respectively (see Chapters 10 and 13). The information collected so far on their efficacy in major depression is limited, but the observations are encouraging.

Psychotherapy

The efficacy of certain forms of psychotherapy in the management of depression is no longer contested. Some authors claim that psychotherapeutic management is as effective as antidepressant medication. Cognitive behavioural therapy (CBT) is a form of therapy used in depression. This therapy, as well as other related therapies, is based on the assumption that behaviour is learned, and that change can be stimulated by the positive experiences resulting from new behaviour. CBT focuses on affect and cognitive regulation skills. In contrast, problem-solving therapy focuses on problem-solving skills. Patients who respond to this type of therapy maintain the treatment gains for up to 2 years after therapy.

Chronic psychotherapy significantly reduces relapse and recurrence in the highest-risk patients, those with recurrent major depressive disorder. Specific CBT strategies can also be used in the management of the main anxiety disorders, such as specific phobias, panic disorder and agoraphobia, social phobia, generalized anxiety disorder, obsessive-compulsive disorder and post-traumatic stress disorder (see below).

Bipolar disorder and its treatment

Bipolar disorder is a form of mood disorder consisting of an alternation of manic phases and depressive episodes. The natural course of the disease is characterized by relapse and recurrence. The goal of treatment is to treat both the acute phase (acute depression or acute mania) and the recurrence of these episodes. The duration of episodes ranges from 2 to 6 weeks. The treatment continuation phase continues for up to 6 months after the remission of acute symptoms. Lifelong treatment may be necessary for a significant number of patients. Bipolar disorder is a clinically heterogeneous disease, so treatment varies with disease subtype.

There is clearly a genetic component to this disease. As for other common and complex diseases, such as diabetes and hypertension, the transmission of bipolar disorder is multifactorial, rather than the result of simple Mendelian inheritance. Linkage studies have suggested the chromosomal regions 4p, 6p, 13q, 15q and 18q.

As with major depression, imaging studies and postmortem morphometric observations in bipolar disorder show neuronal atrophy and loss in cortical areas. Bipolar disorder can be associated with a larger third ventricle, a smaller cerebellum, a smaller temporal lobe and a larger amygdala. The pathophysiology of the disease has not yet been elucidated.

The successful treatment of bipolar disorder remains a challenge in psychiatry. It is generally agreed that patients should be maintained on a mood-stabilizing drug. The most commonly prescribed stabilizers are lithium and the anticonvulsants carbamazepine and sodium valproate.

The discovery of the efficacy of lithium in bipolar disorder represents a landmark in the history of 20th century medicine. Lithium was the first drug for which recurrence-preventing action was demonstrated in mood disorders. It may prevent recurrences not only in bipolar disorder but also in recurrent major depression. This monovalent cation continues to be used for both mainstay treatment for the acute manic phase and prophylaxis for recurrent manic and depressive episodes. The beneficial effects consist of reductions in both the number of episodes and their severity. Long-term lithium treatment is also associated with lower mortality and reduced suicidal behaviour. The drug has efficacy but it also has many side effects that may lead to cessation of treatment. The major side effects include nausea, tremor, fatigue, polyuria and polydypsia. In Europe, the recommended serum lithium range is 0.4–0.8 mmol/L. The risk of lithium intoxication is a drawback of the treatment. Lithium is eliminated through the kidneys, and it should be used with caution in the case of dehydration, sodium deficiency or kidney disease.

Research on the mechanism of action underlying the efficacy of lithium has focused extensively on the hydrolysis of phosphatidylinositol 4,5-bisphosphate (PIP_2). Inositol phospholipids such as PIP_2 are involved in receptor-mediated signal transduction pathways. Several receptor subtypes (e.g. 5-HT$_2$ serotonergic, α_1-noradrenergic, M_1, M_3 and M_5 muscarinic) are coupled to the hydrolysis of inositol phospholipids. The activation of receptors leads to stimulation of phospholipase Cβ. The enzyme catalyses the conversion of PIP_2 to inositol 1,4,5-trisphosphate (IP_3) and diacylglycerol (DAG). IP_3 stimulates the mobilization of intracellular Ca^{2+}, and DAG activates protein kinase C. IP_3 can be phosphorylated and dephosphorylated. Lithium interferes with these processes. At therapeutically relevant concentrations, it inhibits inositol monophosphatase. The effect on protein kinase C may be equally important. Interestingly, it has been recently shown that tamoxifen, a drug that has protein kinase C inhibitory activity, can significantly reduce acute mania. However, the story of lithium—which is still an enigma in psychiatry—continues with even more exciting developments (Box 16.5).

Anticonvulsants such as carbamazepine and sodium valproate have comparable efficacy to lithium and may be better tolerated. There is also evidence that combinations

Box 16.5 Lithium: a story of serendipity and surprises!

A new era in psychiatry started in the second half of the 20th century, and one of the key discoveries triggering this change was the introduction of lithium into therapeutics.

In 1949, the Australian John Cade hypothesized that mental illness is caused by intoxication with a xenobiotic, and that this toxic agent could be eliminated in the patient's urine. In order to explore the effects of uric acid, he injected lithium urate into guinea pigs. This choice was made because of the good solubility of this salt. The effects were surprising: the animals were docile and sedated. Cade immediately thought of treating manic patients with lithium. Following administration of lithium urate, the manic patients showed significantly decreased symptoms. The rest is medical history.

The efficacy of this monovalent cation intrigued researchers for years, and for a while emphasis was placed on its modulatory role in inositol-related biochemical pathways. However, the most recent discoveries suggest that the effects of lithium (and possibly of other mood stabilizers, such as valproate) involve concomitant changes in the expression of numerous genes, e.g. through modulation of the activity of transcription factors such as AP-1. Furthermore, at therapeutically relevant concentrations, lithium is an inhibitor of the enzyme glycogen synthase kinase-3β. This enzyme plays an important role in cytoskeletal dynamics as well as in nuclear transcriptional events. Finally, differential analysis of the transcriptome (i.e. cellular pool of transcribed mRNA) after treatment with lithium suggests that the cation upregulates neuroprotective genes, such as *bcl-2*. Therefore, the emerging view of the effect of lithium is that of action at multiple levels, and significant neuroprotective potential.

Box 16.6 Postnatal depression and seasonal affective disorder

Postnatal depression

Depressive episodes in women after childbirth are relatively common. During the first 6 months after delivery, the prevalence is 12–13%. Risk factors for postnatal depression include: poor marital relationship, past history of psychopathology, low social support, unplanned pregnancy, antenatal parental stress, and depression in fathers. Treatment consists of antidepressant medication and/or cognitive behavioural therapy. Postnatal depression must be distinguished from the very transient period of tearfulness or emotional lability that many mothers experience in the first 1–2 weeks after birth ('baby blues'), which resolves naturally.

Seasonal affective disorder

This type of depression received formal recognition only in the early 1980s. Symptoms of depression affect patients regularly during the autumn or winter months, whereas spontaneous remission is seen in spring and summer. This disorder is correlated with the level of light, and may be connected with an abnormality in the production/secretion of melatonin, a hormone secreted by the pineal gland. As days become shorter and darker, the production of this hormone increases. Many people affected by this disorder respond to bright light therapy. For example, they can be exposed daily for a limited time to a bank of fluorescent lights shielded with a plastic screen. Antidepressant drugs such as selective serotonin reuptake inhibitors (SSRIs) can also be used successfully to treat this disorder.

of lithium with an anticonvulsant drug can help in atypical cases of bipolar disorder, or in patients resistant to treatment. During a depressive episode, it is often necessary to add an antidepressant drug. This, unfortunately, may induce a switch to a manic phase. The antidepressants bupropion and, more recently, lamotrigine, have been shown to be useful in the treatment of depressive episodes, especially in comparison to TCAs, as the latter may induce a switch to a manic phase.

General comments on mood disorders

Mood disorders are among the most prevalent, recurrent and disabling of all illnesses. They cover a wide spectrum, from severe intractable depression to the milder forms, such as seasonal affective disorder and postnatal depression (Box 16.6). Drugs that can be used to treat

mood disorders with some success, were discovered accidentally, not as a result of following a scientific rationale. Drug development has focused heavily on monoaminergic targets, and there is need for more mechanistic diversity. Several major challenges remain: the delayed effect of antidepressants, resistance to treatment and, most of all, an understanding of the pathophysiology of the disease and of its causes. Our understanding of the circuits responsible for the regulation of mood and affect is still rudimentary. Some of these issues are discussed below.

Treatment resistance in depression

Although new-generation compounds are much better tolerated than the original tricyclic drugs, they are not necessarily more efficacious. Furthermore, many patients are resistant to drugs. It is considered that up to 50% of patients who receive drugs still experience symptoms and are somewhat functionally impaired. Combinations of drugs (e.g. lithium and antidepressants) can be attempted, but no optimum strategy to address treatment resistance in depression has been defined yet.

One of the major complications of depressive mood disorders is the increased risk for suicide. The most common biological marker of suicide is a reduced concentration of the 5-HT metabolite 5-hydroxyindoleacetic acid in the CSF of suicide cases versus controls. Although suicide prevention is ideally primary, before the event, most treatment is in fact secondary or tertiary, after initial unsuccessful suicide attempts. Depending on the individual characteristics of the patient, suicide prevention usually includes a pharmacological cocktail (e.g. one of the SSRIs, to raise 5-HT concentrations, perhaps combined with an anxiolytic, mood-stabilizing or antipsychotic agent), supportive psychotherapy and/or ECT. The existence of a significant risk of suicide in a patient necessitates treatment in hospital.

The failure of medication may sometimes be due to the use of inadequate doses. Thus, many patients who receive TCAs are prescribed relatively low doses, and an improvement is seen if doses are increased. At higher doses, plasma monitoring may be required in the case of tricyclic compounds, because of the risk of cardiotoxicity.

Another strategy that can be used is switching to a different class of antidepressant. There is evidence that switching may benefit about 50% of the patients initially unresponsive to medication. One of the problems encountered when attempting to switch to a different antidepressant drug is that withdrawal from the first compound is difficult. It may be more appropriate to add a second compound to the first. Patients with depression with psychotic features have low rates of response to TCAs, but may improve when an antipsychotic drug is added to the treatment (e.g. amitriptyline with perphenazine, or olanzapine with fluoxetine). There is also evidence that lithium added to TCAs, MAOIs or SSRIs leads to an improved response. Finally, maintenance therapy with antidepressant drugs, after the successful treatment of an episode, has been shown to decrease the risk of recurrence.

Delayed onset of antidepressant action: a consequence of autoregulation?

Although drugs such as TCAs and SSRIs block 5-HT reuptake rapidly, their therapeutic action is delayed. A possible explanation for this delay has been suggested, using as an example the SSRIs. It has been suggested that the increase in synaptic 5-HT activates feedback mechanisms mediated by 5-HT_{1A} receptors situated on the cell body, and $5\text{-HT}1_B$ receptors situated on the nerve terminals. The activation of these two types of autoreceptor reduces the firing of 5-HT neurones and decreases the amount of 5-HT released. Long-term treatment with SSRIs desensitizes the inhibitory 5-HT_1 autoreceptors, and 5-HT neurotransmission is ultimately enhanced. The time course of desensitization is similar to the delay

in clinical effect. This explanation is supported by the observation that the addition of pindolol (a drug that blocks 5-HT1_A receptors) to SSRI treatment accelerates and enhances the antidepressant response.

Need for new therapeutic targets

As mentioned earlier, the monoamine theory of depression has certainly served a useful purpose, but the field now needs to move beyond this concept, and it is important to consider, in parallel with the monoamines, the other neurotransmitters that are likely to be dysfunctional in depressive disorders. Evidence suggests that it is possible to target glutamatergic systems (e.g. NMDA receptor antagonists or 4-amino-3-hydroxy-5-methyl-4-isoxazole propionic acid (AMPA) receptor potentiators) or peptidergic systems (CRF receptor antagonists) and obtain significant antidepressant effects. It may be possible in the near future to develop drugs that will address the cause of mood disorders, and not only treat the symptoms during depressive episodes.

Comments on the case history

The unpredictable evolution of depression is illustrated by the case history. Depression emerged unexpectedly, possibly triggered by the stress intrinsic to a high level of activity. However, a genetic susceptibility is also suggested by the family history. The patient responds to an SNRI, and tolerates it well, but makes the mistake of stopping the medication immediately after improvement. Relapse occurs, and it is severe, with added anxiety. This leads to a choice of combination therapy (medication and psychotherapy). It cannot be ruled out that this patient will experience periods of remission and relapse throughout his life.

Anxiety disorders

'The mind is its own place, and in itself can make a heaven of hell, a hell of heaven.'

John Milton (1608–1674)

Anxiety is an unpleasant emotional experience characterized by fear disproportionate to the severity of stressful factors in the environment, or fear without cause. An optimum level of anxiety may improve performance. However, when it is intense and persists for a prolonged period, it is an extremely disabling disorder. Anxiety is categorized into different subtypes (Table 16.6). Some of them are phobic disorders, whereas others do not have a phobic component (Table 16.7). Phobias are characterized by irrational fear and avoidance of objects and situations.

Although included in the class of anxiety disorders, post-traumatic stress disorder is a complex and unique syndrome (Box 16.7).

Anxiety and depression are distinct disorders, but mixed disorders are also frequently encountered. Depression is often co-morbid with generalized anxiety disorder, panic disorder and obsessive-compulsive disorder. Conversely, many types of depression involve a degree of anxiety, as illustrated in the case history, during the second depressive episode.

The prevalence for the various categories of anxiety disorders varies: for example, for phobias it is 3–5%, whereas for post-traumatic stress disorder it is only 1–3%. Anxiety disorders can occur at various ages. Obsessive-compulsive disorder may develop in adolescence or early adulthood, whereas post-traumatic stress disorder can occur at any age, including childhood.

Anxiety manifestations have affective, behavioural and somatic components. The affective component is characterized by the feeling of panic and dread. Behavioural reactions tend to be aimed at avoiding the source of anxiety. Somatic reactions reflect a state of autonomic hyperreactivity, including cardiopulmonary, urinary and gastrointestinal symptoms.

Treatment of anxiety disorders

The management of anxiety disorders can be pharmacological or non-pharmacological.

Benzodiazepines constitute a major first-line treatment for anxiety disorders. Over the last three decades, they have been the most prescribed anxiolytics for both young and old patients. They comprise a large class of related compounds, with sedative, anxiolytic, muscle relaxant and anticonvulsant activity (see Chapter 13). These compounds bind to the $GABA_A$ receptor and act as positive allosteric modulators, that is, they increase the frequency of opening of the ion channel in the presence of the endogenous agonist GABA. The benzodiazepines replaced barbiturates, and became in the 1970s the most prescribed drugs in the world. However, apart from being anxiolytic, benzodiazepines also cause acute sedation. Therefore, benzodiazepines can also be used as hypnotics (see below). Chronically, they have abuse potential and can cause physical dependence. A withdrawal syndrome can emerge upon treatment discontinuation, especially if treatment is stopped without gradual tapering of

Table 16.6 Classification of anxiety disorders (DSM-IV)

Panic disorder with or without agoraphobia (fear of open spaces)

Agoraphobia without history of panic disorder

Specific phobia

Social phobia

Obsessive-compulsive disorder

Post-traumatic stress disorder

Acute stress disorder

Generalized anxiety disorder

Anxiety disorder due to general medical conditions and substance-induced anxiety disorder

Anxiety disorder not otherwise specified

Table 16.7 General characteristics of phobias and of non-phobic anxiety disorders

Phobias

Agoraphobia	Social phobias	Specific (isolated) phobias
Anxiety in situations where escape or help is difficult	Intense fear of embarrassment or humiliation in public or social gatherings	Intense fear provoked by appearance or anticipation of specific situations or objects (e.g. fear of spiders, snakes, heights, water, travelling by plane or by train)
Fear of being alone in public places or in a crowd	Subject feels that other people think them stupid or incompetent	

Non-phobic anxiety disorders

Generalized anxiety disorder	Panic disorder	Obsessive-compulsive disorder
Ill-defined apprehension not related to a specific situation/object lasting for more than 6 months	Recurrent unexpected panic attacks (accompanied by dizziness, nausea, palpitations, chest pain, hyperventilation, sweating, tremor and sometimes incontinence)	Obsessive thoughts (repetitive thoughts that the subject cannot dispel)
Exaggerated worries about health, personal safety, work or finances		Compulsive behaviour (repetitive behaviour that the subject carries out, although realizing that it is irrational, such as repetitive handwashing due to fear of contamination, or checking that the doors are locked)

Post-traumatic stress disorder

Post-traumatic stress disorder is a syndrome that emerges after one or more traumatic events, and involves a series of anxiety symptoms, including emotional numbing, flashbacks and avoidance of reminders of the event. This disorder was associated in the past mainly with the psychological consequences of war, but today it is increasingly recognized as a serious complication after rape, abuse, assault, accidents or natural disasters. In the acute aftermath of a traumatic event, those affected experience hyperarousal, agitation, insomnia and nightmares. These reactions may serve an adaptive role, and may remit in a short time. When they do not remit, they evolve into post-traumatic stress disorder. The presentation of this syndrome is heterogeneous, with symptoms that vary significantly between patients.

Several brain circuits and neurotransmitters are involved in the pathophysiology of this disorder. Catecholamines, serotonin, the hypothalamic–pituitary–adrenal axis (in particular corticotrophin-releasing factor) and corticolimbic circuits are involved in the modulation of fear, anger, arousal and aggression.

There is no established therapy for this syndrome, so different drugs are used, sometimes on a semi-empirical basis, to reduce the flashbacks, anxiety, hyperarousal and depression. Interestingly, compounds from the same pharmacological class appear to have effects on different symptoms. For example, imipramine decreases nightmares and flashbacks, but has no effect on avoidance behaviour. In contrast, amitriptyline reduces avoidance and anxiety. Monoamine oxidase inhibitors such as phenelzine or moclobemide have also been shown to be effective in some patients. Selective serotonin reuptake inhibitors have been shown to be effective in civilian and military trauma victims. Anticonvulsants (carbamazepine and valproate) decrease flashbacks and impulsivity. Overall, approximately 70% of patients get some benefit from pharmacotherapy.

the dose. Recent estimates suggest that 10–30% of chronic benzodiazepine users are physically dependent on the drugs, and 50% of all users suffer withdrawal symptoms.

The $GABA_A$ receptor is probably a pentamer assembled from several subunits that exist in different isoforms: $\alpha(1–6)$, $\beta(1–4)$, $\gamma(1–4)$, $\rho(1–3)$, δ, ε, π and θ. The most abundant $GABA_A$ receptor type is composed of $\alpha_1\beta_2/_3\gamma_2$ subunits. Benzodiazepines enhance the actions of the inhibitory neurotransmitter GABA by binding to a specific recognition site on $GABA_A$ receptors containing α_1, α_2, α_3 and α_5 subunits. Benzodiazepines bind to the α subunits or to the α–γ interface. Two types of benzodiazepine (BZ) binding sites have been described—BZ1 and BZ2—based on the pharmacological profile of native receptors. GABA/BZ receptors have an abundant and heterogeneous distribution in the central nervous system (CNS).

Compounds that bind at benzodiazepine sites and enhance the inhibitory actions of GABA are classified as agonists, those that induce effects opposite to those induced by benzodiazepines are termed inverse agonists, and those that reverse the effects of benzodiazepines (e.g. flumazenil) are benzodiazepine site antagonists. The clinically used benzodiazepines are full agonists. Between the opposite ends of the spectrum (i.e. full agonist and full inverse agonist) are a range of compounds with differing degrees of efficacy, such as partial agonists and partial inverse agonists. Attempts have been made to develop compounds that have the anxiolytic properties of the full-agonist benzodiazepines, but have reduced sedation and dependence (withdrawal) liabilities. Such compounds may interact with all four (i.e. α_1-, α_2-, α_3- and α_5-containing) $GABA_A$ receptor subtypes, and have partial rather than full agonist efficacies. Alternatively, a compound might have comparable binding affinities but different efficacies at the various subtypes, thereby preferentially exerting its effects at subtypes thought to be associated with anxiety (α_2- and/or α_3-containing receptors) rather than the subtype associated with sedation (α_1-containing receptors).

Benzodiazepines differ in terms of pharmacokinetic properties (Table 16.8). These drugs undergo hepatic metabolism. The long half-life benzodiazepines, such as chlordiazepoxide, clorazepate, diazepam and flurazepam, undergo phase I and phase II metabolic transformations. These long half-life compounds are metabolized via phase I reactions (e.g. oxidation) into active compounds with even longer half-lives. Short half-life benzodiazepines, such as lorazepam, oxazepam and temazepam, require only phase II metabolism and are inactivated by hepatic conjugation. Phase II metabolism is less affected by age, so short-acting compounds should be prescribed for the elderly. It is important to be aware of these aspects when prescribing for the elderly, for the management of either insomnia or anxiety. Chronic administration of benzodiazepines in this patient population can be accompanied by serious complications (Table 16.9).

One of the most prescribed anxiolytics is diazepam. For controlling panic attacks, diazepam can be used intravenously. In acute overdose, benzodiazepines are much safer than old anxiolytic/hypnotic drugs such as the barbiturates; this is an important consideration, given that such compounds may be used in suicide attempts. Overdose, in general, leads to prolonged sleep, without depression of respiration or cardiovascular function. However, when benzodiazepines are taken in combination with other CNS depressants, such as alcohol, respiratory depression can become severe. If this occurs, patients can be treated with flumazenil, a benzodiazepine antagonist.

Table 16.8 Pharmacokinetic profiles of commonly used benzodiazepines and non-benzodiazepine drugs

Drug	Onset of action (min)	Elimination half-life (h)	Duration of action	Active metabolites
Diazepam	20–40	20–60	Long	Yes
Flunitrazepam	20–30	11–20	Intermediate	No
Flurazepam	30–60	47–100	Long	Yes
Nitrazepam	20–50	25–35	Long	No
Oxazepam	15–30	8–12	Intermediate	No
Temazepam	45–60	3–25	Intermediate	No
Triazolam	15–30	1.5–5	Short	No
Zaleplon	15–30	1	Short	No
Zolpidem	30	1.5–4.5	Short	No
Zopiclone	15–30	3.5–6.5	Short	Yes

Table 16.9 Complications of chronic benzodiazepine use in the elderly

Psychomotor impairment

Risk of falls

Daytime drowsiness

Intoxication

Amnesia

Depression

Respiratory problems

Abuse and dependence

5-HT$_{1A}$ agonists, such as buspirone, ipsapirone and gepirone, can be used in the treatment of generalized anxiety disorder instead of benzodiazepines. In contrast with the latter, buspirone and related compounds have a delay of action of at least 2 weeks, which makes compliance difficult. Unwanted effects include nausea, headaches and dizziness.

Antidepressant drugs, such as imipramine, can be used to treat panic and social phobias. Side effects include dry mouth, constipation and blurred vision, as discussed above. Clomipramine has shown efficacy in the treatment of obsessive-compulsive disorder. SSRIs, such as fluoxetine, have also been shown to be efficacious in the management of obsessive-compulsive disorder. More recently, new anti-depressants, such as venlafaxine, have shown potential in the treatment of various anxiety disorders.

β-Blockers (e.g. propranolol) do not affect the psychological aspects of anxiety, but reduce the physical symptoms (e.g. tremor and palpitations). They are used in the treatment of social phobias, and also to treat 'stage fright' in performers.

Barbiturates, such as pentobarbitone, have become practically obsolete, because of their narrow therapeutic window and the risk of major cardiovascular and respiratory depression resulting from overdose. Furthermore, their induction of liver metabolic enzymes may lead to dangerous drug interactions, due to changes in the metabolism of co-administered drugs.

It is important to be aware that patients who have anxiety co-morbid with depression tend to discontinue treatment early. It is considered preferable to address the anxiety component first (e.g. using a drug such as venlafaxine, which has a shorter onset of action). Resolution of anxiety improves patients' compliance.

Non-pharmacological approaches are also used in the management of anxiety disorders. Psychological interventions include cognitive therapy, insight-oriented therapy, behavioural therapy and group psychotherapy. Even after pharmacotherapy has been optimized, some patients may still have residual symptoms, and they may benefit from psychotherapy.

Insomnia

Sleep is a physiological process, and is controlled by several neuronal pathways that regulate the degree of wakefulness. The Viennese neurologist von Economo was the first to suggest, in 1930, that prolonged sleepiness is due to injury to neurones in the posterior hypothalamus and rostral midbrain. However, a real understanding of the complex circuitry that controls sleep and wakefulness was possible only during the last two decades of the 20th century. It gradually became possible to correlate the activity of neuronal groups with the different sleep

Box
16.8   The neurobiology of sleep and wakefulness

Sleep is a necessary activity, as its disturbance leads to a decreased quality of life. However, the fundamental role of sleep remains incompletely understood.

During a normal night's sleep, there are usually five consecutive phases of sleep: stages 1, 2, 3 and 4, and rapid eye movement (REM) sleep. These stages progress in a cycle from stage 1 to REM sleep, and then a new cycle starts again with stage 1. A complete cycle lasts 90–120 min on average. The electrical activity of the brain is very different during each stage of this cycle (Fig. 16.4). Almost 50% of the total sleep time is spent in stage 2 sleep, about 20% in REM sleep, and the remaining 30% in the other stages. Babies spend about half of their sleep time in REM sleep.

Stage 1 is light sleep, from which one can be awakened easily. Muscles are relaxed, but sudden muscle contractions (hypnic myoclonia), similar to a startle reaction while awake, are sometimes experienced. These may be preceded by a sensation of starting to fall. In stage 2 sleep, sudden bursts of rapid waves called sleep spindles start appearing on the electroencephalogram trace, on a background of slower electrical activity. In stage 3, extremely slow brain waves called delta waves begin to appear; these dominate in stage 4. Stages 3 and 4 are called deep sleep. There is no eye movement or muscle activity. People awakened during deep sleep do not adjust immediately and may feel disoriented for several minutes. It is during deep sleep that some children experience bedwetting. Sleepwalking can also occur during this phase.

The first REM sleep period usually occurs 70–90 min after the onset of sleep. During this phase, breathing is rapid, irregular and shallow, and the eyes move rapidly in the orbit. There are increases in heart rate and blood pressure, and males develop penile erections. Limb muscles become temporarily paralysed. When people are woken during REM sleep, they often describe dreams.

The first sleep cycles during the night contain relatively short REM periods and long periods of deep sleep. As the night progresses, REM sleep periods increase in length, and deep sleep periods decrease in length. By the morning,

sleep consists almost entirely of stages 1 and 2, and REM sleep.

It is also notable that sleep patterns change as a function of age. Normal ageing is associated with changes in sleep patterns that mirror the neurophysiology of depression: reduced slow-wave sleep, reduced REM sleep latency, and decreased continuity of sleep (i.e. more awakenings). These are accompanied by a blunting of body temperature rhythms and of circadian cortisol variations.

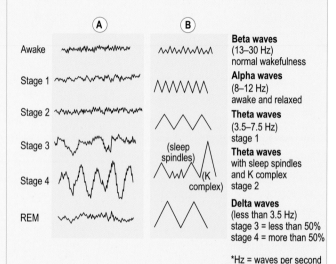

Fig. 16.4 Representation of the profiles of electrical activity of the brain during sleep stages: normal sleep electroencephalogram (A) and diagrammatic representation of types of electrical activity that correspond to sleep stages (B). The wakeful/alert and relaxed/awake electroencephalogram and the rapid eye movement (REM) sleep electroencephalogram are characterized by desynchronized activity (alpha and beta waves), whereas stage 1 is characterized by theta waves, which are slower and stronger than beta waves. Stages 3 and 4 are characterized by the gradual emergence of synchronized activity, represented by the delta waves.

phases (Box 16.8). An arousal system ('the ascending reticular activating system') consisting of monoaminergic and cholinergic neurones has been well described (Fig. 16.5). Cholinergic neurones from the pedunculopontine and laterodorsal tegmental nuclei project to several thalamic nuclei and modulate the activity of thalamocortical neurones. During wakefulness, cholinergic neurones fire rapidly. Their activity decreases during the first stages of sleep. In contrast, during rapid eye movement (REM) sleep, their activity increases again, as a consequence of decreased monoamine-mediated inhibition. The monoaminergic control originates in the locus coeruleus (noradrenaline), raphe nuclei (5-HT) and tuberomamillary nucleus (histamine). Neurones in these nuclei fire

fast during wakefulness, and gradually decrease their activity during sleep. They are almost completely inhibited during REM sleep. Neurones in the ventrolateral preoptic nucleus contain galanin and GABA. In contrast to cholinergic and monoaminergic neurones, they are active during sleep. Reciprocal connections exist between these various nuclei, as well as with other groups of neurones containing neuromodulatory peptides such as orexin/hypocretin. The balance of activity in these circuits is probably a major determining factor in the natural evolution of a sleep–wake cycle.

Insomnia is defined as a disturbance of normal nocturnal sleep patterns that affects daily activities. Patients may have difficulty in initiating sleep, or difficulty in

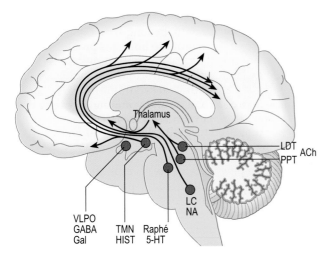

Fig. 16.5 The circuits involved in sleep and wakefulness: the ascending arousal system. Neurones of the laterodorsal tegmental nuclei (LDT) and pedunculopontine tegmental nuclei (PPT) send cholinergic fibres (ACh) to forebrain structures, including the thalamus. Neurones of the tuberomamillary nucleus (TMN) contain histamine (HIST). Neurones of the raphe nuclei contain 5-HT, and neurones of the locus coeruleus (LC) contain noradrenaline (NA). Neurones of the ventrolateral preoptic nucleus (VLPO) contain GABA and galanin (Gal). From Saper et al. (2001).

maintaining sleep (early-morning awakening or frequent nocturnal awakenings).

Insomnia can be transient, short-term or chronic. Transient insomnia can be caused by an acute disturbance or environmental stress (e.g. jetlag). Shiftwork may be associated with transient insomnia. It lasts for less than a week and usually resolves when the cause is eliminated, without intervention, or with only a brief exposure to a short-acting hypnotic drug. Short-term insomnia lasts longer (3–4 weeks) and is often associated with stressors such as illness, or emotional upset caused by bereavement, loss of a job, etc.

Chronic insomnia lasts longer than 3 weeks. It can be associated with a chronic underlying medical condition, with major psychiatric disease (e.g. depression) or with chronic drug abuse. For example, in the case history, the patient suffers from insomnia. When a cause is suspected, it is important to attempt to treat first the underlying problem, and then check if the insomnia persist. Hypnotics can be used intermittently and for limited periods.

The treatment of insomnia has been based for several decades on the use of benzodiazepines. These drugs have replaced barbiturates for the treatment of this condition. Barbiturates, such as pentobarbitone, also act as positive allosteric modulators at the same receptor, but they increase the duration of the opening of the channel. At high doses, barbiturates can open the channel in the absence of GABA.

Benzodiazepines, differ in their pharmacokinetic profiles (see Table 16.8). Some of them have long half-lives,

---

Box 16.9 Benzodiazepine receptors for better sleep

Benzodiazepine 1 (BZ1) receptors are located in brain areas involved in the control of sleep and wakefulness, whereas BZ2 receptors are present in areas involved in memory and cognition. Most benzodiazepine compounds do not differentiate between these two types, and this may account for their unwanted effects. Several non-benzodiazepine hypnotics are now available that have different selectivities for the subtypes of benzodiazepine site, and they offer the promise of being better than the existing drugs. Examples are zopiclone, zolpidem and zaleplon. These are short-acting compounds that act mainly at the BZ1 sites.

Zolpidem is comparable in efficacy to short-acting benzodiazepines such as triazolam. However, it disturbs sleep patterns less. It does not depress respiration, which makes it safer in elderly patients or other patients with respiratory problems. It lacks anticonvulsant and muscle-relaxant properties. There is no evidence that zolpidem induces tolerance, rebound insomnia or withdrawal symptoms.

Zopiclone binds to a site close to the benzodiazepine site on the GABA receptor complex. It induces less sedation and respiratory depression than benzodiazepines. Tolerance is low, and rebound insomnia is more infrequent than with benzodiazepines.

Zaleplon is a very short-acting compound, ideally suited for patients who have difficulty in initiating sleep. Because of its short half-life, it can be taken late at night, without having effects on performance and memory the next day. Its tolerance and abuse potential appear to be low.

Therefore, in clinical practice, non-benzodiazepine compounds may become preferable and safer alternatives to benzodiazepines. It remains to be confirmed whether their dependence and abuse potential is significantly less than that of the old benzodiazepine compounds.

---

and they also have active metabolites, leading to prolongation of the effect of the parent compound. A typical example is diazepam, whose metabolite, *N*-desmethyldiazepam, is active and has a longer half-life than the parent compound. This increases the risks of cumulative effects and a feeling of 'hangover' after use.

Overall, benzodiazepines are much safer drugs than barbiturates and have larger therapeutic windows. Nevertheless, their use is associated with several unwanted effects:

- Change in sleep patterns—they suppress sleep stages 3 and 4. These stages of sleep are restorative, so benzodiazepine use does not lead to good sleep quality. They also suppress REM sleep. A rebound increase in REM sleep, accompanied by frightening dreams, may occur at the end of a period of treatment with benzodiazepine hypnotics.

- Daytime sedation—the use of benzodiazepines may be associated with sedation and a 'hangover' feeling, and impaired psychomotor performance and concentration. This effect is particularly marked with long-acting benzodiazepines.

- Rebound insomnia—this phenomenon may occur at the end of treatment with short-acting or long-acting benzodiazepines. For example, administration of triazolam, for even one night, can lead to rebound insomnia on the night after treatment. This leads to chronic use of the drug and facilitates the development of dependence and the development of a vicious circle.

- Tolerance—the use of benzodiazepines is associated with tolerance, although the rate at which tolerance develops varies (it is faster for short-acting agents). Tolerance leads to the use of increasing doses.

- Physiological dependence—this is a significant problem associated with the long-term use of benzodiazepines. In order to limit this problem, intermittent use of drugs, for short durations, is recommended. Dependence is reflected in the emergence of a withdrawal syndrome (muscle cramps, increased anxiety, nausea and vomiting, sweating, photophobia, tremors and seizures). This syndrome can be minimized by gradual tapering of doses at the end of treatment.

Benzodiazepines can depress respiration and potentiate sleep apnoea. Therefore, in patients with compromised respiratory function, and particularly in elderly patients, benzodiazepines must be used carefully.

More recently, new non-benzodiazepine hypnotics have been developed, and it is hoped that they will offer significant clinical advantages over previous drugs in the treatment of insomnia (Box 16.9).

ADDICTION

17

Chapter objectives

After studying this chapter you should be able to:

1. Define addiction, dependence, tolerance and withdrawal.

2. Describe the characteristics of the main addictive substances and their mechanisms of action.

3. Describe the mechanisms that underlie the development of addiction.

4. Describe the treatments available for addiction.

Introduction

The compulsion of humans to use certain substances in order to obtain a general feeling of wellbeing and pleasure, to relieve sadness or induce euphoria, and to alter their perception of the world, can be traced back to ancient times and remains a characteristic feature of human society. 'If we could sniff or swallow something that would, for five or six hours each day, abolish our solitude as individuals, atone us with our fellows in a glowing exaltation of affection and make life in all its aspects seem not only worth living, but divinely beautiful and significant, and if this heavenly, world-transfiguring drug were of such a kind that we could wake up next morning with a clear head and an undamaged constitution—then, it seems to me, all our problems (and not merely the one small problem of discovering a novel pleasure) would be wholly solved and earth would become paradise,' said the writer Aldous Huxley. Unfortunately, seeking pleasure or consolation through psychoactive substances is far from safe, and the long-lasting consequences can be dramatic. Drug misuse, and addiction to drugs, in its broadest sense, is a problem with considerable negative consequences both for the individual and for society. An example of addiction is illustrated in the case history in Box 17.1, and this also encapsulates some of the misconceptions associated with drug abuse.

Addiction and drug misuse: general comments

'Ecstasy' and cocaine, which is alluded to in the case history, are two examples of drugs that can be misused by people irrespective of age, social background, gender or race. Some drugs are mainly used intermittently, such as 'ecstasy', whereas the use of others becomes part of daily life; there is an irresistible drive to use them on a permanent, regular basis, reflecting a state of strong physical and/or psychological dependence. Some of the substances misused can be quite common, such as nicotine or alcohol. What is dispiriting is the significant percentage of the young that use and abuse drugs (Fig. 17.1). As a preamble to the analysis of substances that are abused, it is useful to define some of the concepts discussed in this chapter.

Addiction is a compulsion to take a drug, with loss of control over drug-taking. It is a chronic relapsing disorder characterized by inability to limit or stop intake. Dependence refers to drug-induced adaptations in cells and tissues after prolonged use, which lead to the need to continue drug intake. Tolerance refers to the necessity to escalate the dose of drug in order to obtain the same effects as those obtained initially. Sensitization, in contrast to tolerance, refers to a gradually enhanced effect of drugs that are abused chronically. The abrupt cessation of drug intake can lead to a withdrawal syndrome, which has both physical and psychological components.

Box 17.1 Case history

Sarah J., a vivacious 17-year-old, went out with her friend James on a Friday night, to meet other friends, drink and dance, and 'have a good time' before the end-of-year examinations. Everything went well until around midnight, when Sarah took two 'ecstasy' pills. A short time after that, she started feeling ill and dizzy. The temperature in the club had been high, and Sarah kept drinking alcoholic drinks and a lot of water, to compensate for the dehydration caused by hours of dancing. About 3 a.m., she felt sick and vomited several times, complaining of a terrible headache. James took her to a friend's house nearby, for a rest, but Sarah's state deteriorated rapidly. She kept vomiting, and drifted in and out of consciousness. James and his friend took her to hospital around 6 a.m. and phoned her parents. The doctors immediately suspected intoxication with ecstasy, and her blood Na^+ level (123 mmol/L) confirmed their suspicion. After a day in hospital, her situation remained critical and the consultant expressed reserved optimism as to her survival. Sarah's state gradually started improving the next day. James is puzzled, and explains that she only took some 'ecstasy' pills, as usual, and cannot see the harm in it. He argues that it was only 'a little bit of fun', and that neither he nor Sarah 'have done any hard stuff like cocaine', as some of his older friends do.

This case gives rise to the following questions:

1. What has led to Sarah's critical state after her use of 'ecstasy'?
2. Is 'ecstasy' a safe drug and what differentiates it from cocaine?
3. What is the incentive that leads to the use of life-threatening drugs?
4. Is it correct to assume that there are 'hard' and unsafe drugs of abuse, in contrast to 'light' and generally safe drugs?
5. What treatment saved Sarah's life after admission to hospital?

Drugs that are abused are subject to regulations defined by law, as described in Box 17.2.

Table 17.1 gives examples of drugs that are misused. These drugs belong to a wide range of pharmacological classes. The main drugs will be discussed first individually, before discussing common mechanisms in the development of addiction.

Opiates

Opium is the dried juice of the unripe seed capsule of the poppy *Papaver somniferum*. The ancient Greeks and Romans were aware of the sedative and euphoria-inducing properties of opium, as well as its analgesic and anti-diarrhoea effects.

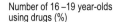

Number of 16–19 year-olds
using drugs (%)

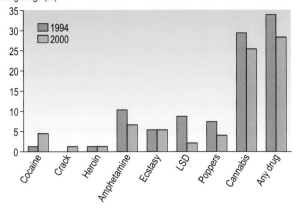

Fig. 17.1 The consumption of drugs of abuse by the 16–19-year-old population in the UK. Data from: British Crime Survey for 2000.

Table 17.1	Examples of drugs of abuse
Drugs	***Molecular targets***
Opiates	Mu (μ) and delta (δ) opioid receptors
Barbiturates and benzodiazepines	GABA$_A$ receptor
Cocaine and amphetamines	Monoamine transporters
Marijuana (cannabis)	CB$_1$ receptor
Nicotine	Nicotinic acetylcholine receptor
Ethanol	GABA$_A$ receptor, NMDA receptor
Phencyclidine	NMDA receptor
Inhalants	Not known
MDMA (ecstasy)	5-HT transporter

NMDA, N-methyl-D-aspartate; 5-HT, 5-hydroxytryptamine; GABA, γ-aminobutyric acid.

Box 17.2 Classification of drugs

In the UK, under the Misuse of Drugs Act 1971, illegal drugs are classified into three main categories: Classes A, B and C. Under the Act, offences include: (1) unlawfully possessing a controlled drug; (2) possessing a controlled drug with intent to supply it; (3) unlawfully supplying (sell/give/share) a controlled drug; (4) allowing premises that you occupy or manage to be used for the smoking or use of drugs; (5) importing or exporting controlled drugs; and (6) producing, cultivating or manufacturing controlled drugs.

Class A includes heroin, methadone, cocaine, crack, ecstasy, LSD, magic mushrooms, and any Class B drug that is injected.
Class B includes amphetamines, barbiturates, codeine and cannabis.
Class C includes mild amphetamines, benzodiazepines and anabolic steroids.

In the 19th century, opium was a commodity available on the market. Morphine (or 'morphia') was introduced in the 1820s, and the hypodermic syringe in the 1850s. The German company Bayer produced heroin in 1898, and described it as a 'heroic drug, that has the ability of morphine to relieve pain, yet is safer'. The number of prescriptions soared, and the Ebert Prescription Survey in the USA in 1885 showed that the ingredients most used in medicines were quinine and morphine. Doctors became aware of the emergence of dependence and withdrawal symptoms, and addiction became defined as a disease. It was in 1934 that the term 'drug addiction' first appeared in the American Psychiatric Association's diagnostic handbook.

Opiate drugs exert their effects by binding to opioid receptors. Of the three opioid receptor types—mu (μ), kappa (κ) and delta (δ)—it is the μ type that is critical for the addictive effects of morphine and heroin. It is the blockade of this receptor type that reduces self-administration of opiates in experimental animals. Agonists at μ receptors activate dopaminergic neurones in the ventral tegmental area (VTA) of the midbrain and enhance dopamine release in the nucleus accumbens. This activation is indirect, through inhibition of GABAergic neurones. The mesolimbic dopaminergic pathway, shown in Figure 17.4, is involved in the reward mechanisms underlying the abuse of several drugs, as will be discussed later in this chapter. Dopamine released from the mesolimbic terminals can modulate the glutamatergic cortical input received by medium-sized spiny output neurones in the nucleus accumbens. After chronic exposure to opiates such as morphine and heroin, functional changes occur in the mesolimbic dopaminergic neurones. Upon cessation of drug intake, decreased dopaminergic transmission in the mesolimbic dopaminergic pathway may underlie the anhedonia and the dysphoria. It has been suggested that it is the need to avoid this strongly aversive state that leads to reinstatement of drug use. It has been suggested that stress is one of the main factors in relapse. Stress responsiveness appears to be influenced by the intensity of the previous exposure to the addictive drug: the more prolonged or intense the exposure, the higher the risk of relapse after a stressful experience.

Heroin is the typical opiate used by addicts. Heroin is diacetylmorphine, and acetylation leads to higher lipid solubility than that of morphine and increased availability to the brain. An overdose of heroin can induce death through respiratory depression. The intravenous administration of opiates such as heroin leads to an intense euphoria, described as a 'rush'. In contrast, cessation of opiate use leads to a withdrawal syndrome that is much feared by opiate addicts. The withdrawal syndrome may only last for a couple of weeks, but the drug craving may continue for many years, and never really fully subsides. The syndrome consists of signs and symptoms that vary in intensity according to the dosage and duration of opiate exposure. The phrases 'cold turkey' and 'kicking the habit', used to describe withdrawal, reflect the gooseflesh and the muscle spasms that occur in the arms and legs, respectively. In the early phase of withdrawal, addicts experience intense agitation and restlessness, anorexia, sweating, rhinorrhoea and tremor. In the later phase, heart rate and blood pressure increase, and there are alternating chills and intense sweating, intense nausea and vomiting, diarrhoea and consequent dehydration. Clonidine and other α_2-adrenergic agonists alleviate symptoms of autonomic hyperactivity during withdrawal, which may be due to excessive release of noradrenaline. Clonidine thus helps to ameliorate some of the more distressing symptoms of heroin withdrawal. A small proportion of patients prescribed clonidine may develop hypotension. Lofexidine is a drug similar to clonidine but with possibly fewer adverse cardiovascular effects. The adrenergic agonists are usually used in combination with several other drugs to provide symptomatic relief. These drugs include paracetamol for bone pain, diphenoxylate or loperamide for control of diarrhoea, and hyoscine to control abdominal cramps. Benzodiazepines such as nitrazepam can be used for the short-term treatment of insomnia during withdrawal.

At present, more than a million people are affected by opiate (mainly heroin) addiction in the USA. They are largely intravenous drug users, and they often suffer from and die of diseases associated with their dangerous and promiscuous lifestyle: human immunodeficiency virus (HIV) infection, hepatitis B or C infection and sexually transmitted diseases. Contrary to the view that opiate addiction occurs only in a limited section of society and affects mainly socially marginalized people, heroin addiction cuts across the social spectrum. Patients enrolled in detoxification programmes include students, lawyers, artists, bankers and doctors. A major hurdle during detoxification remains the intense withdrawal syndrome.

The treatment of opiate-dependent patients consists of a detoxification phase, during which withdrawal symptoms are managed as described above, and a regimen of substitution to prevent relapse. One of the most used regimens is methadone substitution. Methadone is an orally active, long-acting opiate. It acts preferentially at μ receptors, and it also has some weak N-methyl-D-aspartate (NMDA) receptor antagonist activity. Its long half-life leads to a constant level of stimulation of the opiate receptors. Taken orally once a day, methadone suppresses withdrawal symptoms for between 24 and 36h. Because methadone is effective in eliminating withdrawal symptoms, it is the opiate of choice for detoxifying addicts. Methadone reduces the cravings associated with heroin use and blocks the 'high' from heroin. For many addicts, 12 months of maintenance is appropriate, whereas other addicts may require maintenance for years. For most patients, optimal results are achieved with a dose of 60–100 mg/day, although careful titration and use of higher doses may be required in other patients. The lack of development of tolerance to methadone may be due to its NMDA receptor antagonist properties, as it has been suggested that NMDA receptors are involved in the development of tolerance.

Methadone produces no serious unwanted effects. Some patients may experience constipation, water retention, drowsiness and skin rashes. In a survey of the National Institute on Drug Abuse, it was reported that the weekly heroin use of addicts decreased by 69% while they were on methadone maintenance. This allows the patient to reintegrate into normal life and even full-time employment, and thus stops the life of crime that was required to sustain the drug habit. Methadone maintenance programmes help to reduce the risk of infection in addicts resulting from intravenous drug use. Methadone also helps with the management of addiction in convicted addicts. However, the absolute efficacy in terms of relieving opiate addiction remains controversial, as many argue that one addiction is replaced by another, and the core problem remains unsolved. Buprenorphine, a partial agonist at μ receptors, can also be used. It has the advantage of being more difficult to overdose, but its efficacy remains lower than that of methadone, even at high doses. Naltrexone slow-release preparations can also be used in detoxification to provide a constant block of opiate receptors. Overall, it is considered that buprenorphine, or buprenorphine–naloxone combinations, may be valuable for the treatment of addiction, especially in the early phase of treatment, with conversion to methadone maintenance only at a later stage. Another method used for detoxification is accelerated detoxification under general anaesthesia or heavy sedation. This is referred to as ultra-rapid opiate detoxification. It consists of a bolus injection of a high dose of an opiate antagonist (e.g. naloxone) under general anaesthesia or heavy sedation, followed by a slow infusion of a low dose of the antagonist. The procedure lasts for several hours and takes place within an intensive care unit. The patient needs hospitalization for 2–3 days. However, evidence for the efficacy of this treatment is still limited.

Many opiate addicts have multiple addictions: about 40% of patients entering methadone programmes are also users of crack and cocaine, and about one-quarter may also suffer from alcohol addiction. The management of these polyaddictions is complex.

The percentage of addicts who continue to use cocaine after 1 year of methadone maintenance falls to around 30%, suggesting a link between addictions, and highlights a possible role of endogenous opioids in cocaine addiction.

Cocaine and crack

Cocaine is an alkaloid present in the leaves of the shrub *Erythroxylon coca*. In pre-Columbian history, the coca leaves were reserved for the Royal Incas. Their stimulant properties countered fatigue and hunger and boosted physical endurance, especially at high altitude. The Spanish conquistadores introduced coca leaves to Europe, and in 1860 cocaine was isolated by Albert Niemann. A coca leaf contains 0.1–0.8% cocaine. Cocaine use became widespread after its introduction into Europe. Coca Cola was initially sold as a 'brain tonic and cure for all nervous afflictions', and until 1904 contained small amounts of cocaine. There are about two million users of cocaine in the USA, and cocaine is the major cause of strokes and heart attacks in people under the age of 35 years. Recent surveys show that about 8% of 20–24-year-olds in England and Wales have taken cocaine.

The cocaine most commonly used is in the form of a salt, cocaine hydrochloride. The drug inhibits the reuptake of dopamine, noradrenaline and serotonin. It also has local anaesthetic effects. When it is taken systemically, it leads to an increase in the release of dopamine in the nucleus accumbens, through activation of the mesolimbic pathway. Cocaine can be snorted or injected. Its effects reflect its psychostimulant properties. It induces enhanced mood, increases libido and enhances self-confidence. A form of cocaine that can be smoked has been developed: crack cocaine. When cocaine in its salt form is heated, it is converted to the base. This substance makes a cracking noise when heated (hence the name 'crack'), and it vaporizes at relatively low temperatures, so it can be inhaled through a heated pipe. Crack cocaine induces strong sensations of pleasure, which are described by addicts as a 'whole-body orgasm'. The intense stimulation and euphoria are followed by a 'crash', characterized by depression, anxiety, irritability and paranoid delusions. Regular users of crack may develop hallucinations, such as formication (insects crawling under the skin) and a form of delirium. During crack cocaine binges lasting several days, users can consume a large amount of the drug. The habit becomes expensive, and crack users will commit theft or violent crime in order to be able to sustain their consumption of the drug, a pattern of behaviour common in those with 'hard' drug addictions.

Regular ingestion of cocaine by snorting can damage the nasal membranes, and smoking of crack may lead to partial loss of voice. As cocaine is a very strong sympathomimetic, high doses and chronic exposure have significant adverse cardiovascular effects: hypertension, tachycardia and risk of myocardial infarction. Seizures or extreme agitation associated with overdose can be treated with anticonvulsants and dopaminergic antagonists. Recent studies have also shown that cocaine can be rapidly cleared from the body after infusion of butyrylcholinesterase.

There is still a debate about whether cocaine or crack induce tolerance or withdrawal, in a similar manner to heroin. It is well established that regular users experience distressing symptoms if they stop taking the drug. They may feel tired and exhausted but unable to sleep, suffer from diarrhoea and vomiting, and experience intense anxiety. Dependence is not inevitable, and may well be determined by individual characteristics.

Treatment for cocaine addiction is notoriously difficult. As with treatment for opiate addiction, there is first a detoxification phase, and then an abstinence phase, during which relapse must be prevented. In the acute phase, β-receptor blockers such as propranolol may offer symptomatic relief. For the later phase, several categories of drug have been tried, with limited or no success, such as: (1) dopamine receptor antagonists (e.g. haloperidol, flupenthixol and risperidone); (2) dopamine receptor agonists (e.g. pergolide and bromocriptine); (3) dopamine receptor partial agonists (e.g. terguride); (4) dopamine reuptake inhibitors (e.g. amantadine and methylphenidate); (5) monoamine oxidase (MAO) inhibitors (e.g. selegiline); (6) antidepressant drugs (e.g. imipramine, desipramine, fluoxetine and venlafaxine); (7) Ca^{2+} channel blockers (e.g. nimodipine); (8) β-blockers (e.g. propanolol); and (9) opiate antagonists (e.g. naltrexone). One of the most recent and promising new strategies developed to treat cocaine addiction involves use of a vaccine. A cocaine vaccine works by triggering the formation of antibodies against the drug. These bind the drug and prevent it from accessing the brain. The majority of work in the area of vaccines against addiction has been conducted in the field of cocaine and nicotine addiction. Preliminary results are promising, and vaccines for cocaine and nicotine are now in clinical trials. There are certain aspects of the use of vaccines in addicts that still cause concern: (1) lack of protection against a structurally dissimilar drug (which would not be recognized by antibodies); (2) lack of effect of the vaccine on drug craving, which triggers relapse; and (3) the variability between individuals in antibody formation. The induction of passive immunity, by administering the antibody and not the vaccine, has also been attempted. The vaccine and antibody treatments could be combined, for synergism of action.

Cannabis

Cannabis (marijuana) is the most widely abused drug in the UK. Over 8.5 million people have tried it at least once, and approximately 2 million people use it recreationally. Cannabis is the dried female flower of *Cannabis sativa*. Pyrolysis leads to the formation of several dozen compounds that are inhaled when a marijuana cigarette is smoked. The plant contains several psychoactive substances, but the most significant is the terpenoid Δ-9-tetrahydrocannabinol (THC). The content of THC in the cannabis flower is between 2 and 5mg%, whereas the THC content of hashish (resin-soaked flower buds) is closer to 20mg%. More recently, stronger types of cannabis have become available, such as 'super skunk'. Smoking of cannabis is associated with a THC bioavailability of 18%, whereas the consumption of THC in cakes or teas is associated with a bioavailability of about 6%. The effects of marijuana are use- and context-dependent. Overall, cannabis has a mild sedative effect, and the users describe a feeling of relaxation. First-time users may experience feelings of panic or anxiety. The smoking of cannabis leads to decreased blood pressure and bloodshot eyes, a feeling of dizziness and an increased appetite. Memory and coordination can also be transiently affected (See Box 17.3).

The mode of action of THC remained poorly understood until the discovery of cannabinoid-sensitive sites in the central nervous system (CNS). The cannabinoid CB_1 and CB_2 receptors were cloned and identified in the 1990s. A search began after their identification to isolate endogenous cannabinoid ligands. The first was a lipid compound that is an amide of arachidonic acid with ethanolamine, and this was named anandamide. Other endogenous ligands for cannabinoid receptors have subsequently been identified: 2-arachidonoylglycerol, virodhamine, noladin ether and *N*-arachidonoyldopamine. The formation of endogenous ligands such as anandamide is Ca^{2+}-dependent. There is evidence that stimulation of neurotransmitter receptors such as the D_2 dopamine receptor can lead to increased availability of anandamide.

Cannabinoid ligands are hydrophobic compounds, and thus tend to remain associated with lipid membranes. Endocannabinoid signalling appears to be modulated by two processes: carrier-mediated transport into cells and intracellular hydrolysis. The transport is not driven by transmembrane Na^+ gradients, as is the case with other transporters, but instead may depend on facilitated diffusion. The hydrolysis involves several enzymes, such as fatty acid amide hydrolase and monoacylglycerol lipase.

The CB_1 receptor probably mediates most of the effects of cannabinoids on the CNS, whereas the CB_2 receptor is found at the periphery. The CB_1 receptor is present in the neocortex, hippocampus, basal ganglia, cerebellum, thalamus, hypothalamus, midbrain (periaqueductal grey (PAG) and superior colliculus), medulla and spinal cord. The CB_1 receptor is the most abundant G-protein-coupled receptor in the mammalian brain. Activation of CB_1 receptors leads to a series of signalling events: inhibition of N- and P/Q-type voltage-activated Ca^{2+} channels, opening of K^+ channels, and inhibition of adenylate cyclase.

Cannabinoids are involved in the phenomenon called depolarization-induced suppression of inhibition, seen in structures such as the hippocampus and the cerebellum. Thus, when pyramidal neurones in the CA1 region of the hippocampus are firing, it is likely that they release anandamide or 2-arachidonoylglycerol. This may activate CB_1 receptors on the terminals of GABAergic neurones situated in the vicinity, thus inhibiting GABA release. The net result may be a facilitation of long-term potentiation in CA1 neurones. This may seem paradoxical, as cannabinoids have amnesic effects. However, the amnesic effects may involve other circuits and/or mechanisms, distinct from the local depolarization-induced suppression of inhibition. A regulatory role of cannabinoids has also been suggested in the striatum, in terms of modulation of glutamatergic signals from corticostriatal fibres (Fig. 17.2). In this model, intense firing of corticospinal neurones leads to release of glutamate and, through the influx of Ca^{2+}, subsequent activation of the synthesis of endocannabinoids in the medium-sized striatal spiny neurones. These could act retrogradely and stimulate CB_1 receptors on corticostriatal fibres, leading to decreased release of glutamate. This mechanism may underlie long-term depression at this synapse. Thus, cannabinoids can exert complex modulatory

---

Box 17.3 A potted history of 'dope'

Cannabis, or the hemp plant (*Cannabis sativa*), originated in central Asia. The earliest evidence of hemp use comes from the Neolithic age, with pieces of hemp cloth being found in archaeological sites in western China. It is likely that it was cultivated by the Anglo-Saxons from about 400 AD onwards. The economic importance of hemp throughout history as a source of fibre cannot be overstated. Under King Henry VIII of England, a law stipulated that all subjects with arable land should reserve some of it for the cultivation of hemp and flax, which was essential for the rigging of ships. A less fortunate use of hemp was as the fibre that made the hangman's noose! There is evidence, e.g. in the earliest Chinese Pharmacopoeia, that very early on, there was awareness of its effects on consciousness: 'To take too much makes people see demons and throw themselves about like maniacs.' The ancient Indian text, *Artharvarveda*, describes it as a herb that will 'release us from anxiety'. Interestingly, in 1848 a text in the British Pharmacopoeia clearly outlined the effects of cannabis, in particular the antispasmodic and analgesic potential: 'Numerous observers have described the Indian hemp as producing in the natives of the East, who familiarly use it instead of intoxicating spirits, sometimes a heavy, lazy state of agreeable reverie, from which the individual may be easily roused to discharge any simple duty—sometimes a cheerful, active state of inebriation causing him to dance, sing and laugh, provoking the venereal appetite, and increasing the desire for food—and sometimes a quarrelsome drunkenness, leading to acts of violence. During this condition pain is assuaged and spasm arrested.' In Southeast Asia, its traditional use is in the form of 'grass'; that is, its leaves, stalks and flowering tops are smoked, sometimes mixed with tobacco.

---

effects on the CNS, at both inhibitory and excitatory synapses. Some of these may underlie the beneficial effects of cannabinoids, such as the analgesic, antiemetic and antispasmodic effects. It has also been shown that CB_1 receptor antagonists, such as rimonabant, may reduce the potential for relapse in certain addictions, such as alcohol, nicotine and heroin addiction.

One of the most disquieting trends in recreational cannabis use is the increasing number of people who are regular users of cannabis. A recent World Health Organization survey showed that one in five 15-year-olds in the UK smokes cannabis—more than twice the world average. There is also evidence of a strong link between repeated use of cannabis and the development of psychosis in later life. Someone who starts using cannabis at the age of 15 years has more than four times the risk of developing schizophrenia over the next 11 years as someone who starts using cannabis at the age of 18 years. After the age of 18 years, those who have used cannabis at least 50 times

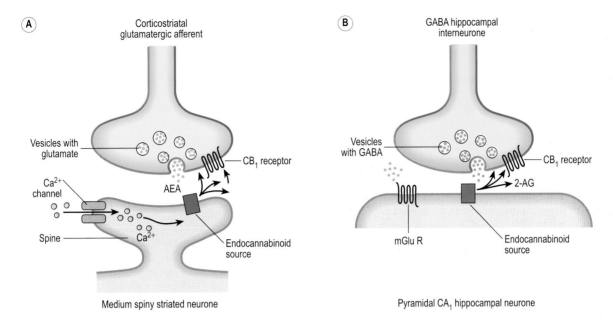

Fig. 17.2 Modulatory effects of cannabinoids. (A) Modulation by anandamide (AEA) of glutamatergic release in the striatum. (B) Modulation by 2-arachidonoylglycerol (2-AG) of GABA release in the hippocampus. mGluR, metabotropic glutamate receptor; GABA, γ-aminobutyric acid.

have a seven-fold risk of developing psychosis over the next 15 years.

Nicotine

Nicotine is the main psychoactive component of tobacco. The Spanish conquistadores were the first to discover the widespread use of tobacco, i.e. the dried leaves of the plant *Nicotiana tabacum*, by the natives in Cuba. Within less than two centuries, tobacco use was well established throughout western Europe, some of its success probably being due to its supposed activity as an aphrodisiac! In parallel, opposition to the habit of smoking developed. For example, King James I of England described smoking as 'a custom loathsome to the Eye, hateful to the Nose, harmful to the Brain, dangerous to the Lungs', showing remarkable insight into the characteristics of the abused substance. Most of the tobacco used in the UK is in the form of cigarettes; a smaller amount is consumed in the form of cigars or pipe tobacco. Addiction to nicotine constitutes one of the most serious health problems worldwide. Over 3 million smoking-related deaths are reported annually. Nicotine is the largest killer in the western world, with smoking-related diseases accounting for 20% of all deaths.

Nicotine was first isolated in 1828. It exerts widespread effects on the autonomic nervous system and also complex effects on the CNS. The effects are mediated by agonist action at nicotinic receptors, which are a particular type of acetylcholine receptor. These have a widespread distribution in the central and peripheral nervous systems. They are ligand-gated ion channels and have a pentameric structure (see Chapter 2), which can result from combinations of 12 different subunits: α2 to α10 and β2 to

β4. The activation of the receptor leads to an influx of Na^+ and K^+ (and to a lesser extent Ca^{2+}) into the neurone, and subsequent depolarization. Nicotine increases both sympathetic and parasympathetic activity. Furthermore, it increases muscle tone, through its effects on nicotinic receptors at the neuromuscular junction. Nicotine also has MAO inhibitory activity. Overall, its effects on the CNS are reflected in mild arousal, a sensation of increased energy and focus, improved memory and concentration.

Nicotinic receptors are located on GABAergic and dopaminergic cells in the VTA, but the two cell types express different combinations of receptor subunits. At doses that are reached in the plasma of smokers, nicotine leads to activation of receptors in the VTA and increased release of dopamine in the nucleus accumbens. The role of dopamine is supported by the observation that the administration of dopamine receptor antagonists, as well as lesion of the dopaminergic mesolimbic pathway, significantly reduces nicotine self-administration. Repeated exposure leads to desensitization, which may underlie nicotine tolerance. Tolerance to nicotine develops rapidly. It disappears almost as quickly as it develops (6–8h), and smokers report that the cigarette they enjoy the most is the one they smoke in the morning! Compounds present in cigarette smoke also act as potent inducers of the P-450 microsomal system, thus affecting the metabolic transformations of other substances. Therefore, several types of drug may have decreased efficacy in smokers (e.g. opiates, anti-anginal drugs and benzodiazepines), necessitating a dose increase.

Attempts to stop smoking lead to symptoms such as craving, irritability, headaches, insomnia and weight gain. The most common approach to dealing with nicotine addiction is the use of a *nicotine replacement therapy*, i.e. nicotine transdermal patches, lozenges, inhalers, gums or sprays, which maintain a certain plasma nicotine level. The drug bupropion, developed initially as an antidepressant, is also used as an aid in the treatment of nicotine addiction. Its primary mechanism of action may involve an increase in dopaminergic and noradrenergic signalling, through inhibition of the reuptake of the amines. Bupropion reduces the withdrawal symptoms and weight gain associated with smoking cessation. Minor side effects include dry mouth and insomnia. The only serious risk with the use of bupropion is the induction of seizures (approximately 0.1% of patients). However, even with bupropion, the abstinence is not maintained for a long time. More than 20 million smokers attempt to quit every year, but less than 10% succeed. Another treatment option for smoking cessation is varenicline, a partial nicotinic receptor agonist, which appears to be at least as effective as nicotine replacement therapy.

Apart from addiction to nicotine *per se*, smoking is also associated with other health risks. The most well-established fact is the significantly increased risk of developing lung cancer. The risk of death is directly related to the number of cigarettes smoked daily and the age when smoking starts. The risk of smokers developing cancers of the mouth, throat and oesophagus is almost 10 times greater than for non-smokers. Other forms of cancer also appear to be more frequent in smokers. Smoking also leads to increased platelet adhesiveness and narrowing of coronary arteries. More than 30% of deaths from coronary heart disease in the UK can be attributed to smoking. Smoking also leads to a high risk of developing chronic obstructive lung disease. Women who smoke give birth to babies that are significantly lighter than those born to women who do not smoke, and these babies are at higher risk of death during the perinatal period. In the last decade, the dangers of passive smoking (i.e. exposure to cigarette smoke without being a smoker) have also become clearer. Passive exposure to cigarette smoke may significantly increase the risk of ischaemic heart disease and asthma.

Alcohol

Alcohol is one of the most commonly used psychoactive substances. Alcohol (ethyl alcohol or ethanol) is a natural product of the fermentation of fruits and cereals. A major part of the alcohol produced and consumed worldwide is derived from fermentation of grapes from various *Viti* species, in particular *Vitis vinifera*, or grain, in the form of wine, beer or spirits.

The pharmacokinetics and pharmacodynamics of alcohol are complex. It is absorbed almost completely from the gastrointestinal tract. About 95% of the amount absorbed is metabolized, and the rest is eliminated in the urine, sweat and breath. Pure alcohol decreases gastric emptying, whereas mixed alcohol (e.g. as found in alcoholic sweetened carbonated drinks such as 'alcopops') is absorbed faster. The absorption of alcohol is slowed by

fat in the food. Alcohol is metabolized by alcohol dehydrogenase, an enzyme whose activity is controlled by the availability of the cofactor nicotine adenine dinucleotide. When alcohol dehydrogenase activity is saturated (at about 10 mg/100 mL blood), the metabolism of alcohol becomes zero-order, which means that even small increases in ingested alcohol will lead to large increases in plasma concentration. Alcohol dehydrogenase shows genetic polymorphism, and this explains the significant variability between individuals in resistance to the intoxicating effects of alcohol. Mild intoxication occurs at a concentration of 30–50 mg of alcohol per 100 mL of blood. When the concentration is higher than 100 mg per 100 mL, most individuals suffer serious neurological symptoms, the most common being slurred speech and disturbed, staggering gait. Aggressive behaviour emerges, and vision and movement are impaired. At higher concentrations, alcoholic coma ensues. Chronic ingestion of alcohol induces the P-450 microsomal system, which leads to pharmacokinetic changes, and increased tolerance to alcohol, but also changes the biotransformation of other drugs (similar to chronic smoking).

Alcohol induces a range of peripheral and central effects. Acute ingestion increases blood pressure and induces peripheral vasodilatation. It reduces the secretion of antidiuretic hormone, and so increases diuresis. It increases the level of blood glucose and inhibits gluconeogenesis. It irritates the gastric mucosa, leading to the development of chronic gastritis in many alcoholics. Heavy drinking sessions ('boozing'), a pattern of drinking common in northern Europe, particularly in the UK, can trigger acute hepatitis. Chronic use of alcohol leads to severe thiamine deficiency, as this compound is used in the metabolism of alcohol, and its absorption is decreased by alcohol itself. This thiamine depletion ultimately leads to Wernicke's encephalopathy and Korsakoff's psychosis (also known as the Wernicke–Korsakoff syndrome). The symptoms include confusion, peripheral neuropathy, ataxia, aphasia, memory loss, confabulation and significant cognitive dysfunction. Fine motor function may also be diminished, and there are vision changes. If alcohol consumption stops and supplementation with thiamine is started, recovery is possible. If treatment is not administered, up to 20% of patients with Wernicke–Korsakoff syndrome will die of it. In the majority of patients, the loss of memory and the cognitive impairment are permanent.

Alcohol also affects pregnancy: the number of miscarriages is significantly higher among alcoholic women, and about 10% of babies born to alcoholics present with the 'fetal alcohol syndrome': mental retardation and microcephaly, low body weight and length, hypotonia, lack of nasal bridge, small eyeballs with short palpebral fissures, and poor motor coordination.

Multiple neurotransmitter systems are involved in the effects of alcohol on the brain. Like other abused drugs, alcohol activates the dopaminergic mesolimbic system, and this is likely to be associated with its rewarding effects. Alcohol increases the firing of dopaminergic cells in the VTA, and as a result increases dopamine release in the nucleus accumbens. Genetic studies have shown a clear association between alcoholism and both the D_2 dopamine receptor and the dopamine transporter. Brain imaging has shown alterations in the D_2 dopamine receptor and the dopamine transporter in the brain of alcoholics. Recent studies suggest that the increased vulnerability to relapse in alcoholic patients is associated with an increased density of D_2 receptors. However, it has been shown that destruction of the dopaminergic mesolimbic pathway does not lead to total cessation of the self-administration of alcohol. Alcohol binds to several neurotransmitter receptors: 5-HT_3, γ-aminobutyric acid (GABA) and NMDA receptors. It facilitates the inhibitory effects of GABA and decreases the stimulatory effects of glutamate. Chronic exposure to alcohol increases the number of NMDA receptors and L-type Ca^{2+} channels. Alcohol intake is also associated with increased release of endogenous opioids.

Alcoholism is a disorder with high heritability (50–60%). It is often co-morbid with other disorders, such as anxiety and depression. Alcoholism can be defined as a chronic and progressive disease characterized by loss of control over the use of alcohol. After chronic use of alcohol, one of the most severe complications of withdrawal is the development of delirium tremens (Box 17.4).

Strategies to treat alcoholism include both pharmacological and non-pharmacological approaches. The most common strategies employed to treat alcoholism are psychosocial interventions and self-help groups, such as 'Alcoholics Anonymous'. Pharmacological treatment can be used to treat three aspects of alcoholism: (1) alleviation of the symptoms of acute withdrawal (e.g. β-blockers and benzodiazepines, which reduce anxiety); (2) anticonvulsant agents for management of seizures during delirium tremens; and (3) aversive drugs such as disulfiram, which irreversibly blocks aldehyde dehydrogenase. Taking disulfiram before ingestion of alcohol disrupts the metabolism of alcohol. Alcohol is metabolized in the liver to acetaldehyde by alcohol dehydrogenase. Acetaldehyde is oxidized to acetate by aldehyde dehydrogenase. Disulfiram reduces the rate of oxidation of acetaldehyde, causing a large increase in the concentration of acetaldehyde. The increased acetaldehyde levels produce unpleasant side effects: vasodilatation, headaches, hypotension, nausea, vomiting and circulatory collapse.

More recently, two new drugs have been introduced for the management of alcoholism: naltrexone and acamprosate. Naltrexone is a long-acting non-selective opiate antagonist that appears to improve abstinence rates and reduces relapse. In the USA, it is the most commonly used pharmacotherapy for alcoholism. Acamprosate (calcium acetyl-homotaurine) exerts its effects through interactions with the NMDA receptors. Like naltrexone, acamprosate reduces relapse and increases abstinence rates. Patient compliance is better with acamprosate than with naltrexone.

Phencyclidine

Phencyclidine (PCP) was introduced in 1950 as an anaesthetic. It soon became obvious that patients experienced

---

Box 17.4 Delirium tremens

The abrupt cessation of intake of alcohol in chronic alcoholics leads to a complex withdrawal syndrome. This often occurs when a person who has developed physical dependence is admitted to hospital, e.g. for accidental injury, and they cannot continue drinking alcohol according to their regular pattern. Symptoms of withdrawal are varied and unfold slowly: some of them may occur as early as 6–8h after the last drink, others at 48–72h, and yet others after 8–10 days. The syndrome is characterized by nervousness and irritability, anxiety, nausea and vomiting, insomnia, palpitations, tremor, sweating and headaches. Confusion and disorientation may follow, and a state of extreme agitation. The patient may become very sensitive to sensory stimulation such as light, sound or touch. Hallucinations (mainly visual) may occur, with the patient complaining of insects crawling under the skin. The delirium may become severe, and some patients may become lethargic or develop seizures of a tonic–clonic type. Associated symptoms include stomach cramps and chest pains and a very irregular heartbeat. Delirium tremens is a medical emergency. First, the blood pressure, fluid and electrolyte balance, and respiration are checked. Seizures require administration of anticonvulsants. Clonidine can be used to decrease anxiety and reduce cardiovascular symptoms. Hallucinations are treated with antipsychotic drugs for as long as necessary. A β-blocker may reduce the symptoms of sympathetic overactivity. It is also important to provide vitamin supplements, in particular thiamine, as alcoholics are usually deficient in thiamine. If the symptoms are severe, the patient may require sedation (e.g. benzodiazepines) for several days. Even after the successful management of a delirium tremens episode, patients may suffer for several months from tiredness, anxiety, depression and fluctuations in mood.

---

psychotic-like symptoms after just one exposure to PCP. The compound was withdrawn from therapeutic use, but remained a popular street drug. PCP is called 'angel dust', because it is often sprinkled on tobacco or marijuana, and then smoked. PCP has a variety of effects on the CNS: anaesthesia, analgesia, psychostimulation, hallucinations and psychotomimetic action. PCP induces very little tolerance. PCP is an NMDA channel blocker. It has a complex toxic profile. Males in particular become agitated, belligerent and violent. The patients present with increased respiration, hypertension and tachycardia, hyperpyrexia, increased secretions, stereotypies and often a blank stare. Blood pressure may fluctuate widely, and seizures are common, with possible conversion to status epilepticus. Experimental studies have shown that chronic use of PCP leads to degenerative changes in neurones, with vacuolization of cells and increased cell death. The toxic syndrome induced by PCP may require patient restraint because of the aggressive behaviour. Sedation can be induced with benzodiazepines. Death may occur due to respiratory and cardiovascular complications, and also to rhabdomyolysis and consequent kidney failure, in a manner similar to intoxication with substituted amphetamines (see below).

Amphetamines

Psychostimulants are abused worldwide, and apart from cocaine, examples include amphetamine and its derivatives. These compounds are indirect agonists at noradrenergic, dopaminergic and serotonergic synapses. They inhibit monoamine reuptake, promote monoamine release, and can also inhibit MAO activity. Administration of amphetamine leads to reduced need for sleep, decreased reaction times, increased motor activity and improved concentration. Amphetamine also increases blood pressure and heart rate and dilates pupils.

The stimulant effects of amphetamines have been known for a long time. Amphetamine was used extensively during World War II to increase resistance to fatigue. Not only soldiers, but also politicians, were users of amphetamine, including Winston Churchill and Adolf Hitler. Amphetamine was presumed to be safe, although the effects of stopping intake were well known: after the rush of energy and euphoric state, and the decreased need to sleep or eat, the users would experience a 'crash', dominated by tiredness and depression. Typically, this would lead to further drug intake. The only amphetamines currently being used for medical purposes are dexamphetamine for narcolepsy and methylphenidate (an amphetamine-related compound) for the treatment of hyperactive children suffering from attention deficit syndrome.

Amphetamines can be snorted, taken orally or prepared for injection. After heroin, amphetamine is the most abused injected drug in the UK. There is particular concern over the use of methamphetamine, which is stronger than amphetamine. It causes an intense and longer-lasting 'high' compared to amphetamine. Its chronic use can lead to strong psychological dependence and bouts of intense depression after the 'high'.

An overdose of amphetamine can lead to cardiac arrhythmia, paranoid ideation, hyperactivity and hyperthermia. Paranoia may be accompanied by hallucinations, and it is known that amphetamine ingestion can precipitate relapse in schizophrenic patients. The combination of hyperthermia and hyperactivity may lead to an acidotic state, convulsions and death. Intense headache and dyskinesias may also occur. The management of amphetamine overdose relies on the use of benzodiazepines and antipsychotics. In the latter category, drugs with an α-adrenergic component are preferred, such as chlorpromazine, in order to counter the increased sympathetic activity. Since amphetamine is a base that is excreted unchanged in the urine, it is possible to acidify urine with ammonium chloride and thus significantly increase the rate of excretion.

Ecstasy—or the beginning of agony?

One of the most abused recreational drugs is a substituted amphetamine: 3,4-methylenedioxymethamphetamine (MDMA), also called 'ecstasy'. MDMA is an amphetamine derivative that is structurally related to the hallucinogenic compound mescaline. Since the mid-1980s, MDMA has become a very popular recreational drug, associated with 'rave' parties. The case history illustrates the dangers associated with the use of this drug. A United Nations survey estimated that between 1995 and 2000 there was a 70% increase in the recreational use of MDMA, reflected in an increase in the number of hospital admissions and deaths associated with this compound. Most deaths are the result of hyperthermia, which leads to breakdown of skeletal muscle (rhabdomyolysis), and associated multiple organ failure. Furthermore, ingestion of large volumes of water in an attempt to decrease the effects of hyperthermia and dehydration (due to hours of dancing, for example) may lead to a typical hyponatraemic syndrome, exacerbated by increased secretion of antidiuretic hormone. The retention of water leads to dilution of the extracellular medium. The subsequent brain swelling is accompanied by signs of increased intracranial pressure. Death may occur as a result of brain herniation. The case history illustrates a typical toxic ecstasy syndrome, which luckily resolved within 48 h, but which may have also ended in the death of the young person involved. Young women are particularly sensitive to the toxic effects of ecstasy. In the case history, the restoration of a normal Na^+ level was probably crucial in saving the life of the patient.

There is increasing concern that the use of ecstasy leads to irreversible brain structural changes. The pharmacodynamic profile of this drug is complex. The acute administration of MDMA leads to increased release of 5-HT in the brain. This effect involves an interaction with the 5-HT reuptake system. MDMA also inhibits MAO activity (with a 10-fold higher potency at MAO_A than at MAO_B). The drug can also increase dopamine release, but its effects may not involve the dopamine carrier, but instead diffusion into the dopaminergic terminal followed by displacement of dopamine from vesicles. Finally, MDMA can also increase acutely the release of noradrenaline. MDMA binds to a variety of receptors; it shows high affinity for $5-HT_2$, α_2-adrenergic, M_1 muscarinic and H_1 histamine receptors, and lower affinity for $5-HT_1$, β-adrenergic and α_1-adrenergic receptors.

Research on monkeys has shown that MDMA has a neurotoxic effect on the 5-HT innervation of the forebrain (Fig. 17.3). The loss of 5-HT fibres may be partly reversible in some brain structures, but it is questionable whether full recovery is ever possible. As illustrated in Figure 17.3, the effects are spectacularly long-lasting. Thus, after only three administrations of ecstasy 7 years before their brain tissue was analysed, the monkeys still showed significantly decreased serotonergic innervation of the striatum and of the hippocampus. Positron emission

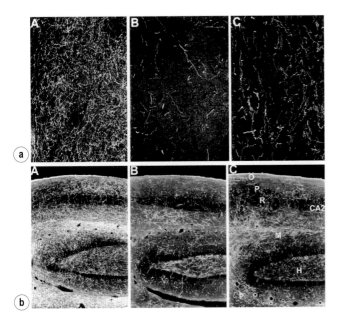

Fig. 17.3 Neurotoxicity of MDMA in monkeys exposed semi-acutely to the drug. (a) Dark-field photomicrograph showing 5-hydroxytryptamine (5-HT) fibres in the caudate nucleus (A) in control animals, (B) 2 weeks after a 3-day exposure to MDMA, and (C) 7 years after a 3-day exposure to MDMA. (b) Dark-field photomicrographs showing 5-HT fibres in the hippocampus (A) in control animals, (B) 2 weeks after a 3-day exposure to MDMA; and (C) 7 years after a 3-day exposure to MDMA. O, stratum oriens; R, stratum radiatum; P, stratum pyramidale; M, the molecular layer, H, hilus. From Hatzidimitriou et al., J Neurosci 1999; 19: 5096–5107.

tomography (PET) studies in chronic ecstasy users confirm that serotonin transmission is altered, raising the possibility that the regular use of ecstasy in humans irreversibly alters serotonergic signalling.

Ecstasy tablets come in a variety of shapes, sizes and colours. Doses and purity vary widely. The effect of the drug occurs after a latent period of 20–60 min, and may last for 3–6 h. MDMA users report a state of relaxation and euphoria. The drug seems to increase empathy and to sharpen emotions. It decreases inhibitions and appears to heighten the perception of sounds and colours.

In the 'UK Drug Situation 2000' report to the European Monitoring Centre for Drugs and Drug Addiction, it was reported that in England and Wales approximately one-third of adults aged 16 to 59 years had used illicit drugs at least once in their lifetime. Among these, ecstasy use has been reported in approximately 10% of individuals under the age of 20 years. In the UK, it has been estimated that about 500 000 young people take ecstasy every weekend.

Hallucinogens

Drugs that induce mental changes similar to psychotic states are called hallucinogens or 'psychedelic' drugs. In 1938, the Swiss chemist Albert Hofmann synthesized the compound lysergic acid diethylamide (LSD), and a few years after its synthesis accidentally ingested some powder, subsequently experiencing the 'mind-expanding' properties of this compound. The effects (also known as 'the trip') were described as a 'dream-like state', during which sensory modalities fused. Hallucinations during which sensory modalities are mixed up are called 'synesthetic'. Interestingly, such hallucinations are sometimes encountered in patients with temporal lobe epilepsy. The sense of time is generally disrupted but memory is unaffected. Feelings of total detachment and depersonalization may occur. Hallucinogens may affect mood, but the type of effect seen is context-dependent and depends on the mindset of the user. Good 'trips' as well as terrifying, bad 'trips' can be experienced by the same user. There is increased sympathetic activity, with increased blood pressure and pulse rate, dilated pupils and increased body temperature.

The structure of LSD and of other hallucinogens, such as the compounds extracted from the psilocybe mushroom (i.e. psilocybin) or the peyote cactus (i.e. mescalin), is very similar to that of serotonin. It is now well established that LSD can activate presynaptic 5-HT receptors and thus decrease the activity of raphe serotonergic neurones. This may underlie at least partly the effects of the hallucinogen, but the compound has a complex pharmacology involving several types of 5-HT receptor. LSD is a very potent compound, 25 μg being sufficient to induce hallucinations. Death from LSD overdose is rare, as the safety range of this compound is wide. When overdose occurs, it manifests as vomiting, respiratory arrest and coma. There is rapid tolerance to the effects of LSD. Hallucinogens may lead to psychological but not physical dependence. Together with cannabis, ecstasy and amphetamine, LSD is among the most popular drugs with club-goers. Experiencing the effects of psychedelic compounds through ingestion of LSD or 'magic mushrooms' (i.e. mushrooms that contain psilocybin) is a common temptation among teenagers in particular, and some of the self-reported effects and consequences are quite disturbing. This is described in Box 17.5, which contains edited fragments of the comments of two people who have taken 'magic mushrooms'.

Solvents

A wide variety of organic compounds that are used as solvents, e.g. in paint, nail varnish remover and glue, as well as cigarette lighter gas or propellent gas used in aerosols, can be abused through inhalation. This is called 'glue-sniffing', and is a form of addiction that affects mainly adolescents. It is quite common in the UK, and it affects especially young people in socially deprived areas. The inhaled solvents are absorbed rapidly and lead to a sensation similar to that of being drunk. Irrespective of their structures (i.e. aliphatic or aromatic hydrocarbons, chlorinated hydrocarbons, acetates, ketones, ether or chloroform), these agents initially produce a stimulating effect, which is followed by depression. The molecular targets activated by solvents to induce these effects are not defined.

Going on 'trips'

'I had a terrible experience yesterday on mushrooms. I had eaten them twice before with no problem... This time, when I ate the 8th, I didn't even finish them all. I felt fine at first. We were going to go to the beach to "people watch". I got up to go to the bathroom first and all of a sudden I felt extreme anxiety. I have never been so scared in my life. I felt like I was fighting with myself. I started screaming at my boyfriend. Everything I saw was changing and I didn't know where I was. I was being really mean to him one second and the next second I was apologizing, trying to tell him I didn't mean it. I could not understand anything that was going on. I had no concept of anything. Even time. I kept asking what time it was. Literally a minute felt like it should have been 2 or 3 hours... He tried to put on some soothing music and I made him take it out. I couldn't even watch commercials with music on television. Now, 24 hours later, I feel extremely sad and not quite myself. I would appreciate it if you could ... tell me what happened. How can I get myself feeling normal again?'

'I took mushrooms at the age of 20 and had a very bad experience. I became suicidal and for about 4 days I was totally wasted. Today at the age of 47 I suffer from severe depression and phobias and have had to have electroshock treatment for a breakdown. Could this be related to that bad experience all those years ago and if so what help could I get, if there is a cure available?'

The effect is short-lived (usually a few minutes), and repeat doses are required every hour. The user can develop hallucinations and delusions, and may slip into a delirious state. Tolerance to solvents can develop very quickly. There is no physical dependence, but there is strong psychological dependence. Chronic exposure to solvents is likely to cause not only neurotoxicity, but also hepatotoxicity and renal toxicity. Accidental death can also be caused by suffocation or choking on vomit, after intense periods of sniffing that may trigger emesis. There is at present no treatment for solvent abuse.

Neurobiology of addiction

Addictions are diseases of the brain with complex and specific neurobiological mechanisms and behavioural manifestations. They can be rightly considered among the most poorly understood chronic diseases of the brain.

The description of the various types of drug that can be misused has highlighted some common cellular aspects underlying addiction. Thus, there is strong evidence that the dopaminergic mesolimbic system, with its origin in the VTA and projection to the nucleus accumbens, plays a major role in addiction (Fig. 17.4).

The dopaminergic mesolimbic system is associated with both natural rewards and the reward induced by addictive drugs. It has been suggested that the powerful effect of addictive drugs may be due to the inability of the brain to distinguish between activation of reward circuitry by natural stimuli such as food or sex, and activation by drugs. Addictive drugs appear to 'hijack' a natural body response and to stimulate the reward circuits with an intensity that is overwhelming and superior to that of natural stimuli. Although addictive drugs belong to a variety of pharmacological classes, many of them can increase the levels of dopamine in the nucleus accumbens. Some of them act directly in the VTA, and others activate endogenous opioid pathways that ultimately lead to activation of the VTA dopaminergic neurones (e.g. alcohol and nicotine). Dopaminergic cells in the brain have a complex response to rewarding stimuli. When the reward is still new and unanticipated, the dopamine neurones fire intensely. After a prolonged period of repeated exposure to the reward, dopaminergic neurones fire in anticipation of the reward. If a predicted reward is not presented, the firing of cells is suppressed. If, on the contrary, the reward exceeds expectation, the firing of the cells is amplified.

However, it is likely that other brain structures are also involved in the addiction process. In particular, the craving for a drug long after withdrawal symptoms have vanished, and the relapse upon exposure to certain cues, strongly suggest the involvement of structures such as the amygdala, cortex and hippocampus. Experimental evidence shows that drug-associated cues can elicit activation of these areas, as well as of the nucleus accumbens.

It also seems likely that prolonged exposure to drugs triggers complex and long-lasting changes in gene expression. Among the various cellular factors regulated by drugs of abuse, two have received particular attention: the cyclic AMP response-element-binding protein (CREB) and the transcription factor ΔFosB. CREB is a transcription factor that regulates the expression of genes containing a cyclic AMP-responsive element in their regulatory regions. It has been shown, for example, that chronic opiate or cocaine exposure leads to a significant increase in the expression of CREB in several brain regions. Interestingly, transgenic animals with a mutated CREB gene show decreased dependence after chronic opiate administration. However, changes in CREB are reversed within a week of the cessation of drug intake. Therefore, it is likely that they are involved only in the subacute changes induced by abused drugs, and the withdrawal phase in particular. In contrast, ΔFosB is a much stronger candidate for a role in long-term changes. ΔFosB is a member of the Fos family of transcription factors. As shown in Figure 17.5, the acute administration of a drug of abuse induces a complex pattern of upregulation of members of the Fos-related antigen (Fras) family of proteins in the nucleus accumbens. The upregulation is transient, apart from certain ΔFosB isoforms, which are much more stable. Upon chronic exposure, the modifications in these isoforms, although discrete at the beginning, begin to take on increasing importance,

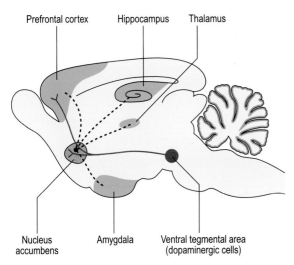

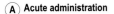

Fig. 17.4 Pathways involved in addiction. The projection from the ventral tegmental area illustrates the mesolimbic pathway and the mesocortical pathway. Dotted lines show connections of the nucleus accumbens to other structures.

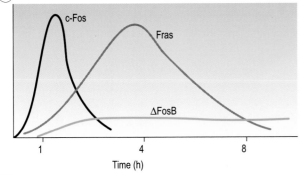

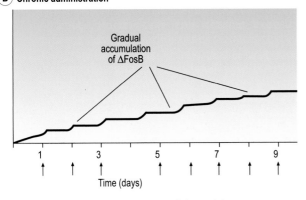

Fig. 17.5 Regulation of genes by drugs of abuse. (A) Acute administration of drugs of abuse leads to a marked transient increase in c-Fos, a smaller but more durable increase in certain Fos-related antigens (acute Fras), and a small but very long-lasting increase in ΔFosB. (B) Upon chronic exposure, the effect on ΔFosB becomes cumulative (bottom panel).

and the cumulative effect is significant. As a result, ΔFosB persists in the brain for a long time. Finally, it has been shown experimentally that drugs of abuse, such as cocaine and amphetamine, can induce significant and long-lasting structural changes, such as increased branching of dendrites and an increased number of dendritic spines on neurones in structures such as the prefrontal cortex and nucleus accumbens. Such structural changes can be seen for a very long time after cessation of drug intake.

Addiction and rehabilitation: general issues

In the treatment of addiction, there are three stages at which intervention can play an important role: (1) during the active use of the drug; (2) to alleviate the symptoms of withdrawal; and (3) to prevent relapse. The concept that addiction is a disease of the brain, with complex physical and emotional aspects, is relatively recent. Multiple drug addiction is a common problem. Addicts may use, at the same time, varying combinations of alcohol, cocaine, crack, methadone, PCP and glue. Each of these drugs, as discussed above, has its own characteristics, and sometimes their negative effects can be synergistic. Cocaine and heroin can lead to tolerance. However, under certain conditions, drugs of abuse, such as amphetamine, can lead to the opposite phenomenon, that of sensitization, i.e. an enhancement of the effects of the drug. Ethanol and opiates lead to physical dependence, whereas cocaine and amphetamine do not. It is becoming increasingly clear that cues associated with drug-taking play a major role in relapse, either a short time after abuse, or after a long period of abstinence. Places, people or the paraphernalia associated with drug abuse can trigger relapse. Stress also appears to act as a triggering factor for relapse in many addictions.

The life of an addict can lead to extreme physical and moral degradation, as described by the autobiographies or diaries of addicts: 'I wake to the feeling of something warm dripping down my chin. I lift my hand to feel my face. My four front teeth are gone. I have a hole in my cheek, my nose is broken and my eyes are swollen nearly shut… I look at my clothes and my clothes are covered with a colourful mixture of spit, snot, urine, vomit and blood.' There are at present very few efficient ways of treating addiction, and in future the answer may lie in an approach based on a better understanding of the changes induced in the brain by chronic consumption of drugs. It has been suggested that in the brain of an addict, homeostasis has been replaced by 'allostasis', i.e. a totally different set point, and efficiently treating addiction will require better characterization of all the neurotransmitter changes involved in this allostatic transformation.

Index